The MGH Textbook
of Anesthetic Equipment

The MGH Textbook of Anesthetic Equipment

Warren S. Sandberg, MD, PhD
Professor of Anesthesiology,
Surgery and Biomedical Informatics,
Chair of Department of Anesthesiology,
Vanderbilt University School of Medicine,
Nashville, Tennessee

Richard D. Urman, MD, MBA
Assistant Professor of Anesthesia,
Harvard Medical School,
Director of Procedural Sedation Management,
Department of Anesthesiology,
Perioperative and Pain Management
Brigham and Women's Hospital,
Boston, Massachusetts

Jesse M. Ehrenfeld, MD, MPH
Assistant Professor of Anaesthesia,
Harvard Medical School,
Director of Anesthesia Informatics Fellowship,
Director of Anesthesia Clinical Research Center,
Department of Anesthesia, Critical Care, and Pain
Medicine,
Massachusetts General Hospital,
Boston, Massachusetts

ELSEVIER
SAUNDERS

1600 John F. Kennedy Blvd.
Ste 1800
Philadelphia, PA 19103-2899

THE MGH TEXTBOOK OF ANESTHETIC EQUIPMENT, FIRST EDITION ISBN: 978-1-4377-0973-5
Copyright © 2011 by Saunders, an imprint of Elsevier Inc.

Notice

Library of Congress Cataloging-in-Publication Data

The MGH textbook of anesthetic equipment / [edited by]
Warren Sandberg, Richard D. Urman, Jesse M. Ehrenfeld. -- 1st ed.
    p. ; cm.
  Other title: Massachusetts General Hospital textbook of anesthetic equipment
  Other title: Textbook of anesthetic equipment
  Includes bibliographical references.
  ISBN 978-1-4377-0973-5
1. Anesthesiology--Apparatus and instruments. 2. Anesthesia--Equipment and supplies. I. Sandberg, Warren, MD. II. Urman, Richard D. III. Ehrenfeld, Jesse M. IV. Massachusetts General Hospital. V. Title: Massachusetts General Hospital textbook of anesthetic equipment. VI. Title: Textbook of anesthetic equipment.
  [DNLM: 1. Anesthesiology--instrumentation. WO 240 M617 2010]
  RD78.8.M54 2010
  617.9'60028--dc22

                                                              2010002825

Executive Publisher: Natasha Andjelkovic
Developmental Editor: Brad McIlwain
Publishing Services Manager: Debbie Vogel/Anitha Raj
Project Manager: Annie Victor
Design Direction: Steven Stave

Printed in the United States of America
Last digit is the print number: 9 8 7 6 5 4 3 2 1

Contents

Contributors

Young Ahn, MD
Clinical Fellow in Anaesthesia, Harvard Medical School; Department of Anesthesia, Critical Care and Pain Medicine, Massachusetts General Hospital, Boston, Massachusetts

Anuja Antony, MD, MPH
Assistant Professor, University of Illinois at Chicago; Clinical Research Fellow, Massachusetts General Hospital, Harvard Medical School, Boston, Massachusetts

William G. Austen Jr, MD
Chief, Division of Plastic and Reconstructive Surgery, Massachusetts General Hospital, Harvard Medical School, Boston, Massachusetts

Arna Banerjee, MD
Assistant Professor of Anesthesiology and Surgery, Vanderbilt University Medical Center; Medical Co-Director, Surgical ICU, VA Tennessee Valley Healthcare System, Nashville, Tennessee

Sergio D. Bergese, MD
Director of Neuroanesthesia, Department of Anesthesiology, The Ohio State University, Columbus, Ohio

Arnold Berry, MD, MPH
Professor of Anesthesiology, Emory University School of Medicine, Atlanta, Georgia

John A. Carter, MBBS, FRCA
Consultant in Anaesthesia and Critical Care Medicine, Department of Anaesthesia, Frenchay Hospital, Bristol, UK

Jennifer A. Chatburn, MD
Clinical Fellow in Anesthesia, Harvard Medical School; Department of Anesthesia, Critical Care and Pain Medicine, Massachusetts General Hospital, Boston, Massachusetts

Marianna P. Crowley, MD
Assistant Professor, Harvard Medical School; Anesthetist, Massachusetts General Hospital, Boston, Massachusetts

Paul D. Davis, BSc
Principal Physicist, Department of Clinical Physics and Bioengineering, Southern General Hospital, Glasgow, UK

Harold J. DeMonaco, MS
Director, Innovation Support Center, Massachusetts General Hospital, Boston, Massachusetts

Ali Diba, BM, FRCA
Consultant Anaesthetist, Anaesthetic Department, Queen Victoria Hospital NHS Foundation Trust, East Grinstead, UK

Richard P. Dutton, MD, MBA
Professor of Anesthesiology, University of Maryland Medical Center, Baltimore, Maryland

Jane Easdown, MD
Associate Professor of Anesthesiology and Associate Residency Director, Vanderbilt University Medical Center, Nashville, Tennessee

Jesse Ehrenfeld, MD
Assistant Professor of Anaesthesia, Harvard Medical School; Director of Anesthesia Informatics Fellowship, Director of Anesthesia Clinical Research Center, Department of Anesthesia, Critical Care, and Pain Medicine, Massachusetts General Hospital, Boston, Massachusetts

Stephanie Ennis, NP
Nurse Practitioner, Cardiology Service, Massachusetts General Hospital, Boston, Massachusetts

Roy K. Esaki, MD, MS
Resident, Department of Anesthesia, Stanford University School of Medicine, Palo Alto, California

Jeffrey M. Feldman, MD
Division Chief, General Anesthesiology, Children's Hospital of Philadelphia, Philadelphia, Pennsylvania

Gayle Fishman, BSN, MBA
Vice President of Clinical Services, Massachusetts Eye and Ear Infirmary, Boston, Massachusetts

Michael G. Fitzsimons, MD
Assistant Professor of Anaesthesia, Harvard Medical School; Department of Anesthesia, Critical Care and Pain Medicine, Massachusetts General Hospital, Boston, Massachusetts

Rick Hampton, BS
Wireless Communications Manager, Partners HealthCare System, Boston, Massachusetts

Deborah Harris, LMS, FRCA
Consultant in Anaesthesia and Intensive Care Medicine, North Bristol NHS Trust, Bristol, UK

Vanessa Henke, MD
Department of Anaesthesia, Critical Care and Pain Medicine, Massachusetts General Hospital, Boston, Massachusetts

Robert Holzman, MD
Senior Associate in Anesthesiology, Children's Hospital Boston; Associate Professor of Anaesthesia, Harvard Medical School, Boston, Massachusetts

Yandong Jiang, MD, PHD
Assistant Professor of Anaesthesia, Harvard Medical School; Department of Anesthesia, Critical Care, and Pain Medicine, Massachusetts General Hospital, Boston, Massachusetts

Robert M. Kacmarek, PhD
Professor of Anaesthesia, Harvard Medical School; Director of Respiratory Care, Massachusetts General Hospital, Boston, Massachusetts

Jacob Kaczmarski, MD
Staff Physician, Baptist Hospital of Miami, Miami, Florida

Sachin Kheterpal, MD, MBA
Assistant Professor of Anesthesiology, University of Michigan Medical School, Ann Arbor, Michigan

M. Ellen Kinnealey, BSN
Advanced Infusion Systems Specialist, Massachusetts General Hospital, Boston, Massachusetts

Rebecca Lintner, MD
Assistant Professor of Anesthesiology, Mount Sinai School of Medicine, New York, New York

Thomas E. MacGillivray, MD
Assistant Professor of Surgery, Harvard Medical School; Division of Cardiac Surgery, Massachusetts General Hospital, Boston, Massachusetts

George Mashour, MD, PhD
Director, Division of Neuroanesthesiology,
Assistant Professor of Anesthesiology and
Neurosurgery, University of Michigan
Medical School, Ann Arbor, Michigan

Rafael Montecino, MD
Clinical Assistant Professor of Surgery,
Leavenworth VA Medical Center, University
of Kansas, Lawrence, Kansas

Beverly Newhouse, MD
Assistant Clinical Professor of Anesthesiology
and Critical Care, University of California–
San Diego Medical Center, San Diego,
California

Jordan L. Newmark, MD
Clinical Fellow in Anaesthesia, Harvard
Medical School; Department of Anesthesia,
Critical Care and Pain Medicine,
Massachusetts General Hospital, Boston,
Massachusetts

Michael Oleyar, DO, JD
Michigan State University College of
Osteopathic Medicine, East Lansing,
Michigan

Eric Pierce, MD, PhD
Assistant Professor, Harvard Medical School;
Vice-Chair, Anesthesia Quality Assurance
Committee, Massachusetts General Hospital,
Boston, Massachusetts

Erika G. Puente, MD
Professor of Anesthesiology, Surgery and
Biomedical Informatics
Chair, Department of Anesthesiology,
Vanderbilt University School of Medicine

Warren S. Sandberg, MD, PhD
Professor of Anesthesiology, Surgery and
Biomedical Informatics
Chair, Department of Anesthesiology,
Vanderbilt University School of Medicine,
Nashville, Tennessee

F. Jacob Seagull, PhD
Assistant Professor, Division of General
Surgery, University of Maryland Medical
School, Baltimore, Maryland

Nathaniel M. Sims, MD
Assistant Professor of Anaesthesia,
Harvard Medical School; Department of
Anesthesia, Critical Care and Pain Medicine,
Massachusetts General Hospital, Boston,
Massachusetts

Reuben Slater, FANZCA
Staff Anaesthetist, St. Vincent's Hospital,
Melbourne, Australia

Demet Suleymanci, MD
Research Fellow, Department of Anesthesia,
Critical Care, and Pain Medicine, Massachusetts
General Hospital, Boston, Massachusetts

Sugantha Sundar, MD
Assistant Professor of Anaesthesia, Harvard
Medical School, Beth Israel Deaconess
Medical Center, Boston, Massachusetts

Richard D. Urman, MD, MBA
Assistant Professor of Anethesia, Harvard
Medical School; Director of Procedural
Sedation Management, Department of
Anesthesiology, Perioperative and Pain
Management, Brigham and Women's Hospital,
Boston, Massachusetts

Lisa Warren, MD
Instructor in Anesthesia, Harvard Medical
School; Director, Ambulatory and Regional
Anesthesia, Department of Anesthesia,
Critical Care, and Pain Medicine,
Massachusetts General Hospital, Boston,
Massachusetts

Matthew B. Weinger, MD
Professor of Anesthesiology, Medical
Simulation, and Biomedical Informatics,
Vanderbilt University Medical Center;
Senior Physician Scientist, Geriatric Research
Education and Clinical Center, VA Tennessee
Valley Healthcare System, Nashville,
Tennessee

Zhongcong Xie, MD
Associate Professor of Anaesthesia, Harvard
Medical School, Boston, Massachusetts

Zhipeng (David) Xu, MD, PhD
Research Fellow of Anaesthesia, Harvard
Medical School, Boston, Massachusetts

Chunbai Zhang, MD, MPH
Chief Resident, Occupational and
Environmental Medicine and Epidemiology,
Harvard School of Public Health, Boston,
Massachusetts

Gilat Zisman, BS
Post-Doctoral Researcher, Department of
Anesthesiology, The Ohio State University,
Columbus, Ohio

Preface

Medical technology has changed at a rapid pace over the past 30 years and continues to evolve quickly as new devices and techniques change and facilitate the way we practice anesthesiology. For example, a mere 15 years ago, ultrasound was a luxury in anesthesia. Today portable ultrasound has become a de facto standard of care for central venous catheter placement and for regional anesthesia. There are numerous examples of the profusion of such 'ancillary' anesthesia equipment, with completely new classes of equipment appearing almost overnight. On the other hand, some aspects of technology – such as the anesthesia machine – seem to be fairly constant. However, a closer examination reveals that this is not really correct as modern equipment only appears to function like its predecessors. Learning to operate, diagnose and troubleshoot all of this equipment competes aggressively with the patient- and disease-oriented components of anesthesiology practice.

Our goal in writing this book was to help clinicians better understand the underlying principles behind the equipment they use on a daily basis. In this firstst edition, we cover all of the equipment used in the operating room from the anesthesia machine to airway devices, physiologic monitors, and equipment used for point-of-care testing. We also included chapters on anesthesia information management systems, alarms, challenges encountered working outside of the operating room, and equipment for use in unusual environments such as a field hospital.

We begin this book with a chapter on simulation in anesthesia. This was deliberate – complexity in anesthesia practice has increased to the point where simulation must play a larger role in the education of future anesthesiologists, including education about the use of equipment and management of equipment in failure mode. It is increasingly problematic to learn how to use equipment 'on the fly' with actual patients.

Recognizing that technology evolves rapidly, we sought to illustrate fundamental principles succinctly, rather than provide a completely comprehensive review of each available device within every category. This book represents the collective wisdom of almost one hundred experts in the fields of anesthesiology, biomedical engineering, and technology. We are grateful to all of our contributors whose efforts, insight, and expertise made this book the most accessible and up-to-date work of its kind.

We would like to thank a number of individuals without whom this book would not have come to fruition. They include Dr Elisabeth H. Sandberg, Dr Katharine M. Nicodemus, Dr David C. Ehrenfeld, and Dr Zina Matlyuk-Urman. Additionally, we would like to thank our families and colleagues for their tireless support, and the generations of trainees, from whom we have learned as much as we have taught, for their inspiration. Special thanks to the Elsevier editorial team, especially Natasha Andjelkovic and Bradley McIlwain.

We hope you find this book useful and wish you well in your journey through the world of clinical anesthetic equipment.

Warren S. Sandberg, MD, PhD
Vanderbilt University
Richard D. Urman, MD, MBA
Harvard University
Jesse M. Ehrenfeld, MD, MPH
Harvard University

Chapter 1

Anesthesia Equipment and Patient Safety

Arna Banerjee, L. Jane Easdown, and Matthew B. Weinger

Anesthesia Safety: Is It a Model or a Myth?

Anesthesia has been touted as being one of the safest specialties in medicine. In 1999, the Institute of Medicine (IOM) published a report on medical errors in U.S. hospitals, which noted that anesthesiology had made substantial improvements in patient safety.[1] One impetus for reducing medical errors in the 1970s and the 1980s was the soaring cost of medical malpractice. Anesthesiologists responded by establishing national practice standards for patient monitoring, deliberately analyzing adverse events, improving the safety of anesthesia machines, fostering the widespread adoption of new technologies (e.g., pulse oximetry), improving provider training in crisis event management, and creating an independent foundation whose sole purpose was to advance anesthesia patient safety (the Anesthesia Patient Safety Foundation or APSF). Deaths in anesthesia have decreased from 2 deaths per 10,000 anesthetic procedures in the 1980s to about 1 death per 200,000 to 300,000 in 2000.[2] These numbers have been validated by surveys conducted in the Netherlands, France, and Australia.[3-5] A 2003 report from the Center for Quality Improvement and Patient Safety of the Agency for Healthcare Research and Quality (AHRQ) found 1369 complications from anesthesia in 1,933,085 patients at risk of 0.71 per 1,000 discharges.[6] This rate compares favorably to other rates of hospital complications as shown in Table 1–1.[6] Not all anesthesiologists believe that anesthesiology is as safe as these data suggest—even in young, healthy patients. For instance, in 2002, Lagasse published an extensive review of the literature in which he concluded that anesthesiology mortality was still in the range of 1 in 10,000.[7] Similar contention has been made by other authors.[8] It can be very difficult to separate errors or mishaps in anesthesia from surgical mishaps or patient disease. In studies reviewed by Lagasse, the definitions for death in which anesthesia was "associated," "related,"

"contributory," or "preventable" varied widely as did the time windows for defining the perioperative period (24 hours to 30 days). Many of these studies had small numbers and involved single healthcare sites. An alternative way of understanding patient safety in anesthesia is to study "opportunities for error." This more probabilistic approach focuses on events and their likelihood of causing patient harm. A key advantage of an event, rather than injury focus, is that data can be collected prospectively and the analysis is less likely to be affected by hindsight or outcome bias. For example, Weinger and colleagues introduced the concept of "nonroutine events" (or NRE) and showed that NRE, which represent any deviation in optimal care, occurred in 25% to 35% of all anesthetics in three different academic medical centers.[8] Moreover, an NRE data collection system captured seven times more patient injuries than a traditional anesthesia quality assurance reporting system.[9] They concluded that anesthesiology is complex and errors still occur, resulting in poor patient outcomes.

Role of Equipment in Anesthesia Safety

In 1978 Cooper et al applied the critical incident technique first described by Flanagan to understand anesthesia incidents. A critical incident was defined as: a human error or equipment failure that could have led (if not discovered or corrected in time) or did lead to an undesirable outcome, ranging from increased length of stay to death.[10] In this study, 139 anesthesiologists were interviewed and 1089 preventable incidents were reported. Seventy incidents were deemed a critical event with a substantial negative outcome. They reported that 30% of critical incidents reported by clinicians were related to equipment problems. Nineteen percent were reported instantly, while 11% were reported retrospectively. Twenty-eight percent of these demonstrated inadequate knowledge or familiarity with specific equipment or use of a relatively new technique or device.

Table 1–1 Patient Safety Indicators: Comparison Between Medical and Surgical Subspecialties[6]

Patient Safety Indicators	No. of Events	Risk Pool	Rate per 1000 Discharges at Risk	Match Rate %
Accidental puncture or laceration	11,810	5628 112	3.32	75
Birth trauma, injury to neonate	4740	720 021	6.53	96
Complications of anesthesia	1369	1933 085	0.71	74
Decubitus ulcer	41,440	1932 676	21.51	56
Foreign body left during procedure	536	6572 845	0.09	69
Iatrogenic pneumothorax	3919	5861 689	0.67	66
Obstetric trauma, cesarean birth	1138	191 227	6.97	99
Obstetric trauma, vaginal birth with instrumentation	12,518	51,225	224.21	95
Obstetric trauma, vaginal birth without instrumentation	51,223	591 752	86.61	99
Postoperative hemorrhage or hematoma	3494	1695 495	2.06	69
Postoperative hip fracture	1068	1397 898	0.77	51
Postoperative physiological and metabolic derangement	799	801 702	1	44
Postoperative pulmonary embolism or deep vein thrombosis	15,704	1689 662	9.34	61
Postoperative respiratory failure	2275	633 855	3.58	37
Postoperative sepsis	2592	229 853	11.25	33
Postoperative wound dehiscence	843	411 099	2.05	55
Selected infection resulting from medical care	11,449	5752 102	1.99	63
Transfusion reaction	30	6572 845	0.004	80

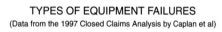

TYPES OF EQUIPMENT FAILURES
(Data from the 1997 Closed Claims Analysis by Caplan et al)

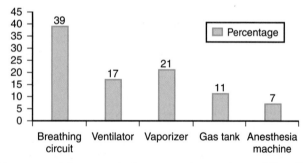

Figure 1–1 Adverse anesthetic outcomes from equipment failures.[11]

The American Society of Anesthesiologists (ASA) Closed Claims Project (CCP) was initiated in 1985 to collect information about anesthesia-related adverse outcomes. A total of 8496 closed insurance claims have been collected and analyzed. An analysis in 1997 found that only 2% of the claims were related to equipment issues (Figure 1–1). Death or brain damage occurred in 76% of these cases. Misuse of equipment was judged to have occurred in 75% of the cases and true equipment failure in 24%. Overall, 78% of claims were deemed preventable by appropriate use of monitoring.[11] Subsequent studies have called into question the validity of this finding since the reviewers were not blinded to case outcome.

Subsequent studies in anesthesia showing similar results are summarized in (Table 1–2).

Similar studies have been conducted in other countries. The Australian Incident Monitoring Study issued results on 2000 critical incidents in 1993. One hundred and seventy-seven (9%) were due to equipment problems and of these 107 (60%) were due to failures of the anesthesia gas delivery system.[13] The National Reporting and Learning System database from the United Kingdom reported similar results. Of 12,606 incidents reported to the National Patient Safety Agency, 13% were related to equipment failures. Of those incidents, 81% caused little or no harm, 18% produced moderate harm, and only 1.2% resulted in severe harm or death.[14]

As of May 2009, the ASA Closed Claims Database had 71 claims of a total 2945 claims from 1995 to 2003 due to problems with anesthesiology equipment. Eighteen of these claims were for gas delivery equipment. These included one anesthesia machine problem (unspecified), five vaporizer problems, three ventilator problems, and four breathing circuit problems. There were another five claims involving supplemental oxygen equipment or other devices attached to the patient's endotracheal tube. There were an additional two claims involving malfunctioning Ambu bags. Most equipment problem claims resulted in temporary or nondisabling injuries (66%). There were 8 (11%) permanent and disabling injuries and 16 (23%) deaths. Payment was made in 52 (73%) of these claims, with a median payment (in 2007 inflation adjusted dollars) of $137,525 (range $2720 to $2,825,750).[15] Over time, gas delivery problems appear to be decreasing as a proportion of total claims. These types of incidents represented 3% of all claims in the 1970s, 2% in the 1980s, and 1% in the period 1990 to 2003.[16]

In Canada, medical device problems reported to the Health Protection Branch were studied to determine the problems associated with anesthesia devices.[17] While only 2.3% of new

Table 1–2 Studies Examining the Incidence of Human Error in Anesthesia Mishaps[12]

Authors	Year	Type of Study Design	No. of Cases	% Equipment-Related
Cooper JB et al	1978	Retrospective critical incident reporting	359	14% as a result of failure
Craig and Wilson	1981	Retrospective critical incident reporting	81	12% related to failure
Cooper JB et al	1984	Retrospective critical incident reporting	1089	11% as a result of failure
		Also instant reporting	239	19%
Keenan and Boyan	1985	All anesthesia-related cardiac arrests	27	
Utting JE	1987	Deaths or cerebral injury cases reported to medical defense unit of UK	1501	28% of technique errors
Kumar V et al	1988	Voluntary QA reporting	129	19% related to failure
Cheney FW et al	1989	ASA closed claims study analysis	869 lawsuits	?
Chopra V et al	1992	Voluntary QA reporting	549	21% related to failure
Caplan RA et al	1997	ASA closed claims study of gas delivery equipment claims	72	24%
Weinger et al	2007	Prospective videotaped anesthetics	407	45% as judged by at least two expert reviewers of the actual videotape; usability or failure was considered to be a contributory factor in a nonroutine anesthesia event

devices were classified as anesthesia devices, these devices produced 8.6% of problem reports and 37.5% of alerts. The percentages of recalls and problem reports were also higher in the anesthesia (10.2%) than in other (4.9%) devices.

Why Is It Important to Know Your Equipment If the Mortality Has Decreased Tenfold in the Last Decade?

Although the most recent gas delivery system closed claim was for an event in 2003, equipment failures have been reported in the literature after that and even in 2008. New equipment continues to be introduced and errors reported. If the goal of the APSF, "no patient will be harmed during anesthesia," is to be realized, then any error occurring due to equipment misuse or malfunction is unacceptable. Safety can plateau or even diminish without constant effort at improvement. Included in Table 1–3 are recent examples in the literature of equipment problems.

The Nature of Errors

Although anesthesia is deemed safe, there are still reports of poor patient outcomes due to equipment failure or misuse. Detailed literature exists on the types of errors and mistakes that occur during the perioperative period and the complex human and organizational factors which lead to it.[10, 22-23] The practice of anesthesiology incorporates many sophisticated types of medical equipment both to deliver therapy and to monitor the effects of anesthesia and surgery on patient physiology. Safe anesthesia requires a comprehensive understanding of equipment both for routine cases and during clinical crisis. The following chapters provide key knowledge about commonly used anesthesia equipment; the goal is to prevent misuse, reduce use errors, facilitate failure detection and recovery, and enable clinicians to help manufacturers to design even better equipment in the future.

The complexity of anesthesia has been compared with that of managing nuclear power plants, military campaigns, or airline flight operations. In fact, the induction and emergence phases of general anesthesia can be compared with the "take off and landing" of an aircraft.

Errors involving disasters in power plants (Chernobyl) or factories (Bhopal) have been examined in great detail.[24] Although a single event or person may have been initially implicated in each of these disasters, careful analysis has consistently revealed an array of complex organizational problems and system factors interacted over time to produce the accident. Anesthesiology critical events show similar patterns. However, healthcare errors typically involve only one patient and if the outcome is poor, rarely garner public attention.

Most investigations of patient safety in anesthesia have attributed human error as being responsible for 70% to 80% of critical events. However, this is not a useful statistic. Even most outright equipment failures are inevitably due to human errors—failures of design, installation, maintenance, etc. Moreover, as described above, the clinician who ultimately pushes the wrong button is but one factor in a complex chain of events that can lead to an adverse event. Reason suggested that: "Individual unsafe acts are hard to predict but organizational and contextual factors that give rise to them are both diagnosable and manageable.[22]"

Errors by individuals do occur and can be characterized further according to Reason. There are slips and lapses that result from inattention during routine management. Mistakes, rule-based or knowledge-based, imply deviation from a plan. An example of a rule-based mistake would be the failure of an anesthesiologist to provide a proper rapid sequence induction to secure a patient's airway leading to aspiration of stomach contents. Rule-based mistakes may result in misapplication of a rule or not understanding the full rationale for its use. Knowledge-based mistakes occur when an event or experience is outside the experience of the provider. This causes the diagnosis and management to be complicated by poor mental

Table 1–3 Recent Examples in the Literature of Equipment Failure

Title	Synopsis	Date	Reference Citation
A surprising twist: an unusual failure of a keyed filling device specific for a volatile inhaled anesthetic Michael F. Keresztury, MD	Two cases were described where keyed filling devices for sevoflurane were inadvertently screwed onto isoflurane bottles. The mishaps were possible because the collars on sevoflurane and isoflurane bottles are mirror images of each other. The particular keyed filling device was designed with a flexible outer sleeve and could be screwed onto the wrong bottle while slightly gouging its soft plastic collar. The keyed filling adapters for sevoflurane and isoflurane could each be manipulated to fit the other's bottle. A manufacturer (Southmedic, Inc., Barrie, Canada) has modified their keyed filling adapters to prevent this unusual circumstance from recurring.	2006	[18]
An insidious failure of an oxygen analyzer Bryan Harris, MD and Matthew B. Weinger, MD, MS	The authors reported a case of oxygen analyzer malfunction that was diagnosed by the failure of the patient to adequately breathe oxygen as a measure of end-tidal oxygen concentration. Those involved with the care of the patient did not notice a warning icon, compliant with international standards, at the time.	2006	[19]
Aestiva ventilation mode selector switch failures Dietrich Gravenstein, MD; Harshdeep Wilkhu, MD; Edwin B. Liem, MD; Stuart Tilman, MD; Samsun Lampotang, PhD	Three cases of previously unreported failures of the Bag-Ventilator Switch in Aestiva/5 anesthesia machines (GE Healthcare/Datex-Ohmeda, Madison, Wis.) were described by the authors. Each failure mode produced a large breathing-circuit leak. Examination of the switches revealed a cracked toggle actuator, residue build-up, and cracked selector switch housing as causes for the failures. When a leak with no visible cause develops, consider advancing the mode selector switch fully to its mechanical limit or consider that the toggle actuator or its anchoring mechanism may have failed.	2007	[20]
APSF newsletter: dear sirs, misplaced valve poses potential hazard (Vanderbilt University Med Ctr)	A problem is in the AGSS (active gas scavenging system) option which produces, when the evacuation hose becomes occluded, sustained airway pressures (PEEP) of up to 40 cm. This condition was exacerbated by high fresh gas flows during mechanical ventilation. The AGSS is designed to have an opening in the bottom of a plastic receiver, providing relief of both positive and negative excess pressures. In what appears to be an assembly error, a negative pressure relief valve (similar to a circle system one-way valve) was installed in this opening (see photos below 1 and 2). This provided relief of excess negative pressure (too much evacuation suction), but no positive pressure relief. This valve is used appropriately in the passive system, but the passive system also has a positive pressure relief in the upper portion of the receiver unit.		[21]

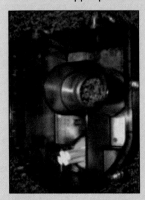

Bottom view of the active scavenging reservoir without valve (correct configuration).

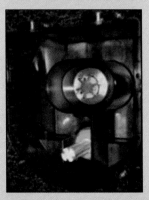

Bottom view of the active scavenging reservoir with valve in place (incorrect configuration).

modeling and false hypotheses. In this situation the practitioner is prone to have fixation or "cognitive lockup" going down the wrong diagnostic pathway or fixating on one cause to the denial to all other clues. Violations imply a deviation from a standard and must be managed in a social context. An example would be the complete disregard for doing a complete machine check in the morning before starting a case.

Conditions that predispose front-line personnel to make operational errors are called latent failure modes and lead to latent errors. Most hazardous systems are well designed to prevent single point failures; it is the occurrence of multiple unlikely events that culminate in a critical event. Prevention of latent errors (failures of design that lead to the occurrence of errors) is where we need to focus through better communication and teamwork, better design and maintenance of equipment, and planning for coordination of patient care.

Use Error Versus Device Failure

A use error is an "act or omission of an act that results in a different medical device response than intended by the manufacturer or expected by the user.[25]" Use errors can be subject to budgetary constraints, regulatory demands, and limits of technology. It may become necessary to compromise complexity for simplicity for use in complex environments. Monitoring devices may have an array of alarms to increase vigilance but unfortunately, many alarms are confusing and distracting. Equipment designers often do not interface with users and proper feedback mechanisms often do not exist. A report by the International Electrotechnical Committee (IEC), a body that regulates and standardizes electrical and electronic devices, made the following comment:

"Medical practice is increasingly using medical devices for observation and treatment of patients. Use errors caused by inadequate medical device usability have become an increasing cause for concern. Many of the medical devices developed without applying a usability engineering process are nonintuitive, and difficult to learn and to use. As healthcare evolves, less skilled users, including patients themselves, are now using medical devices, and medical devices are becoming more complicated.[25]"

What Sorts of Problems Can Occur Directly as a Result of Equipment Failure?

Equipment malfunction may be due to poor equipment design, poor user interface, or poorly designed displays or alarms. Sometimes equipment used in the operating room is used in an other environment—ICU or home care—and is inappropriate for the educational level or pace of use. Included is a table of the most common equipment errors (Table 1–4).

Current Methods for Training New Users of Anesthesia Equipment

The Food and Drug Administration (FDA) regulates the manufacture, distribution, importation, and use of medical devices in the United States. The FDA regulates the "labeling" of all medical devices. Labeling includes specific indications for use, all on-device markings, and all instructions

Table 1–4 Common Equipment Errors
Breathing circuit disconnections
Breathing circuit leaks or defective valves
Breathing circuit misconnection
Breathing circuit control error (e.g., failure to adjust APL valve)
Inadvertent gas low control errors
Gas supply problems
Vaporizer control errors (under-dose/over-dose)
Intravenous drug dose errors (including infusion and syringe pumps)
Intravenous drug/fluid delivery system problems
Ventilator missetting or malfunction
Misuse of monitors
Laryngoscope malfunction
Scavenging system problems
Other (e.g., soda lime exhaustion, sensor failure, blood warmer malfunction, etc.)

for use (including user manuals and quick reference guides). While modern medical devices intended for patients' use often include well-designed training materials, this is much less common for devices intended for clinicians. In fact, with the recent exception of very high risk devices (e.g., carotid stenting), the FDA does not mandate clinician training before device use.

Conventionally, new anesthesia equipment is introduced through an "in-service" session. An in-service is an educational session during which the company demonstrates the equipment to intended users. These efforts are usually voluntary, superficial, and inadequate because they do not allow the individuals to practice with the device nor do they include an assessment of user understanding or competency. Moreover, in-services typically occur only once with installation and are not repeated for personnel who are away from work or who join the facility thereafter. Device manufacturers have manuals for use but 48% of anesthesiologists do not read the manual and 60% do not follow a manufacturer's checklist before using new equipment.[26]

Unfortunately, there are no laws or regulations regarding responsibility for assuring equipment use competency. There is one federal statue, the Safe Medical Devices Act of 1990, but this is directed toward the manufacturer and not the hospital or practitioner. Responsibility is diffusely disbursed among clinicians, facilities, and industry. The APSF has recently advocated mandatory training and certification before introduction of new critical care equipment into patient care.

Is Conventional Training Enough?

Dalley et al showed that after a standard introduction to complex and unfamiliar anesthesia equipment, clinicians were unable to self-assess their competence to use that equipment. They concluded that providers were likely to make multiple errors, which interacting with latent design faults may produce critical incidents.[27] Similar findings were seen by Larson et al.[28] Their study was performed during a nationally attended anesthesia meeting held at a large academic medical center. Anesthesia providers were observed performing anesthesia machine checkouts on an anesthesia machine with five preset faults. Regardless of experience, most anesthesia providers were unable to uncover a majority of the machine faults (Table 1–5).

In another recent study, eight simulated scenarios were developed, which included equipment failures or misuse.[29] Second to fourth year residents completed the scenarios. A four item scoring checklist for each scenario was employed to evaluate completed items. Performance increased with experience but no perfect scores were obtained as shown in Table 1–6.

Management of some types of machine problems may require annual review to assure continued competency. A simulation-based training environment may be helpful to develop and maintain these skills.

How Should We Introduce New Equipment into the Operating Room and Train Anesthesia Personnel?

An APSF Board of Director's Workshop was convened in 2007 to discuss the attitudes, evidence, comparisons, and recommendations for training on the use of complicated new equipment.[26] Seventy-two participants from medicine, nursing, technical, administrative, regulatory, insurance, governmental, aviation, and safety industries participated (Table 1–7).

Table 1–5 Detection of Equipment Failure by Anesthesia Providers

Years of Experience	Number of Faults Detected
0-2 yr	3.7 faults
2-7 yr	3.6 faults
7 yr	2.3 faults

Larson E, Nuttall G, Ogren B, et al. A prospective study on anesthesia machine fault identification. Anesthesia Analgesia 2007;104(1):154.[28]

Table 1–6 Detection of Equipment Failure by Anesthesia Residents - by Year of Training

Residents (n = 43)	Score	Range (Maximum Possible Score of 32)
CA – 1 (n = 13)	21.8 ± 3.9	14–26
CA – 2 (n = 14)	23.86 ± 2.0	21–26
CA – 3 (n = 16)	24.7 ± 3.1	19–30

Waldrop W, Murray D, Kras J. Simulation training for anesthesia equipment failure. Anesthesiology 2007;107:A1110.[29]

Table 1–7 Goals, Findings, and Recommendations of the APSF Workshop

Goals and Findings of the APSF Workshop

▸ **THE PROBLEMS AND SHORTCOMINGS OF CONVENTIONAL TRAINING**

Conventional "in-service" programs are thought to be superficial and inadequate. They usually do not require advanced preparation, are not mandated, do not allow individual practice, and do not test for learning or application skills. They are frequently abandoned for lack of time. These programs typically occur only once when new equipment is installed and do not account for personnel who are away from work or new personnel.[30]

▸ **LIMITATIONS AND IMPEDIMENTS OF MANDATORY TRAINING**

There are no published trials of mandated vs nonmandated training. Most believe that it would greatly benefit the specialty, but there is a need to establish baseline practices and to convince the staff that this is necessary and valuable. The most difficult obstacle is to figure out how to mandate the program to so many different categories of clinician

▸ **DESCRIBE NEW APPROACHES TO TRAINING THAT MIGHT BE MORE SUCCESSFUL**

Focus on new technology. Development of an in-house training program would be beneficial (train users and then have them train others, thus demonstrating understanding, and create superusers as resource personnel). Simulation and hands-on training show greater promise.

▸ **CONSIDER ANALOGOUS END POINTS AND SUCCESSES FROM AVIATION MODEL**

Aviation safety is regulated by the airline industry. As pilots die of their own deficiencies, they too support the efforts of regulating training. Mandatory retraining is derived from actual complications encountered in the previous year. If possible e-learning is also used in the aviation industry.

▸ **EXPLORE THE REGULATORY AND THE MEDICOLEGAL AND REGULATORY PRESSURES DRIVING SUCH EFFORTS**

Most believe that the Joint Commission would be the most appropriate regulatory body to oversee training for advanced medical devices. This training should be further tied in to the credentialing process and not be optional.

▸ **PROMOTE DISCUSSION AND TARGET EFFORTS AT IMPLEMENTATION**

Most believe that we should require mandatory training on all new equipment, but keep it focused on the critical aspects. To change culture and increase competency, a sense of accountability and responsibility needs to be instilled in the practitioners. We need to partner with other bodies, such as NPSF, Joint Commission, NQF, IHI, CMS, and insurance companies, to implement this training.

APSF Recommendations

Although existing literature does not describe frequent adverse anesthesia events owing to the anesthesia professional's lack of understanding of equipment, the APSF believes that the logic is compelling to require confirmation of competency before using unfamiliar and/or complex anesthesia equipment that can directly affect patient safety. In this regard, the APSF believes that each facility should develop a required, formal process to ensure that anesthesia professionals have received appropriate training and/or demonstrated competence in the use of such medical devices.

Manufacturers should refine and initially offer this training. This required process for administering training and/or demonstrating competence should be efficient, timely, and pertinent in addressing new critical features and relevant failure modes. The most effective manner to successfully accomplish this training and testing is not known and requires deliberate investigation.

SIMULATION AS A METHOD TO TRAIN FOR EQUIPMENT COMPETENCY

Simulation is used in most industries that handle hazardous materials, involve risk of injury, and face uncommon critical situations or in which operational errors have high costs. Thus simulation training and testing is ubiquitous in nuclear power, process control, aviation, military, and maritime industries. *Simulation* can be defined as a situation or environment created to allow persons to experience a representation of a real event for the purpose of practice, learning, evaluation, testing, or to gain an understanding of systems and human factors. The first medical simulation mannequin, Sim One, was developed in 1960 by Dr. Stephen Abrahamson at the University of Southern California. It was not until the 1980s that computer-controlled mannequins were created for anesthesiology training at two separate university centers: at the University of Florida at Gainesville by Drs. Nik Gravenstein and Mike Good and at Stanford University by Dr. David Gaba. These early innovators spawned a robust industry that now has international implications across most medical, nursing, and ancillary care disciplines. The advantages of simulation for medical training are obvious. It is possible to train in a totally safe environment where mistakes are not costly to real patients, to observe and evaluate performance, to create a reliable curriculum and to train teams in emergency management, communication skills, and especially the use of new equipment (Figure 1–2). The simulation lab can become an operating room (OR), intensive care unit (ICU), bed on a floor, or an emergency department (ED) bay (Figure 1–3). With the appropriate props, all clinical scenarios can be simulated. Although there are not yet rigorous studies showing that simulation training leads to better patient outcomes, anecdotal evidence and face validity have moved the field forward. Students enjoy experiential learning and there is good evidence that simulation learning is more profound than passive learning (e.g., lectures) (Figure 1–4). The biggest impediment to simulation is that it is very costly to build, outfit, staff, and maintain simulation facilities. Beyond training, simulation can be used to evaluate skills and behaviors, credential personnel, and evaluate equipment. Simulation is now a part of the Israeli national board examination for all anesthesiologists.[30]

The ABA has introduced simulation as a method to demonstrate maintenance of certification (MOCA) and the ASA has begun to endorse simulation centers for delivery of high quality simulation training (Figure 1–4).[31] It seems inevitable that full-scale simulation will be an integral part of all anesthesiologists' training, certification, and MOCA in the near future.

USE OF SIMULATION FOR DEVICE DESIGN AND USABILITY TESTING

Simulation for device design and usability testing is a more recent development. A few prospective trials have demonstrated the value of simulation in medical device design and evaluation. Such usability studies are carried out to ensure safe use of anesthesiology equipment in the simulated clinical environment.[32] Kushniruk et al have made use of simulation to test out the effectiveness of new healthcare information systems and medication ordering systems.[33] In another study, a new infusion pump was tested in simulation by 13 nurses during three scenarios. As a result of observations made during the simulation, changes were made to the hardware and software program, making it safer for patient use.[34] The FDA has asked that companies seeking premarket clearance for clinical use of their products add to their application proof that the device can be used safely by typical users working under the normal range of conditions. Most manufacturers do usability studies in their own centers and then in clinical trials. Not all

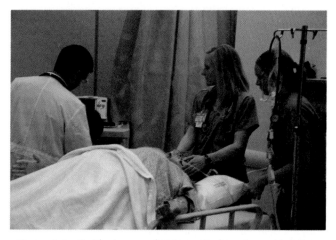
Figure 1–3   Residents responding to a critical event in a simulation.

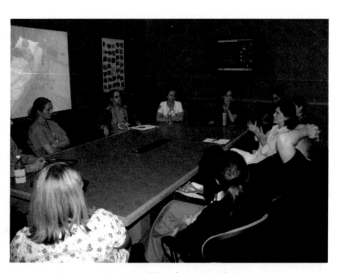
Figure 1–2   Team debriefing a simulation event.

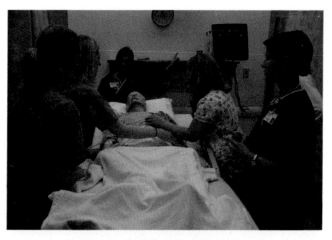
Figure 1–4   Multidisciplinary team training.

clinical scenarios can arise during this testing, however. Using simulation to test devices under stressful conditions is very useful and centers such as the Center for Medical Simulation in Boston have worked with device manufacturers on just such studies.[31]

Dalley et al introduced a new anesthesiology delivery system with a new circuit design, fresh gas flow delivery, and ventilator control to 15 anesthesiology residents.[27] In a randomized, controlled, prospective study they investigated the value of the addition of a simulator session compared with a traditional in-service one. Each group was tested in a second simulation involving an emergency situation. The group who had used the new anesthesia machine in a simulation scenario solved the emergency problem in less time and made fewer errors. Both groups made serious mistakes despite assessing themselves as competent in using the new machine.

Simulation was also used to evaluate the prototype of a new system for administering anesthesiology medications.[35] The new system included special trays of medications with prefilled syringes, which were color- and bar-coded. Before administering the drug, the barcode would be read and the system audibly enunciated the name of the drug. Ten anesthesiologists performed simulated clinical scenarios with each system and then were asked to rate the new system for its acceptability, practicality, ease of use, propensity for error, and overall safety. Medication set up time was shorter with the new system. Three drug omissions occurred with the traditional system. With the new system, one event was prevented; the wrong drug was picked up for use but the auditory clue caused the provider to realize the error. The anesthetists believed the system was safe and clinically useful.

Simulation has also been used to study the use of anesthesiology monitoring. Lampotang et al demonstrated that the use of pulse oximetry and capnography shortened the time to detection and treatment of hypoxemia in a clinical scenario.[36] This study is not ethical to do in human subjects since this type of monitoring is mandatory in the clinical setting. Overall there are many reasons why simulation can be useful to test medical devices but the most important one is that it does not impact patient safety.

In 2006 the APSF Committee on Technology launched an Anesthesia Workstation Training Initiative.[37] The committee noted the increasing complexity of anesthesiology equipment and the paucity of literature on how best to train providers for safe and effective use. Technology training has been mandated by a few institutions in the United States and Europe. Olympio et al at Wake Forest University conducted a pilot project to train providers before introduction of a new and more complex electronic anesthesia workstation. Over a 2-month period, the learners had to complete four training components: attend a lecture, a hands-on workshop, a 30-minute simulation, and take a competency examination. Of 195 eligible participants, 54% completed the training. Most or many participants said that the hands-on and simulation components were the most valuable and endorsed more of these kinds of training experiences (especially if conducted close to the clinical areas). However, only 14% of faculty completed this training. Of note, while required by the department chair, residents and nurse anesthetists, the training was voluntary for faculty. This is unfortunate since faculty members are the ones who are called on should an equipment event occur. All authors emphasize the need for continual in-service for

new techniques and devices and a real appreciation for the inherent hazards of working with the unfamiliar.

Equipment safety in a complex system involving both humans and machines, human error is always a factor. What can manufacturers and clinicians use to improve equipment safety? A task checklist is one way to ensure systematic review of key portions of a task. Checklists can support teamwork and are authority neutral. The Food and Drug Administration and the ASA first endorsed a checklist for anesthesiology machine checkout in 1986. The FDA machine checklist has been revised and abbreviated but is still recommended.[38] In another study, a checklist was developed for preoperative preparation for administering general anesthesia for a cesarean delivery.[39] Twenty experienced anesthesiologists in a high-fidelity simulator prepared for induction both using and not using this checklist. On average, without the list, the participants missed one third of the items, but no items were missed when using the checklist. The simulation study made modifications to the checklist to make it easier to use in the clinical setting.

The ASA Committee on Standards and Practice parameters recently recommended that all practitioners receive training and demonstrate competence before use of any anesthesia workstation. They also recommended the use, the completion and documentation of a pre-use checkout before an anesthesia provider uses an anesthesia workstation on patients. The APSF has advocated that training be mandatory and implemented at the local level.

SIMULATION AS A QUALITY IMPROVEMENT TOOL

Simulation can be used to examine errors made in the clinical setting. During simulation scenarios, other problems may arise which are not anticipated. As reported by DeAnda,[40] during a simulation session many other events can occur which are not expected. Analysis of these events can help to determine human errors or problems with equipment. Simulation has been used to observe the use of standard operating procedures (SOP).[41] Although the use of SOP is often evaluated by survey, one group of anesthesiologists was studied performing an SOP, rapid sequence induction, using simulation. They demonstrated more automatic functions than they described in the survey. The authors felt that using both a questionnaire and simulation could lead to better evaluation and improvement of SOP. Anderson et al studied the effect of using a disposable laryngoscope, which had been mandated for use by the United Kingdom Department of Health, to prevent prion infection.[42] They demonstrated in simulation that the recommended disposable laryngoscope was more difficult to use than reusable ones, a problem not anticipated when the mandate was put into effect.

Conclusion

Anesthesiology is generally very safe, but poor patient outcomes still occur because of device failures and use errors. These are most commonly associated with equipment design flaws. An excellent understanding of all equipment (but especially new devices) is essential for safe patient care. The ASA and the APSF have advocated standardized, mandatory training and certification before the clinical use of new equipment in the anesthesiology workstation. Simulation is an excellent tool for studying new devices and to train providers in its safe and effective use.

Further Reading

1. Cooper, J.B., Newbower, R.S., Kitz, R.J., 1984. An analysis of major errors and equipment failures in anesthesia management: considerations for prevention and detection. Anesthesiology 60 (1), 34–42.
2. Reason, J., 2005. Safety in the operating theatre — part 2: human error and organisational failure. Qual Saf Health Care 14 (1), 56–60.
3. Perrow, C., 1999. Normal accidents—living with high risk technologies. Princeton University Press, Princeton, NJ.
4. Wiklund, M.E., Wilcox, S.B. (Eds.), 2005. Designing usability into medical products. Taylor & Francis, Boca Raton, FL.
5. Sinz, E.H., 2007. Anesthesiology national CME program and ASA activities in simulation. Anesthesiol Clin 25, 209–223.

References

1. Kohn, L., Corrigan, J., Donaldson, M., 2000. To err is human: building a safer health system. Institute of Medicine, Washington, DC.
2. Clergue, F., 2008. What next targets for anaesthesia safety? Curr Opin Anesthesiol 2 (3), 360.
3. Leape, L., 2009. Errors in medicine. Clinica Chimica Acta 404 (1), 2–5.
4. Lienhart, A., Auroy, Y., Péquignot, F., et al., 2006. Survey of anesthesia-related mortality in France. Anesthesiology 105 (6), 1087–1097.
5. Arbous, M., Grobbee, D., van Kleef, J., et al., 2001. Mortality associated with anaesthesia: a qualitative analysis to identify risk factors. Anaesthesia 56 (12), 1141–1153.
6. Zhan, C., Miller, M., 2003. Excess length of stay, charges, and mortality attributable to medical injuries during hospitalization. JAMA 290, 1868–1874.
7. Lagasse, R.S., 2002. Anesthesia safety: model or myth? A review of the published literature and analysis of current original data. Anesthesiology 97 (6), 1609–1617.
8. Weinger, M., Slagle, J., 2002. Human factors research in anesthesia patient safety: techniques to elucidate factors affecting clinical task performance and decision making. J Am Med Inform Assoc 9 (6 suppl. 1), s58.
9. Oken, A., Rasmussen, M., Slagle, J., et al., 2007. A facilitated survey instrument captures significantly more anesthesia events than does traditional voluntary event reporting. Anesthesiology 107 (6), 909.
10. Cooper, J.B., Newbower, R.S., Kitz, R.J., 1984. An analysis of major errors and equipment failures in anesthesia management: considerations for prevention and detection. Anesthesiology 60 (1), 34–42.
11. Caplan, R., Vistica, M., Posner, K., et al., 1997. Adverse anesthetic outcomes arising from gas delivery equipment: a closed claims analysis. Anesthesiology 87 (4), 741–748.
12. Weinger, M.B., 1999. Anesthesia equipment and human error. J Clin Monit Comput 15 (5), 319–323.
13. Webb, R., Russell, W., Klepper, I., et al., 1993. Equipment failure: an analysis of 2000 incident reports: the Australian incident monitoring study. Anaesth Intensive Care 21 (5), 673–677.
14. Catchpole, K., Bell, M., Johnson, S., 2008. Safety in anaesthesia: a study of 12,606 reported incidents from the UK National Reporting and Learning System. Anaesthesia 63 (4), 340–346.
15. Posner, K. On behalf of the ASA closed claims project. May 18, 2009 (personal communication).
16. Eisenkraft, J., 2009. Hazards of the anesthesia workstation. ASA Refresher Courses in Anesthesiology 37 (1), 37.
17. Gilron, I., 1993. Anaesthesia equipment safety in Canada: the role of government regulation. Can J Anaesth 40 (10), 987–992.
18. Keresztury, M., Newman, A., Kode, A., et al., 2006. A surprising twist: an unusual failure of a Keyed filling device specific for a volatile inhaled anesthetic. Anesth Analg 103 (1), 124.
19. Harris, B., Weinger, M., 2006. An insidious failure of an oxygen analyzer. Anesthesia Analgesia 102 (5), 1468.
20. Gravenstein, D., Wilkhu, H., Liem, E., et al., 2007. Aestiva ventilation mode selector switch failures. Anesth Analg 104 (4), 860.
21. Berry, J.M., 2004. Misplaced valve poses potential hazard. APSF Newsletter. 8. website: http://www.apsf.org/assets/documents/spring2004.pdf#page=8.
22. Reason, J., 2005. Safety in the operating theatre — part 2: human error and organisational failure. Qual Saf Health Care 14 (1), 56–60.
23. Weinger, M., Englund, C., 1990. Ergonomic and human factors affecting anesthetic vigilance and monitoring performance in the operating room environment. Anesthesiology 73 (5), 995–1021.
24. Perrow, C., 1999. Normal accidents: living with high-risk technologies. Princeton University Press, Princeton, NJ.
25. IEC 62366 ed 1.0, 2007 Medical devices- application of usability enginering to medical devices.
26. Olympio, M.A., 2008. Formal training and assessment before using advanced medical devices in the operating room. APSF Newsl 22 (4), 6–8.
27. Dalley, P., Robinson, B., Weller, J., et al., 2004. The use of high-fidelity human patient simulation and the introduction of new anesthesia delivery systems. Anesth Analg 99 (6), 1737–1741.
28. Larson, E., Nuttall, G., Ogren, B., et al., 2007. A prospective study on anesthesia machine fault identification. Anesth Analg 104 (1), 154.
29. Waldrop, W., Murray, D., Kras, J., 2007. Simulation training for anesthesia equipment failure. Anesthesiology 107, A1110.
30. Ziv, A., Rubin, O., Sidi, A., et al., 2007. Credentialing and certifying with simulation. Anesthesiol Clin 25 (2), 261–269.
31. Sinz, E., 2007. Anesthesiology national CME program and ASA activities in simulation. Anesthesiol Clin 25 (2), 209–223.
32. Wiklund, M.E., Wilcox, S.B. (Eds.), 2005. Designing usability into medical products. Taylor & Francis, Boca Raton, FL.
33. Kohn, L., Corrigan, J., Donaldson, M., 2000. To err is human: building a safer health system. Institute of Medicine, Washington, DC.
34. Lamsdale, A., Chisholm, S., Gagnon, R., et al., 2005. A usability evaluation of an infusion pump by nurses using a patient simulator. Proceedings of the Human Factors and Ergonomics Society 49th annual meeting.
35. Merry, A.F., Webster, C.S., Weller, J., et al., 2002. Evaluation in an anaesthetic simulator of a prototype of a new drug administration system designed to reduce error. Anaesthesia 57, 256–263.
36. Lampotang, S., Gravenstein, J.S., Euliano, T.Y., et al., 1998. Influence of pulse oximetry and capnography on time to diagnosis of critical incidents in anesthesia: a pilot study using a full-scale patient simulator. J Clin Monit 14, 313–321.
37. Olympio, M.A., 2006. A report on the training inititaive of the committee of technology. APSF Newsletter 21 (3), 43–47.
38. U.S. Food and Drug Administration. Anesthesia apparatus checkout recommendations (website): http://www.asahq.org/clinical/fda.htm. Accessed July 2010.
39. Hart, E.M., Owen, H., 2005. Errors and omissions in anesthesia: a pilot study using a pilot's checklist. Anesth Analg Jul 101 (1), 246–250.
40. DeAnda, A., Gaba, D.M., 1990. Unplanned incidents during comprehensive simulation. Anesth Analg 71, 77–82.
41. Zaustig, Y.A., Bayer, Y., Hacke, N., et al., 2007. Simulation as an additional tool for investigating the performance of standard operating procedures in anaesthesia. Br J Anaesth 99 (5), 673–678.
42. Anderson, K., Gambhir, S., Glavin, R., et al., 2006. The use of an anaesthetic simulator to assess single-use laryngoscopy equipment. Int J Qual Health Care 18, 17–22.

Chapter 2

Medical Gases: Properties, Supply, and Removal

Jesse M. Ehrenfeld and Michael Oleyar

In the United States, the supply and sale of medical gases and medical gas delivery systems are regulated by the Food and Drug Administration (FDA). Most other industrialized nations also regulate gases used for medicinal purposes—including Canada (by Health and Welfare Canada), the United Kingdom (by the Medicines and Healthcare products Regulatory Agency), and the European Union.[1] Requirements for the manufacturing, labeling, filling, transportation, storage, handling, and maintenance of cylinders and containers for the storage of medical gases have been published by the U.S. Department of Transportation. The Department of Labor and the Occupational Safety and Health Administration (OSHA) regulates matters affecting safety and health of employees in all industries, including employee safety when dealing with waste anesthetic gases.[2] Other safety measures, either voluntary or regulated, are published by The National Fire Protection Association (NFPA),[3] the Compressed Gas Association (CGA), Canadian Standards Association (CSA), and the International Standards Organization (ISO).

While regulatory measures are designed to ensure the safe and consistent manufacturing and use of medical gases, occasional accidents have been reported during their delivery.[4] Unfortunately, these incidents have the potential to harm both patients and health care providers alike, especially anesthesiologists. Therefore proper precautions should be taken and backup systems must be put into place to minimize the impact of an adverse event. While regulatory measures play a large part in ensuring the safety supply of medical gases, perhaps even more important is the vigilant anesthesia provider, who should always be mindful of medical gases and their safe delivery.

Physical principles of medical gases must be considered by anesthesia providers as each gas has its own unique properties, which can affect storage, delivery, and use. Medical gases may be found throughout the hospital, especially in anesthetizing locations such as operating rooms. Anesthesia providers must be aware of the sources of medical grade gas to ensure an adequate supply when delivering to patients. The three most common medical grade gases (oxygen, nitrous oxide, and air) are typically supplied via a large central source. Alternatively, these and other gases may be supplied via gas cylinders, most often "E" size cylinders mounted on the anesthesia machine. A waste anesthetic gas (WAG) scavenging system and a medical suction system for surgical and anesthetic use are also provided centrally.

Physical Principles of Medical Gases

Common Gas Laws

Medical gases may be stored either as liquefied gases (oxygen, nitrous oxide, carbon dioxide) or compressed gases (oxygen, air). The state in which a gas may be stored is dependent on the physical properties, and the relationship between pressure, volume, and temperature. These relationships are described by the Common Gas Laws (Table 2–1), also see chapter 27. Although the SI unit of pressure is the pascal (see Appendix I), anesthesiologists often measure and report pressure as kilopascals (kPa),

Table 2–1 Common Gas Laws		
Gas Law	**Formula**	**Relationship**
Boyle's law	$P_1V_1 = P_2V_2$	Pressure and volume
Charles' law	$V_1/T_1 = V_2/T_2$	Volume and temperature
Gay-Lussac's law	$P_1/T_1 = P_2/T_2$	Temperature and pressure
Ideal gas law	$PV = nRT$	Pressure, volume, and temperature

P, pressure; *V*, volume; *T*, temperature; *n*, number of moles; *R*, universal gas constant.

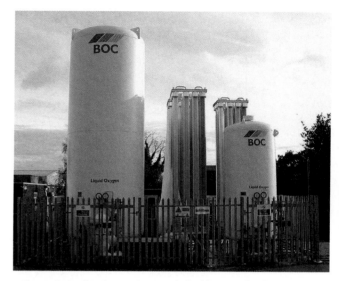

Figure 2–1   A twin vessel cryogenic liquid system (CLS) installation.

centimeters of water (cm H_2O), pounds per square inch (psi), or millimeters of mercury (mm Hg). 1 kPa = 7.5 mm Hg and 1 mm Hg = 1.35 cm H_2O.

Critical Pressure and Critical Temperature

Critical pressure and critical temperature are two important concepts that impact how medical gases are stored (also see, chapter 27). The critical temperature of a gas is defined as the temperature above which a particular gas is unable to be liquefied through the application of pressure. The critical pressure of a gas is defined as the pressure where a gas is able to be liquefied at the critical temperature of that particular gas.

The critical temperature of oxygen is −118° C, and, therefore, oxygen exists as a compressed gas at room temperature.[5] The critical temperature of nitrous oxide is 36.5° C and therefore at room temperature nitrous oxide exists as a liquefied gas. To create liquid oxygen, one must first cool the oxygen below its critical temperature and then pressurize it. To maintain oxygen as a liquid, highly specialized containers, which are insulated and refrigerated, must be used.

Medical Gases

Oxygen

Medical grade oxygen is at least 99% pure. The commercial synthesis of oxygen begins with the liquefaction of compressed air. Factional distillation is then used to separate oxygen from liquid air by taking advantage of the differences in the boiling points of oxygen and nitrogen. During this process, nitrogen evaporates, first leaving liquid oxygen behind, which can then be evaporated and collected. In the medical environment, oxygen can be supplied as either a compressed gas from room temperature cylinders or as liquid oxygen from a cryogenic liquid system (CLS) container (Figure 2–1). Although the systems required to supply and store liquid oxygen are more involved and expensive than regular oxygen cylinders, they often are more economical in facilities in which higher volumes of oxygen are used. This is because liquid storage is less bulky and less costly than the equivalent capacity of high pressure gaseous storage.

Liquid Oxygen Storage Systems

A typical cryogenic liquid oxygen storage system consists of one or more cryogenic storage tanks (Figure 2–1), one or more vaporizers, a pressure control system, and the piping necessary

to support all of the requisite fill, vaporization, and supply functions (Figure 2–2). As previously mentioned, liquid oxygen must remain below its critical temperature of −118° F and pressurized to remain as a liquid. Because the temperature gradient between liquid oxygen and the surrounding environment is significant, keeping liquid oxygen well insulated from the surrounding heat is critically important.[5] To accomplish this, cryogenic tanks are constructed in principle like a thermos bottle to shield the inner vessel from ambient heat. Vaporizers attached to the system convert liquid oxygen into a gaseous state. Downstream, a pressure control manifold then adjusts the gas pressure that is provided to the outgoing pipelines. Most cryogenic liquid systems include a backup system, which often consists of another smaller sized liquid oxygen container or a separate manifold of oxygen cylinders. In the event of an oxygen supply failure, anesthesia providers may be required to play a critical role in ensuring patient safety.[6]

Oxygen Concentrators

Oxygen concentrators, which can generate pure oxygen from atmospheric air, are occasionally used as the primary oxygen source in some remote locations. These devices work through the adsorption of atmospheric nitrogen by a molecule sieve. To ensure adequate delivery of oxygen, the oxygen output concentration should be carefully monitored when these devices are used. Most include a pressurized reservoir, which allows a stable supply of oxygen, even when demand on the system peaks. The size of the adsorption bed is the main determinant of the maximum output of the device, and a number of different sized oxygen concentrators are commercially available. Remote military bases may use large industrial-sized units, which can supply enough oxygen for an operating room, whereas smaller portable units (Figure 2–3) are often used to provide home oxygen therapy.

The Dangers of Oxygen

Although oxygen is essential for life, the anesthesia provider must be aware of potential toxicities of oxygen. Exposure to high fractional concentration of oxygen for an extended time

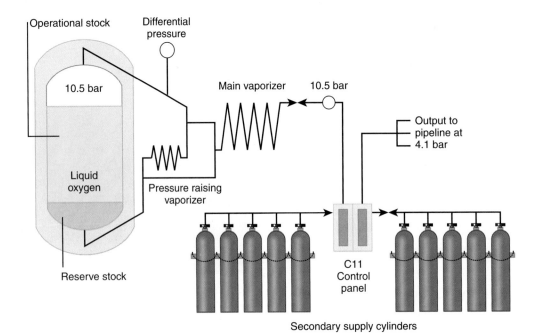

Figure 2–2   A simplified schematic of a single vessel cryogenic liquid system.

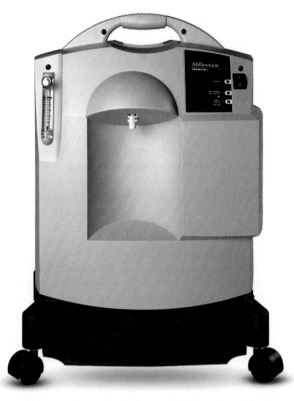

Figure 2–3   The Millenium Respironics Oxygen Concentrator—a portable oxygen concentrator for home use. *(Image courtesy Respironics, Inc. and its affiliates, Murrysville, Pa.)*

may lead to lung injury via hyperoxia-induced necrosis and apoptosis.[7] Oxygen is also extremely flammable and can act as an oxidizer for operating room fires.[8] A change in oxygen concentration from 21% to 23% poses a fire threat even for substances that are not normally considered flammable, which reinforces the importance of adequate ventilation.[5]

Liquid oxygen can be splashed on items such as clothing, making them a fire hazard. Liquid oxygen may also cause freeze burns on direct contact, as it is −118° C. Nevertheless, oxygen is an essential drug used by every anesthesiologist. The physical properties of oxygen are summarized in Table 2–2.

Nitrous Oxide

Joseph Priestley first described nitrous oxide preparation in 1772, and it is still prepared using the same principles.[9] Nitrous oxide is synthesized commercially by heating ammonium nitrate and separating nitrous oxide from other compounds such as nitric oxide. Nitrous oxide exists primarily in the liquid phase at room temperature, and it is typically stored in large H-cylinders, which are cross-connected via an auto-switching manifold. Nitrous oxide storage banks typically have a smaller number of cylinders compared with oxygen supply systems because of the lower overall consumption of nitrous oxide and the higher content of liquefied gas. Nitrous oxide is often also found on the anesthesia machine in smaller E-cylinders. Because pressure within a storage cylinder remains stable around 745 psig at constant temperatures, in order to determine the amount of nitrous oxide left inside a given cylinder the cylinder must be weighed and compared against its tare weight.[10] As liquid nitrous oxide is removed from a cylinder and approaches its critical temperature of 36.5° C,[11] nitrous oxide reverts to the gaseous form. As nitrous oxide vaporizes from liquid to gas, heat is absorbed from the surrounding environment, which can lead to the formation of frost on the outside of the metallic gas cylinder.

Nitrous oxide has been used in clinical anesthesia for more than 150 years, although in the last 50 years there has been increasing concern over potential toxicity to patients, anesthesia providers, and the environment.[12] Some choose to avoid nitrous oxide in patient care over concerns of postoperative nausea and vomiting, infection, pulmonary complications, endothelial dysfunction, and air-space expansion.[13]

Table 2–2 Physical Properties of Common Pressurized Gases

	Oxygen	Nitrous Oxide	Carbon Dioxide	Xenon	Nitric Oxide	Carbon Monoxide	Helium
Physical state in cylinder	Gas	Liquid	Liquid	Gas	Gas	Gas	Gas
Molecular weight	32	44	44	131	30	28	4 (He)
Melting point (°C)	N/A	–90.81	–56.6	–112	–164	–205	N/A
Boiling point (°C)	–183	–88.5	–78.5*	–108	–152	–192	–269
Clinical temperature (°C)	–118.4	36.4	30	16.6	–93	–140	–268
Relative density, gas (air=1)	1.04	1.5	1.52	4.5	1	1	0.14
Relative density, liquid (water=1)	N/A	1.2	0.82	N/A	1.3	N/A	N/A
Vapor pressure at 20°C (bar)	N/A	50.8	57.3	N/A	N/A	N/A	N/A
Solubility [in] water (mg/mL)	N/A	2.2	2000	644	67	30	1.5
Appearance/Color	Colorless	Colorless gas	Colorless gas	Colorless gas	Colorless gas	Colorless gas	Colorless gas
Odor	None	Sweetish	None	None	Pungent	None	None
Other data		Gas/vapor heavier than air. May accumulate in confined spaces, particularly at or below ground level	Gas/vapor heavier than air. May accumulate in confined spaces, particularly at or below ground level	Gas/vapor heavier than air. May accumulate in confined spaces, particularly at or below ground level. Note that due to its density, Xe will flow through standard flowmeters more slowly. A conversion factor of 0.468 should be applied	Currently supplied in N_2 at less than 1000 ppm	Currently only supplied at mixtures of less than 0.3% in air and helium	Use the appropriate conversion chart when using oxygen flowmeters

N/A, Not applicable.
Note: all values STP.
Mixed gases, e.g., Heliox, will have different physical properties. For exact values, please contact the manufacturer.
*Sublimation

Other concerns relate to the potential occupational hazards to anesthesia providers—because levels in operating rooms have occasionally been found to measure above national guidelines.[14] Main occupational concerns include vitamin B_{12} depression, genetic damage, and reproductive compromise,[15] although there is no definitive evidence for any of these side effects among hospital workers or anesthesiologists. Finally, nitrous oxide is also known to be a potent greenhouse gas, and some have discussed the possibility of nitrous oxide contributing to global warming.[16] The physical properties of nitrous oxide are summarized in Table 2–2.

Medical Air

Air is a nonflammable, colorless, odorless gas that makes up the natural atmosphere of the earth. Air consists primarily of nitrogen, oxygen, and water vapor—with small amounts of carbon dioxide and other elements mixed in. Medical air may be supplied from either a central plant or a series of cylinders connected by an autoswitching manifold. Hospitals with a central plant typically have two compressors to ensure that the supply is not interrupted during service or maintenance. Having two compressors also allows the system to handle periods of peak demand. An air intake first brings air through a series of filters into a compressor. Most systems include an air cooler to cool the compressed air. From the compressor, air then passes through a one-way valve into a reservoir, where a constant pressure is maintained. Upon leaving the reservoir, another series of filters and separators removes particulate matter and impurities such as oil droplets from the pressurized air supply. A set of driers containing chemical desiccant then eliminates excess humidity from the air and a final bacterial filter removes any contaminants.

Entonox

Entonox is a 50:50 mixture of nitrous oxide and oxygen that is stored at a pressure of around 2000 psig in metallic cylinders. While used mostly for dental and obstetric analgesia, dressing changes,[17] and transport of patients with long bone fractures, some recent studies have suggested broadening its use for procedures such as bone marrow biopsy[18] and extracorporeal shock wave lithtripsy.[19] Entonox is typically self-administered to patients while under medical supervision via a two-stage pressure regulator that is connected to a demand valve. Because Entonox is a mixture of gases, although the critical temperature of nitrous oxide is 36.5° C, nitrous oxide usually remains in gaseous phase. At temperatures below −5.5° C (the pseudocritical temperature), it is possible for a liquid phase to form below the gas containing 80% nitrous oxide and 20% oxygen. Because of this phenomenon, Entonox cylinders are typically stored in environments where the temperature is greater than 10° C to prevent the administration of a hypoxic mixture of gases.

Anesthesiologists should be aware of the potential for spreading infectious and/or communicable diseases via the Entonox apparatus should it be connected to the anesthesia machine. Because of the potential for cross-infection, a new Entonox apparatus must be used with each patient or a special antimicrobial filter must be placed on the tubing.[20]

Nitric Oxide

Nitric oxide, a poisonous gas whose clinical utility has only recently been established, has found increasing use for treatment of pulmonary dysfunction in the intensive care unit and operating room and is currently being studied as a possible therapeutic agent for treatment of acute myocardial infarction.

Inhaled nitric oxide (iNO) has a profound impact on pulmonary vascular tone. Although the only current Food and Drug Administration–approved use of iNO is the treatment of hypoxic respiratory failure due to pulmonary hypertension in neonates, inhaled nitric oxide is occasionally used to treat pulmonary hypertension in adults.[21]

Nitric oxide is stored in a nonliquefied form as a gaseous blend of nitric oxide (800 ppm) and nitrogen at a cylinder pressure of 2000 psig at 21° C. Administration occurs by injecting nitric oxide into a ventilator breathing circuit via a monitoring unit (NOx Box, Nodomo unit, iNOvent), which operates at 55 to 60 psig. The usual initial dose of nitric oxide is 5 to 20 ppm. Monitoring the levels of inspired nitric oxide, nitrogen dioxide levels, and methemoglobin levels is essential because methemoglobinemia is a well-known toxicity of iNO use.[22] Patients should be slowly weaned off inhaled nitric oxide in decrements of 5 ppm over 6 to 8 hours and under no circumstances should nitric oxide ever be abruptly discontinued. The physical properties of nitric oxide are summarized in Table 2–2.

Heliox

Helium-oxygen mixtures (heliox) have been used for medicinal purposes for almost 100 years. Helium is an inert gas, which also has no odor, color, or taste and does not support combustion or react with biological membranes.[23] Helium is 86% less dense (0.179 g/L) than room air (1.293 g/L). Administration may be conducted using either an endotracheal tube or face-mask with a reservoir bag.

Treatment with heliox takes advantage of the low density of helium to improve respiratory mechanics in a number of pathological states by reducing the Reynolds number associated with flow through the airways, thereby increasing laminar flow and breathing efficiency. This technique is particularly effective in obstructive conditions.[24] In addition to increasing laminar flow, heliox also facilitates gas diffusion, which may enhance alveolar ventilation in some circumstances.[23] Heliox has been studied and reported by some to be effective in a variety of respiratory conditions, such as upper airway obstruction, status asthmaticus, decompression sickness, postextubation stridor, bronchiolitis, ARDS, and COPD,[25] although more recent studies failed to show an improvement in reintubation rates when using heliox.[26] It is important to note that heliox mixtures have the potential to decrease the work of breathing in patients with increased airway resistance, but administration does not "treat" airway resistance and is not a substitution for alleviating obstruction.

Heliox is supplied in compressed medical gas cylinders, which are typically provided in sizes E, H, and G. Helium and oxygen are usually blended to provide concentrations of 80/20, 70/30, or 60/40. Gas regulators manufactured and designed specifically for the delivery of helium must be used to deliver the gas accurately and safely. The high costs and technical challenges of delivering heliox, combined with a lack of overwhelming evidence demonstrating clinical benefit, has limited everyday use of heliox.[27] The physical properties of heliox are summarized in Table 2–2.

Xenon

Xenon is a noble gas, sharing nontoxic and physiologically inert properties with helium. It is found in the atmosphere in a concentration of 0.00005 ppm (50 cubic meters of air contains 4 mL of xenon).[28] Xenon is a more potent anesthetic gas than nitrous oxide with a minimum alveolar concentration (MAC) of approximately 71%.[29] It is poorly soluble in the blood with a blood/gas distribution coefficient of 0.115, which means it has rapid onset and offset. Administration is similar to other inhaled anesthetics, but special regulators are required to accurately determine administration values, as xenon gas is approximately five times denser than air.

Xenon is a gas still in the experimental phases for medical use. Xenon has anesthetic properties, which have been known since 1939 but were not reported until 1946 when Lawrence published a paper on xenon anesthesia in mice. Since then, multiple reports of successful use as an anesthetic have been published, and many benefits over nitrous oxide have been described such as better circulatory stability, better end-organ perfusion, and reduced neurocognitive dysfunction after general anesthesia.[30] Environmental advantages of its use have also been documented. Unlike the fluorinated hydrocarbons in use, xenon does not deplete the ozone layer.

Xenon has advantages as a noble gas anesthetic, but still is not a major part of the anesthesiologist's armamentarium. A major prohibitive factor is the high cost associated with a complicated production and delivery process. Current cost estimates show xenon anesthesia as costing roughly 10 times as much as conventional anesthesia. Closed circuit apparatuses with unique gas detector systems have been designed as a way to recycle gas and reduce costs and may help lead to greater use of xenon as an anesthetic in the future.[31,32] The physical properties of Xenon are summarized in Table 2–2.

Medical Gas Supply and Storage

Although medical gases each have unique properties, universal safety measures apply to their supply and storage. Medical gases are stored in different types of cylinders, ranging in size from 1.2 L to 7900 L, which are fitted with different types of valves.[33] Cylinders are mostly made of steel alloys or aluminum. Before being placed into use, each medical gas cylinder is tested by visual inspection and with a hydraulic stretch test to ensure that the vessel will maintain its integrity when subjected to test pressures that reach at least 1.66 times the rated service pressure. Once tested, each medical gas cylinder is permanently stamped with a symbol that indicates its contents, service pressure, manufacturer's symbol, serial number, owner's symbol, test date, and testing facility. After a cylinder has been tested and filled, a cylinder label and a separate batch label (Figures 2–4 and 2–5) will be affixed indicating the contents of the cylinder, directions for use, batch number, fill, and expiration date. This information is important, should the cylinder be involved in a recall or accident.

Table 2–3 summarizes the color codes, state in cylinders, and pressure for different medical gases.[34] It is important to remember that cylinders may contain contents under high pressures, and safety measures should always be taken to prevent catastrophe. Extreme temperatures and rapid temperature changes must also be avoided to prevent cylinder damage and/or leakage.

Valves: Common valves types include pin index valves (Figure 2–6), bullnose valves (Figure 2–7), hand-wheel valves (Figure 2–8), and integral valves.[33] The valve types on any given cylinder will typically vary according to the cylinder size. Smaller cylinders (Type E cylinders), which are commonly used as backup reservoirs on an anesthesia machine, usually have pin indexed valves (Figure 2–6). Large bulk cylinders, which supply hospital pipelines (Type H cylinders), are usually fitted with bullnose valves (Figure 2–7). The bullnose valve includes a noninterchangeable screw thread system, with a different number of threads per inch for each medical gas.

Opening/closing cylinders: Small cylinders (Type E) usually have a spindle, which may be opened or closed with a wrench. The correct-sized wrench is usually permanently attached to the back of the anesthesia machine to prevent removal. Larger cylinders (Type H) include a hand-wheel valve (Figure 2–8), which may be used to open or close the valves without any additional equipment.

Cylinder filling: Medical gas cylinders should not be overfilled—because of the risk of accidental explosion and/or damage with overpressurization. It is important to keep in mind that the pressure inside a cylinder will vary with the ambient temperature—and a cylinder filled to a given pressure at one temperature might not withstand the pressure changes associated with a drastic increase in ambient temperature. Each cylinder will have a service pressure stamped on it. To prevent damage or possible explosion, cylinders should never be filled above the service pressure. For cylinders that contain liquefied gases, the filling limit is based on the filling density or percent ratio of weight of a gas in the cylinder to the weight of the water in the cylinder. For both nitrous oxide and carbon dioxide, the filling density is 68%.

Safety pressure release valves: All medical gas cylinders are fitted with a safety pressure release valve, which allows the gas inside to escape, should the internal pressure rise too high. Three types of safety release valves are commonly used; spring-loaded pressure relief valves, discs that rupture at a predefined pressure, or metallic plugs that melt at high temperatures. Note: on cylinders with pin-indexed valves, the safety pressure release is located directly below the conical depression for the screw clamp. Care should therefore be taken not to damage this valve while mounting cylinders with pin-indexed valves onto the back of the anesthesia machine.

Calculating a cylinder's contents: It is possible to determine the contents of a medical gas cylinder that contains a compressed gas (such as oxygen or air) using Boyle's law ($P_1V_1 = P_2V_2$) where P_1 stands for the atmospheric pressure, V_1 the volume of gas at atmospheric pressure, P_2 the pressure in the cylinder, and V_2 the water capacity of the gas in compressed state (see also Common Gas Laws section). Therefore the pressure in an oxygen or air cylinder (which can be directly measured by use of a

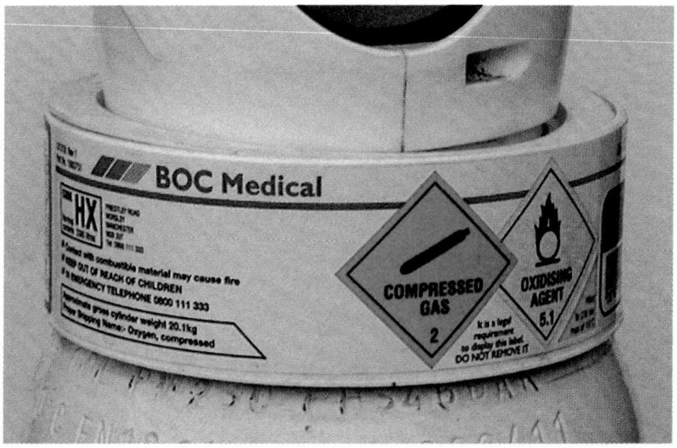

Figure 2–4 Cylinder label.

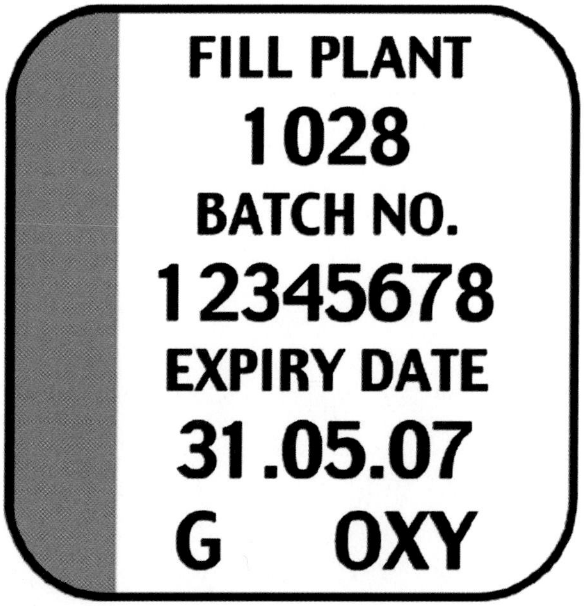

FILL PLANT
1028
BATCH NO.
12345678
EXPIRY DATE
31.05.07
G   OXY

Figure 2–5 Batch label.

Table 2–3 **Medical Gas Cylinders**[34]

Gas	Formula	Color (U.S.)	Color (International)	PSI at 21° C	State in Cylinder	E-Cylinder Capacity (L)
Oxygen	O_2	Green	White	1900-2200	Gas	660
Carbon dioxide	CO_2	Gray	Gray	838	Gas and Liquid <31° C	1590
Nitrous oxide	N_2O	Blue	Blue	745	Gas and Liquid < 37° C	1600
Helium	He	Brown	Brown	1600-2000	Gas	500
Nitrogen	N_2	Black	Black	1800-2200	Gas	660
Air		Yellow	White and Black	1800	Gas	600

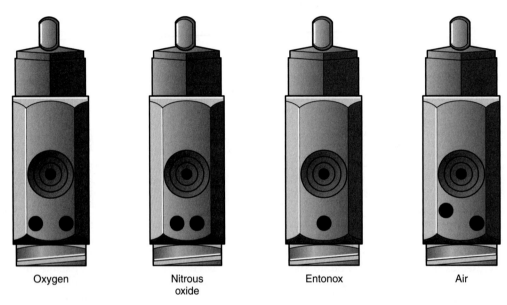

Oxygen   Nitrous oxide   Entonox   Air

Figure 2–6   Pin index safety system for different gases. Two pins in the hanger yoke of anesthesia machine are aligned with two corresponding holes on the cylinder head to prevent mounting of wrong cylinder.

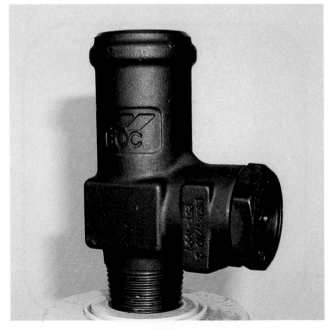

Figure 2–7   Bullnose cylinder valve.

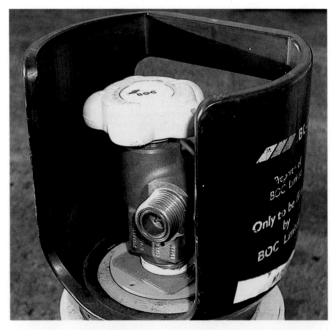

Figure 2–8   Medical gas cylinder with hand-wheel valve.

Table 2–4 Relative Sizes and Specifications of Commonly Used Oxygen Cylinders

Cylinder Size	C	CD/DD	D	E	F	HX	G	J	ZX
Nominal cylinder pressure at 15° C (bar)	137	230	137	137	137	230	137	137	300
Valve type	Pin index	Integral	Pin index	Pin index	Bull nose	Integral	Bull nose	Side spindle Pin index	Integral
Contents (liters)	170	460	340	680	1360	2300	3400	6800	3970
Water capacity (liters)	1.2	2	2.32	4.68	9.43	10	23.6	47.2	10
Dimensions (mm)	430 × 189	520 × 100	535 × 102	865 × 102	930 × 140	940 × 140	1320 × 178	1520 × 229	940 ×143
Empty weight (kg)	2.0	3.0	3.4	5.4	14.5	15	34.5	68.9	10

Table 2–5 Relative Sizes and Specifications of Commonly Used Nitrous Oxide Cylinders

Cylinder Size	C	D	E	F	G	J
Norminal cylinder pressure at 15° C (bar)	44	44	44	44	44	44
Valve type	Pin index	Pin index	Pin index	Handwheel 11/16"×20 tpi	Handwheel 11/16"×20 tpi	Handwheel 11/16"×20 tpi
Contents (liters)	450	900	1800	3600	9000	18,000
Dimensions (mm)	430 × 189	535 × 102	865 × 102	930 × 140	1320 × 178	1520 × 229
Empty weight	2.0	3.4	5.4	14.5	34.5	68.9

Table 2–6 Relative Sizes and Specifications Of Commonly Used Entonox Cylinders

Cyilnder Size	D	CD	ZD	F	HX	G	ZX
Nominal cylinder pressure at 15° C (bar)	137	137	260	137	137	137	260
Valve type	Pin index	Integral	Integral	Side spindle pin index	Integral	Side spindle pin index	Integral
Contents (liters)	500	440	794	2000	2200	5000	3970
Dimensions (mm)	535 × 102	520 × 100	465 × 90	930 × 140	940 × 140	1320 × 178	940 × 143
Empty weight (kg)	3.4	2.7	3.1	14.5	15.5	34.5	10

Entonox, a mixture of 50% oxygen and 50% nitrous oxide, exists as a gas. The pseudocritical temperature of Entonox in pipelines at 4.1 bar is below –30° C. Nitrous oxide in an Entonox cylinder however begins to separate out from Entonox if the temperature falls below –6° C. A homogenous mixture is again obtained when the temperature is raised above 10° c and the cylinder is agitated.

pressure gauge) is directly proportional to the volume of gas remaining.

For liquefied gases, such as nitrous oxide and carbon dioxide, it is not possible to estimate the contents of the cylinder by measuring pressure because the pressure inside the cylinder will stay constant until all the liquid has evaporated. To determine how much gas remains in a cylinder of liquefied gas, one must weigh the cylinder. By subtracting the tare weight (the weight of an empty cylinder, which is permanently stamped on the outside) from the total cylinder weight, one can estimate the contents of liquefied gas remaining.

Temperature: Liquid oxygen stored in medical gas cylinders is −118° C and can cause immediate tissue damage on contact. It is therefore important to avoid direct contact with liquefied gases stored in cylinders.

Cylinder sizes: Tables 2–4 to 2–8 give details for oxygen, nitrous oxide, Entonox, carbon dioxide, and heliox. The water capacity of the various cylinder sizes is given in Table 2–4.

Medical Gas Cylinder Safety

Medical gas cylinders should always be properly stored and secured to prevent damage and/or injury. Cylinders should never be dropped because a cracked pressurized cylinder can turn into a high speed projectile. All cylinders should be stored away from open flame and in a dry, cool environment.

Table 2–7 Relative Sizes and Specifications of Commonly Used Carbon Dioxide Cylinders

Cylinder Size	C	E	VF	LF
Nominal cylinder pressure at 15° C (bar)	50	50	50	50
Valve type	Pin index	Pin index	Handwheel 0.86"×14 tpi	Handwheel 0.86"×14 tpi
Contents (liters)	450	1800	3600	3600
Dimensions (mm)	430 × 89	865 × 102	930 × 140	930 × 140
Empty weight (kg)	2.0	5.4	14.5	14.5

Table 2–8 Relative Sizes and Specifications of Commonly Used Heliox21 Cylinders

Cylinder Size	F	HX
Nominal cylinder pressure at 15° C (bar)	137	200
Valve type	Bullnose	Integral
Contents (liters)	1200	1780
Dimensions (mm)	930 × 140	940 × 140
Empty weight (kg)	14.5	15.5

Table 2–9 Factors Contributing to Pollution of the Operating Room

1. Use of breathing systems with high flow anesthetic techniques
2. Poorly fitting masks
3. Failure to turn off gases at the end of anesthetic
4. Filling anesthetic vaporizers without key systems
5. Volatile agent spills
6. Leaks in the anesthesia machine and/or breathing circuit
7. Ineffective waste anesthetic gas scavenging

All individuals who are expected to handle medical gas cylinders should receive training and education about their proper use and storage. Medical gas cylinders should (1) always be opened slowly to prevent rapid temperature rise from adiabatic expansion and (2) always be kept closed when not in use. Although medical gas cylinders are one of the simplest pieces of equipment used in the operating room, they have the potential to be one of the most dangerous if not used and handled properly.

Medical Gas Pipeline Network and Manifold

The main oxygen supply in the operating room, and for the anesthesia machine, is the hospital pipeline. This system delivers oxygen at 55 pounds per square inch gauge (psig) and comes from one of two sources:

1. A primary liquid oxygen tank (with either a manifold of compressed gas cylinders or a smaller secondary liquid oxygen tank as a backup)
2. Two redundant banks of compressed gas cylinders (with a smaller bank of compressed gas cylinders as a backup)

A hospital should always have at least a 2-day supply of oxygen on-hand, and a backup supply with at least a 1-day supply. The specific total amount required will, of course, depend on the particulars of a hospital, its patient care volume, and specific needs.

The high pressure oxygen source connects to the hospital pipeline through a two stage pressure regulator. In hospitals where a manifold of oxygen cylinders is used, only one of the two oxygen banks will supply the main pipeline at any time. Once the first bank becomes exhausted, the second bank will automatically switch over. This allows the depleted cylinders to be changed out, without having to disrupt the whole system. The entire system is typically monitored by a centralized manned control station where visual indicators show the status of the two banks at all times.

All of the main hospital gas supplies and manifolds (Figure 2–9) are typically physically located outside of the hospital itself. A series of gas supply pipelines take gas from the manifold to the required delivery points around the hospital campus. Safety standards for both oxygen and other positive-pressure medical gases require the use of copper tubing to prevent the spontaneous combustion of organic oils. The supply networks are designed with pressure monitors and shut off valves (Figure 2–10) throughout the system to allow isolation of problem areas for maintenance or emergency repairs. Supply lines typically have the contents and flow direction labeled at regular intervals.

Medical gas outlets: All hospital pipelines will end in terminal wall outlets. These color-coded outlets come in one of two varieties: (1) Diameter index safety system (DISS) outlets or (2) noninterchangeable quick coupling connectors.

DISS: The DISS was developed to prevent accidental wrong connections among different medical gases (Figures 2–11, 2–12). The connector system makes it physically impossible to connect the wrong hose to the wrong pipeline. Each connector is made up of a body, nipple, and nut. The body has two concentric bores, which match specific shoulders on the matching nipple. The diameters of the bores are different for each gas, making then noninterchangable. Only appropriately matched parts will fit together and allow a complete connection.

Noninterchangable quick connectors: Quick connectors allow flow meters, hoses, machines, and other pieces of equipment to be quickly connected/disconnected without using any tools or large amounts of force. Each quick connector is made up of a pair of gas-specific male and female pieces. The two components are then locked together by a releasable spring mechanism. Different shapes prevent hoses from being placed into the wrong outlet. While quick connectors may be easier to use than DISS connections, they tend to leak with a higher frequency.

Medical Gas Delivery to the Anesthesia Machine

Whether using medical gas from a central hospital supply or free standing cylinders, anesthetic gases are delivered in the operating room using an anesthesia machine. It is essential that the anesthesia machine be properly attached to its gas

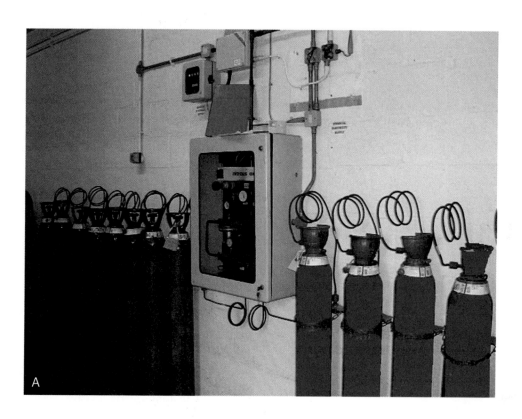

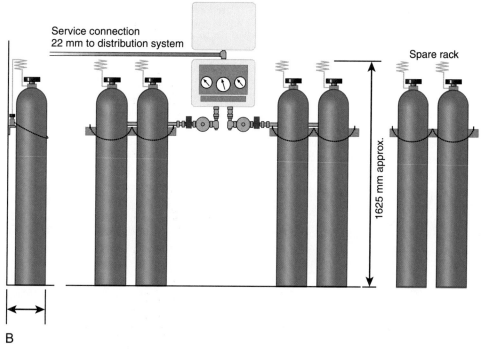

Figure 2–9   A nitrous oxide cylinder manifold **(A)**, with schematic shown below **(B)**.

sources—because incorrect connections can lead to disaster. As discussed previously, the valves for each medical gas are unique and have been designed to prevent improper connections. However, the connections between the anesthesia machine and the wall supply should be checked daily to ensure there is no physical damage or disconnect. Additionally, the pressures in the anesthesia machine should be checked to ensure that there is an adequate quantity of medical gas

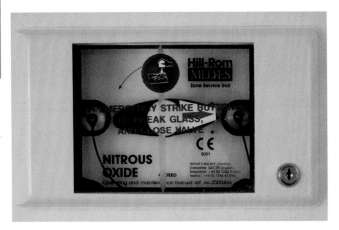

Figure 2–10 A typical medical gas control valve, which may be used to isolate the medical gas supply to a specific operating room or group of operating rooms.

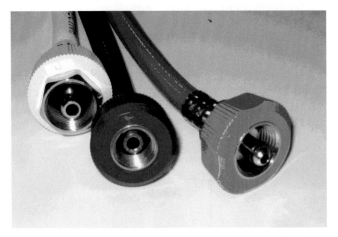

Figure 2–11 Medical gas hoses employing the diameter index safety system. Note that each color-coded hose has a different connection diameter, which matches the corresponding wall terminus (see Figure 2–12).

available.[35] Vigilance must always be practiced, especially in unfamiliar anesthetic delivery areas, because wrong gases can be mistakenly delivered.[36]

Medical Gas Removal and Waste Gas

Medical gas removal is just as important as medical gas delivery. Anesthetic gases and the excess vapors that leak into the surrounding environment during surgical procedures are considered waste anesthetic gases. The number of health care professionals in the United States who are potentially exposed to waste anesthetic gases has been estimated to be in the range of 250,000 individuals annually.[2] For a number of years, there have been questions about the potential relationship between exposure to trace concentrations of waste anesthetic gases and the possible development of adverse health effects. The *potential* effects of exposure to waste anesthetic gases include symptoms such as headaches, fatigue, nausea, dizziness, and irritability. Some also claim that exposure to waste anesthetic gas increases the risk of sterility and/or miscarriages among operating room personnel. However, the topic remains controversial and the evidence that trace anesthetic gases are harmful is at best suggestive, rather than conclusive.

It is nonetheless recommended to scavenge waste anesthetic gases to reduce the potential for excess contamination/exposure. Medical gas removal is therefore an important consideration for the well-being of not just the patient, but also the patient's healthcare providers. Design for removal systems is similar to design for delivery systems, and vacuum removal is an important component of the overall system design.

Vacuum

A vacuum is defined as a volume of space that has no matter in it. This results in a space having a much lower (negative) pressure than atmospheric pressure. Vacuums are important because they are used to create suction. Suction can then be used within the operating room to remove gases, liquids, and solid materials from both patients and the environment.

Hospitals typically provide a vacuum to each patient care location via a pipeline system, which is capable of delivering a vacuum of close to 300 mm Hg at each terminus. Vacuum pipelines are typically constructed the same way medical gas supply lines are (copper tubing) but are usually larger in diameter. A vacuum is created placing two pumps in parallel with a reservoir between them to (1) even out the vacuum and (2) remove any debris from the system. Filters, before and after the wall connection, are important to prevent major leakage of harmful or

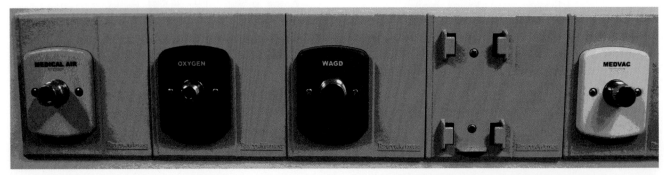

Figure 2–12 Terminal wall outlet. Note that the different diameters match the corresponding flexible gas hoses (Figure 2–11).

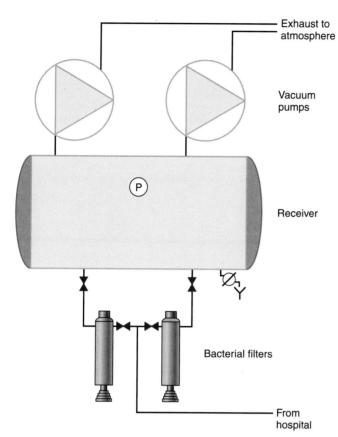

Figure 2–13   Main components of a medical vacuum plant.

contaminated materials into the central vacuum system. A diagram of a typical hospital vacuum plant is shown in Figure 2–13.

Scavenging Systems

A scavenging system is designed to vent excess anesthetic gas from the ventilator and breathing circuit. Most systems collect waste gas from across a ventilator's relief valve. Waste anesthetic gas is then transferred via special tubing into the scavenging interface. These tubes are intentionally made into a different size and appearance, so that they cannot be accidentally connected to the breathing circuit. The scavenging interface prevents excessive positive or negative pressure from coming into contact with the breathing system. Most scavenging systems employ an active, central vacuum to remove excess gas—although some rely on the pressure of the waste gas itself to move excess anesthetic through the scavenging system, i.e. a passive system. Occlusion of a scavenging system can lead to excess positive pressure being transmitted into the breathing circuit and therefore must be avoided.

All hospitals should have a standing program for management of waste anesthetic gases, including a documented maintenance schedule for the ventilation system in the operating room, postanesthesia care units, and the anesthesia machines (Table 2–9).

Conclusion

Medical gases are a critical element of the practice of anesthesiology, but also a potential source of harm for patients and anesthesia providers alike. It is therefore critical that

personnel who work in the operating room understand how to properly use, maintain, and store medical gases. Although the practice of anesthesiology is constantly changing, such as a recent trend toward increased use of total intravenous anesthetics (TIVA),[14] our medical gases and their delivery will always be an important part of perioperative care.

Suggested Further Reading

American Society of Anesthesiologists. *Waste anesthetic gases: information for management in anesthetizing areas and the postanesthesia care unit (PACU)* (website): http://www.asahq.org/publicationsAndServices/wasteanes.pdf. Accessed October 5, 2009.

Davey, A., Diba, A., Ward, C.S. (Eds.), 2005. Ward's anaesthetic equipment, ed 5. Elsevier Saunders, Philadelphia.

Eichhorn, J.H., 1981. Medical gas delivery systems. Int Anesthesiol Clin 19 (2), 1–26.

References

1. Safe handling of compressed gases in containers. 2008. Compressed gas association, vol. P1, Eleventh ed. 1–25. Available online at http://www.cganet.com/customer/publication detail.aspx? id-p-1.
2. OSHA. Safety and health topics: waste anesthetic gases (website): http://www.osha.gov/SLTC/wasteanestheticgases/index.html. Accessed October 3, 2008.
3. National Fire Protection Association, 2005. Standards for health care facilities. National Fire Protection Association, Quincy, MA.
4. Schumacher, S.D., Brockwell, R.C., Andrews, J.J., et al., 2004. Bulk liquid oxygen supply failure. Anesthesiology 100 (1), 186–189.
5. Harvard Intranet. Information specific to liquid oxygen (website): http://safety.seas.harvard.edu/services/oxygen.html. Accessed October 5, 2009.
6. Weller, J., Merry, A., Warman, G., et al., 2007. Anaesthetists' management of oxygen pipeline failure: room for improvement. Anaesthesia 62 (2), 122–126.
7. Barazzone, C., Horowitz, S., Donati, Y.R., et al., 1998. Oxygen toxicity in mouse lung: pathways to cell death. Am J Respir Cell Mol Biol 19 (4), 573–581.
8. Caplan, R.A., Barker, S.J., Connis, R.T., et al., 2008. Practice advisory for the prevention and management of operating room fires. Anesthesiology 108 (5), 786–801, quiz 971-982.
9. Bicentenary of nitrous oxide 1972. Br Med J 2 (5810), 367–368.
10. Rousseau, G.F., Carr, A.S., 2000. Reserve nitrous oxide cylinders on anaesthetic machines. A survey of attitudes and equipment at a large DGH. Anaesthesia 55 (9), 883–885.
11. Wiberg, E., Wiberg, N., Holleman, A.F., 2001. Inorganic chemistry, English, Academic Press, San Diego, CA.
12. Sanders, R.D., Weimann, J., Maze, M., 2008. Biologic effects of nitrous oxide: a mechanistic and toxicologic review. Anesthesiology 109 (4), 707–722.
13. Myles, P.S., Leslie, K., Peyton, P., et al., 2009. Nitrous oxide and perioperative cardiac morbidity (ENIGMA-II) trial: rationale and design. Am Heart J 157 (3), 488–494, e481.
14. Irwin, M.G., Trinh, T., Yao, C.L., 2009. Occupational exposure to anaesthetic gases: a role for TIVA. Expert Opin Drug Saf 8 (4), 473–483.
15. Wronska-Nofer, T., Palus, J., Krajewski, W., et al., 2009. DNA damage induced by nitrous oxide: study in medical personnel of operating rooms. Mutat Res 666 (1-2), 39–43.
16. Parker, N.W., Behringer, E.C., 2009. Nitrous oxide: a global toxicological effect to consider. Anesthesiology 110 (5), 1195, author reply 1196.
17. Jones, A.P., Allison, K., Wright, H., et al., 2009. Use of prehospital dressings in soft tissue trauma: is there any conformity or plan? Emerg Med J 26 (7), 532–534.
18. Gudgin, E.J., Besser, M.W., Craig, J.I., 2008. Entonox as a sedative for bone marrow aspiration and biopsy. Int J Lab Hematol 30 (1), 65–67.
19. Mazdak, H., Abazari, P., Ghassami, F., et al., 2007. The analgesic effect of inhalational Entonox for extracorporeal shock wave lithotripsy. Urol Res 35 (6), 331–334.
20. Chilvers, R.J., Weisz, M., 2000. Entonox equipment as a potential source of cross-infection. Anaesthesia 55 (2), 176–179.
21. Hillier, S.C., 2003. Recent advances in the treatment of pulmonary hypertension. Curr Opin Anaesthesiol 16 (3), 331–336.
22. Taylor, M.B., Christian, K.G., Patel, N., et al., 2001. Methemoglobinemia: toxicity of inhaled nitric oxide therapy. Pediatr Crit Care Med 2 (1), 99–101.
23. Harris, P.D., Barnes, R., 2008. The uses of helium and xenon in current clinical practice. Anaesthesia 63 (3), 284–293.

24. Kass, J.E., Terregino, C.A., 1999. The effect of heliox in acute severe asthma: a randomized controlled trial. Chest 116 (2), 296–300.

25. Allan, P.F., Thomas, K.V., Ward, M.R., et al., 2009. Feasibility study of noninvasive ventilation with helium-oxygen gas flow for chronic obstructive pulmonary disease during exercise. Respir Care 54 (9), 1175–1182.

26. Rodrigo, G., Pollack, C., Rodrigo, C., et al., 2002. Heliox for treatment of exacerbations of chronic obstructive pulmonary disease. Cochrane Database Syst Rev 2, CD003571.

27. Valli, G., Paoletti, P., Savi, D., et al., 2007. Clinical use of Heliox in asthma and COPD. Monaldi Arch Chest Dis 67 (3), 159–164.

28. Marx, T., Schmidt, M., Schirmer, U., et al., 2000. Xenon anaesthesia. J R Soc Med 93 (10), 513–517.

29. Luttropp, H.H., Thomasson, R., Dahm, S., et al., 1994. Clinical experience with minimal flow xenon anesthesia. Acta Anaesthesiol Scand 38 (2), 121–125.

30. Derwall, M., Coburn, M., Rex, S., et al., 2009. Xenon: recent developments and future perspectives. Minerva Anestesiol 75 (1-2), 37–45.

31. Meyer, J.U., Kullik, G., Wruck, N., et al., 2008. Advanced technologies and devices for inhalational anesthetic drug dosing. Handb Exp Pharmacol 182, 451–470.

32. Dingley, J., Findlay, G.P., Foex, B.A., et al., 2001. A closed xenon anesthesia delivery system. Anesthesiology 94 (1), 173–176.

33. Davey, A., Diba, A., Ward, C.S. (Eds.), 2005. Ward's anaesthetic equipment, Elsevier Saunders, Philadelphia.

34. BOC-Healthcare. *Medical gas cylinder data chart* (website): http://www.bochealthcare.co.uk/images/local/content_pages/safety/cylinder_chart/cylinder_data_med309965.pdf. Accessed October 5, 2009

35. Wicker, P., Smith, B., 2006. Checking the anaesthetic machine. J Perioper Pract 16 (12), 585–590.

36. Ellett, A.E., Shields, J.C., Ifune, C., et al., 2009. A near miss: a nitrous oxide-carbon dioxide mix-up despite current safety standards. Anesthesiology 110 (6), 1429–1431.

Chapter 3

Anesthesia Machine: A Practical Overview

Jeffrey M. Feldman

I recall the first time I administered anesthesia. The attending anesthesiologist injected the thiopental and muscle relaxant and the patient peacefully closed their eyes and stopped breathing. He then turned to me and said: "What are you going to do now?"

Of course, I was not completely unprepared to deliver this first anesthetic. The preoperative evaluation process was just a modified version of taking a history and performing a physical exam. I set up the room according to a straightforward protocol given to me by a more experienced person. I had even already developed some endotracheal intubation skills. In contrast, the anesthesia machine beside me was completely new. Sure, it had some resemblance to the ventilators I had seen used in the intensive care unit (ICU), but it was obviously different. Fortunately, a more experienced person guided my hand as I adjusted flows, administered potent anesthetic vapors, and adjusted the ventilator. As I reflect on the experience, I now understand how little I knew about the anesthesia machine that I relied upon to keep the patient safe and comfortable.

The anesthesia machine is essential to the practice of anesthesiology. We use it in some fashion for almost every patient we anesthetize. At the same time, the manner in which the machine interacts with the patient is complex. This chapter is intended to help the reader to develop an intuition for how the anesthesia machine can be used most effectively to anesthetize patients. Although specific machine designs will be used to illustrate the concepts, the intention is not to focus on a particular machine design. Virtually all modern anesthesia

machines can be used safely and effectively if the anesthesia provider understands the capabilities and limitations of the machine. The most commonly used design of a machine with a circle system and anesthetic vaporizer will be the focus of this chapter (Figure 3–1).

The ultimate goal of this chapter is to help the novice to use the anesthesia machine safely and effectively. By the end of the chapter, the reader will understand how to set the fresh gas flow, deliver anesthetic vapor effectively, and use the ventilator. Machine checkout and common causes of patient injury and machine failure are also reviewed. The engineering of the machine will not be discussed because that information is readily available in other sources. Hopefully, the information in this chapter will stimulate the curiosity to explore some of the suggested references at the end of the chapter, which will lead to mastery of the anesthesia machine.

What Is an Anesthesia Machine?

Simply put, an anesthesia machine is designed to deliver fresh gas (typically oxygen and air or nitrous oxide) and anesthetic vapor to a patient through a breathing circuit and allow for spontaneous, manual, or mechanical ventilation. Much of the design is focused on minimizing the waste of anesthetic vapors and preventing contamination of the operating room (OR) environment with anesthetic gases. There are typically monitoring functions built into the machine that verify

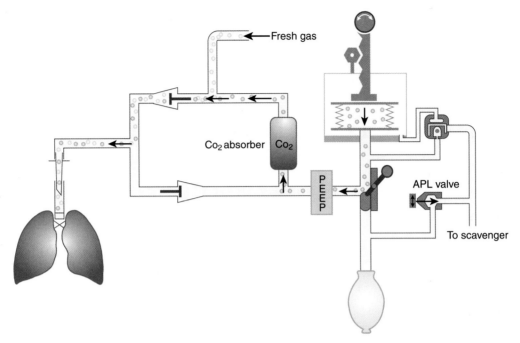

Figure 3–1 Schematic of standard anesthesia machine during inspiration. Source of fresh gas and anesthetic vapor (*blue circles*), bellows ventilator, circle breathing circuit, and scavenging system. *Orange circles* depict previously exhaled gas.

proper machine function and help to detect potentially unsafe conditions. Various anesthesia machine designs are available, all of which have differing capabilities, but the basic function of the machine is universal.

The ideal anesthesia machine design would provide instantaneous control of concentrations of oxygen and anesthetic vapor delivered to the patient, and have the capabilities of an intensive care ventilator. Further, the machine would be easy to use and never break down or malfunction. It would be entirely safe without any potential to injure a patient. Unfortunately, the ideal anesthesia machine does not exist, so the informed clinician must understand the capabilities and limitations of the machine(s) they use for patient care.

Fresh Gas Flow

All anesthesia machines provide controls to select and adjust the fresh gas that is introduced into the anesthesia circuit. Typically, these controls are mechanical flowmeters with valves that can be opened to precisely control the flow of pressurized gases into the breathing circuit. Newer machines may have electronic flowmeters but the basic function is the same. There is always an oxygen flowmeter and usually additional flowmeters for nitrous oxide and air. Specialty anesthesia machines can also have flowmeters for helium and carbon dioxide but the use of these gases is beyond the scope of this chapter.

So how should fresh gas flow be adjusted? The operator can make choices about the *types of gases to deliver* and the *flow rate of each gas* to be delivered.

Which Types of Gases Should Be Mixed in the Fresh Gas Flow?

The oxygen flow setting is probably the most used control on the anesthesia machine. The novice may decide to only administer oxygen to a patient and feel comfortable that the

patient will be as safe as possible. Selecting the anesthetic gases to be delivered should, however, be carefully considered (Table 3–1).

If oxygen alone is delivered, the patient will receive 100% oxygen in the inspired gas. Although oxygen is generally considered beneficial, there are disadvantages to delivering only oxygen to the patient. Oxygen toxicity is classically described as a disadvantage to delivering high oxygen concentrations, especially in neonates who are at risk for retinal disease in the presence of high oxygen concentration. It is arguable whether or not exposure to high oxygen concentrations for the relatively brief periods during anesthesia leads to complications of oxygen toxicity. Nevertheless, it is accepted practice to reduce the oxygen concentration especially for neonates.

There are disadvantages to delivering 100% oxygen that are more commonly applicable to the anesthetized patient. It is well documented that 100% oxygen will lead to absorption atelectasis—a common cause of lung dysfunction during and after anesthesia.[1] Pulse oximetry is typically used to assess oxygenation during anesthesia, but only estimates oxyhemoglobin saturation. In the presence of an enriched oxygen concentration, the oxyhemoglobin saturation may be 100% despite the presence of significant ventilation perfusion mismatch. Using an increased oxygen concentration will potentially hide an oxygenation problem that could otherwise be identified by the pulse oximeter as a reduced oxyhemoglobin saturation.[2] Oxygen also supports combustion and it must be avoided in high concentrations when there is a risk of fire (e.g., airway surgery) or by open delivery (e.g., nasal cannula) during head and neck surgery.[1,3]

There are situations when the patient's medical condition dictates the need for inspired gas consisting of 100% oxygen. Most commonly, 100% oxygen is used during induction of, and emergence from, general anesthetic to reduce the risk for significant hypoxemia if there are problems maintaining an adequate airway. Patients with critical lung disease due to

Table 3–1 Which Gas Should Be Delivered During Anesthesia?

Gas	Advantages	Disadvantages
O₂	• Reduce risk of hypoxemia during ○ Induction and emergence ○ One lung ventilation ○ ARDS or other lung injury • Reduce risk of wound infection?	• Absorption atelectasis • Increases the risk of fire especially during airway surgery • O₂ toxicity especially for neonates • Reduces utility of pulse oximeter to assess the alveolar to arterial O₂ gradient
Nitrous Oxide	• Increases MAC at high concentrations • Enhances uptake of anesthetic vapor during induction by the second gas effect	• Increases the volume of air-containing spaces within the body • Increases risk of postoperative nausea and vomiting • Increases risk of fire especially during airway surgery
Air	• Contains 21% O₂ and can be used as the sole gas if lung function is normal • Physiological	• Reduces inspired O₂ concentration if high inspired O₂ concentration is required

Note: Advantages and disadvantages of typical balance gases used during anesthesia are described. Administering 100% O₂ can have many disadvantages and should not be used by default.

ARDS or an acute lung injury often require 100% oxygen to maintain an acceptable oxyhemoglobin saturation. Lung isolation procedures where only one lung is ventilated can facilitate surgery, but are associated with pulmonary shunt and ventilation perfusion mismatch often requiring 100% oxygen. There is some debate in the surgical literature about the potential for increased oxygen concentrations to reduce the risk of postoperative wound infection, but the evidence is not sufficiently conclusive to guide anesthetic practice.

If gas exchange in the lungs is normal, oxyhemoglobin should be 100% saturated with oxygen when only 21% oxygen is present in the inspired gas. Given the disadvantages of using 100% oxygen and the fact that it is not required to maintain adequate oxygen delivery, oxygen is typically mixed with another gas by the anesthesia provider.

Oxygen is mixed with nitrous oxide when a reduced inspired oxygen concentration is acceptable and the anesthetic properties of nitrous oxide are desired. Nitrous oxide is a relatively weak anesthetic agent and will increase the effective delivered MAC, but is most useful at concentrations of at least 50% and ideally 70%. When nitrous oxide is used, the ratio of nitrous oxide to oxygen flow should provide concentrations of N₂O and O₂ of 50% each or even 70%:30%, respectively. These ratios can be achieved with a variety of total flow settings and the rationale for selecting a particular magnitude of flow will be discussed below. Nitrous oxide can be especially useful during inhalation inductions with a potent anesthetic, such as sevoflurane, where the so-called second gas effect enhances the uptake of the potent anesthetic vapor. Nitrous oxide is often avoided for different reasons. It is not desirable when there are confined air spaces in the body where expansion of the air space in the presence of N₂O is not desired. Examples include bowel surgery especially for intestinal obstruction or ear, eye, or intracranial surgery. There is arguable evidence that N₂O increases the incidence of postoperative nausea and vomiting which can be the reason for avoiding N₂O. Like oxygen, N₂O also supports combustion and it should be avoided if there is a risk of fire.

Air is the most common gas delivered with oxygen when N₂O is not administered. Air does not have any anesthetic properties but is an ideal balance gas for reducing the inspired oxygen concentration. Air contains 21% oxygen and can be used as the only fresh gas supplied to the patient assuming

Table 3–2 Ratios of O₂ and Air Flows and Resulting Inspired O₂ Concentration

Air Flow Setting	O₂ Flow Setting	Resulting Inspired O₂ Concentration
1	0.5	47%
1	1	60.5%
2	0.5	37%
2	1	67.6%
5	0.5	28%

Note: Air and O₂ are often mixed to achieve a certain inspired O₂ concentration. Since air already contains 21% O₂, it does not take much additional O₂ flow to significantly enrich the inspired O₂ concentration. If the goal is to limit the inspired O₂ concentration, the total flow of O₂ mixed with the air must be considered. Some examples are given below. The inspired O₂ concentration monitor will measure the inspired O₂ concentration that results from the air and O₂ flow settings. The equation for calculating the inspired O₂ concentration in mixtures of air and O₂ is:
$$O_2 \text{ Concentration (\%)} = 100 \times (1.0 \times O_2 \text{ L/min}) + (0.21 \times \text{Air L/min})/(O_2 \text{ L/min} + \text{Air L/min})$$

that ventilation is adequate and there is no lung pathology impairing gas exchange. Due to the oxygen already present in air, not much additional oxygen flow is needed to significantly enrich the inspired oxygen concentration (Table 3–2). This is an important consideration when it is important to minimize the inspired oxygen concentration such as when there is potential for an OR fire. Some anesthesia machines are only equipped with oxygen and nitrous oxide flowmeters. This configuration is a significant limitation and leaves the anesthesia provider with only the ability to deliver 100% oxygen or oxygen and nitrous oxide. When the risk of fire is a concern, this type of anesthesia machine should not be used.

It is useful to have an intuition for which gases to select to achieve a desired inspired oxygen concentration. Fortunately, inspired oxygen concentration monitors are standard on most anesthesia machines and considered a standard of care in much of the world. The inspired oxygen monitor should be used, especially by the novice, to confirm that the desired oxygen concentration has been achieved or to guide adjusting the gas flows accordingly.

How Much Flow Should Be Set for Each Gas?

In the previous section, the considerations for selecting the types of gases in the fresh gas were discussed. The combination of flows of each of the gases set to be delivered will determine the concentrations of each of the gases that result. Many combinations of flows can be used that will result in the same concentrations of gases in the circuit. For example, it would seem that 50% O_2 and 50% N_2O could be achieved by using equal flows of each gas at any setting, the only difference being the magnitude of the total flow. However, as we will see, as the total flow is lowered, the actual concentrations that result will be influenced by the patient's oxygen consumption. There are other implications that should be considered when selecting the actual gas flow setting. The total flow set to be delivered is dictated in part by the desired concentrations of the individual gases, but also by 1) the *desired rate of change* of gas and anesthetic vapor concentration and 2) the *desire to minimize the waste of anesthetic vapor and gases* by rebreathing exhaled gases.

Fresh Gas Flow and the Rate of Change of Gas and Vapor Concentrations

In our standard anesthesia machine, the gases delivered by the flowmeters pass through the anesthetic vaporizer and enter the anesthetic circuit as a mixture of vapors and gases. That mixture then combines with the existing gases in the breathing circuit to determine the combination of gases delivered to the patient. It is often desirable to change the concentrations of gases and vapor in the circuit rapidly. The most notable examples are during induction and emergence when the inspired anesthetic vapor concentration must be increased and decreased respectively. Although the actual factors that determine the rate at which the inspired concentration delivered to the patient changes are complex, the total fresh gas flow and the volume of the breathing circuit are major factors.

The rate of change of gas concentrations in the anesthetic circuit can be estimated by dividing the total volume of the circuit by the total fresh gas flow. The resulting number is the time constant, or the time it takes for the concentration of gases in the system to reach 63% of the final concentration. For example, consider the case where the total volume of the anesthetic system is 5 liters. If the total fresh gas flow is 5 liters per minute, the time constant is one minute, and it will take four time constants (4 minutes) for the concentrations in the system to reach 98% of the concentrations in the fresh gas. Similarly, if the fresh gas flow is 1 liter per minute, the time constant will be 5 minutes and it will take 20 minutes to reach 98% of the concentrations in the fresh gas. This estimation process is useful to gain an intuition for the impact of the total fresh gas flow and the volume of the circuit on the rate of change of concentration. It is not entirely accurate since the actual time depends upon a complex relationship of the geometry of the anesthetic system, the volume delivered to the patient with each breath and the ventilator settings. A complete explanation of these relationships is beyond the scope of this chapter. Suffice it to say that the higher the fresh gas flow, the more rapidly the concentrations of gases in the circuit will change and based upon the time constant estimation, relatively high fresh gas flows are needed to effect a rapid change in concentrations (Figure 3–2).

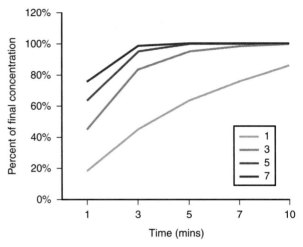

RATE OF CHANGE OF CONCENTRATION
IN CIRCLE SYSTEM AT DIFFERENT
FRESH GAS FLOWS
(5 liter circuit volume)

Figure 3–2   Concentration time plot that indicates predicted rate of change of anesthetic agent concentration from 0 to 1 MAC at different fresh gas flows.

Total Fresh Gas Flow and the Conservation (Waste) of Anesthetic Gases

Before the introduction of the circle anesthesia circuit, anesthetic vapors were delivered in an open circuit configuration. Patients inhaled the anesthetic gases and exhaled gases never returned to the patient. This design was inherently wasteful as any anesthetic vapors that were exhaled were basically lost, primarily as contaminants, into the OR environment. In an effort to reduce the amount of waste, the circle circuit was designed to allow for exhaled gases to return to the patient. *The total amount of fresh gas flow determines how much of the exhaled gases return to the patient.* This important fact will be used to explain the concepts of an Open Circuit, Closed Circuit, and Minimal (Low) Fresh Gas Flow approach to fresh gas delivery (Table 3–3).

Using the Circle System as an "Open Circuit"

The concept of the open circuit is fairly intuitive. In essence, if the total fresh gas flow is so great that it supplies all of the inspired gas to the patient, then none of the exhaled gas returns to the patient, i.e., all of the exhaled gas leaves the circuit as waste. The open circuit is desirable when a rapid change in inspired gas concentration is desired since the inspired gas concentrations will equal those in the fresh gas flow, and any changes in gas or vapor concentrations will be reflected in the inspired gases rapidly (Table 3–3).

So how much fresh gas is needed to achieve an open circuit? A general rule of thumb is that total fresh gas flow in excess of minute ventilation[2] will result in an open circuit, i.e., no rebreathing of exhaled gases. The exact amount of fresh gas needed to achieve an open circuit will vary between anesthesia machine designs. Breath to breath monitoring of fresh gas and vapor concentrations is common in modern anesthesia practice. Inspired gas concentration monitoring

Table 3–3 Examples of Fresh Gas Flow Settings That Can Be Used to Create Open and Closed Circuit Configurations

Functional Circuit Configuration	O₂ Only Flow (L/min)	O₂/Nitrous Oxide Flow (L/min)	O₂/Air Flow (L/min)	Comments
Open Circuit	7	2/5	1/6	Assumes minute ventilation of 7 L/min or less. No requirement for increased O₂ concentration.
Closed Circuit	0.4	—	—	Only O₂ is given to match O₂ consumption (assumed 400 mL/min) once concentrations of other gases and vapors are achieved.
Minimal Flow				
Induction	7	2/5	1/6	Higher flows reflect need to change concentration in the circuit rapidly and make up for rapid uptake of anesthetic from the lungs.
Maintenance	0.4	0.4/1.0	0.2/1.0	Based on estimated O₂ consumption of 400 mL/min Air adds to available O₂. Use inspired O₂ monitor to ensure that inspired O₂ concentration is not decreasing.

Note: Sample flows for open, closed, and minimal flow conditions using a circle anesthesia system to care for an adult patient. Minute ventilation assumed to be 7 L/min and O₂ consumption 400 mL/min.
When using a closed or minimum flow configuration during maintenance, increase O₂ flow for greater O₂ consumption, decrease flow when O₂ consumption is less. Use the inspired O₂ concentration monitor to guide settings and prevent hypoxemia.
Note: Open circuit—Can be used during induction or maintenance
Closed circuit—Best during maintenance of anesthesia
Minimal flow—Adequate for all phases of anesthesia, but requires interactive alteration of gas flows

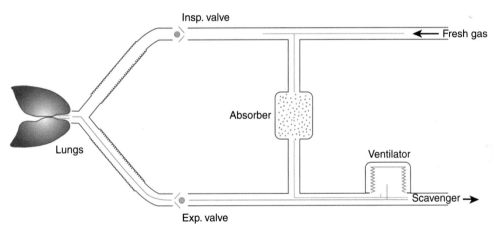

Figure 3–3 Schematic of circle system at end exhalation in open circuit condition. Fresh gas flow exceeds minute ventilation so that none of the exhaled gas returns to the patient. Once the bellows fills, the gas leaving via the scavenging system consists of all of the exhaled gas and additional fresh gas depending upon the total fresh gas flow.

can be used to confirm that an open circuit configuration exists since the inspired gas and vapor concentrations will equal the concentrations set to be delivered by the flowmeters and vaporizer.

It is interesting to note that the open circuit can be useful in the event of a failure of the carbon dioxide absorbent material. Since no exhaled gases return to the patient when fresh gas flow is sufficient to create an open circuit, CO_2 absorption is not required. When using a properly functioning circle system, the inspired carbon dioxide should be zero. If the CO_2 absorbent becomes saturated and can no longer absorb carbon dioxide, inspired CO_2 will increase and the capnogram will indicate inspired carbon dioxide throughout inspiration. The definitive solution is to replace the absorbent material, but increasing the fresh gas flow to exceed minute ventilation

will "open the circuit " and eliminate the inspired CO2 until the absorbent can be replaced.

Using the Circle System as a "Closed Circuit"

Delivering anesthesia via a closed circuit is an interesting and challenging activity. The basic concept is to deliver only enough fresh gas and anesthetic vapor to replace what is used by the patient. In essence, this means setting the oxygen flowmeter to deliver only enough oxygen to meet the metabolic demands or oxygen consumption, and only enough anesthetic vapor to replace the amount of vapor taken up by the body. Delivering anesthesia by closed circuit is not particularly convenient. A leak proof anesthesia circuit is required

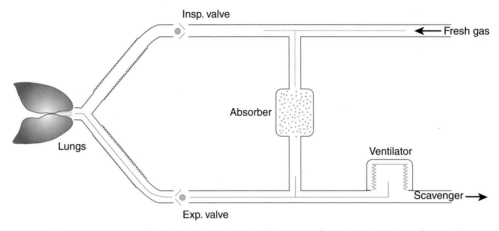

Figure 3–4 Schematic of circle system at onset of inspiration showing closed circuit configuration. Note that all exhaled gas returns to the patient after passing through the CO_2 absorbent. No gas exits via the scavenging system. This condition occurs when fresh gas entering the system exactly matches the O_2 and anesthetic vapor used by the patient. Note that the bellows does not fill to the top of the bellows chamber. This is done on purpose to serve as a visual indicator of proper fresh gas flow setting. If there is too much fresh gas, the bellows will rise with each breath. If there is inadequate fresh gas, the bellows will fall with each breath.

and a means to add anesthetic vapor rapidly to the inspired gas despite a low total fresh gas flow intended to only match oxygen consumption.[3] Due to the practical constraints, the details of performing closed circuit anesthesia are primarily of historical interest although the science and methods are well described. Anyone interested in developing a thorough understanding of the circle system will benefit from learning about closed circuit anesthesia (Figure 3–4; see also Chapter 4).[4]

Using "Minimal or Low Fresh Gas Flow" with a Circle System

Determining the total magnitude of fresh gas flow to provide at any given time is a balance between providing enough fresh gas flow to effect a change in inspired gas or vapor concentrations at the desired rate, and conserving gases and vapors by returning as much of the exhaled gas to the patient as possible. The open circuit and closed circuit conditions exemplify the opposite extremes of these two goals. Low flow anesthesia is a term often used to describe the use of reduced fresh gas flows to conserve gas without the challenges of a true closed circuit anesthetic. "Minimal flow anesthesia" may be more descriptive of the goals since it indicates the lowest flow needed to achieve the desired balance between rate of change of concentrations and conservation.

Initial delivery of anesthetic vapor to a patient requires a fairly high total gas flow if a rapid induction is desired. A minimal flow anesthetic would require much higher fresh gas flows in this phase of the anesthetic to achieve the desired goal of a rapid induction than during the maintenance phase of anesthesia. These relationships can be observed during induction by comparing the vaporizer setting with the measured concentrations of inspired and expired anesthetic vapors. If the fresh gas flow is high enough to approach an open circuit, the inspired concentration of vapor should approximate the vaporizer setting. The expired vapor concentration will initially be much lower than the inspired concentration but as induction proceeds, the difference between inspired and expired concentrations will diminish to reflect a reduced amount of uptake of anesthetic vapor. As the anesthetic vapor

delivery continues, the rate of uptake of anesthetic vapor by the body will diminish, and the difference between inspired and expired anesthetic concentrations will become small. The total fresh gas flow can then be reduced to minimize waste by returning exhaled gas to the patient.

It is possible to approach a closed circuit configuration during maintenance of anesthesia by reducing the total amount of oxygen to approximate oxygen consumption. It is important to ensure that total oxygen flow equals the sum of oxygen consumption and any leaks from the circuit. If an aspirating (sidestream) gas analyzer is being used to sample gas from the breathing circuit, the volume removed must be replaced by the fresh gas flow unless it is returned to the breathing circuit via a return circuit. The volume of oxygen provided is the total flow from the oxygen flowmeter and 21% of the flow from the air flowmeter if it is being used. If air or nitrous oxide are being delivered, it is difficult to approximate a true closed circuit and some exhaled gas will be wasted.

Special Case: Sevoflurance and Minimal Flows

The total fresh gas flow required when administering sevoflurance has been somewhat controversial. Sevoflurance is known to interact with carbon dioxide absorbents, primarily those containing sodium, barium, or potassium hydroxide, to produce Compound A*, which has been shown to be nephrotoxic to animals. The degree of nephrotoxicity is directly related to the total concentration of Compound A and duration of exposure. Although the nephrotoxic potential in humans does not seem to be clinically important, there are recommendations to limit the exposure to Compound A. Specifically, the labeling for sevoflurance approved by the Food and Drug Administration indicates that fresh gas flow should never be less than 1 L/min and not less than 2 L/min for more than 2 MAC-hours. Fresh gas flow is used in this

*Compound A is short for fluoromethyl-2-2-difluoro-1-(trifluoromethyl) vinyl ether

case to limit the exposure to Compound A by ensuring that a certain amount of fresh gas continuously enters the circuit, washing out exhaled gas and any products of chemical decomposition within the circuit.

Is It Possible to Deliver Too Little Oxygen?

An adequate supply of oxygen is essential to safe anesthetic care. Unfortunately, patients have died or been permanently injured as a result of hypoxia during anesthesia. For that reason, modern anesthesia machines are designed with a variety of safeguards to ensure the availability of oxygen. Even with all of these safeguards, it is still possible to deliver too little oxygen when using a minimal or low flow anesthetic technique.

The first safeguard monitors oxygen supply pressure to the anesthesia machine and sounds an alarm if oxygen pressure falls below a preset minimum. This alarm will sound regardless of whether the machine is supplied from a piped or a cylinder source and is a safety feature required by international standards. Some oxygen flowmeters are designed to provide a minimum oxygen flow at all times, typically about 175 mL/min. Some machines allow for air alone, which contains 21% oxygen, to be administered without any minimum oxygen flow. Another safeguard required by the standards organizations is an interlock between the oxygen and nitrous oxide flowmeters, which ensures a ratio of gases that cannot provide less than 21% oxygen in the fresh gas. All anesthesia machines in use should have this feature.

Since the minimum concentration of oxygen supplied by the flowmeters is always 21%, no matter which gases are used, how then is it possible to provide too little oxygen? The important concept here is that the concentration of oxygen, and the total amount of oxygen, are two different things. If 21% oxygen is supplied, but the total amount of oxygen is less than the patient's oxygen consumption, then the concentration of oxygen in the breathing circuit will diminish. Consider, for example, a mixture of oxygen and nitrous oxide of 300 mL/min and 700 mL/min, respectively. This would be a minimal flow approach, whereby the oxygen flow is set to approximate oxygen consumption, and the total nitrous oxide flow would be set to achieve an effective concentration of nitrous oxide. The concentration of oxygen in the fresh gas flow would be 30%. If, however, the patient's oxygen consumption was greater than 300 mL/min, then insufficient oxygen would be supplied. The result would be a gradual decrease in the inspired oxygen concentration in the breathing circuit as the patient consumed more oxygen than was being supplied, leading ultimately to hypoxemia.

This observation underscores the importance of the last safeguard to adequate oxygen delivery—continuous monitoring of inspired oxygen concentration. This safeguard is mandated by both anesthesia machine design standards and patient monitoring standards. Every anesthesia machine must be equipped with the capability to monitor the inspired oxygen concentration delivered to the patient. Alternatively, one can use a separate monitoring system or device to provide that capability. In any event, a functioning inspired oxygen monitor must be used during every anesthetic procedure. Not only will this device facilitate a minimal fresh gas flow technique and confirm adequate oxygen delivery, but it will also ensure that the gas actually delivered to the anesthesia machine from the pipeline or cylinder is indeed oxygen.

Vaporizers

Modern anesthesia vaporizers are designed to turn liquid anesthetic into a vapor that can be mixed with gases and delivered to the patient in a controlled concentration. In general, modern anesthesia vaporizers are highly reliable devices. The user can be comfortable that the vapor concentration set to be delivered will indeed be the concentration that leaves the vaporizer and enters the circle system. Periodic calibrations should be performed as part of a preventive maintenance schedule to ensure proper function.

The most important consideration when using a vaporizer is that the concentration set to be delivered will not be identical to the concentration actually delivered to the patient. This difference is due to the volume of the breathing circuit and the rate of fresh gas flow as discussed previously. Since the actual difference between set and delivered concentrations is difficult to predict, monitoring the concentration of anesthetic vapors in the breathing circuit is useful to both understand how well the vapor is being delivered, and how deeply the patient is anesthetized.[4] Anesthetic vapor monitors measure both inspired and expired anesthetic concentrations in the breathing circuit. The inspired concentration can be compared with the concentration set to be delivered by the vaporizer to appreciate the relationship between fresh gas flow and the rate of change of vapor concentration. The expired anesthetic concentration is the better indicator of how deeply the patient is anesthetized because it is a reflection of the concentration of anesthetic in the alveolus. At the beginning of an anesthetic procedure, fresh gas flow is typically set relatively high and the inspired vapor concentration approaches the set concentration on the dial, while the expired concentration starts out low and gradually approaches the inspired concentration. As the expired concentration reaches the desired value (typically 0.5-1 MAC), the fresh gas flow rate can be reduced to conserve anesthetic vapor. The vapor, however, will continue to be taken up by the patient so that continued monitoring of expired vapor concentration should be used to assure adequate depth of anesthesia.

The specifics of vaporizer designs are well described in many other references and will not be reviewed in detail here. Historically, vaporizers have been passive devices that are filled with liquid anesthetic agents and designed to mix anesthetic vapor with fresh gas at a specific concentration that is selected by the anesthesia professional. The term applied to these vaporizers is 'variable bypass vaporizers' since they direct a variable amount of fresh gas through the vaporizing chamber to achieve a specific concentration in the effluent from the vaporizer. Since vaporization is a temperature dependent process, modern anesthesia vaporizers are temperature compensated to ensure that the accuracy of the vaporizer is not influenced by ambient temperature. More recently, alternate vaporizer designs have been introduced that require electrical power, for example, vaporizers designed to deliver Desflurane.

Desflurane is unique among the potent anesthetic vapors because it boils (vaporizers) at or around room temperature (22.8° C) and also because the MAC value is 3 to 6 times greater than the other potent anesthetics. As a result, delivering desflurane using a variable bypass vaporizer would vaporize so much anesthetic that it would be impossible to compensate for the cooling effect of the vaporization process. As a result, modern desflurane vaporizers are heated to a constant temperature to ensure that the vapor can be delivered at a constant and reliable concentration.

Scavenging Systems

Scavenging systems are designed to prevent the anesthetic vapors from contaminating the OR environment and exposing OR personnel to the anesthetic gases and vapors. Specific designs are well described and will not be reviewed here. From a user's perspective, it is important to ensure that the scavenging systems are connected appropriately. Typically, there are two connections to the scavenging system, one to the breathing circuit and another to a suction supply in the operating room. The breathing circuit connection carries any excess gas in the breathing circuit to the scavenging system. Recall from our previous discussion of closed circuit anesthesia that any amount of gas that exceeds what the patient consumes will be wasted and must escape from the circuit via the scavenging system. The only condition when the scavenging system is not needed is during closed circuit anesthesia delivery.

The suction connection to the scavenging system carries waste gases away from the OR to a central suction system in the hospital. Most scavenging system designs include an adjustment for the amount of suction applied to the scavenging system. Depending upon the system, there are different approaches to adjusting the amount of suction and the user must be familiar with the method required for the equipment being used. Often there is a flowmeter or some other indicator of the amount of suction with a guide to the proper setting. Scavenging systems also have safety features that prevent suction from being applied to the breathing circuit leading to negative pressure applied to the patient's lungs. Scavenging systems are also designed to vent excess gases to the room if suction becomes ineffective rather than expose the patient to excessive pressure in the circuit if the gases cannot escape.

Traditionally, the suction connection has been identical to the suction supply that is used for patient care in the operating room. More modern OR construction uses a separate waste anesthesia gas device (WAGD) suction that may or may not be distinct from the OR suction (i.e., there may or may not be separate piping to the central hospital suction). One motivation for a separate WAGD system is to be able to use special suction pumps that reduce the risk of fire. Although flammable anesthetics are no longer in use, the gases leaving the anesthesia machine often contain high concentrations of oxygen, which increases the fire hazard.

The Anesthesia Ventilator

For many years after the introduction of ether anesthesia, there was no need for an anesthesia ventilator. One of the great advantages of ether anesthesia was the ability to anesthetize the patient without depressing the respiratory drive to a dangerous degree. It was not until the introduction of muscle relaxants and opioids into anesthesia practice that the need for an anesthesia ventilator became compelling. Anesthesia providers at that time would manually ventilate patients by squeezing a bag attached to the breathing circuit. Manual ventilation, however, became tiresome and inconvenient,

especially for long procedures, as it was difficult to provide all the aspects of care when the hands were continuously occupied. The early anesthesia ventilators were essentially automated bag squeezers that used pressurized gas to move a bellows and mimic manual ventilation by delivering a set tidal volume at a set rate. In recent years, a major focus of modern anesthesia machine design has been to incorporate enhanced modes of ventilation that reproduce the capabilities of an intensive care unit ventilator.

At present, there are a variety of anesthesia ventilator designs in use. The capabilities of these ventilators range from basic volume ventilators to devices that approach the capabilities of an intensive care ventilator. Many patients who require anesthesia have normal lung function and do not require a very sophisticated ventilator. There are, however, certain patient populations that require careful attention to mechanical ventilation. These patients include people with ARDS or other low lung compliance conditions (e.g., obesity) where high inspiratory pressures may be needed for effective ventilation. Pediatric patients are another population who require precise ventilation since even small errors in volume delivery can be a significant percentage of the desired tidal volume.

Why Not Use an ICU Ventilator Instead of an Anesthesia Machine?

ICU ventilators offer a wide variety of ventilator modes and can ventilate even the most challenging patients. The technology is mature and readily available. Why bother to redesign anesthesia ventilators to enhance their capabilities when ICU ventilators are readily available? The primary limitation of ICU ventilators for delivering anesthetic vapors is their inherent open circuit configuration. The virtually unlimited pressure and flow capabilities of these ventilators is made possible by an unlimited supply of inspired gas, which is available to the breathing circuit directly from regulated pipeline or cylinder gas supplies. The gas that is delivered to the patient provides both the patient's needs, and the pressure and flow required for adequate ventilation. The basic design of the ICU ventilator does not allow for exhaled gas to return to the patient and therefore wastes all exhaled anesthetic gas and vapor. There have been examples where vaporizers were added to ICU ventilators but the inherent open circuit configuration made vapor delivery impractical and wasteful.

In contrast to the ICU ventilator, anesthesia ventilators separate the gas delivered to the patient from the power to the ventilator to conserve the anesthetic agent. As a result, the volume of gas available to generate inspiratory pressure and flow is limited by the total volume of the ventilator chamber. This volume is typically about 2 L and must satisfy the tidal volume to be delivered, any volume lost via leaks in the circuit, and the pressure and flow required to ventilate effectively. Once the ventilator chamber is empty, it does not matter how much pressure is exerted by the ventilator, no gas will flow to the patient. This basic need to separate patient gas from the ventilator power makes it challenging to design anesthesia ventilators that can mimic the function of an ICU ventilator. In contrast to the ICU ventilator, which has an unlimited supply of gas, the anesthesia ventilator is limited by the capacity of the patient gas chamber whether it be a bellows or a piston.

Basic Anesthesia Ventilator Design

As noted previously, the early anesthesia ventilators were essentially devices that automated the process of manual ventilation. Many ventilators such as this are still in use today. The clinician switches between using a manual bag or using the ventilator. Typically, a manual switch is moved, directing the exhaled patient gas either to the bag for manual ventilation, or to the ventilator for automated ventilation. A bellows is used to separate the drive gas from the patient gas. These basic ventilators are pneumatically powered such that regulated high pressure supply gas is used to move the bellows, producing the desired inspiration and exhalation. Traditional anesthesia ventilators are typically designed as volume ventilators (i.e., the clinician selects both the volume to be delivered to the patient and the respiratory rate. Some of these ventilators are enhanced with the ability to provide positive end-expiratory pressure (PEEP) and pressure, rather than volume, targeted ventilation.

Unfortunately, the basic anesthesia ventilator design has some important limitations. These limitations prevent accurate volume delivery and development of enhanced modes of ventilation. As surgical procedures have become more ambitious, and sicker patients have presented for anesthesia care, the need for better ventilator capabilities has become apparent.

What Are the Limitations of the Basic Anesthesia Ventilator?

A fundamental limitation of the basic anesthesia ventilator is the inability to accurately deliver the set tidal volume to the patient. This limitation is important when using volume controlled ventilation. There are two reasons why tidal volume is not delivered accurately—the compliance of the breathing system and the interaction between fresh gas flow and tidal volume (Figure 3–5).

Compliance in general is the ratio of volume to pressure. For every positive pressure ventilator circuit, there is a compliance factor that expresses the volume of gas that will be compressed in the circuit as pressure builds. This portion of the volume is "stored" in the circuit during inspiration and is not delivered to the patient. Expansion of the tubing connecting the ventilator to the patient is often considered a source of compliance but modern circuit tubing does not expand significantly under pressure. It is gas compression that is the primary reason for breathing system compliance. The length of the circuit is a major factor in determining the circuit compliance. Breathing circuits that are designed to expand or contract in an accordion-like fashion can have very different compliances depending upon the length of the circuit.

The compliance factor can be determined by occluding the end of the circuit and injecting a known volume of gas into the circuit. The gas can be injected with a calibrated syringe or, in the case of a modern anesthesia machine, the ventilator is designed to add the volume to the circuit and measure the resulting pressure. The ratio of the volume delivered by the ventilator into the occluded circuit to the pressure created is the compliance factor expressed in mL/cm H_2O. It is important that this compliance test be performed with the circuit configuration that will be used for the patient.

The compliance factor influences the ability of a ventilator to deliver tidal volume accurately. During inspiration, gas from the ventilator is moved into the patient's lungs by creating positive pressure in the breathing circuit. As the set tidal volume leaves the ventilator, pressure builds in the circuit, gas

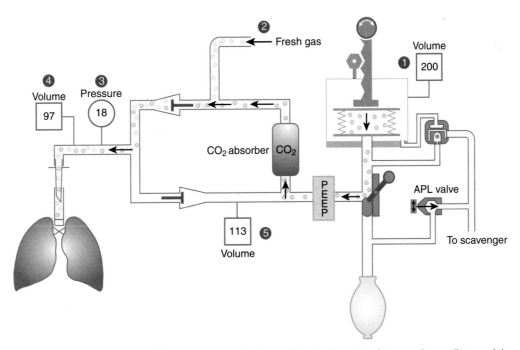

Figure 3–5   Changes in volume that occur around the circuit as a result of compliance in the system between the ventilator and the patient. Example shown for pediatric patient. *(1)* The set tidal volume is delivered at the ventilator. *(2)* Fresh gas adds to the delivered tidal volume. *(3)* Pressure increases in the circuit. *(4)* Compliance reduces the volume delivered to the patient. *(5)* The exhaled volume measurement is influenced by the compliance of the breathing circuit and will overestimate the actual delivered volume. The volume delivered to the patient's airway is unpredictable and typically not measured. The difference between set and delivered tidal volume can be significant in pediatric patients and all patients where high airway pressures are required.

is compressed, and a portion of the set tidal volume does not reach the patient.

Older anesthesia ventilators are designed so that the ventilator will deliver the set tidal volume into the breathing circuit. Compliance, however, reduces the tidal volume that ultimately reaches the patient. The typical compliance of the breathing system between the ventilator and the patient can be in the range of 5 to 7 mL/cm H_2O. At normal inspiratory pressures of 15 to 20 cm H_2O, compliance might only reduce tidal volume by 100 mL, which may not be critical in the average healthy adult patient. However, when increased inspiratory pressures (e.g., 40 cm H_2O) are needed, or when tidal volumes are small (pediatric patients), the inability of the ventilator to compensate for the compliance of the breathing system makes it difficult to provide precise ventilation to these patients. These are, however, the very patients who require precise ventilation to ensure adequate gas exchange.

The tidal volume delivered to the patient is influenced not only by the compliance of the breathing system, but also by fresh gas flow. When using a circle system, changes in fresh gas flow will alter the delivered tidal volume. The degree to which fresh gas flow alters tidal volume depends upon respiratory rate and I:E ratio (inspiratory time) and total fresh gas flow and can be difficult to predict. If fresh gas flow is reduced without a compensatory increase in set tidal volume, minute ventilation will be reduced and hypoventilation and hypoxemia are possible. Likewise, an increase in fresh gas flow without reducing set tidal volume can cause hyperventilation and even excessive pressure with the potential for barotrauma. Once the ventilator has been set to deliver a particular tidal volume, any change in fresh gas flow will alter the volume that the patient receives. The interaction between fresh gas flow and tidal volume becomes important again for patients with poor lung compliance or pediatric patients that require small tidal volumes.

Another consequence of breathing system compliance is the inaccuracy it introduces into tidal volume monitoring. Tidal volume monitoring can be inaccurate since the flow sensor used to measure tidal volume is typically located at the expiratory valve. During exhalation, both exhaled gas and the gas that was compressed in the breathing circuit during inspiration pass through the flow sensor. As a result, the sensor will indicate a tidal volume that is greater than the volume the patient actually received. For example, if the breathing circuit compliance is 1.5 mL/cm H_2O, and the peak inspiratory pressure is 30 cm H_2O, the tidal volume measurement will be overestimated by 45 mL. Depending upon the compliance of the circuit, the inspiratory pressure and the actual desired tidal volume, the difference between measured and delivered tidal volume can be significant, especially for pediatric patients.

To this day, it is not uncommon to bring an ICU ventilator into the operating room and provide intravenous anesthesia for patients who are difficult to ventilate. The increasingly sophisticated anesthesia ventilators that have been developed in recent years are, however, eliminating the need to bring an ICU ventilator into the operating room.

What Are the Features of the Modern Anesthesia Ventilators?

When using volume controlled ventilation, the goal of modern ventilator design is to deliver a volume to the patient that is as close as possible to the volume set to be delivered. To achieve this goal, the ventilator must be able to compensate for both the compliance of the breathing system and the influence of fresh gas flow on tidal volume, independent of changes in lung compliance. Some bellows ventilators use a flow sensor at the inspiratory limb to control the volume delivered by the ventilator. The ventilator output is controlled by the flow sensor such that the set volume is delivered to the breathing circuit independent of changes in fresh gas flow or the compliance of the system between the ventilator and the flow sensor. These designs are an improvement over traditional designs but only ensure set tidal volume delivery to the inspiratory limb of the circuit where the sensor is in place. There is no compensation for compliance of the breathing circuit downstream from the flow sensor.

Newer bellows ventilators and piston anesthesia ventilators measure the compliance of the breathing system during the preanesthesia checkout with the circuit occluded. The compliance measurement is then used to determine how much additional volume must be added to each breath to deliver the set volume to the patient's airway. The influence of fresh gas on delivered volume is eliminated in the piston design by altering the configuration of the circle system and including a valve, which prevents fresh gas from entering the patient circuit during mechanical inspiration. Other designs eliminate the fresh gas flow interaction by using an inspiratory flow sensor to detect changes in fresh gas flow. Anesthesia ventilators that measure the breathing circuit compliance typically provide improved exhaled volume measurement since the measured volume is corrected using the circuit compliance measurement (Figure 3–6).

Efforts to improve the design of anesthesia ventilators have been directed toward improving the accuracy of volume ventilation so that the patient reliably receives a tidal volume that is as close as possible to the set tidal volume. Another important improvement in anesthesia ventilator design has been to make multiple modes of ventilation available to the clinician in the operating room, especially modes that support spontaneous ventilation.

Selecting the Ventilation Mode: Volume Control, Pressure Control, and Pressure Support Ventilation

Volume controlled ventilation (VCV)[5] by definition is designed to deliver a constant tidal volume despite changes in the patient's pulmonary compliance. During volume controlled ventilation, inspiratory pressure varies and is dependent on the set tidal volume, PEEP, inspired gas flow rate, gas flow resistance, and respiratory system compliance. Increasing inflation pressure indicates decreased pulmonary compliance or obstruction of the breathing circuit (e.g., occluded ETT) (Figure 3–7).

The disadvantages of VCV include the potential to produce very high inflating pressures with the associated risk of barotrauma. This is an important consideration for adult patients with poor lung compliance and pediatric patients who may be exposed to high airway pressures for any number of reasons from a surgeon leaning on the patient's chest, to a mainstem intubation, to a cough that coincides with the inspiratory cycle of the ventilator. In all of these cases, in volume mode, the ventilator will continue to deliver

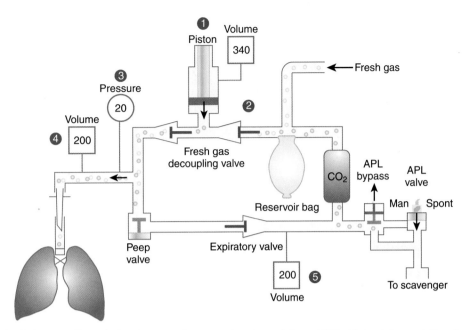

Figure 3–6   Schematic of piston ventilator design demonstrating accurate volume delivery. *(1)* Ventilator delivers additional volume to compensate for the compliance of the breathing system. *(2)* Fresh gas decoupling valve prevents fresh gas from entering the breathing circuit during inspiration. *(3)* Pressure increases in the circuit. *(4)* Desired tidal volume is delivered to the patient's airway. *(5)* Exhaled tidal volume measurement is compensated for compliance. Note: Even in the most modern anesthesia machine, the exhaled flow sensor is typically accurate to +/–10% of the actual value and will rarely agree exactly with the set tidal volume.

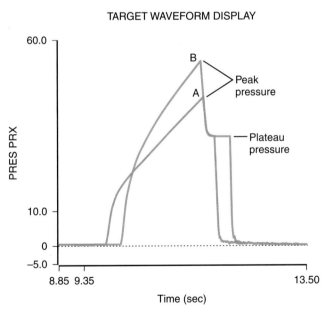

Figure 3–7   Typical pressure-time waveform during volume controlled ventilation. Peak and plateau pressure are both visible as a result of inspiratory pause, which ceases flow once the set tidal volume is delivered until the inspiratory time ends. The inspiratory pause is set to be longer in breath *B* compared with breath *A*, which increases the inspiratory flow to deliver the set tidal volume in a shorter time. The increased inspiratory flow increases the pressure generated by the resistance of the endotracheal tube. Since tidal volume and lung compliance have not changed, the plateau pressure is unchanged. Plateau pressure is the better measure of the pressure required to ventilate the patient because it is a combination of the lung-thorax compliance and the volume delivered. Peak pressure is not the pressure in the patient's lungs.

volume until it reaches either the target volume or the maximum pressure setting. Some modern anesthesia ventilators offer the ability to preset the maximum pressure when using volume controlled ventilation to reduce concern for barotrauma. If the inspiratory pressure limit is set to 40 cm H_2O, the ventilator will maintain pressure for the duration of inspiration, but cease to deliver gas once the pressure limit of 40 cm H_2O is reached. It is important to note that if the pressure limit is reached before the end of inspiration, the set tidal volume will not be delivered. The pressure limit should therefore be used as a safety net to prevent excessive pressure due to transient changes in lung compliance and not as a routine part of the ventilation strategy to limit the pressure of each breath. With proper monitoring of inspiratory pressure, including the use of appropriate limits and alarms, changes in the patient's pulmonary mechanics can be observed and the risk of barotrauma minimized. When an uncuffed endotracheal tube is used, VCV may not be desirable since any leaks that occur during inspiration will reduce the volume delivered to the patient.

Pressure controlled ventilation (PCV) differs from VCV in that the inspiratory pressure is constant and tidal volume changes as lung compliance changes. As a result, a decrease in the compliance of the patient's respiratory system, ventilator circuit, or tracheal tube will cause a reduction in delivered tidal volume. An increase in compliance, conversely, will result in an increased tidal volume (Figure 3–8). Alarm settings for volume and minute ventilation can be useful to help detect changes in volume delivery during PCV. Once baseline adequate ventilation is established at a set inspiratory pressure, upper and lower limits for tidal volume or minute ventilation alarms can be set close to the current baseline value.

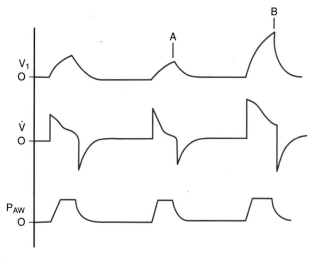

Figure 3–8 Pressure, flow, and volume waveforms during PCV. Note how lung compliance influences tidal volume, whereas the pressure waveform does not change. **A,** Indicates a reduced tidal volume resulting from reduced lung compliance relative to baseline, and **(B)** indicates an increased tidal volume resulting from increased lung compliance.

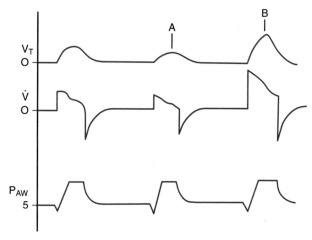

Figure 3–9 Pressure, flow, and volume waveforms during PSV. Changes in delivered volume are directly related to patient effort and lung compliance. **A,** Represents a decrease in lung compliance (or patient effort); **B,** represents an increase in lung compliance (or patient effort).

Any significant variation in lung compliance will cause a change in delivered volume and trigger the associated alarm.

PCV can be useful when using a traditional anesthesia ventilator that is not designed to deliver tidal volume accurately. Once the pressure required to deliver the desired tidal volume for a given circuit configuration is determined, the patient will receive that pressure independent of circuit compliance, changes in fresh gas flow, or small leaks around the endotracheal tube. The ventilator will deliver sufficient gas to reach the desired inspiratory pressure automatically compensating for compliance. As fresh gas flow is increased or decreased, the ventilator will deliver less, or more, gas to reach the set inspiratory pressure. Furthermore, since inspiratory pressure is set, excessive inflating pressures and barotrauma are avoided.

Pressure support ventilation (PSV) is widely used in the intensive care unit to support spontaneous ventilation for intubated patients. The primary advantage of PSV is the ability to use varying degrees of pressure support to reduce the work of breathing for the intubated patient. The tidal volume that results for a given breath is determined by the amount of patient effort, the set inspiratory pressure, and the patient's lung compliance (Figure 3–9).

For the anesthetized patient, the work of breathing imposed by an endotracheal tube or laryngeal mask airway and a circle system is an obstacle to allowing spontaneous ventilation. Anesthesia ventilators are now available with the capability to provide PSV. In PSV mode, the ventilator will detect the onset of a spontaneous breath typically by measuring inspiratory flow. Once the inspiratory flow exceeds a set trigger threshold, the ventilator will provide sufficient flow to achieve the set inspiratory pressure. If the trigger threshold is set too low, it is possible for "auto-triggering" to occur whereby the ventilator provides inspiratory pressure without a spontaneous effort by the patient. If the trigger threshold is set too high, the ventilator will not detect an inspiratory effort. Inspection of the pressure waveform can identify whether or not the trigger threshold is set appropriately.

Not surprisingly, studies comparing PSV during anesthesia to unsupported spontaneous ventilation have demonstrated increased tidal volume, reduced end-tidal carbon dioxide and work of breathing, and increased oxygenation.[5,6] PSV can support safe spontaneous ventilation despite the imposed work of breathing by the circle system and the respiratory depressant effects of anesthetic agents. Clinical advantages may be improved gas exchange, ability to titrate anesthetic depth (especially narcotics) based upon respiratory efforts, and facilitating the emergence process.

An important caveat is to remember the influence of anesthetic agents and opioid analgesics on the carbon dioxide response curve. Anesthetized patients typically require an elevated P_{CO_2} to breathe spontaneously. PSV may be useful to increase the volume and effectiveness of individual breaths, thereby improving oxygenation and offsetting the impact of work of breathing on P_{CO_2}; however, the minimum P_{CO_2} that can be attained will be limited by the apneic threshold as spontaneous breathing efforts must be maintained.

Modern anesthesia ventilators provide backup ventilation features that can be used if there is a risk of apnea during PSV. Synchronized intermittent mandatory ventilation (SIMV) can be combined with PSV to ensure that a minimum amount of minute ventilation will be provided. Depending upon the capabilities of the ventilator, SIMV can be used as either a volume or pressure controlled synchronized mode or both. When SIMV and PSV are used together, the patient will receive the preset SIMV breaths in synchrony with spontaneous efforts and will receive pressure support for additional breaths that exceed the SIMV rate. Should the patient cease to breathe, the SIMV breaths will continue to be delivered. Another backup mode that is available uses the pressure support settings to generate positive pressure breaths. Breaths are delivered at a preset minimum rate using the pressure support settings for both inspiratory and expiratory breaths. Although pressure support settings can be used as a safety net if apnea should occur during PSV, these backup modes should not be relied upon as a primary mode of controlled ventilation. In general, pressure support settings provide adequate tidal volumes when the patient is making spontaneous efforts.

Table 3–4 Guidelines for Selecting the Mode of Ventilation

Ventilation Mode	Description	Indications	Comments for Safe Use
Volume Controlled Ventilation (VCV)	Delivers a constant tidal volume with each breath. Pressure will vary with changes in lung compliance and resistance.	• Consistent tidal volume is desired • Excess pressure is not a major concern • No circuit leaks	• Assess inspiratory plateau pressure generated for desired volume. • Set pressure limit above plateau pressure to limit maximum possible pressure with changes in compliance or resistance.
Pressure Controlled Ventilation (PCV)	Delivers a constant inspiratory pressure with each breath. Volume will vary with changes in lung compliance and resistance.	• Small leaks in circuit (e.g., uncuffed endotracheal tube) • Older anesthesia ventilators not capable of accurate volume ventilation • Patients with respiratory distress syndrome requiring increased inspiratory pressures	• Exhaled tidal volume monitoring is important. • Set tidal volume or minute ventilation alarm just below desired value to facilitate recognizing reduced tidal volume.
Pressure Support Ventilation (PSV)	Detects inspiration and augments spontaneous breath by adding preset pressure during inspiration. Can also provide a set amount of expiratory pressure (PEEP).	• Patients breathing spontaneously during anesthesia	• Exhaled volume should be monitored and inspiratory pressure adjusted to achieve desired tidal volume. A minimum exhaled volume of 5 mL/kg is desirable. • Set trigger threshold appropriately based upon pressure and volume monitoring. • If apnea occurs, consider changing to controlled or mixed mode of ventilation.
VCV or PCV + PSV	VCV or PCV breaths are provided at the preset respiratory rate. Spontaneous efforts can trigger these breaths. Spontaneous breaths that exceed the preset rate trigger PSV breaths.	• Minimum mandatory ventilation is desired • Patients capable of spontaneous ventilation who are at risk for apnea or inadequate spontaneous efforts	• Same as PCV, VCV, and PSV modes depending upon which modes are selected.

Note: Commonly available modes of ventilation are listed along with indications for use for the anesthetized patient. Volume and pressure controlled ventilation can also be referred to as volume or pressure limited or volume or pressure targeted ventilation.

Pressure support settings will generate tidal volumes but the total volume may not be adequate in the absence of a patient effort (Table 3–4).

How Do You Know You Are Ventilating the Patient Effectively?

Setting the ventilator properly is the first step toward ensuring effective ventilation. Monitoring the ventilator function and the interaction of the ventilator with the patient is important to ensure that the intended ventilation is occurring. Several monitoring devices are commonly used toward that end.

Capnography, measurement of inspired and expired carbon dioxide, is one of the most important methods for ensuring proper ventilation and is required during every anesthetic procedure by ASA standards. There is no question that capnography has saved lives by serving as an immediate monitor of gas moving in and out of the patient's lungs. The typical capnogram measured using a circle anesthesia system should indicate that inspired CO_2 is zero and with each breath there is exhaled CO_2. An inspired CO_2 of zero confirms that the circle system is functioning properly to eliminate CO_2 rebreathing. Exhaled CO_2 documents the integrity of the patient's airway and is typically reported as the end-tidal value ($ETCO_2$) or the CO_2 concentration at the end of exhalation and most reflective of alveolar CO_2. The primary limitation of capnography is the unpredictable gradient between end-tidal CO_2 and arterial CO_2. If tidal volume is inadequate, the gradient between end-tidal and arterial CO_2 is increased and the end-tidal value can appear normal despite significant hypercarbia. Capnography is a necessary part of patient monitoring but not sufficient to ensure adequate ventilation. Capnography may be built into the anesthesia machine or it will be available from the bedside patient monitor.

Most anesthesia machines have the ability to measure tidal volume directly. A flow sensor is placed at the expiratory valve to measure exhaled flow and calculate tidal volume for each breath. Different technologies are used for these flow sensors and all are influenced by the concentrations of the exhaled gases. As a result, the inherent accuracy is +/−10% at best. Modern anesthesia machines that correct the exhaled volume measurements for circuit compliance provide more accurate volume monitoring than traditional machines. One should not expect the measured exhaled tidal volume to match the set tidal volume exactly. Despite the accuracy limitations, exhaled tidal volume monitoring is useful for confirming that the intended ventilation is occurring.

Pressure monitoring is also useful to evaluate ventilator function and is built into all anesthesia machines in use today. Typically, a pressure waveform is displayed indicating the cyclical changes in inspired and expired pressure. Numerical values for pressure are also displayed. Both peak and plateau pressures are typically provided along with PEEP. During pressure controlled ventilation, one would expect the inspired pressure to be constant breath to breath. During VCV, pressure can fluctuate as lung compliance changes. A primer on pressure monitoring is beyond the scope of this chapter but new users should familiarize themselves with the pressure monitoring capabilities of the anesthesia machine.

The final guarantor of adequate ventilation is the pulse oximeter, which measures oxyhemoglobin saturation. If the oxygen saturation approaches 100% and the F_{IO_2} is low (30% or less), one can have confidence that the ventilation is adequate. Since the pulse oximeter measures oxyhemoglobin saturation and not Pa_{O_2}, it is possible to have a significant unrecognized alveolar to arterial oxygen gradient at higher inspired oxygen concentrations. Assessing the effectiveness of mechanical ventilation using the pulse oximeter requires lower inspired oxygen concentrations. Arterial blood gas analysis is required to document the gradient between alveolar and arterial P_{O_2} if enriched oxygen is delivered in the inspired gas.

Avoiding and Troubleshooting Anesthesia Machine Problems

When used properly, the anesthesia machine is a highly reliable device capable of delivering anesthetic vapors safely and providing effective mechanical ventilation. Since the anesthetized patient is dependent upon the anesthesia machine to sustain life, problems with the anesthesia machine can have grave consequences. Indeed, there are numerous reports of patient injury and death related to improper use or failure of the anesthesia machine.

There are a variety of strategies that should be used to minimize the risk of patient injury related to the anesthesia machine. Preventive maintenance is essential. All anesthesia machine manufacturers have recommendations for preventive maintenance to be performed on a semiannual and/or annual basis. Whether the preventive maintenance is performed by an outside organization or by the hospital clinical engineering staff, it is essential to safe practice.

Anesthesia machines must also meet accepted safety standards. Obsolete anesthesia machines should not be used, and the definitions of obsolescence, both absolute and relative, are nicely described in a guideline published by the American Society of Anesthesiologists (Table 3–5).[7] Even when the most modern, well-maintained, anesthesia machine is used, there is still the potential for patient injury due to improper setup or failure of components. The final protection for the patient is therefore the checkout process that should be performed by the anesthesia provider before anesthetizing a patient.

Preanesthesia Checkout Procedures

Failure to check anesthesia equipment before use can lead to patient injury and has also been associated with an increased risk of severe postoperative morbidity and mortality.[8,9] In the past, anesthesia machine designs were sufficiently uniform that one checkout procedure could be applied to almost all anesthesia machines. Modern anesthesia machines have enough design differences that checkout procedures need to be customized to some degree for each type of anesthesia machine. Every anesthesia machine manufacturer publishes recommendations for equipment checkout before use. Recommendations for checkout procedures have also been published by the ASA.[10]

Table 3–5 Defining Anesthesia Machine Obsolescence
ABSOLUTE CRITERIA
1. Lack of essential safety features
2. Presence of unacceptable features
3. Adequate maintenance no longer possible
RELATIVE CRITERIA
1. Lack of certain safety features
2. Problems with maintenance
3. Potential for human error
4. Inability to meet practice needs
Note: Criteria specified in the American Society of Anesthesiologist's guidelines for determining anesthesia machine obsolescence.

The ASA preanesthesia checkout recommendations describe the minimum number of steps that need to be followed when checking the anesthesia machine and are based upon the following requirements for safe delivery of anesthesia.

- Reliable delivery of oxygen at any appropriate concentration up to 100%
- Reliable means of positive pressure ventilation
- Backup ventilation equipment available and functioning
- Controlled release of positive pressure from the breathing circuit
- Anesthesia vapor delivery (if intended as part of the anesthetic plan)
- Adequate suction
- Means to conform to standards for patient monitoring

Recommended checkout procedures are organized into those steps that need to be performed at the start of each day, and before anesthetizing each individual patient (Table 3–6). Properly trained anesthesia technicians and clinical engineers can assist with these checkout procedures, but it is the responsibility of each anesthesia provider to ensure that the anesthesia machine is functioning properly before each use. It is beyond the scope of this chapter to review checkout procedures for the variety of anesthesia machines in use. Every anesthesia department should have clearly described checkout procedures for the anesthesia machines in use in that department. The ASA publishes sample checkout procedures for a variety of anesthesia machines currently available.[6]

Although it is important to ensure proper function of the anesthesia machine, the preanesthesia checkout procedure must include confirmation of a backup supply of oxygen and means to ventilate the patient. If a backup method for oxygenation and ventilation is assured, no patient should suffer injury or death due to a problem with the anesthesia machine.

Specific Anesthesia Machine Problems

A complete troubleshooting guide for every anesthesia machine is beyond the scope of this chapter but there are some specific conditions that warrant mention. Anesthesia machines require supplies of compressed gases and electrical power to function properly. Loss of gas supplies or electrical power can result in complete failure of the anesthesia machine but proper attention to detail can allow for continued function until power is restored or another machine is made available.

Table 3–6 Anesthesia Machine Preuse Checkout Procedures
Summary of Checkout Recommendations by Frequency and Responsible Party

TO BE COMPLETED DAILY

Item to Be Completed	Responsible Party
Item 1: Verify auxiliary O_2 cylinder and self-inflating manual ventilation device are available and functioning.	Provider and tech
Item 2: Verify patient suction is adequate to clear the airway.	Provider and tech
Item 3: Turn on anesthesia delivery system and confirm that AC power is available.	Provider or tech
Item 4: Verify availability of required monitors, including alarms.	Provider or tech
Item 5: Verify that pressure is adequate on the spare O_2 cylinder mounted on the anesthesia machine.	Provider and tech
Item 6: Verify that the piped gas pressures are ≥50 psig.	Provider and tech
Item 7: Verify that vaporizers are adequately filled and, if applicable, that the filler ports are tightly closed.	Provider or tech
Item 8: Verify that there are no leaks in the gas supply lines between the flowmeters and the common gas outlet.	Provider or tech
Item 9: Test scavenging system function.	Provider or tech
Item 10: Calibrate, or verify calibration of, the O_2 monitor and check the low O_2 alarm.	Provider or tech
Item 11: Verify CO_2 absorbent is not exhausted.	Provider or tech
Item 12: Breathing system pressure and leak testing.	Provider and tech
Item 13: Verify that gas flows properly through the breathing circuit during both inspiration and exhalation.	Provider and tech
Item 14: Document completion of checkout procedures.	Provider and tech
Item 15: Confirm ventilator settings and evaluate readiness to deliver anesthesia care. (anesthesia timeout)	Provider

TO BE COMPLETED BEFORE EACH PROCEDURE

Item to Be Completed	Responsible Party
Item 2: Verify patient suction is adequate to clear the airway.	Provider and tech
Item 4: Verify availability of required monitors, including alarms.	Provider or tech
Item 7: Verify that vaporizers are adequately filled and, if applicable, that the filler ports are tightly closed.	Provider
Item 11: Verify CO_2 absorbent is not exhausted.	Provider or tech
Item 12: Breathing system pressure and leak testing.	Provider and tech
Item 13: Verify that gas flows properly through the breathing circuit during both inspiration and exhalation.	Provider and tech
Item 14: Document completion of checkout procedures.	Provider and tech
Item 15: Confirm ventilator settings and evaluate readiness to deliver anesthesia care. (anesthesia timeout)	Provider

Before discussing specific problems, the most important point to emphasize is that the anesthesia provider's first duty is to provide continuous care and attention to the patient. If a situation should arise that puts the function of the anesthesia machine into question, the anesthesia provider should not be distracted from patient care by troubleshooting activities. The first step if a machine malfunction is suspected is to ensure adequate ventilation and oxygenation using a backup method of ventilation. Every operating room should have a cylinder supply of oxygen and ventilation device (e.g., Mapleson circuit) immediately available. Anesthesia may need to be provided using intravenous anesthetics if the anesthesia machine cannot be used. Once the patient's safety and anesthetic depth is assured, attention can be directed to troubleshooting the anesthesia machine, but attention to troubleshooting should never occur at the expense of attending to the patient.

Loss of Compressed Gases

Compressed gases are supplied to the anesthesia machine typically from a central pipeline supply with cylinders mounted on the anesthesia machine for backup. There may be locations where anesthesia is provided that do not have piped gas supplies and cylinders are the only supply. Oxygen is always provided to the machine and typically nitrous oxide and air are also connected. The implications for loss of compressed gases depend upon how the ventilator on the anesthesia machine is powered and the capacity of the cylinders connected to the anesthesia machine.

From the perspective of gas supply, there are two basic types of ventilator designs in use today—those that use pneumatic or compressed gases and those that use electrical power. Pneumatic anesthesia ventilators use compressed gases to move a bellows that delivers anesthetic gases to the patient during inspiration. Oxygen is the primary drive gas, but it is sometimes mixed with air from the atmosphere to reduce the oxygen required to power the ventilator. These ventilators use a small amount of electrical power for the timing and control circuits that determine the ventilator mode and rate. The other type of ventilator uses electrical power to move a piston that delivers anesthetic gases to the patient. This ventilator does not require any compressed gas supply to power the ventilator, only to provide the anesthetic gases in the breathing circuit. The type of ventilator being used will determine how the machine will function if compressed gas supplies are lost. Ventilators requiring compressed gas to power the ventilator will not function nearly as long on a cylinder supply as ventilators using electrical power.

Oxygen supply failure is the most important problem to consider. Other gases supplied to the anesthesia machine (air, nitrous oxide) are important to anesthetic care, but are not required to keep the patient safe if the gas supply fails. When using a machine with pipeline oxygen supply, the oxygen cylinder mounted on the anesthesia machine should be checked daily for adequate pressure (>1000 psi for an E cylinder) and then the valve on the cylinder should be turned off. Closing the valve is very important to keeping the backup oxygen supply available. If the pipeline supply should fail, every anesthesia machine is designed to sound a loud audible alarm when the oxygen supply pressure falls. If the cylinder valve is open when the pipeline supply fails, the machine will take oxygen from the cylinder and in many machines, there will not be an audible alarm until the cylinder is empty and there is no oxygen supply available. More modern anesthesia machines are designed to identify specifically when the pipeline supply fails and notify the user even if the cylinder supply is being used. Nevertheless, it is prudent to turn off the oxygen cylinder after checking it so that pipeline failure will result in a clear notification to the user and the cylinder can be turned on.

When only a cylinder supply of gas is available, either due to failure of the pipeline supply or a location where pipeline supply is not available, the anesthesia provider must know how long the gas supply will last. The duration of the cylinder supply in minutes will depend upon the volume of gas in the cylinder and the total volume used per minute. For example, a full E cylinder of oxygen will contain 660 L of oxygen at 1900 psig. If the fresh gas flow of oxygen is 5 L/min, then the oxygen supply will last 132 minutes if the patient is breathing spontaneously (i.e., the anesthesia ventilator is not used). Anesthesia machines that use pneumatic ventilators will use the available gas in the cylinder more rapidly if mechanical ventilation is required, and depending upon the ventilator settings and inspiratory pressure required, the gas supply may be depleted quite rapidly. If a pneumatic ventilator is being powered by an E cylinder of oxygen, plans for replacing or fixing the gas supply should begin as soon as possible after the supply fails. Anesthesia machines that use an electrically powered ventilator can provide mechanical ventilation without altering the duration of the cylinder supply. If an E cylinder of oxygen is not full, the volume of oxygen is directly proportional to the pressure in the cylinder; so when the pressure is 950 psis, there is half the original volume or 330 L.

Loss of Electrical Power

All anesthesia machines require some amount of electrical power. Older machines relied less on electrical power and more on compressed gases, whereas for some of the newer machine designs, the electrical power needs have increased and compressed gases are not as heavily used. Battery backup supplies are typically built into most anesthesia machines. It is important that the anesthesia machines be kept plugged in at all times, even for spare machines that are rarely used. This will ensure that the batteries remain fully charged. Older machines may have batteries that require periodic discharging

as part of their maintenance but the service procedures for the anesthesia machine should accommodate that consideration.

The duration of the electrical power will depend upon the size of the battery supply and how the machine is used. Many machines can deliver fresh gas and anesthetic vapors even without any electrical power, although the monitoring and alarm functions will not function. Each machine is designed differently so it is important to check the manual for the individual machine to understand the implications of complete loss of electrical power.

Preparing the Anesthesia Machine for Use with Patients Suspected to Be Susceptible to Malignant Hyperthermia

Malignant hyperthermia is a rare genetic condition whereby susceptible patients can develop a life-threatening hypermetabolic state upon exposure to potent inhaled anesthetic vapors and succinylcholine. Patients who are considered susceptible to malignant hyperthermia (family history, positive testing, rare forms of muscular dystrophy) may require anesthetic care including mechanical ventilation. The anesthesia machine can serve as a ventilator for these patients but even small amounts of anesthetic vapor remaining in the machine must be eliminated. For many years, recommended steps for preparing the machine before use with one of these patients included:[11]
1. Removing the vaporizers
2. Flushing with oxygen at 10 L/min for 5 minutes
3. Replacing the fresh gas outlet hose
4. Replacing the breathing circuit and carbon dioxide absorbent.

More recently, it has been demonstrated that new anesthesia machines require substantially more time (60 minutes or more) to flush anesthetic vapors from the machine.[12] Alternative recommendations for these machines include replacing the ventilator components with clean components, autoclaving the ventilator components to eliminate any anesthetic vapor that has been absorbed by the materials, or using a carbon filter to eliminate anesthetic vapor from the inspired gases.[13] No single best approach has yet been determined, but every department should have a policy for preparing the machine for these patients based upon the types of machines in use and recommendations in the literature.

Specific Hazards Related to the Anesthesia Machine

The safety record of the anesthesia machine is quite good overall but there is no question that patient injury can occur related to malfunctions or improper use of the machine. The goal here is not to provide a comprehensive review of machine hazards but there are some that deserve special mention.

Awareness During General Anesthesia

Awareness is one of the most common fears expressed by patients. There are circumstances (e.g., trauma) where little to no anesthesia can be administered, leading to a greater likelihood of awareness. Problems with anesthesia vaporizers can also play a role. With the exception of desflurane, which is administered using an electronic vaporizer, there are rarely alarms to indicate that a vaporizer is empty. Anesthetic agent monitoring may or may not be built into the anesthesia machine, but is very useful for confirming vaporizer function. The anesthetic provider must observe the measured concentration at intervals since alarms for the absence of vapor, or a lower limit of vapor concentration, are typically not enabled. Although anesthetic agent monitoring is not required by the monitoring standards, it is very valuable for ensuring delivery of anesthetic vapors.

Since most anesthetic vaporizers are mechanical, information about the vaporizer setting or even that it has been turned on is not transferred to the monitoring system. There are some electronic vaporizer designs in use where monitors are built in or can communicate with the vaporizer to help monitor for proper function. In the future, the electronic designs should become more common and it will be easier to prevent awareness due to lack of anesthetic vapor. Once the vaporizer is turned on to a specific setting, if that information is available electronically, an alarm can be set to identify significant variance of vapor concentration from the set value.

Pressure Injuries

Too much pressure in the breathing circuit can lead to hemodynamic compromise and barotrauma to the lungs. Pressure monitoring is required during anesthesia, and alarms for both high pressure and continuous pressure will identify potentially hazardous conditions where there is too much or sustained pressure in the breathing circuit. These alarms should be enabled and set close enough to the desired values to be sensitive indicators of change, but not so close that they alarm too frequently. Preventing injury due to excessive pressure begins with the preanesthesia checkout procedure.

One special case to be aware of is the potential for the oxygen flush to harm the patient. This flush button provides a virtually unlimited source of high pressure gas at high flow. If this button is pressed when the APL valve is closed or when the ventilator is in the inspiratory cycle, it is possible to add a great deal of gas to the lungs at high pressure. This flush valve should only be used when the APL valve is open during manual ventilation or only briefly between breaths during mechanical ventilation. Some of the newer designs do not allow fresh gas to enter the breathing circuit during inspiration, thereby eliminating the concern that the oxygen flush could injure the patient.

Lack of Pressure

Inadequate or absent spontaneous ventilation is the most common life-threatening consequence of anesthetizing a patient. The ability to provide positive pressure ventilation is the only way to prevent the morbidity or mortality that will result from respiratory impairment. It is essential therefore that the anesthesia machine and breathing circuit be functional and able to provide positive pressure ventilation at whatever pressure is necessary to keep the patient safe.

Leaks and disconnections are a common cause of machine failure that leads to an inability to provide effective positive pressure ventilation. Leaks in particular can be difficult to identify especially when the patient is apneic and there is a pressing need to provide ventilation. The time to troubleshoot these leaks and disconnects is not once the patient is anesthetized. The preanesthesia checkout procedure should include testing to ensure that positive pressure can be maintained in the breathing circuit. Since it is possible for a leak to develop after the breathing circuit has been checked, a separate means for providing positive pressure ventilation and oxygen should be readily available in every location where anesthesia care is provided.

Future Possibilities

The anesthesia machine has evolved significantly in recent years. Most notably, anesthesia ventilator design has advanced to the point where the most modern anesthesia ventilators approach the capabilities of intensive care ventilators while preserving the ability to deliver anesthetic vapors using a circle system. Anesthetic vapor delivery remains a significant limitation of most anesthesia machine designs. The set vapor concentration is not the same as the delivered concentration, and the difference between the two depends upon complex interactions between the fresh gas flow, circuit volume, and configuration and patient uptake. Machine designs are available that provide a high degree of control over delivered vapor concentration. In the future, we can expect machine designs that provide both high quality mechanical ventilation and moment to moment control of vapor delivery.

Future anesthesia machines are also likely to use a different approach to scavenging and recovery of wasted anesthetic vapors. The anesthetic agents are fluorocarbons that contribute to green house gases and ozone degradation. These environmental considerations are likely to stimulate development of recovery systems that prevent the vapors from entering the atmosphere. Whether or not these recovery systems will actually provide useful anesthetics for reuse or just a more controlled method for disposal remains to be seen.

Finally, intravenous anesthesia continues to be increasingly used either for deep sedation during minor procedures or general anesthesia. Although there is technology for managing infusions of intravenous anesthetics, that technology has yet to be integrated with the existing anesthesia machines that are designed to provide anesthetic vapor and mechanical ventilation. Future machines will likely integrate not only the ability to deliver inhaled or intravenous anesthetics, but also the ability to monitor the delivered concentrations and effects of these agents.

The information in this chapter is intended to be a foundation for understanding proper use of the different anesthesia machines currently available. There are differences between machines, and the user's guide and training tools from the manufacturer should always be consulted. The anesthesia machine of today is a sophisticated device that can be used to provide high quality, safe anesthetic care when used by a skilled and knowledgeable professional.

1. Fires in the operating room are a significant cause of morbidity and mortality. Estimates of the number of annual operating room fires in the United States run into the hundreds, and enriched O_2 delivered by the anesthetist is the primary root cause.
2. Minute ventilation is defined as the product of respiratory rate and tidal volume.

3. O_2 consumption is approximately 350 mL/min in the average adult, which is lower than the usual fresh gas flow.

4. Anesthetic vapor monitoring during anesthesia delivery is not mandated by standards, but is recommended. In contrast, monitoring O_2 and CO_2 concentrations is considered standard of care.

5. Other terms used to describe this mode of ventilation include volume and pressure limited or targeted ventilation.

6. Sample preanesthesia checkout procedures. http://www.asahq.org/clinical/checklist.htm. Accessed June 29, 2009.

References

1. Duggan, M. 2005. Cavanaugh BP. Pulmonary atelectasis. Anesthesiology 102, 838–854.
2. Jones, J.G., Jones, S.E. 2000. Discriminating between the effect of shunt and reduced V/Q on arterial oxygen saturation is particularly useful in clinical practice. J Clin Monit Comput 16, 337–350.
3. Caplan, R.A., Barker, S.J., Connis, R.T. 2008. Practice advisory for the prevention and management of operating room fires. A report by the American Society of Anesthesiologists task force on operating room fires. Anesthesiology 108, 786–801.
4. Lowe, H.J., Ernst, E.A. 1981. The quantitative practice of anesthesia. Use of closed circuit. Williams and Wilkins, Baltimore.
5. Brimacombe, J., Keller, C., Hormann, C. 2000. Pressure support ventilation versus continuous positive airway pressure with the laryngeal mask airway. Anesthesiology 92, 1621–1623.
6. von Goedecke, A., Brimacombe, J., et al., 2005. Pressure support ventilation versus continuous positive airway pressure ventilation with the Proseal laryngeal mask airway: a randomized crossover study of anesthetized pediatric patients. Anesth Analg 100, 357–360.
7. American Society of Anesthesiologists. Guidelines for determining anesthesia machine obsolescence (website): http://www.asahq.org/publicationsAnd Services/machineobsolescense.pdf. Accessed June 29, 2009.
8. Cooper, J.B., Newbower, R.S., Kitz, R.J. 1984. An analysis of major errors and equipment failures in anesthesia management: considerations for prevention and detection. Anesthesiology 60, 34–42.
9. Arbous, M.S., Meursing, A.E., van Kleef, J.W., et al., 2005. Impact of anesthesia management characteristics on severe morbidity and mortality. Anesthesiology 102, 257–268.
10. Subcommittee of ASA Committee on Equipment and Facilities. Recommendations for preanesthesia checkout procedures, 2008.
11. Beebe, J.J., Sessler, D.I. 1988. Preparation of anesthesia machine for patients susceptible to malignant hyperthermia. Anesthesiology 69, 395–400.
12. Prinzhausen, H., Crawford, M., O'Rourke, J., et al., 2006. Preparation of the Drager Primus anesthetic machine for malignant hyperthermia-susceptible patients. Can J Anaesth 53, 885–890.
13. Gunter, J.B., Ball, J., Than-Win, S. 2008. Preparation of the Drager Fabius anesthesia machine for the malignant-hyperthermia susceptible patient. Anesth Analg 107, 1936–1945.

Suggested Additional Materials

1. The Virtual Anesthesia Machine. This is a definitive web-based interactive simulation of anesthesia machine function. The website contains a variety of instructional materials and simulation of different machine designs. Much of the content is available free of charge. http://vam.anest.ufl.edu.

2. *Understanding Anesthesia Equipment* by Jerry Dorsch and Susan Dorsch is the definitive textbook on anesthesia equipment. Details of the design of many different anesthesia machines are well described. This is a good source for in-depth information about individual anesthesia machines.

3. *Quantitative Practice of Anesthesia: Use of Closed Circuit* by Harry Lowe and Edward Ernst is a complete reference on the details of closed circuit anesthesia. The text is out of print, but can be found in libraries and from specialty printers that can reproduce the text.

Chapter 4

Principles and Practices of Closed Circuit Anesthesia

Robert S. Holzman and Rebecca N. Lintner

History, Philosophy, and General Comments

Very low flow and closed circuit anesthetic techniques are predicated upon a practical method for the absorption of carbon dioxide and therefore the prevention of CO_2 rebreathing. Between 1935 and 1950, most anesthesiologists were quite familiar with closed circuit anesthetics using cyclopropane and Waters' granular 4 to 8 mesh pellets.[1] Low flow and closed circuit anesthesia eliminate the spillover of oxygen and explosive gases into an operating room with electrocautery and static electricity.

The practice of closed circuit anesthesia became less common following the introduction of halothane in the 1950s and was replaced by the semiclosed circle absorption technique using a variety of fresh gas flows (FGF), often 5 L/min or greater. Yet the basic principles are easy in concept and implementation: the closed circuit technique emphasizes *the maintenance of a constant anesthetic state by the addition of gases and vapors to the breathing circuit at the same rate that the patient's body redistributes, stores, and eliminates them.* While the open or semiclosed anesthetic relies on *progressively diminishing delivered concentrations* to maintain a desired alveolar and arterial concentration of anesthetic, the closed circuit anesthetic approach emphasizes the *amount of vapor or gas needed* to maintain that constant alveolar and arterial concentration.

The successful use of potent inhalation agents in a closed circuit requires the repeated administration of a calculated unit dose at sequential time intervals that increase by the square of time. The clinical skills needed are identical to those required for any anesthetic practice—vigilance, diligence, and attention to detail. Moreover, a sound fund of knowledge about physiology, pharmacology, and equipment remains the basis for the close adjustments required for the care of each individual patient. The calculations are simple: when the patient plus the anesthesia machine are viewed as interdependent, a combined "prime" for the breathing circuit and the patient followed by a unit dose for the patient can be delivered at predictably lengthening time intervals to attenuate the surgical stress response and keep the patient at basal levels of oxygen consumption (Appendix A).

The advantages of this concept include:

1. The patient constantly providing information about his metabolic state using the anesthesia machine as a monitor of metabolic oxygen consumption ($\dot{V}_{O_2}$). The quantitative nature of the practice also evaluates carbon dioxide production ($\dot{V}_{CO_2}$), cardiac output, and free water requirements.
2. A relative humidity of 40% to 60% without additional connections or the use of valveless breathing systems used at partial rebreathing flows. Thus, mucociliary function may be better preserved.
3. Heat is conserved from the patient and supplied because of the exothermic reaction of the carbon dioxide absorbent.
4. Adequacy of the circulation can be assessed by monitoring $\dot{V}_{O_2}$.
5. Adequacy of neuromuscular blockade can be assessed by monitoring the ventilator bellows or the rebreathing bag.
6. Economy—decreasing the total milliliters of anesthetic agent administered using low flow techniques can save hundreds of millions of dollars annually in the United States, and upwards of half a billion dollars worldwide.
7. Environmental responsibility—with a lower total amount of chlorinated hydrocarbon anesthetics used, the contribution we make to ozone layer depletion will be less. Chlorine-free anesthetics such as desflurane can be used less expensively.

8. The use of nitrous oxide for the administration of anesthesia or analgesia accounts for 3% to 12% of global nitrous oxide release. With a lower total amount of nitrous oxide used, ozone layer depletion will be decreased.

Only with flows less than 2.0 L/min does the rebreathing fraction reach 50% or more. It is useful, therefore, to start with some definitions:

Low flow technique: less than 1.0 L/min (where the rebreathing fraction is >50%)

Minimal flow technique: 0.5 L/min

Closed circuit technique: a fresh gas flow not to exceed the gas loss via patient uptake plus system leaks. May be *nonquantitative* (with the administration of volatile anesthetic agent according to clinical assessment) or *quantitative* (with the administration of volatile anesthetic agent according to calculated values based on prime dose plus unit dose administered according to the square root of time model).

Clinical Practice Using the Closed Circuit Technique

Proper equipment for a closed circuit technique includes an anesthesia machine and the appropriate circuit delivery components, which typically are a circle system passing through a carbon dioxide absorber.

CO_2 Absorption

Understanding the chemistry of CO_2 absorption is the basis of confidence in the closed circuit technique. CO_2 absorption is a chemical reaction of a base neutralizing an acid. The acid is carbonic acid formed by the reaction of CO_2 and water; the base is the hydroxide of an alkali or alkaline earth metal. The end products of the exothermic reaction are water, heat, and a carbonate. The most common absorbent is soda lime; Baralyme (barium hydroxide) is no longer available. A 1.13 kg canister of soda lime should last approximately 15 hours with 0% breakthrough or 16.3 hours with only 0.5% CO_2 breakthrough.

Machine Construction

The ideal machine will have a leak-free gas delivery system, breathing circuit, and ventilator. Low gas flow capability (i.e., low-flow calibrated flowmeters) is highly desirable, and a mechanical ventilator tidal volume that is not related to the circuit volume. A tight system (i.e., leak less than 100 mL/min at 30 cm H_2O pressure) is required.

Anesthetic Uptake

The uptake of volatile agents is rapid in the first few minutes of the anesthetic and therefore attaining a clinically satisfactory alveolar concentration may be more problematic. The less soluble the agent, such as the newer agent desflurane (introduced in 1992) and sevoflurane (introduced in 1995), the less this is a problem. Although experience has been gained worldwide with closed circuit administration of sevoflurane, current FDA regulations and the package insert state "to minimize exposure to compound A, sevoflurane exposure should not exceed 2 minimal alveolar concentration (MAC) hours at flow rates of 1 to less than 2 L/min. Fresh gas flow rates less than 1 L/min are not recommended," so we will restrict this discussion to desflurane.

The anesthetic potency of desflurane is low, with an MAC between 4% and 8%, depending on the age of the patient; a comparatively high alveolar concentration is therefore required for maintenance. Desflurane is metabolized at a virtually negligible rate of approximately 0.02%. The wash-in of desflurane is so rapid that within 10 minutes after induction the inspired desflurane concentration is about 85% of the fresh gas concentration. Even with extremely low fresh gas flows, the difference between inspired and fresh gas concentration is comparatively small and the desflurane concentration can be readily increased.

While one may get started with an intravenous or mask induction, during the first 10 to 20 minutes, a semiclosed circuit fresh gas flow of several liters should be used, and then reduce the flow thereafter. A closed circuit requires a reasonable atmospheric seal and most patients would prefer not to have a tight-fitting mask while conscious. Moreover, a volatile agent induction at closed circuit flows is impractical because the fresh gas flow rate will not be sufficient to vaporize an induction dose.

Vapor Delivery Techniques

It doesn't matter whether the agent is vaporized in a vaporizer or in the circuit itself by liquid injection; similar mean circuit concentrations will be produced according to the technology of the vaporizer and the settings determined by the anesthetist or to the gas laws at standard temperature and pressure (STP).

Vaporizer Techniques

Once the patient is induced and the trachea intubated, high flow rates (e.g., FGF of 4 to 6 L/min) should be used for the first 10 to 15 minutes to (1) flush and prime the circuit and functional residual capacity (FRC) and (2) to provide for early uptake in the rapid saturation phase. The FGF is then decreased progressively over the first half hour (in adults) to approximately 250 mL/min O_2 and 250 mL/min N_2O (unless N_2O is not used as an agent). The N_2O can then be decreased according to the adequacy of circuit volume, best detected by the rise of ventilator bellows to "almost fill" or the rebreathing bag to "almost full." The setting on the vaporizer typically used at this time is *that setting required to maintain an adequate end-tidal anesthetic level, typically 1.3 MAC*. It would not be unusual, for example, to have the vaporizer set to 4% and read an end-tidal level of 1.5%. Fifteen to 30 minutes before the end of the surgery, the N_2O (if used) and agent may be shut off with only the oxygen flowing at the closed circuit rate; it is usually possible to "coast" in this fashion for the last 15 to 30 minutes of the case. If a rapid change in circuit vapor concentration is required, flows may be transiently increased. Care should be taken, however, that if the vaporizer is already set high, when flows are increased, much higher blood vapor concentrations will result in a short time.

Injection Techniques

The liquid anesthetic agent can be introduced into either limb of the breathing circuit and will vaporize in a fashion predicted by the gas laws. Usually the expiratory limb is chosen because of the greater distance and volume of gas between the injection port and the patient. This affords an additional buffer of circuit volume at the expense of a longer time interval to the desired alveolar concentration of anesthetic agent.

Free Water Requirements

Water is required for the elimination of heat generated during metabolic activity, and water loss is normally 100 mol for every 100 kcal expended. Free water requirements are ultimately proportional to caloric demands, which are decreased when patients are anesthetized. Basal water requirements can therefore be calculated in relation to basal metabolic demand:

1. The consumption of 1000 mL of oxygen generates 4825 calories.
2. If $\dot{V}O_2$ is equal to $10 \times kg^{3/4}$ (mL/min) in adults, then heat production per hour is:

3. $$\frac{10 \times kg^{3/4} \times 4825 \times 60}{1000}$$

4. The calories required for 1 mL of water to evaporate are 63 cal. This plus 540 calories are required to achieve the heat of vaporization (total 603 cal/mL of water). This modifies the above equation to: mL water/hour =

$$\frac{10 \times kg^{3/4} \times 4825 \times 60}{1000 \times 603} \approx 5 \times kg^{3/4}$$ which parallels basal

oxygen consumption once again.[2]

Physiological Aspects of Closed Circuit Anesthesia

Monitoring $\dot{V}O_2$, $\dot{V}CO_2$, Cardiac Output, and Respiratory Mechanics

With the volume of the system constant and the oxygen concentration maintained in a steady state as monitored by an oxygen analyzer, *the oxygen flow required becomes a monitor of oxygen consumption*. Basal oxygen consumption ($\dot{V}O_2$), CO_2 production ($\dot{V}CO_2$), free water requirements, and the cardiac output can be estimated by the "3/4 power law" (Brody's number).

For example, if Brody's number was calculated for a 70 kg adult:

Body weight (kg)		70.0
Brody's No.	$kg^{3/4}$	24.2
Oxygen consumption ($\dot{V}O_2$) (mL/min)	Brody's No. × 10	242.0
CO_2 production ($\dot{V}CO_2$) (mL/min)	Brody's No. × 8	193.6
Free water requirement (mL/hr)	Brody's No. × 5	121.0
Cardiac output (dL/min)	Brody's No. × 2	48.4

The minimum flow rate of 250 mL/minute established for anesthesia machines,[3] when calculated for a 70 kg adult, is equal to $10.5 \times kg^{3/4}$. Oxygen consumption calculated from Brody's number might underestimate the true oxygen consumption at the start of the case due to patient anxiety and the release of endogenous catecholamines. Given a steady-state relationship established between the anesthesia machine and the patient, an *increase* in mean circuit oxygen concentration reflects an excess of O_2 supply compared with metabolic demand. Likewise, a *decrease* in mean circuit oxygen concentration reflects an increase in the patient's oxygen demand.

The rate of CO_2 production will be related to the rate of oxygen consumption by the respiratory quotient (RQ = 0.8 normally) and can aid in the calculation of minute ventilation requirements.

For example, if we calculate the minute volume required for normocarbia:

Brody's No.	$kg^{3/4}$	24.2
Minute CO_2 production (mL/min)	Brody's No. × 8	193.6
Normocarbia (% atm)	5%	
V_A for normocarbia (mL/min)	$\dot{V}CO_2/.05$	3872.0

Ventilatory requirements significantly out of proportion to "normal" or expected amounts may accompany a hypometabolic or hypermetabolic state, such as hypothyroidism or malignant hyperthermia.

Human studies have verified subgroups of patients compensating for an oxygen debt, for example, following the release of an aortic cross clamp after aortic aneurysmorrhaphy. This was monitored by a decrease in mean circuit O_2 concentration accompanied by an increase in cardiac output.[4,5] Intriguingly, the linear correlation between body mass and oxygen consumption established with painstaking detail in animal models by Brody[6] is the basis of the concept of oxygen debt in experimental models[7] and the early studies of survival of critical illness in humans.[8]

For anesthesia machines with a ventilator bellows, the bellows themselves become a sensitive monitor of diaphragm activity when filling just before the next ventilatory cycle, as respiratory efforts can easily be detected by watching bellows movement. Moreover, the bellows of a low-flow system more accurately reflects the expiratory flow rate because the patient's exhalation volume provides the bulk of the gas in the bellows—the rate of ascent of the bellows directly reflects the exhalation flow rate of the patient. Bronchospasm or impaired exhalation is more easily detected and the fill rate of the bellows more easily monitors the success of therapeutic interventions. Finally, movement of the bellows is a sensitive monitor of the degree of neuromuscular blockade because the diaphragm recovers from neuromuscular blockade before the peripheral muscles.

Defense Against Humidity and Temperature Loss

Gases entering the breathing system (and therefore the patient) are anhydrous. In contrast, at the normal body temperature of 37° C, the saturated vapor pressure is 47 mm Hg. Thus humidification of respiratory gases has been recommended for the prevention of pulmonary damage, maintenance of

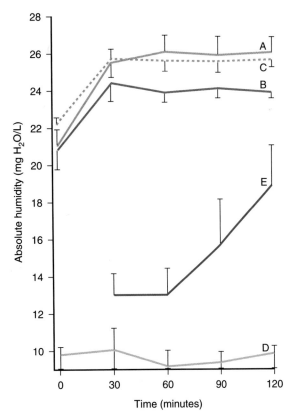

Figure 4–1 Absolute humidity in various breathing circuits with varying fresh gas flows.[29] Group **A,** Children and partial rebreathing Bain circuit; Group **B,** Adults and partial rebreathing Bain circuit; Group **C,** Same as Group **B** with inspired humidity measured distal to the FGF; Group **D,** Adults and semiclosed circle system; Group **E,** Adults and a closed circuit system.

normal ciliary motility, and for the maintenance of body temperature. Humidification well within the recommended range of 14 to 30 mg H_2O/L is readily achievable in a short time using a closed circuit technique and compares favorably with other partial rebreathing ventilation methods or the use of heat and moisture exchangers (Figure 4–1).

Similarly, advantage can be taken of the exothermic reaction of CO_2 absorption by soda lime during a closed circuit anesthetic, as heat is liberated at the rate of 13,700 calories per mole of water produced. In addition, a lower fresh gas flow rate will allow the patient to not lose heat to the incoming bulk of cold, dry fresh gas.

Pediatric Considerations

Energy requirements of children are greater than those of adults, even more than would be predicted by the exponential nature of Brody's equation. Sarrus and Rameaux proposed that metabolic values in homeotherms were likely an exponential function more than 150 years ago.[9,10] They went on to suggest that not only was oxygen consumption related to heat production and surface area, but it was also related to respiratory rate, heart rate, pulse volume, and body size. Among many authors who extended this proposition, Kleiber[11] reasoned that *if heat loss is proportional to surface area, then heat production must also be proportional to surface area, since homeothermia dictates that heat production equals heat loss.*

To complicate matters a little further, in children, RQ may be influenced by the anesthetic. For babies weighing less than 10 kg, a reduced V_{CO_2} in relation to $\dot{V}_{O_2}$ has been noted, yielding respiratory quotients that sometimes were lower than 0.7. This may result from partial inhibition of brown adipose tissue function caused by halothane.[12,13] In an in vitro model, halothane, isoflurane, and enflurane were approximately equipotent inhibitors of thermogenesis, with concentrations of approximately 0.7% resulting in 50% inhibition.[14]

Additional challenges may occur when using a closed circuit technique during pediatric anesthesia.

- The use of *cuffless endotracheal tubes* with a variable leak from 15 to 30 cm H_2O will result in volume loss to the atmosphere and decreased volume return to the breathing circuit. Throat packs may be used to seal the leak without using a larger tube or a cuffed tube. On the other hand, small-sized cuffed endotracheal tubes are perfectly safe when attention is given to not exceeding an intracuff pressure of approximately 25 mm Hg, or a pressure just sufficient to prevent an air leak.
- *Flowmeters,* even when calibrated to 50 mL/min FGF, may be insufficiently precise for delivering very low fresh gas flow rates.
- *Relatively small arterial doses* in comparison to the breathing circuit and ventilator prime doses compel practitioners to precisely calculate pediatric dosing requirements for the closed circuit lest an overdose occur. Couto da Silva found that pediatric patients typically required higher volume and more frequent dosing of volatile agents than predicted on theoretical grounds,[15] which parallels Lindahl's recommendation of increasing the constant "k" multiplier of Brody's number by 40% for children.[16]

Potential Problems

Because gases that would ordinarily be flushed out continuously during the administration of higher FGF anesthetics remain within the breathing circuit, accumulation of toxic substances is of potential concern during closed circuit practice.

Accumulation of Gases

Metabolic by-products of *halothane* have been detected in very low concentrations in the closed circuit; however, they do not appear to be of clinical significance.[17] *Ethrane, isoflurane,* and *desflurane* have not been found to have significant metabolic by-products. Sevoflurane produces a variety of degradation products with the use of soda lime and baralyme. In the short term (cases up to 12 MAC hours in duration), compound A accumulation does not appear to be a clinical problem.[18-21] Mean compound A concentrations in the inspiratory and expiratory limbs of the circle are significantly different at FGF rates of 0.5 and 2.0 L/min. The quadrupling of the FGF rate was not associated with a significant difference in compound A volume within the circle in one study,[22] while in general there appears to be some FGF dependence of compound A circuit concentrations.[23]

The FRC (of an adult) contains about 2 L of *nitrogen,* and the breathing circuit contains about 4 L of nitrogen. In addition, tissue nitrogen is released into the breathing circuit as progressive denitrogenation occurs.[24] The amount of nitrogen dissolved in tissues of the average adult is about 1 to 1.5 L. Even if all this nitrogen were to pass into the functional residual capacity and recreating system, its inspired concentration would increase to, at most, 10% to 15%.

Acetone, methane, and other gases have also been detected in the breathing circuit, prompting the suggestion that the closed circuit should be flushed briefly but periodically with higher FGFs. Methane, up to 100 parts per million (ppm), is excreted in expired gas. Intestinal organisms produce it. Blood methane levels of 2000 ppm (0.02%) have been recorded without apparent clinically significant effect. Acetone is produced by hepatic metabolism and may accumulate in patients with preoperative starvation or increased production (diabetes, cirrhosis). Concentrations greater than 50 ppm may cause nausea, vomiting, and slow emergence from anesthesia.

Carbon monoxide production occurs endogenously during the degradation of red cell hemoglobin to bile pigments when a carbon atom is separated from the porphyrin nucleus and is subsequently catabolized by heme oxygenase. Any disturbance leading to accelerated destruction of RBCs and accelerated breakdown of other hemoproteins would lead to increased production of CO. Hematomas, intravascular hemolysis of RBCs, blood transfusion, and ineffective erythropoiesis all will elevate carboxyhemoglobin (COHb) concentration in blood. In females, COHb levels fluctuate with the menstrual cycle; the mean rate of CO production in the premenstrual, progesterone phase is almost doubled. Neonates and pregnant women also show a significant increase in endogenous CO production related to increased breakdown of RBCs. COHb formation as a hemoglobin breakdown product occurs with a normal physiological range of 0.4% to 0.8% (somewhat higher findings in urban dwellers).

There is a constant rise of carboxyhemoglobin during a closed circuit anesthetic, approximately 0.05 g/100 mL of blood over 6 hours in adults.[25] The rate of rise is equal in smokers and nonsmokers, although their baselines are different. During ventilation with high flows, carboxyhemoglobin levels decrease. Patients for whom this may be a potential problem are those with anemia, severe coronary artery disease or peripheral vascular disease, or increased levels of endogenous carbon monoxide production such as pregnant women, newborns, those with hemolytic disease, and porphyria cutanea. *Prolonged exposure of desflurane, enflurane, and isoflurane to desiccated CO_2 absorbents may result in anesthetic degradation, leading to the production of CO.* The use of dry absorbent produces more CO than standard absorbent with normal amounts of water. Increased temperature increases CO production, as does the use of higher anesthetic concentrations. To minimize exposure to CO from the degradation of anesthetics in the breathing system, *only an absorbent with the full complement of water should be used.*

Physiological Monitoring Considerations
Carbon Monoxide Toxicity Monitoring

Pulse oximetry is inadequate as a safety monitor with regard to COHb monitoring, since the commonly employed sensors do not differentiate between O_2Hb and COHb with the two wavelengths of light used. Under anesthesia, alterations in mental status or the development of respiratory distress cannot be detected. Skin color is not accurate since COHb has a red color and mild acidosis increases skin perfusion. Thus unexplained ECG signs of *myocardial hypoxia* (ST segment changes, T wave inversion, rhythm disturbances) or an *unexpected acidosis* or base deficit despite normovolemia should prompt further diagnosis. CO saturation *can* be measured with blood gas analyzers employing light of at least five different wavelengths. The detection of CO in the circle system can be performed by electrochemical devices used in toxicological studies; however, there are numerous technical challenges in relating ambient air CO levels to blood CO levels, let alone tissue levels such as brain or myocardial CO.

Sidestream Bulk Gas Monitoring

Sidestream respiratory gas monitoring potentially complicates the use of closed circuit techniques because of sample gas withdrawal and therefore circuit volume loss at rates from 50 to 200 mL/minute, depending on the specifications of the particular gas analyzer. Mainstream infrared analysis without bulk gas withdrawal is one solution. An alternative is the return of sampled gas from the exhaust valve of the capnograph back to the breathing circuit. Adding fresh gas at identical gas composition to offset the loss of circuit gas is a third option. This is of questionable clinical significance in adult patients, but may become important for children.[26]

Emergence

As a corollary to the "quantitative" uptake and distribution concepts of closed circuit practice, the rate of decline of residual agent will be related to the duration of the anesthesia itself (i.e., after 121 minutes of anesthesia (11^2), another unit dose will result in approximately 23 minutes of anesthesia ($12^2 - 11^2 = 144 - 121$). To the extent that one does not inject during that time, one can "coast" to the next square of time interval, with an expected decrease in end-tidal agent concentration. FGF will be another means of affecting the end-tidal agent concentration, in that a higher FGF will "flush" residual agent in the ventilatory portion of the system. If the patient is waking up too fast, the FGF can be reduced and the agent will equilibrate from tissue stores. The usual clinical signs of emergence should be followed such as patient movement, pupil size, vital signs, respiratory tidal volume (if breathing spontaneously), abdominal tone (if muscle relaxants are not used), and end-tidal agent levels. The Bispectral Index (BIS) or the Entropy monitor may also be helpful.

A charcoal shunt on the inspiratory limb may be used to facilitate emergence while maintaining a closed circuit. A reservoir containing 50 g of activated charcoal (carbon processed to make it extremely porous and thus have a very large surface area available for adsorption) can be incorporated into the inspiratory limb of the circuit to *adsorb* volatile anesthetic agents (without adsorbing oxygen or nitrous oxide). Inspiratory levels of volatile agents are reduced with incorporation of the charcoal shunt.

Closed Circuit Anesthetic Record Keeping

Recording the output setting of the vaporizer at closed circuit flows is meaningless other than to satisfy the curiosity of the anesthetist about the unreliability of vaporizer output and low FGF.

At FGFs below 1 L/min, one should record inspired and expired agent concentrations on separate lines of the anesthesia record when an agent-specific vaporizer is used. Alternatively, with injection methods, one may simply wish to record only the end-tidal agent level.

Cost Containment Considerations

Closed circuit anesthesia is one of the easiest ways to reduce anesthesia costs. The costs of inhalation anesthesia are primarily related to the agent selected, the concentration delivered, the duration of the anesthetic, and the total FGF rate. As a rough guideline for adult practice, the agent used in milliliters per hour is approximately the FGF in liters per minute times three times the percent of the agent. Therefore an FGF of 5 L/min with 2% isoflurane uses approximately 30 mL/hr of liquid isoflurane; an FGF of 1 L/min and 2% isoflurane uses approximately 6 mL/hr of liquid isoflurane.

Appendix A
Quantitative Calculations for Dosing the Closed Circuit by Injection Techniques
DOSING FREQUENCY

In 1954, Severinghaus suggested that the rate of rise and uptake of anesthetic gases and oxygen was predictable according to a square root of a time-based model, visually expressed as the familiar tissue uptake curve. These calculations became the basis for the "square root of time" model for quantitative dosing of the closed circuit:

$$\text{Administration rate} = \text{Uptake} = kt^{-1/2}$$

Lowe confirmed this mathematical model pharmacologically with halothane arterial blood concentration analysis and also pointed out that the time *between* injections is the sequence of odd integers (1, 3, 5, 7… minutes).[27] This is best illustrated by the overlaying of a typical vapor delivery curve on the above tissue distribution curve, which in either event should achieve a constant alveolar concentration (Figure 4–2).

Identical areas under the curve at square root of time progressively lengthening intervals are responsible for the clinical "steady state," when the gas machine, breathing circuit, patient's lungs, heart, and end organs are viewed as a unitary delivery and uptake "system." The amount of anesthetic vapor required to fill this system is the sum of what is required to fill the ventilatory portion and arterial transport system at time "0" (the *prime dose*) and the amount required to be added

as the anesthetic is absorbed, distributed, and biotransformed through body tissues until time t (the *unit dose*). This is the amount that is constant at each additional "square root of time" unit (Figure 4–3).

Knowledge of the physical properties of the inhalation agents is important for calculating the unit dose (Table 4–1). Sevoflurane is excluded because of current Food and Drug Administration regulations regarding its use at closed circuit flows; current recommendations are not to use it at less than 1 L of total fresh gas flow for up to 2 MAC hours.

DOSE REQUIREMENTS

Because any alveolar anesthetic concentration (C_A) can be considered a fraction or a multiple (*f*) of MAC, the following equation applies:

$$C_A = f\text{MAC (in mL of vapor / dL)}$$

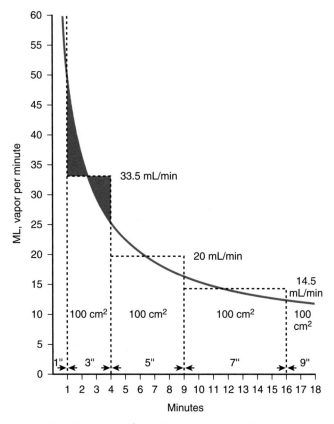

Figure 4–3 The amount of anesthetic vapor required as it is absorbed, distributed, and biotransformed is constant at each square root of time.

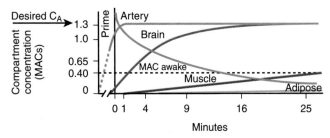

Figure 4–2 Overlay of a typical vapor delivery curve on a tissue distribution curve; both strategies satisfy the goal of a constant alveolar concentration.

Table 4–1 Physical Properties of Inhaled Agents				
Agent	**mL vapor/mL liquid at 37° C**	**MAC at 37° C**	**Λ B/G at 37° C**	**Vapor Pressure at 20° C**
Halothane	240	0.75	2.4	242
Enflurane	210	1.7	1.9	180
Isoflurane	206	1.3	1.5	250
Desflurane	195	4.6	0.42	735

Equilibrium is expected to occur in normal alveoli, therefore, the systemic arterial and blood anesthetic concentration (C_a) can be calculated from the alveolar concentration (C_A) provided pulmonary shunts are excluded because $\lambda B/G$ values equate vapor concentrations between gas and blood phases:

$$C_a = C_A \times \lambda B/G = fMAC \times \lambda B/G \text{ (in mL of vapor/dL)}$$

The anesthetic arterial concentration C_a (mL/dL) and the cardiac output Q (dL/min) determine the rate at which tissues become saturated with anesthetic molecules. Their product, C_aQ, represents the amount of anesthetic delivered to the tissues:

$$C_aQ = fMAC \times \lambda B/G \times Q$$

This "unit dose" is, however, only one part of the story; for a priming dose, the arterial unit dose at time 0 must be added to a "ventilatory prime (V_{vent})," which is a *physical* but not a *physiological* participant in the "anesthetic system" of machine, breathing circuit, and patient.

$$\text{Prime (mL of vapor)} = (C_aQ) + (V_{vent}XfMAC)$$
$$= fMAC((Q \times \lambda B/G) + (V_{circ} + FRC))$$

To rapidly attain a desired alveolar and arterial anesthetic concentration, an initial amount of anesthetic vapor, adequate to provide a *ventilatory prime* plus an *arterial prime*, must be introduced into the breathing system.

VENTILATORY PRIME

The amount of anesthetic agent needed to achieve the *ventilatory* component of the prime dose is the product of the system's volume times the desired alveolar concentration, $fMAC$. The system's volume (V_{vent}) is the sum of the circuit volume (V_{circ}) plus the patient's FRC. For most adults, V_{vent} is about 100 dL.

$$\text{Ventilatory prime} = V_{vent} \times \text{desired alveolar concentration}$$
$$= V_{vent} \times C_A$$
$$= V_{vent} \times fMAC$$
$$\approx 100\, fMAC \text{ for the usual adult patient}$$

ARTERIAL PRIME

The amount of anesthetic necessary to achieve the *arterial* component of the prime dose is the product of the desired arterial concentration times the amount of blood circulating through the lungs during the first minute of anesthesia, or cardiac output, Q.

$$\text{Arterial prime} = \text{desired arterial concentration} \times Q$$
$$= fMAC \times \lambda B/G \times Q$$
$$= C_aQ$$

C_aQ represents the mL of vapor needed to "fill" the arterial delivery system with the desired concentration. It also represents the amount of agent presented to all the tissues in the body per minute as long as C_a and Q remain constant.

PRIME DOSE

The sum of the arterial prime and the ventilatory prime is called the prime dose, and is the amount of agent that must be introduced to attain the appropriate *initial* C_a.

$$\text{Prime dose} = \text{arterial prime} + \text{ventilatory prime}$$
$$= C_aQ + V_{vent} \times fMAC$$
$$C_aQ + 100\, fMAC \text{ for the usual adult patient}$$

For adults, the ventilatory prime of the breathing circuit is approximately equivalent to the arterial prime; *under these circumstances, the combined prime dose then becomes approximately 2 C_aQ.*

The prime dose is introduced once during the anesthetic and C_a is kept constant by subsequently delivering into the circuit the amount of agent taken up by all the tissues in the body. For example, the prime dose required by a 100 kg patient receiving isoflurane ($f = 1.3$, MAC = 1.3, $V_{vent} = 100$ dL, and Q = 2 kg $^{3/4}$ or 63.25 dL/min) is:

$$(1.3)(1.3)(63.25)(1.5) + (100)(1.3)(1.3) =$$
$$160 + 169 \text{ mL vapor} =$$
$$329 \text{ mL vapor}$$
$$\text{and } 329 \text{ mL vapor/206 mL vapor/mL}$$
$$\text{isoflurane liquid} = 1.6 \text{ mL liquid}$$

For a "pediatric" example, if we wished to determine a unit and prime dose for a 30 kg 8-year-old at 1.3 MAC, using isoflurane with an adult circle system:
$$\text{Prime}_{(vent)} = 1.3 \times 1.3 \text{ mL/dL} \times 100 \text{ dL} =$$
$$169 \text{ mL of isoflurane vapor}$$
$$\text{Prime}_{(vent)} = 1.3 \times 1.3 \text{ mL/dL} \times 1.5 \times 25.6 \text{ dL} =$$
$$65 \text{ mL of isoflurane vapor}$$

The liquid equivalent would be 169 + 65 = 234 mL of vapor/206 mL of vapor/mL of liquid, or 1.1 mL of isoflurane liquid, of which the unit dose (for subsequent dosing intervals related to the square root of time) would be 65 mL of vapor, or 0.3 mL of liquid.

While the prime dose should be sufficient to establish the desired arterial concentration at time 0, C_a can remain constant only if anesthetic is introduced into the circuit at the same rate at which it is lost to tissues. A unit dose must be delivered between 0-1, 1-4, 4-9… minutes. If the arterial blood content falls, it will draw on the "reservoir" of the ventilatory prime, which will then require repriming.

References

1. Waters, R.M., 1926. Advantages and technique of carbon dioxide filtration with inhalation anesthesia. Anesth Analg 5, 160.
2. Lowe, H.J., Ernst, E.A., 1981. The quantitative practice of anesthesia: use of closed circuit. Williams and Wilkins, Baltimore.
3. Standard specification for minimum performance and safety requirements for components and systems of anesthesia gas machines. American Society for Testing and Materials, West Conshohocken, Pa.
4. Van der Zee, H., Verkaaik, A., 1990. Cardiovascular implementations of respiratory measurements. Acta Anaesthesiol Belg 41, 167–175.
5. Verkaaik, A.P.K., Erdmann, W., 1990. Respiratory diagnostic possibilities during closed circuit anesthesia. Acta Anaesthesiol Belg 41, 177–188.
6. Brody, S., 1945. Bioenergetics and growth. Reinhold, New York.
7. Crowell, J., Smith, E., 1964. Oxygen deficit and irreversible hemorrhagic shock. Am J Physiol 206, 313.
8. Shoemaker, W., Montgomery, E., Kaplan, E., et al., 1973. Physiologic patterns in surviving and nonsurviving shock patients: use of sequential cardiorespiratory variables in defining criteria for therapeutic goals and early warning of death. Arch Surg 106, 630–636.
9. Robiquet, T., 1839. Rapport sur un memoire adresse a l'Academie royale de medecine par MM Sarrus et Rameaux. Bull Acad Roy Med Belg 3, 1094–1100.
10. Sarrus, R., 1838. Application des sciences accessoires et principalement des mathematiques a la physiologie generale (correspondance manuscrite). Bull Acad Roy Med Belg 2, 538.
11. Kleiber, M., 1932. Body size and metabolism. Hilgardia 6, 315–353.
12. Dicker, A., Ohlson, K., Johnson, L., et al., 1995. Halothane selectively inhibits nonshivering thermogenesis. Possible implications for thermoregulation during anesthesia of infants. Anesthesiology 82, 491–501.

13. Lindahl, S., 1989. Oxygen consumption and carbon dioxide elimination in infants and children during anaesthesia and surgery. Br J Anaesth 62, 70–76.

14. Ohlson, K., Mohell, N., Cannon, B., et al., 1994. Thermogenesis in brown adipocytes is inhibited by volatile anesthetic agents. A factor contributing to hypothermia in infants? Anesthesiology 81, 176–183.

15. Couto da Silva, J.M., Tubino, P.J., Garcia Vieira, Z.E., et al., 1984. Closed circuit anesthesia in infants and children. Anesth Analg 63, 765–769.

16. Lindahl, S., Hulse, M., Hatch, D., 1984. Metabolic correlates in infants and children during anaesthesia and surgery. Acta Anaesthiol Scand 28, 52–56.

17. Eger, E.I.I., 1979. Dragons and other scientific hazards. Anesthesiology 30, 1 (editorial).

18. Bito, H., Ikeda, K., 1994. Closed-circuit anesthesia with sevoflurane in humans. Anesthesiology 80, 71–76.

19. Hanaki, C., Fujii, K., Morio, M., et al., 1987. Decomposition of sevoflurane by soda lime. Hiroshima J Med Sci 36, 61–67.

20. Morio, M., Fujii, K., Satoh, N., et al., 1992. Reaction of sevoflurane and its degradation products with soda lime. Toxicity of the byproducts. Anesthesiology 77, 1155–1156.

21. Strum, D.P., Johnson, B.H., Eger, E.I.D., 1987. Stability of sevoflurane in soda lime. Anesthesiology 67, 779–781.

22. Munday, I.T., Foden, N.D., Ward, P.M., et al., 1994. Sevoflurane degradation in a circle system at 2 different fresh gas flow rates. Anesthesiology 81, A433.

23. Frink E.J., Jr., Isner, R.J., Malan T.P., Jr., et al., 1994. Sevoflurane degradation product concentrations with soda lime during prolonged anesthesia. J Clin Anesth 6, 239–242.

24. Philip, J., 1990. Nitrogen buildup in a closed circuit. Anesthesiology 73, A465 (abstract).

25. Strauss, J.M., Bannasch, W., Hausdorfer, J., et al., 1991. Die Entwicklung von Carboxyhamoglobin wahrend Langzeitnarkosen im geschlossenen Kreis-system. Anaesthetist 40, 324–327.

26. Bengtson, J.P., Bengtsson, J., Bengtsson, A., et al., 1993. Sampled gas need not be returned during low-flow anesthesia. J Clin Monit 9, 330–334.

27. Lowe, H.J., 1972. Dose regulated penthrane methoxyflurane anesthesia. Abbott Laboratories, Chicago.

28. Olympio, M., 2005. Absorbent comparisons table 3. APSF Newsl 20, 29.

29. Rayburn, R., Watson, R., 1980. Humidity in children and adults using the controlled partial rebreathing anesthesia method. Anesthesiology 52, 291–295.

Chapter 5

Manual and Mechanical Ventilators

Demet Sulemanji, Robert M. Kacmarek, and Yandong Jiang

The maintenance of appropriate ventilation and oxygenation is an essential aspect of the provision of anesthesia. Numerous approaches to ventilatory support are available to the anesthesia care provider during the administration of anesthesia. The purpose of this chapter is to provide an in-depth overview of manual ventilators, automatic ventilators, jet ventilators, and the terminology used to provide ventilatory support. The principles associated with the application of PEEP and the overall capabilities of the newest generation of anesthesia ventilators will also be presented.

Manual Ventilators

Manual ventilators are the mainstay for the provision of ventilatory support in all care settings. Although they are not the ideal approach for continuous ventilatory support they are commonly used for the transition from spontaneous breathing to ventilatory support and for support during emergency airway management. In general, manual ventilators are composed of three parts: (1) A self-refilling bag; (2) A non-rebreathing valve; and (3) an oxygen/air inlet and oxygen reservoir (Figure 5-1).

1. **The self-refilling bag:** This component acts as a reservoir for the O_2 and/or air that is directed to the patient when the bag is compressed during inhalation. During exhalation, the bag automatically recoils to its inspiratory position or it passively expands as O_2/air refills the reservoir. The bag may be made of silicone rubber, chloroprene rubber, butyl rubber, or polyvinyl chloride (Figures 5-2 through 5-5). All rubber bags can be reused after sterilization. The polyvinyl chloride bags are for single use only. Most new designs are latex-free.
2. **Non-rebreathing valve:** This valve ensures that exhaled gas does not mix with the fresh gas entering the self-refilling bag and allows exhaled gas to enter the atmosphere. All manual ventilators allow the attachment of a positive end-expiratory pressure (PEEP) valve to the expiratory port to ensure that varying levels of PEEP can be applied during manual ventilation. During inspiration the non-rebreathing valve ensures that fresh gas from the self-refilling bag directly enters the patient without leaking and that the patient only receives gas from the bag during inspiration. With most manual ventilators, patients are able to breathe spontaneously directly from the self-refilling bag via the non-rebreathing valve. However, inspiratory effort may be excessive depending on the opening pressure of the non-rebreathing valve and the amount of PEEP applied to the system. If PEEP is applied, the patient must decompress the applied PEEP before they can spontaneously inhale gas from the self-inflating bag.

Non-rebreathing valves are formed by two parts: the body, and the unidirectional valve or valves. The body of the valve is usually T-shaped and consists of an *inspiratory port* that directs the gas from the bag to the patient, an *expiratory port* that allows the gas from the patient to leave the valve, and a *patient port* that serves as a connector for masks, endotracheal tubes, or other airway devices (Figure 5-6). Unidirectional valves ensure that the patient inhales the fresh gas in the bag by closing the expiratory port during inspiration, and that the exhaled gas leaves the system without being mixed with the fresh gas by closing the inspiratory port during exhalation. More than one unidirectional valve may be used for this purpose. A number of designs of unidirectional valves are currently in use, all operating by similar principles: a spring, a duckbill, or a flap mechanism.
Spring valve: With this design, a ball or a disc is attached to the spring. In its resting state or during exhalation, the spring seats the ball or the disc on the inspiratory port. In this position, the exhaled gas from the patient port is

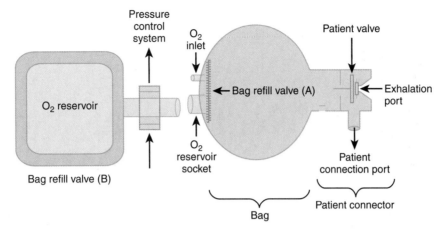

Figure 5–1 Schematic presentation of manual ventilator parts; A self refilling bag, A non-rebreathing valve, and an oxygen/air inlet and oxygen reservoir. *From http://www.scielo.br/img/revistas/jbpneu/v34n4/en_a05fig01.gif*

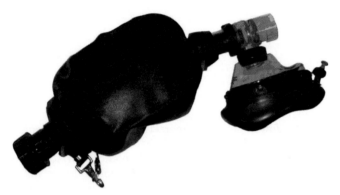

Figure 5–2 Non-disposable Military Ambu bag and face mask. This model is made of butyl rubber. http://www.ambu.com/RespiratoryCare/ Respiratory_Care.aspx?GID=GROUP51&ProductID=PROD986

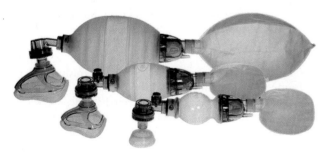

Figure 5–3 The Laerdal system in adult, child and infant sizes. The versions shown all have oxygen reservoir bags attached. The child and infant versions show overpressure safety valves fitted.

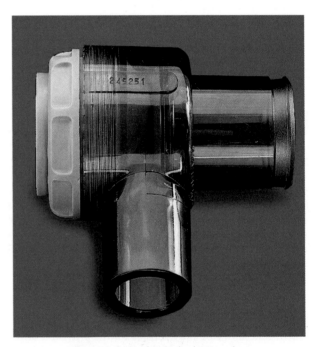

Figure 5–4 Ambu single-shutter valve.

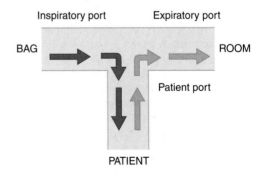

Figure 5–5 Illustration of the body of the nonrebreathing valve in a manual ventilator. All consists of **an inspiratory port** that directs the gas from the bag to the patient, **an expiratory port** that allows the gas from the patient to leave the valve, and **a patient port** that serves as a connector for the airway devices (masks, endotracheal tubes, etc.).

directed out of the expiratory port. During inhalation, when the bag is compressed, the fresh gas from the self-refilling bag moves the ball or the disc back, so that it blocks the expiratory port and fresh gas is directed to the patient port (Figures 5-7 and 5-8).

Duckbill valve: During inhalation, fresh gas flow from the self-refilling bag opens the duckbill valve, allowing the fresh gas to enter the inspiratory port. When the valve is open, it also prevents gas from entering the expiratory port. When fresh gas flow ceases, the duckbill

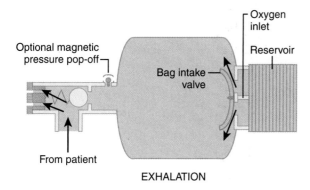

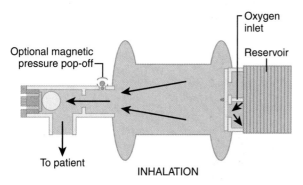

Figure 5–6   Spring valve operation during inhalation and exhalation phases. *Fig: Steven Mcpherson, Respiratory Care Equipment, 5th ed., 1995, USA, Mosby-Year Book Inc., pp130, Fig 6-2.A*

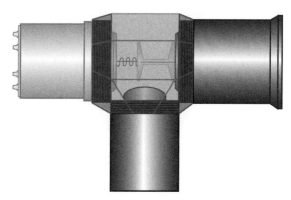

Figure 5–7   The Ruben Valve is an example of spring valve mechanism. from www.intersurgical.com/utils/GetFile.aspx?FileID=2659

valve returns to its closed state and exhalation begins. The exhaled gas flow from the patient is directed to the expiratory port maintaining the valve closed (Figures 5-9 and 5-10).

Flap Valve: During inhalation, the opening of the flap valve by the fresh gas flow from the self-inflating bag closes the expiratory port and directs the fresh gas to the patient. At the end of inhalation, the flap returns to its original position, which allows exhaled gas to exit through the expiratory valve. Various designs of this valve are available by positioning the flap on its edge or centrally, or combining it with a diaphragm (e.g., diaphragm-flap valve, mushroom-flap valve, fish-mouth-flap valve)[1] (Figures 5-11 and 5-12).

3. **Oxygen/air inlet and oxygen reservoir:** The gas inlet to the reservoir is generally located at the other side of the self-refilling bag from the non-rebreathing valve end. However, in some older designs the gas inlet is part of the non-rebreathing valve assembly. The gas inlet normally has a unidirectional valve, which opens during exhalation when the bag is refilling and closes during inhalation when the bag is compressed.

Oxygen may be delivered into the system in two ways; through a nipple as part of the inlet valve assembly or via an oxygen reservoir. Oxygen reservoirs are either bags (closed reservoir) or lengths of large bore (22 mm internal diameter) tubing (open reservoir) that allow the accumulation of oxygen during the inhalation phase and release the stored oxygen into the self-refilling bag during the exhalation phase when the bag is refilling (Figure 5-13). The addition of an oxygen reservoir to the system significantly increases the achievable inspired oxygen concentration.

Two security valves are placed between the reservoir and the gas inlet; one is a "pressure relief valve," which opens at a threshold pressure, preventing the bag from being over-filled. This valve limits the exposure of the patient's airway to high pressure. The other is the "air intake" valve; it opens when subatmospheric pressure is established in the self-refilling bag by its normal elastic recoil allowing air to enter and refill the reservoir. This preserves the ability to provide ventilation even when the oxygen tank is empty.

Positive end-expiratory pressure (PEEP) valves may be added to the system simply by inserting the PEEP valve into the expiratory port of the manual ventilator. Some of the newly designed models have built-in PEEP valves with adjusting dials (Figures 5-14 and 5-15).

Automatic Ventilators

Historically, anesthesia ventilators were designed to relieve the anesthesia care provider from continuously squeezing the bag, thus the design of the ventilator was quite simple. As technology advanced, and critical care management of patients improved, anesthesiologists increasingly have been required to provide anesthesia to critically ill patients with a variety of severe cardiopulmonary problems. As new airway devices such as the laryngeal mask were introduced into anesthesia practice, the need for ventilation modes beyond the standard volume control became critical. To meet these new demands, anesthesia ventilators have been designed to allow a comparable range of operation as seen on ICU ventilators. Most new anesthesia ventilators are equipped with a wide selection of modes, the ability to apply PEEP, and the capability of monitoring patients in the same manner as in the ICU.

Classification

Today's anesthesia ventilators can be classified according to their application, power system, and cycling mechanism.

Application Type

Ward et al[2] have classified anesthesia ventilators into four different groups: mechanical thumb ventilators, minute volume dividers, bag squeezers, and intermittent blowers.

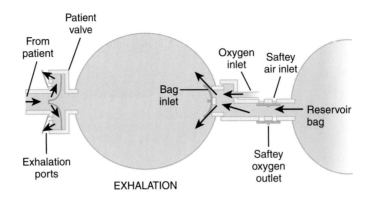

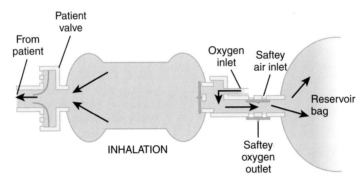

Figure 5–8 Duckbill valve operation during inhalation and exhalation phases. *Fig: Steven Mcpherson, Respiratory Care Equipment, 5th ed., 1995, USA, Mosby-Year Book Inc., pp131, Fig 6-4.A*

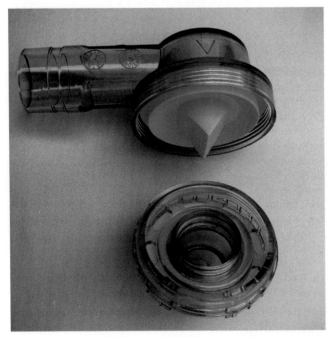

Figure 5–9 The Laerdal valve

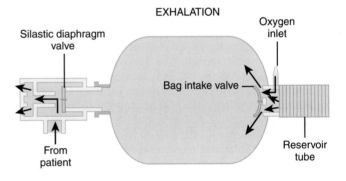

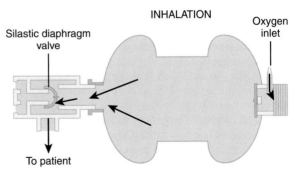

Figure 5–10 Flap valve operation during inhalation and exhalation phases. *Fig: Steven Mcpherson, Respiratory Care Equipment, 5th ed., 1995, USA, Mosby-Year Book Inc., pp136, Fig 6-11.A*

■ **Mechanical thumb ventilators:** This type of ventilator delivers pressurized gas from a cylinder or the wall outlet to the patient as a continuous flow through a simple T-piece breathing system. Either the thumb of the anesthesia care provider or a mechanical thumb (a pneumatic valve) rhythmically occludes and opens the end of the

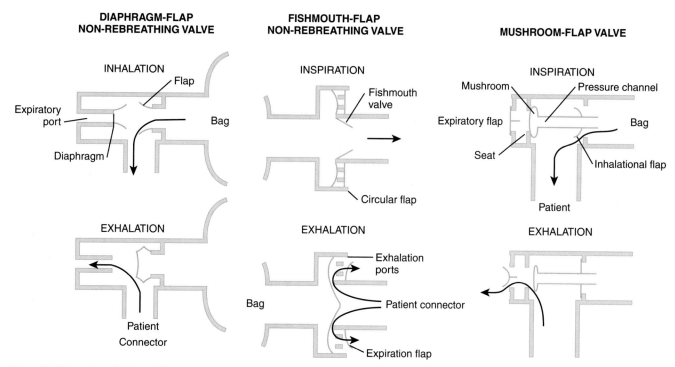

DIAPHRAGM-FLAP NON-REBREATHING VALVE

INHALATION

Flap

Expiratory port

Bag

Diaphragm

EXHALATION

Patient Connector

FISHMOUTH-FLAP NON-REBREATHING VALVE

INSPIRATION

Fishmouth valve

Circular flap

EXHALATION

Exhalation ports

Bag

Patient connector

Expiration flap

MUSHROOM-FLAP VALVE

INSPIRATION

Mushroom

Pressure channel

Expiratory flap

Bag

Seat

Inhalational flap

Patient

EXHALATION

Figure 5–11   Various designs of flap valves; Edge mounted flap valve, centrally mounted flap valve, diaphragm flap valve, mushroom flap valve, fishmouth flap valve. From *Dorsch JA, Dorsch SE, Understanding Anesthetic Equipment, 5th edition, 2007, USA, Lippincott Williams & Wilkins, pp 285, Fig 10-6(edge m), 10-7(centrally m), pp 286 Fig 10-10(diaphragm flap), pp 287, Fig 10-11(mushroom flap), 10-12(fishmouth flap).*

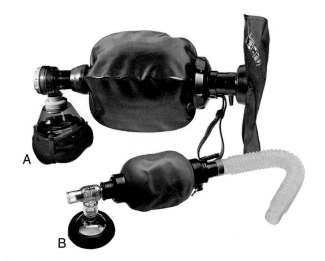

Figure 5–12   AMBU re-usable adult **A,** and paediatric **B,** resuscitators.

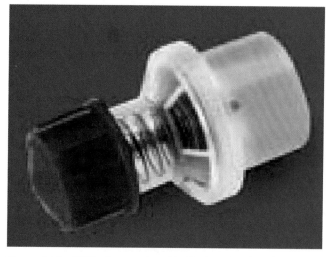

Figure 5–13   PEEP valves may be added by inserting the valve into the expiratory port of the manual ventilator. From http://www.ambu.co.uk/SiteBuilder/ecmedia.nsf/ViewImagesById/iA388B913FFED2487C1256DDC0043ED4E/$File/PEEP_valve_w.jpeg

T-piece, which creates the intermittent positive pressure to ventilate the patient. The use of this early design ventilator is currently limited to ventilation of neonates or during emergencies since it requires a high fresh gas flow, which is wasted and lost to the atmosphere during exhalation resulting in higher costs of ventilation. In addition, ventilation is unregulated (i.e., the anesthesiologist has no idea of the pressures or volumes of gas delivered to the patient's airways) (Figure 5-16).

- **Minute volume divider ventilators:** In this simple design, a specific volume of fresh gas equal to the patient's minute volume is delivered to the ventilator per minute. This volume is then divided by the

number of the breaths, and the resultant tidal volume is delivered to the patient. Gas entering the ventilator is collected in a reservoir. The alternate opening and closing of two linked valves directs the gas from the reservoir to the patient and the exhaled gas from the patient to the atmosphere. These ventilators are very rarely found in U.S. anesthesia practice (Figure 5-17).

- **Bag squeezer ventilators:** This application was inspired by the anesthesia care provider's hands squeezing the breathing bag. Until recently, these ventilators were the most common type found on anesthesia machines.

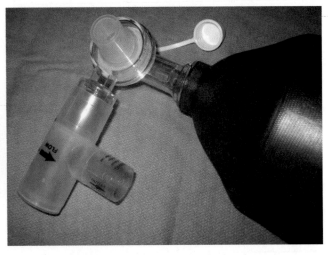

Figure 5–14 A PEEP valve is shown as attached to the expiratory port of a manual ventilator.

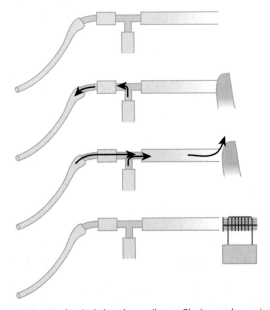

Figure 5–15 Mechanical thumb ventilator. Closing and opening one end of the t-shaped mechanism by the anesthesiologist's thumb or a mechanical thumb delivers intermittent positive pressure to ventilate the patient. *From; Davey A, Diba A, Ward CS, Ward's Anesthetic Equipment, 5th edition, 2005, UK, Elselvier Health Sciences. pp 247, Fig.11.4*

These ventilators may be subgrouped according to their bellows type and driving mechanism, as outlined below.

Bellows Type

The most typical design of an anesthesia ventilator is "a bag in the bottle," that is a bellows (bag) inside a cylinder. The bellows is filled with gas that moves to and from the patient, whereas the cylinder is filled with the driving gas that compresses the bellows, moving gas to the patient. The bellow's movement is easily observed through the cylinder. The bellows may be ascending or descending according to its movement during exhalation.

■ **Ascending:** Ascending bellows rise during exhalation. The bellows is attached to the system from its base; exhaled gas coming from the patient fills the bellows

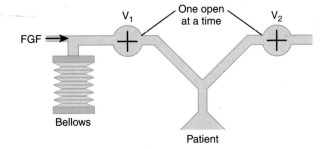

Figure 5–16 Minute volume divider type ventilator, working principle. *From; Davey A, Diba A, Ward CS, Ward's Anesthetic Equipment, 5th edition, 2005, UK, Elselvier Health Sciences. pp 249, Fig.11.6*

and generates the ascending motion. During inhalation, the driving gas surrounding the bellows pushes the bellows downward and the gas inside the bellows moves toward the patient. During exhalation, the expired gas refills the bellows and the next cycle starts. If there is any disconnection of the circuit, the bag does not fill providing an instant visual alert for the anesthesiologist. Because of this design, ascending bellows ventilators provide an obligate amount of PEEP, usually 2 to 3 cm H_2O applied to the exhalation port of the bellows so that the exhaled gas will force the bellows to rise.

■ **Descending:** Descending bellows fall during patient exhalation and ascend during inhalation. The bellows is attached to the system from the top and usually is weighted to facilitate its descending motion during exhalation. If there is a leak or disconnection of the system, the bellows will still descend during exhalation, and the negative pressure produced by the weight of the bellows allows room air to enter the system. Since the movement of the bellows appears normal despite the leak, the bellows movement may be deceiving to the anesthesiologist. Early models of anesthesia ventilators used descending bellows but due to the high risk of complications all ventilators produced after the 1980s have ascending bellows for improved safety.[3] However, recent models of anesthesia ventilators (e.g., Drager Julian, Datascope Anestar) have again integrated descending bellows into their design but they have also added safety features: these include built-in end-tidal carbon dioxide monitors; software, sensors and monitors to identify bellows failure and activate alarms; and a negative pressure relief valve to prevent the development of negative pressure in the system (Figure 5–18).

Drive Mechanism and Circuit Design Type

■ **Double circuit pneumatically driven:** In these ventilators, a pneumatic force created by the driving gas compresses the bellows so that the bellows empties its contents—exhaled gas that has been passed through the CO_2 absorbent, gas from flowmeters, and gas from the vaporizer—into the inspiratory limb of the breathing circuit. The driving gas may be oxygen, air, or both. This pressurized gas from the ventilator power outlet directly enters the space between the inner wall of the container and the outer wall of the bellows. To reduce oxygen consumption when 100% oxygen is the driving

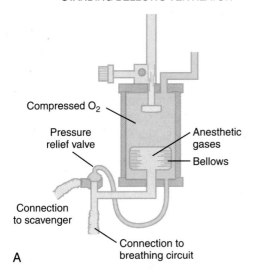

STANDING BELLOWS VENTILATOR

Compressed O₂

Pressure
relief valve

Anesthetic
gases

Bellows

Connection
to scavenger

Connection to
breathing circuit

A

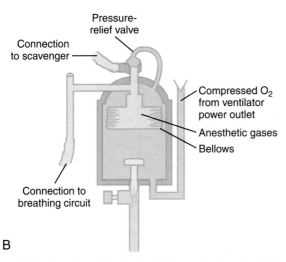

HANGING BELLOWS VENTILATOR

Pressure-
relief valve

Connection
to scavenger

Compressed O₂
from ventilator
power outlet

Anesthetic gases

Bellows

Connection to
breathing circuit

B

Figure 5–17 Ascending (standing) and descending (hanging) bellows ventilators. *From Morgan GE, Mikhail MS, Murray MJ, Clinical Anesthesiology, 4th ed, 2006, USA, McGraw-Hill Companies Inc. Fig 4.12*

force, a **venturi** device may be used to entrain room air and conserve the amount of oxygen driving the ventilator (Figure 5-19 and 5-20).

- **Single circuit piston design:** In these ventilators, a piston replaces the bellows and drives the gas to be inhaled by the patient into the breathing circuit. There is minimal or no requirement for driving gas. The piston may be pneumatic or powered by an electric motor. Most new designs are equipped with electric motors (Figures 5-21 and 5-22).

- **Intermittent blower ventilators:** Most of these ventilators are microprocessor controlled and use either a pneumatically timed oscillator or an electronically timed and activated proportional flow valve to adjust the size of the tidal volume and frequency of ventilation. As a result precise control over the ventilatory pattern is established. Another advantage of this design is the low internal compliance of the gas delivery system. With these ventilators the driving gas pathway is short

and of low volume. This increases the efficiency of these ventilators compared with all other designs. This design is not only used for anesthesia, but also common in intensive care unit (ICU) ventilators, and in basic and sophisticated automatic resuscitators (Figure 5-23).

Power Type

Anesthesia ventilators are classified as either low power or high power ventilators.

- **Low power:** This design is intended to produce only the limited pressure required to ventilate patients with normal compliance and resistance. These ventilators do not have the capacity to deliver the required tidal volumes for patients with increased resistance and/or low compliance. Therefore, when these ventilators are used it is essential that patients are continuously monitored by capnography and expired tidal volume or minute volume to ensure adequate ventilation is always provided. Advantages of low power ventilators are their simple design, low cost, and the fact that the low airway pressures established are less likely to cause lung damage than high airway pressures. Low power ventilators were common in anesthesia practice in the past. Today they are replaced by high power ventilators.

- **High power:** In contrast to low power ventilators, these ventilators have the ability to deliver appropriate tidal volumes to patients with low compliance and/or high resistance. They produce the high gas pressures needed to overcome changes in resistance and compliance. The primary disadvantage of these ventilators is the potential for developing the high inspiratory pressures that may cause lung damage. Thus, in these ventilators, high pressure alarms and pressure-relief valves are essential design features. All new anesthesia machine ventilators are high power ventilators.

Cycling Type

Anesthesia machine ventilators, as with all forms of mechanical ventilators, can be cycled from inspiration to expiration or from expiration to inspiration by one of the following variables; volume, pressure, time, or flow.

- **Volume cycling:** An inspiratory volume-cycled ventilator ends the inspiratory phase when a preset gas volume is delivered. This is the most common mode of ventilation. An expiratory volume-cycled ventilator ends the expiratory phase when the gas entering the bellows reaches a preset volume and initiates inhalation.

- **Pressure cycling:** An inspiratory pressure-cycled ventilator ends the inspiratory phase and initiates the expiratory phase when a preset airway pressure is reached. An expiratory pressure-cycled ventilator initiates the inspiratory phase when a preset expiratory airway pressure is reached.

- **Time cycling:** An inspiratory or expiratory time-cycled ventilator terminates the inspiratory or expiratory phase after a predetermined time period. Most modern ventilators are time cycled.

- **Flow cycling:** An inspiratory flow-cycled ventilator terminates the inspiratory phase when inspiratory flow decreases to a preset level.

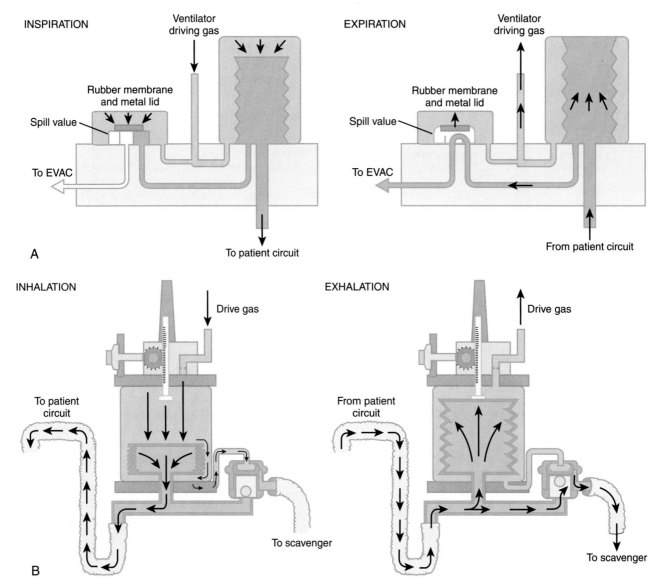

Figure 5–18   Double circuit pneumatic ventilator designs. (A:Datex-Ohmeda, B: Drager) *From Morgan GE, Mikhail MS, Murray MJ, Clinical Anesthesiology, 4th ed, 2006, USA, McGraw-Hill Companies Inc., pp 79 , Fig 4.29*

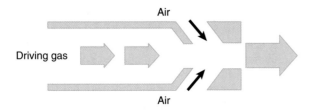

Figure 5–19   Venturi device consists of a constriction in the driving gas flow channel, resulting in an increase in gas velocity which creates a negative pressure entraining a second gas into the system. *From Dorsch JA & Dorsch SE, Understanding Anesthetic Equipment, 5th edition, 2007, USA, Lippincott Williams & Wilkins, pp 314, Fig 12.2*

Ventilation Modes

Modern anesthesia machines and modern ICU ventilators are equipped with a variety of ventilation modes. These modes can be globally categorized as volume or pressure targeted modes. With volume ventilation, the ventilator is programmed to deliver a precise tidal volume with each breath. However, the airway pressure required to deliver this tidal volume can vary greatly, depending upon the patient's compliance and resistance. With pressure targeted ventilation, a target gas delivery pressure is established, which cannot be exceeded. As a result tidal volume may vary from breath to breath, again depending upon the patient's compliance and resistance. In addition, with volume ventilation the gas flow pattern is defined (square or decreasing ramp) and the peak inspiratory flow or inspiratory time is set by the anesthetist. With pressure ventilation, the impedance to gas delivery along with the patient's inspiratory efforts determine the gas delivery pattern and tidal volume. Impedance to gas delivery is heavily influenced by surgical maneuvers such as intraabdominal insufflation.

In general, patients allowed to spontaneously breathe experience less distress with properly set pressure ventilation than volume ventilation.

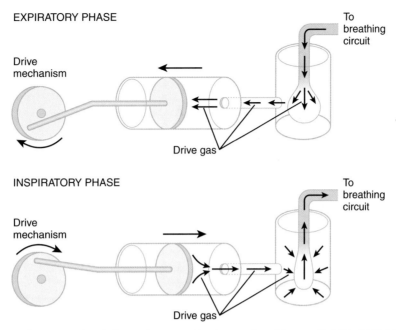

Figure 5–20   A piston driven ventilator; operation during expiratory and inspiratory. *From Morgan GE, Mikhail MS, Murray MJ, Clinical Anesthesiology, 4th ed, 2006, USA, McGraw-Hill Companies Inc., pp 77, Fig 4.27*

- **Volume control:** This is the most commonly used ventilation mode in anesthesia practice. The ventilator controls the inspiratory flow and delivers a preset tidal volume. Inspiratory flow and volume are constant but peak inspiratory pressure may vary. The patient should be a passive recipient of mechanical ventilation. In addition, in newer anesthesia ventilators, as an optional feature, the breath delivery can be synchronized with the patients' inspiratory efforts by the adjustment of a sensitivity control.

- **Pressure control:** With this mode of ventilation, inspiratory flow rapidly accelerates to try to reach the set target pressure, then flow rapidly decreases as airway pressure approaches that set on the ventilator. Pressure is constant every breath but volume may vary from one breath to another. The major advantage of pressure control is the control of airway pressure. The patient should be a passive recipient of mechanical ventilation. In addition, in newer anesthesia ventilators, as an optional feature, the breath delivery can be synchronized with the patients' inspiratory efforts by the adjustment of a sensitivity control. As mentioned above, tidal volume and minute ventilation produced by a given pressure setting can vary dramatically depending on the surgical manipulation.

- **SIMV:** The ventilator delivers a mandatory set breath rate in volume or pressure control. The patient, however, is allowed to trigger these breaths (proper setting of the sensitivity). If no triggering occurs within a manufacturer's defined time period, the ventilator delivers a controlled mandatory breath. In between these mandatory breaths, the patient can breathe spontaneously around baseline pressure (positive end-expiratory pressure [PEEP]). In some ventilators pressure support can be applied to these spontaneous breaths. This mode is usually preferred when patients are allowed to spontaneously breathe or during the weaning period.

- **Pressure support:** This mode is similar to pressure control except that the patient must trigger every breath and the breath is terminated when flow decreases to a predetermined level. That is, the patient essentially controls all aspects of gas delivery except the setting of peak airway pressure. In this mode respiratory rate, inspiratory time, and tidal volume are determined by the patient. Patients should be monitored closely during pressure support ventilation since no breaths will be initiated if the patient's inspiratory effort stops. If the patients become apneic, the ventilator automatically activates a backup mode.

- **Autoflow:** This mode of ventilation is considered a dual mode of ventilation (i.e., it combines features of both volume and pressure ventilation[4]). Gas delivery is in a pressure ventilation format but a target tidal volume is set. During each breath the ventilator evaluates the tidal volume delivered and adjusts the pressure control level up or down for the next breath to try to ensure that the target tidal volume is delivered. There is a potential that the ventilator may need to adjust the pressure control level each and every breath.

- **CPAP:** Continuous positive airway pressure is not a true mode of ventilation since all it entails is the adjustment of baseline end expiratory pressure. The patient still provides all of the work of breathing but at an elevated baseline pressure. Essentially this is the application of PEEP to the noninvasively ventilated patient (Figure 5-24).

Positive End-Expiratory Pressure (PEEP) Valves

PEEP improves oxygenation by keeping alveoli from collapsing, restoring the functional residual capacity and decreasing the physiological shunt. With older anesthesia ventilators and manual ventilators, PEEP application in the operating

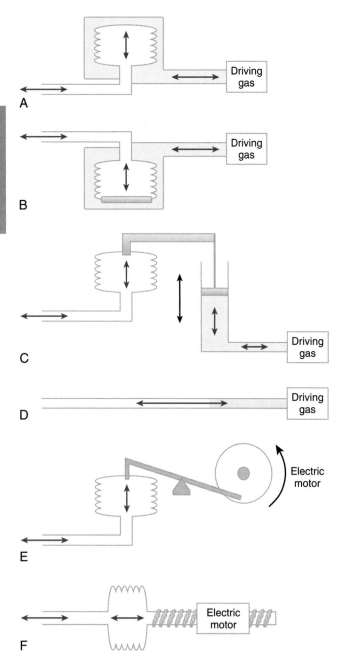

Figure 5–21 Bag squeezer ventilator types. a) Ascending bellows b) Descending bellows c) pneumatic piston with bellows assembly d) pneumatic piston e-f) electric motor driven designs *From; Davey A, Diba A, Ward CS, Ward's Anesthetic Equipment, 5th edition, 2005, UK, Elselvier Health Sciences. pp 252, Fig.11.8*

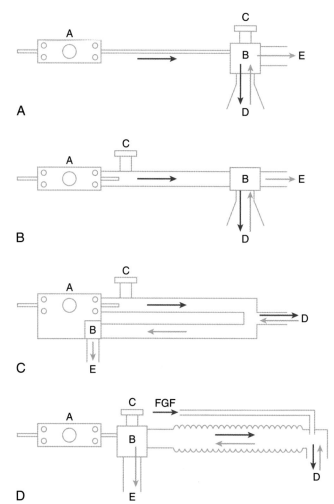

Figure 5–22 Intermittent blower ventilator types. a) basic resuscitator, b) sophisticated resuscitator c) intensive care ventilator d) anesthetic ventilator for Mapleson D system. A: resuscitator/ventilator, B: patient valve, C: overpressure relief valve, D: patient pathway, E: expiratory pathway *From; Davey A, Diba A, Ward CS, Ward's Anesthetic Equipment, 5th edition, 2005, UK, Elselvier Health Sciences. pp 263, Fig.11.15*

room is achieved by the use of detachable valves. Modern anesthesia ventilators allow PEEP to be set as a ventilatory parameter. PEEP valves generate positive end-expiratory pressure when placed in the expiratory limb of the breathing system. They may be unidirectional or bidirectional flow valves. PEEP, however, is only produced when gas flows through the valve in the correct direction. Any incorrect placement of a unidirectional PEEP valve opposing gas flow causes obstruction resulting in the patient "not being ventilated" if incorrectly placed in the inspiratory limb and the potential of severe barotrauma if incorrectly placed in the

expiratory limb.[5] Misplacement of a bidirectional PEEP valve opposing gas flow in either limb does not cause occlusion but no PEEP will be generated. Anesthesia care providers should pay close attention to the correct placement of these easy-to-install PEEP valves and ensure effective ventilation following valve placement.

Because modern ventilators have in-built PEEP valves, this eliminates the potential serious errors related to the misplacement of PEEP valves by anesthesia personnel.[6] Depending on the manufacturer, these valves may be magnetic one-way valves, spring-loaded adjustable valves, or electronic valves. Magnetic and spring-loaded valves establish PEEP by the force exerted on the valve disk by the magnet or the spring. Electronic valves create a pressure threshold (usually by pneumatic pressurization of the expiratory valve) that allows expiratory flow to occur only when airway pressure equals or exceeds the selected PEEP level.

In descending bellows or piston ventilators, PEEP can be set at zero if desired; however, with ascending bellows ventilators a minimum of 2 to 4 cm H_2O PEEP is always established.

Ventilatory modes			
Mode	Initiation	Limit	Cycle
Volume control ventilation	Time	Volume	Volume/time
Pressure control ventilation	Time	Pressure	Time
Intermittent mandatory ventilation	Time	Volume	Volume/time
Synchronized intermittent mandatory ventilation	Time/pressure	Volume	Volume/time
Pressure support ventilation	Pressure/flow	Pressure	Flow/time

Figure 5–23 Ventilatory Modes Dorsch JA & Dorsch SE, *Understanding Anesthetic Equipment, 5th edition, 2007, USA, Lippincott Williams & Wilkins, pp 316, Tb 12.1*

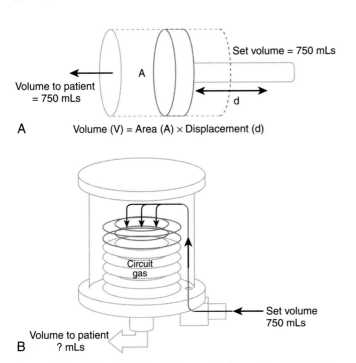

Figure 5–24 **A.** Piston, **B.** Bellows driving mechanisms - Since the tidal volume is equal to the surface area of the piston times the distance the piston moves to ventilate the patient, the set tidal volume can accurately be delivered to the patient whereas with a bellows mechanism, the set tidal volume is equal to the driving gas volume around the bellows which makes it difficult to deliver accurate tidal volumes, even more difficult with increased airway resistance or decreased compliance. *From; Drager, Medical Insight*

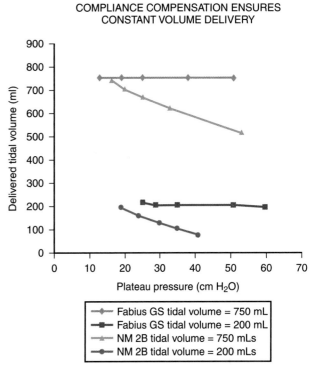

Figure 5–25 Comparison of compliance compensation with a piston ventilator (Fabius GS) and a traditional bellows ventilator Narkomed 2B). As the airway pressure increases, tidal volume delivery to the airway stays constant with Fabius GS while it decreases with Narkomed 2B. *From; Drager Website*

Alarms

Alarms are indispensable aspects of all anesthesia ventilators. The most important alarms on a ventilator are the disconnection alarms since breathing circuit disconnection is one of the leading causes of anesthesia accidents.[7,8] The disconnection alarms should always be active when the ventilator is in use. Low peak inspiratory pressure, low exhaled tidal or minute volume, and low exhaled end-tidal carbon dioxide alarms alert the anesthesiologist to potential disconnection. Other typical ventilator alarms include high peak inspiratory pressure, sustained high inspiratory pressure, subatmospheric pressure, low minute volume, high respiratory rate, reverse flow (indicates incompetent expiratory valve), and low oxygen supply pressure.

New Features

Recent advances in ventilator technology have affected anesthesia ventilators and ICU ventilators. Modern ventilators are quite sophisticated and sensitive to patient inspiratory efforts. They also have electronic controls, highly flexible ventilation settings and modes, and the ability to deliver accurate tidal volumes, even at very small set values. This is especially important for pediatric patients.[9,10] The operational capabilities of new anesthesia ventilators are almost equivalent to that of ICU ventilators.[11,12]

Piston: Pistons have largely replaced bellows in modern ventilators. The major advantage of this design is accuracy of tidal volume. When the tidal volume is set, the piston moves the distance necessary to deliver the required volume into the breathing circuit. Since the cross-sectional area of the piston is fixed, the volume delivered by the piston is directly proportional to the linear movement of the piston. In bellows ventilators, the driving gas volume is equal to the set tidal volume; however, the pressure in the breathing circuit varies between patients or even breaths, thus the compression level of the bellows varies and the delivered tidal volume may not be accurate. This is a common problem when small tidal volumes are needed or inspiratory pressures are high (Figure 5-25).

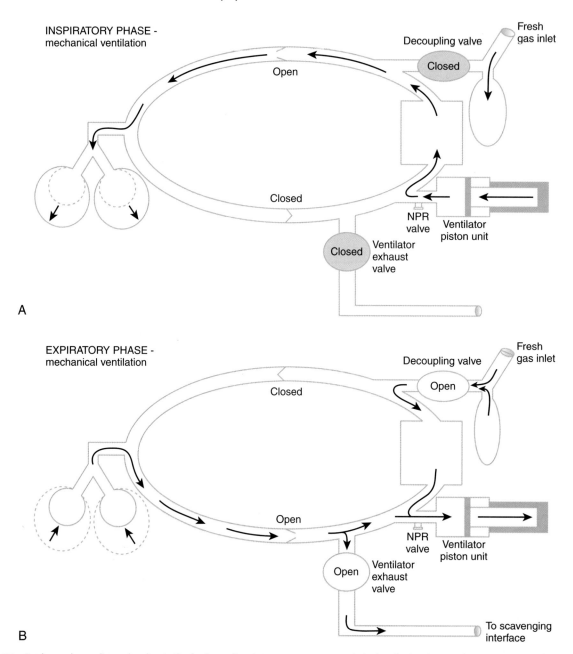

INSPIRATORY PHASE -
mechanical ventilation

Decoupling valve

Fresh
gas inlet

Closed

Open

Open

Closed

NPR
valve

Ventilator
piston unit

Closed

Ventilator
exhaust
valve

A

EXPIRATORY PHASE -
mechanical ventilation

Decoupling valve

Fresh
gas inlet

Open

Closed

Open

NPR
valve

Ventilator
piston unit

Open

Ventilator
exhaust
valve

To scavenging
interface

B

Figure 5–26 Fresh gas decoupling valve diverts the fresh gas flow into a separate reservoir during the inspiratory phase. Operation of the decoupling valve during inspiration and expiration is illustrated. *From; Brockwell RC, Andrews JJ. Understanding your anesthesia workstation. ASA Refresher Courses Vol 35: Chapter 2: 15-29, Fig 4.*

In addition, the connection between the piston and the drive motor is rigid, so the position of the piston and the volume delivered is always known whereas in bellows ventilators the position of the bellows at the end of inspiration is not known nor is the amount of delivered tidal volume.

Another advantage is that the control of the piston is based on pressure sensors instead of flow sensors as in bellows ventilators. This ensures better compensation for breathing system compliance (Figure 5-26). The increased precision possible with piston-driven ventilators allows adjustable flow delivery and is a better base for bringing advanced ICU ventilation modes to the operation room.

Fresh gas decoupling: In traditional anesthesia ventilators, while the preset tidal volume is being delivered to the patient, the fresh gas flow continues to enter the circle system. Because the ventilator exhaust valve is closed at this point, no gas can escape the system. Therefore, the tidal volume is attributed not only to the preset tidal volume but also to the continuous fresh gas flow during the inspiratory phase; this is referred to as "fresh gas coupling." Thus increasing the fresh gas flow also increases the tidal volume, minute volume, and peak inspiratory pressure. Traditionally anesthesiologists have remembered (or not remembered!) to adjust the set ventilation volumes when adjusting fresh gas flows. To prevent the potential hyperventilation and more

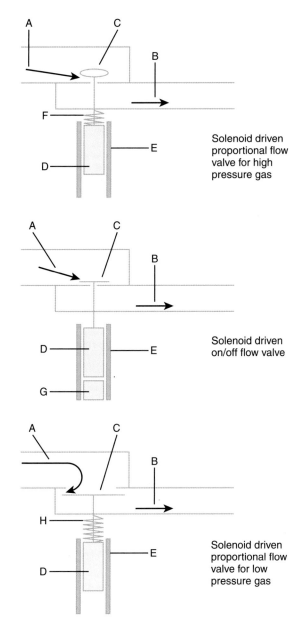

Solenoid driven proportional flow valve for high pressure gas

Solenoid driven on/off flow valve

Solenoid driven proportional flow valve for low pressure gas

Figure 5–27 Electronic Valves. A: gas input, B: gas output, C: valve, D: ferromagnetic core, E: solenoid coil, F-H: spring, G: magnet. *From; Davey A, Diba A, Ward CS, Ward's Anesthetic Equipment, 5th edition, 2005, UK, Elselvier Health Sciences. pp 253, Fig.11.9.*

importantly barotrauma or volutrauma, a "decoupling valve" is added to new ventilators to divert the fresh gas flow into a separate reservoir during the inspiratory phase. The decoupling valve is placed between the fresh gas source and the circle breathing system. Fresh gas decoupling is designed to be used with piston—or descending bellows—ventilators since both systems refill under slight negative pressure and thus the fresh gas in the reservoir is drawn into the breathing circuit for the next inspiration.[13] Since ascending bellows ventilators refill under positive pressure, they do not allow the use of decoupling valves (Figure 5-27).

Electronic flow valves: Modern anesthesia ventilators have electronic flow valves as a major component in their driving gas pathway. These include structurally and

functionally three different valve types[2]: Proportional flow valves, which, by changing the size of the valve opening, control the inspiratory phase (tidal volume and inspiratory time), ventilation rate, and the pressure waveform profile; on/off valves, which simply switch flow on or off; and low-pressure proportional flow valves, which allow a high gas flow at low pressure and are mainly used as expiratory and PEEP valves (Figure 5-28).

Microprocessors: New generation anesthesia ventilators are equipped with programmable microprocessors that control the electric signal to the above mentioned electronic flow valves and process feedback from flow and pressure sensors. Ventilator control by microprocessors facilitates the inclusion of a variety of ventilatory mode and parameter options, helps improve the accuracy of gas delivery, and the quality of ventilation (e.g., leak and compliance testing, compensating for compliance changes), ensures accurate application of PEEP and enhances safety (e.g., detecting problems, adjustable alarm limits, data recording).

Current Models

Contemporary anesthesia "workstations" each have unique ventilators. However, all share a common goal of overcoming the limitations of conventional anesthesia ventilators. Modern ventilators have user-friendly screens on which capnography waveforms, pressure-volume, or flow-volume loops and other ventilatory data are displayed, data trends are recorded and all ventilatory settings are easily controlled.

GE-Datex-Ohmeda and Drager-Siemens are the two major companies manufacturing anesthesia ventilators in both the United States and in global markets. Datascope is another vendor providing anesthesia machines in the U.S. market. The ventilators on the most common GE and Drager anesthesia workstations are briefly described below:

Drager E-Vent (Fabius GS, Fabius Tiro): This ventilator is an electrically driven and electronically controlled piston ventilator, which offers manual/spontaneous and volume control modes as standard modes and pressure control, pressure support, synchronized volume, and controlled ventilation with pressure support (SIMV/PS) modes as optional. Fresh gas decoupling, compliance compensation, presence of high pressure, and negative pressure relief valves are some of the special features for this model. (*Please see the table* [Figure 5-29] *for operating specifications and their comparison with other models* [Figure 5-30].)

Drager E-Vent Plus (Apollo, Primus): This ventilator is an electrically driven and electronically controlled high speed piston ventilator. Ventilation modes include volume control, pressure control, optional synchronization with volume or pressure control and pressure support. To activate synchronization in pressure or volume modes, the trigger sensitivity control must be adjusted. However, in the pressure support mode, synchronization is automatically activated. Decelerating flow control, optimal flow in the presence of changing inspiratory resistance, adjustable flow trigger in the synchronized volume mode and adjustable PEEP are the features that help this ventilator be almost equivalent to intensive care ventilators with

	Datex-Ohmeda 7800	Datex-Ohmeda-SmartVent 7900	Datex-Ohmeda-7100	Datex-Ohmeda S/5 ADU	Drager AV2+	Drager E-vent	Drager Divan	Drager E-vent Plus	Drager Turbovent
Power	Pneumatic	Pneumatic	Pneumatic	Pneumatic	Pneumatic	Electric motor	Electric motor	Electric motor	
Design type	Double-circuit ascending bellows	Double-circuit ascending bellows	Double-circuit ascending bellows	Double-circuit ascending bellows	Double-circuit ascending bellows	Piston	Piston	Piston	Turbine
Control	Electronic	Microprocessor	Electronic	Microprocessor	Electronic	Microprocessor	Microprocessor	Electronic	Electronic
Modes	VCV	VCV, PCV (SIMV, PSV options)	VCV, PCV	VCV, PCV, SIMV	VCV, PLV	VCV, PCV	VCV, PCV, SIMV	VCV, PC optional SIMV and PS	VC, VC with autoflow, PC, SIMV (V, P), CPAP, PS
Inspiratory flow (L/min)	10–100	1–120 (80 max sustained)	2–70	≤80	10–100	10–75	5–75	0–150	0–180
Tidal volume (mL in VCV)	50–1500	20–1500	45–1500	20–1400	20–1500	20–1400	10–1400	20–1400	20–1500
Pressure limit (cmH2O in VCV)	20–100	12–100	12–99	6–80	15–120	18–70	10–80	10–70	8–51
Inspiratory pressure (cm/H2O in PCV)	NA	5–60	5–50	5–40 (above PEEP)	NA	5–60	7–70	5–70	3–51
Ventilator rate	2–100	4–100	4–65	2–60	1–99	4–60	3–80	3–80	3–80
I:E ratio	2:1 to 1:9	2:1 to 1:8	2:1 to 1:6	2:1 to 1:4.5	4:1 to 1:4.5	4:1 to 1:4	5:1 to 1:5	5:1 to 1:5	4:1 to 1:4
Inspiratory pause	25%	NA	5–60%	0–60%	NA	0–50%	0–60%	0–60%	
PEEP (cmH2O)	0–20 (optional)	4–30	4–30	5–20	2–15	0–20	0–20	0–20	3–36

Figure 5–28 Operating specifications of various anesthesia ventilator models. All in one table. *Modified from Morgan GE, Mikhail MS, Murray MJ, Clinical Anesthesiology, 4th ed, 2006, USA, McGraw-Hill Companies Inc., pp 80, Tb. 4.4.*

respect to performance options. (*Please see the table [Figure 5-29] for operating specifications and their comparison with other models (Figures 5-31 to 5-34)*
Drager Turbo-Vent (Zeus): This anesthesia ventilator is electronically powered but turbine driven. A turbine blower located in the inspiratory limb generates target ventilation with constant and precise feedback of inspiratory pressure, flow, and PEEP. With the blower-drive mechanism, spontaneous breathing is possible at any time and inspiratory flow is delivered as high as 180 L/min. The use of a turbine allows the application of new ventilation modes: "volume mode with Autoflow" and "continuous positive airway pressure." In "volume mode with Autoflow," the level of inspiratory flow is determined in such a way that the lowest inspiratory pressure is used to guarantee the set volume based on a breath by breath feedback control loop.[14] Other modes available on this ventilator are volume control, pressure control, synchronized volume, and pressure modes and pressure support. Pressure support is provided as a standard mode. (*The Zeus workstation is a closed circuit system and currently not*

available in the United States. Please see the table [Figure 5-29] for operating specifications and their comparison with other models.*)
Datex-Ohmeda Smart Vent 7900 (Aestiva, Excel SE, Modulus SE, S5 Avance): This ventilator is a pneumatically driven and microprocessor-controlled ventilator with a double circuit ascending bellows. It was the first modern anesthesia ventilator to offer pressure-control mode and an integrated electronic PEEP control. Other modes on this ventilator are volume control, optional synchronized intermittent mandatory ventilation, and optional pressure support modes. Tidal volume is automatically compensated for compression losses, changes in fresh gas concentration, and small leaks within the absorber and bellows by using sensors placed at the absorber, and the inspiratory and expiratory limbs of the circuit. Additionally, this ventilator automatically corrects for lower density gases (helium) and has a cardiopulmonary bypass mode, which turns off the volume and apnea alarms. (*Please see the table [Figure 5-29] for operating specifications and their comparison with other models [Figures 5-35 and 5-36].*)

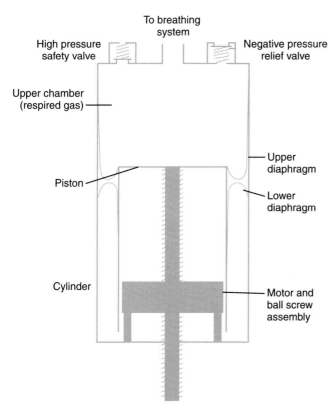

Figure 5–29 Piston assembly of Drager E Vent. During inspiration the piston moves upward, during expiration downward. *From; Dorsch JA & Dorsch SE, Understanding Anesthetic Equipment, 5th edition, 2007, USA, Lippincott Williams & Wilkins, pp 337, Fig.12.21.*

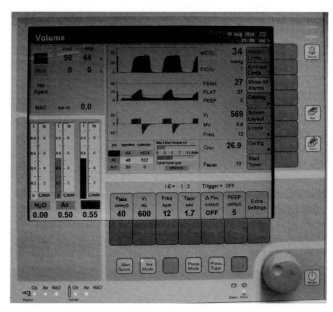

Figure 5–30 Apollo anesthesia workstation; screen displays all ventilatory data on breath by breath basis.

Datex-Ohmeda S/5 ADU ventilator: This ventilator is a pneumatically driven and microprocessor controlled ventilator with a double circuit ascending bellows design. Spontaneous/manual, volume-control, pressure control, and synchronized intermittent mandatory ventilation modes are available with integrated electronic PEEP. Tidal volume compensation for changes in fresh gas flow, and breathing circuit compliance losses are assessed by a D-Lite sensor at the Y-piece of the circuit (as opposed to sensors placed at the absorber and both inspiratory and expiratory limbs as in the Smart Vent 7900). (*Please see the table* [Figure 5-29] *for operating specifications and their comparison with other models* [Figure 5-37].)

Jet Ventilators

Jet ventilators generate tidal volume by employing the Venturi effect. The tidal volume is the combination of two flows: one is the volume directly from the jet ventilator, delivered via a jet ventilation catheter, and the other is the volume entrained from room air due to the Venturi effect. At the tip of the catheter, the jet stream of fresh gas creates a pressure gradient and the pressure gradient generates a negative pressure entraining flow.

The jet catheter may be inserted into an endotracheal tube placed in the natural glottis or inside a laryngeal mask airway supraglottically or via a direct cricothyroid membrane puncture. In microlaryngeal surgery and some other rare settings, the jet ventilation catheter may be introduced orally or nasally and then into the trachea without any other adjunct airway devices.

The jet ventilator can precisely control the pressure, I:E ratio, FIO_2, frequency, temperature and humidity of the gas delivered. At the distal end of the catheter, airway pressure is measured. Therefore adequate ventilation can be easily achieved, and PEEP can be monitored and precisely controlled. See Figure 5-38 for a schematic illustration of jet ventilator function. (Also see Figure 5-39.)

The manual jet ventilator is used less frequently. However, transcrico-thyroid membrane jet ventilation is still an effective backup method in case mask ventilation and tracheal intubation is not possible and oxygenation is urgently required. In such cases, the volume delivered with this technique is primarily from the jet, since the upper airway most likely is at least partially obstructed. Of major concern with this approach is the fact that airway pressure and tidal volume are unknown. See Figure 5-40 for an illustration of a manufactured manual jet ventilator.

Manual jet ventilators can be constructed in an emergency from readily available supplies found in any anesthesia cart. For ventilation via a cricothyroid catheter, this can consist of only a stopcock, a length of oxygen supply tubing, and the supplemental oxygen flowmeter of the anesthesia machine (Figure 5-41).

1993 FDA Anesthesia Apparatus Checkout Recommendations[15]

This checkout has 14 steps for 8 different systems in the anesthesia workstation. Here we have only included the checkout recommendations for *Manual and Automatic Ventilation Systems*:

Step 12. Test ventilation systems and unidirectional valves.
   a. Place a second breathing bag on the Y-piece.
   b. Set appropriate ventilator parameters for the next patient.
   c. Switch to automatic ventilation mode.
   d. Turn ventilator on and fill bellows and breathing bag with O_2 flush.

APOLLO MECHANICAL VENTILATION INSPIRATION

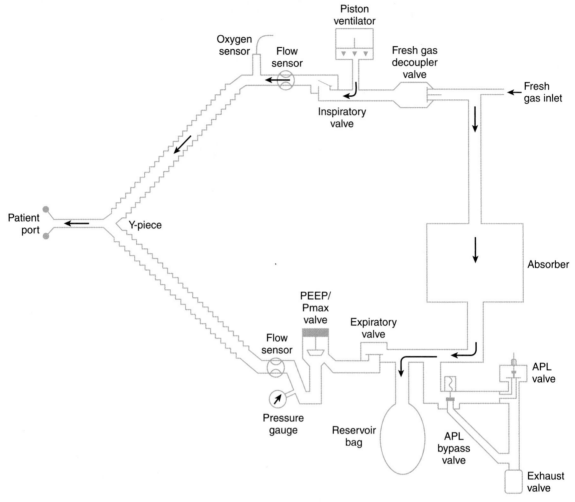

Figure 5–31   Drager E Vent Plus and Apollo workstation-during inspiration *From; Dorsch JA & Dorsch SE, Understanding Anesthetic Equipment, 5th edition, 2007, USA, Lippincott Williams & Wilkins, pp 345, Fig. 12.30*

e. Set O_2 flow to minimum and other gas flows to zero.

f. Verify that during inspiration the bellows delivers appropriate tidal volume and that during expiration the bellows fill completely.

g. Set fresh gas flow to approximately 5 L/min.

h. Verify that the ventilator bellows and simulated lungs fill and empty appropriately without sustained pressure at end expiration.

i. Check for proper action of unidirectional valves.

j. Exercise breathing circuit accessories to ensure proper function.

k. Turn ventilator off and switch to manual ventilation (bag-*adjustable pressure limiting valve-*) mode.

l. Ventilate manually and assure inflation and deflation of artificial lungs and appropriate feel of system resistance and compliance.

m. Remove second breathing bag from Y-piece.

In 2008, ASA Committee on Equipment and Facilities has updated the "Pre-anesthesia Checkout Procedures" mainly due to the evolution of anesthesia delivery systems and the fact that one checkout procedure is not applicable to all anesthesia delivery systems currently on the market.[16]

Recommended steps include:

To Be Completed Daily, Item to Be Completed	Responsible Party
Item 1: Verify auxiliary O_2 cylinder and self-inflating manual ventilation device are available and functioning	Provider and tech
Item 2: Verify patient suction is adequate to clear the airway	Provider and tech
Item 3: Turn on anesthesia delivery system and confirm that AC power is available	Provider or tech
Item 4: Verify availability of required monitors, including alarms	Provider or tech
Item 5: Verify that pressure is adequate on the spare O_2 cylinder mounted on the anesthesia machine	Provider and tech
Item 6: Verify that the piped gas pressures are ≥50 psig	Provider and tech
Item 7: Verify that vaporizers are adequately filled and, if applicable, that the filler ports are tightly closed	Provider or tech

APOLLO MECHANICAL VENTILATION EARLY EXHALATION

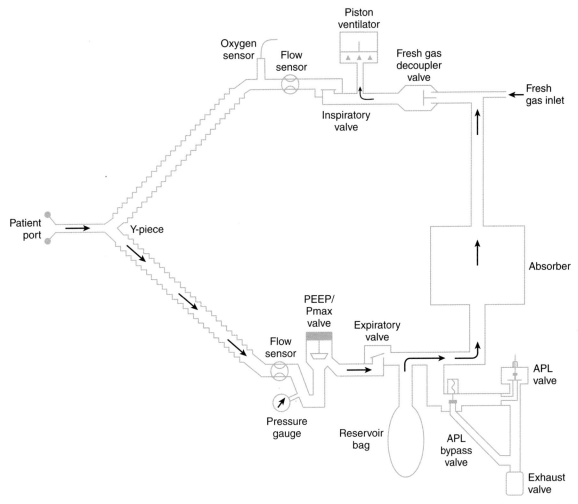

Figure 5–32   Drager E Vent Plus and Apollo workstation-during early exhalation. *From; Dorsch JA & Dorsch SE, Understanding Anesthetic Equipment, 5th edition, 2007, USA, Lippincott Williams & Wilkins, pp 346, Fig. 12.31*

To Be Completed Daily, Item to Be Completed	Responsible Party
Item 8: Verify that there are no leaks in the gas supply lines between the flowmeters and the common gas outlet	Provider or tech
Item 9: Test scavenging system function	Provider or tech
Item 10: Calibrate, or verify calibration of, the O_2 monitor and check the low O_2 alarm	Provider or tech
Item 11: Verify CO_2 absorbent is not exhausted	Provider or tech
Item 12: Breathing system pressure and leak testing	Provider and tech
Item 13: Verify that gas flows properly through the breathing circuit during both inspiration and exhalation	Provider and tech
Item 14: Document completion of checkout procedures	Provider and tech
Item 15: Confirm ventilator settings and evaluate readiness to deliver anesthesia care (anesthesia timeout)	Provider

APOLLO MECHANICAL VENTILATION LATE EXHALATION

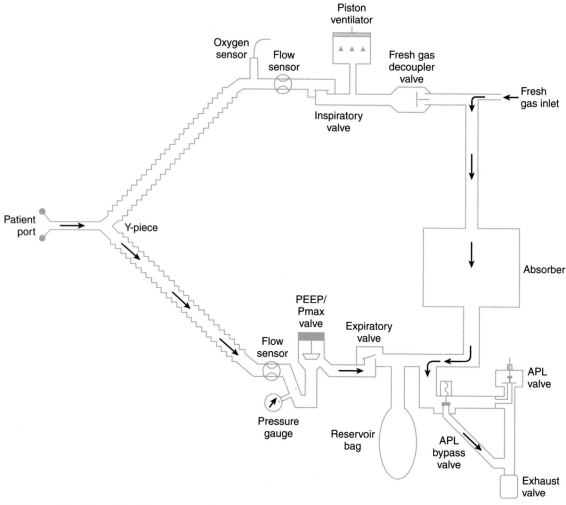

Figure 5–33   Drager E Vent Plus and Apollo workstation-during late exhalation. *From; Dorsch JA & Dorsch SE, Understanding Anesthetic Equipment, 5th edition, 2007, USA, Lippincott Williams & Wilkins, pp 347, Fig.12-32*

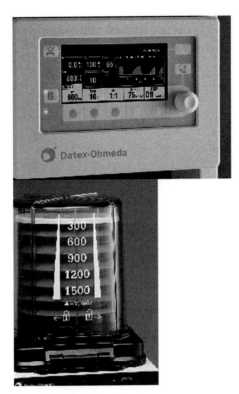

Figure 5–34   Datex-Ohmeda Smart Vent 7900. *From http://www.gehealthcare.com/euen/anesthesia/docs/AN2842.pdf*

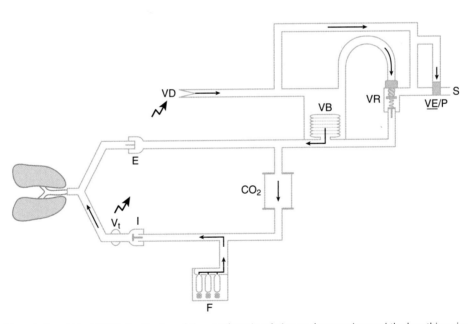

Figure 5–35   Datex-Ohmeda Smart Vent 7900. Positioning of the ventilator in relation to the vaporizer and the breathing circuit. From *http://www. apsf.org/assets/documents/circuit.ppt*

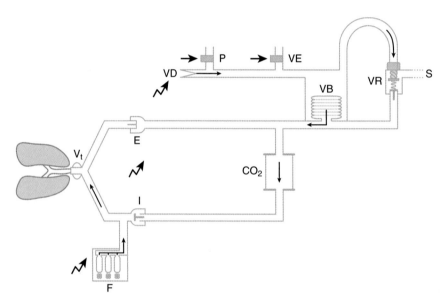

Figure 5-36 **Datex-Ohmeda S/5 ADU ventilator.** Positioning of the ventilator in relation to the vaporizer and the breathing circuit. From *http://www.apsf.org/assets/documents/circuit.ppt*

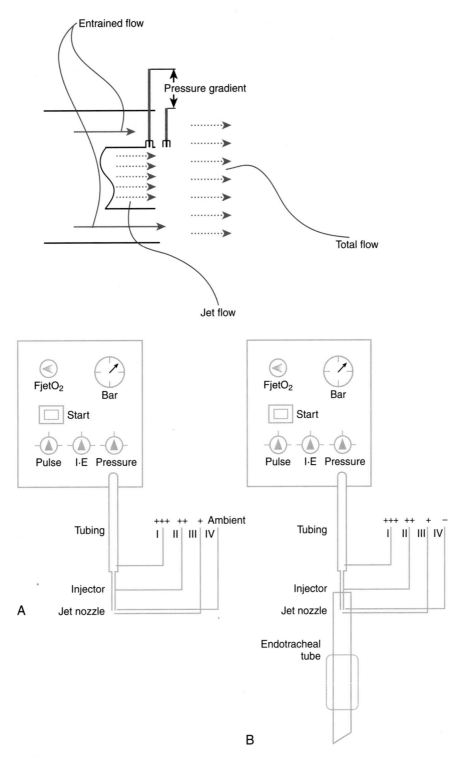

Figure 5–37 Jet Ventilator. Illustrating measurements of pressures during jet ventilation with the injector outside (**A.**) and inside an endotracheal tube (**B.**) Depending on the size of the tube directing the gas flow, pressures are increasingly positive (+, ++, +++). Around the jet nozzle pressures are ambient (**A.**) or subatmospheric (**B.**) depending on the injector's location. From *http://images.google.com/imgres?imgurl=http://www.mdconsult. com/das/book/body/0/0/1365/f4-u1.0-B0-323-02845-4..50006-8..gr17.jpg&imgrefurl=http://www.mdconsult.com/das/book/body/0/0/1365/I4-u1. 0-B0-323-02845-4..50006-8--f17.fig&usg=___Po_eWOLJI47MkQis8pl181icBo=&h=417&w=600&sz=190&hl=en&start=13&um=1&tbnid=IJeaZSH99 ZFvnM:&tbnh=94&tbnw=135&prev=/images%3Fq%3Djet%2Bventilation%26um%3D1%26hl%3Den%26rlz%3D1W1GPEA_en%26sa%3DG. Marx: Rosen's Emergency Medicine, 7th ed.*

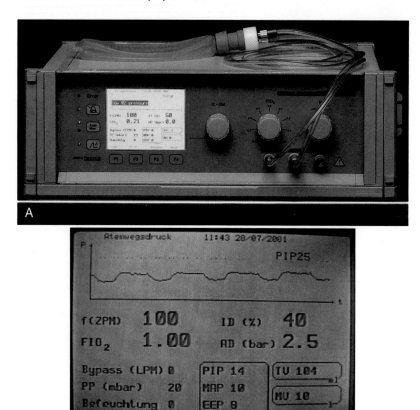

Figure 5–38 **A,** Monsoon Universal Jet ventilator, Acutronic Medical Systems AG; **B,** Ventilator display.

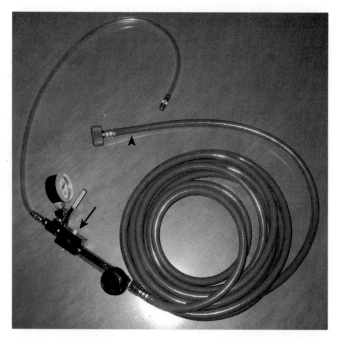

Figure 5–39 Jet ventilator. Black triangle shows the high-pressure ventilation tubing that attaches to standard wall oxygen outlet with 50 psi working pressure. Ventilation block (white arrow) is used to control oxygen flow through tubing to a catheter, which is inserted in the airway.

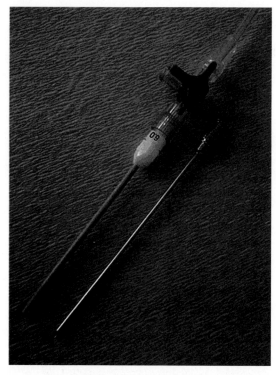

Figure 5–40 A three-way stopcock connected to a 15-G transtracheal airway catheter with a length of 7.5 cm and an inner diameter of 2 mm and an oxygen supply. Inspiration and expiration are adjusted by opening or closing the nonconnected hole of the stopcock. *From http://www3. interscience.wiley.com/cgi-bin/fulltext/118497821/PDFSTART*

Further Reading

Davey, A.J., 2005. Automatic ventilators. In: Davey, A., Diba, A., Ward, C.S. (Eds.), Ward's anesthetic equipment, ed 5. Elsevier Saunders, Philadelphia. *You will find further detailed information and many illustrations about anesthesia ventilators in this book. It is a UK edition, so it may give you a perspective of devices used in UK anesthesia practice.*

Hess, D.R., Kacmarek, R.M., 2002. Traditional modes of mechanical ventilation; Hess DR, Kacmarek RM. New modes of mechanical ventilation. In: Hess, D.R., Kacmarek, R.M. (Eds.), Essentials of mechanical ventilation, ed 2. McGraw-Hill, New York. *Essentials of mechanical ventilation is a highly recommended resource for the basics of mechanical ventilation where you will also find detailed information on both traditional and new mechanical ventilation modes.*

Online Resources

www.simanest.org

http://vam.anest.ufl.edu

Both websites offer a variety of anesthesia equipment simulations; very useful educational tools.

http://www.ambu.com/RespiratoryCare/Respiratory_Care.aspx?GID=GROUP51&;ProductID=PROD862

This is a video link showing an assembly of a manual ventilator (Ambu mark IV).

http://www.youtube.com/breathsim

Dr Julian Goldman has several online videos where he uses simulation (Breath-Sim) and animation to illustrate principles of gas flow, capnography, and spirometry in the anesthesia breathing system.

References

1. Dorsch, J.A., Dorsch, S.E., 2007. Anesthesia ventilators. In: Dorsch, J.A., Dorsch, S.E. (Eds.), Understanding anesthetic equipment, ed 5. Lippincott Williams & Wilkins, Philadelphia.
2. Davey, A.J., 2005. Automatic ventilators. In: Davey, A., Diba, A., Ward, C.S. (Eds.), Ward's anesthetic equipment, ed 5. Elsevier Saunders, Philadelphia.
3. Anesthesia ventilators with descending bellows, 1996. the need for appropriate monitoring. Health Devices 25 (10), 391 Available at www.mdsr.ecri.org. Accessed December 15, 2008.
4. Hess, D.R., Kacmarek, R.M., 2002. New modes of mechanical ventilation. In: Hess, D.R., Kacmarek, R.M. (Eds.), Essentials of mechanical ventilation, ed 2. McGraw-Hill, New York.
5. PEEP valves in anesthesia circuits. Health Devices 1983;13(1):24. Available at www. mdsr.ecri.org. Accessed December 12, 2008.
6. Eisenkraft, J.B., 2005. Problems with anesthesia gas delivery systems. In: Schwartz, A.J., Matjasko, M.J., Gross, J.B. (Eds.), ASA refresher courses in anesthesiology, vol. 33. Williams & Wilkins, Lippincott, Philadelphia.
7. Caplan, R.A., Vistica, M.F., Posner, K.L., et al., 1997. Adverse anesthetic outcomes arising from gas delivery equipment. Anesthesiology 87, 741.
8. Brockwell, R.C., Andrews, J.J., 2005. Inhaled anesthetic delivery systems. In: Miller, R.D. (Ed.), Miller's anesthesia, ed 6. Churchill Livingstone, Philadelphia.
9. Stayer, S., Olutoye, O., 2005. Anesthesia ventilators, better options for children. Anesthesiol Clin North America 23 (4), 677–691.
10. Bachiller, P.R., McDonough, J.M., Feldman, J.M., 2008. Do new anesthesia ventilators deliver small tidal volumes accurately during volume-controlled ventilation? Anesth Analg 106 (5), 1392–1400.
11. Jaber, S., Tassaux, D., Sebbane, M., et al., 2006. Performance characteristics of five new anesthesia ventilators and four intensive care ventilators in pressure-support mode: a comparative bench study. Anesthesiology 105 (5), 944–952.
12. Katz, J.A., Kallet, R.H., et al., 2000. Improved flow and capabilities of the Datex-Ohmeda Smart Vent anesthesia ventilator. J Clin Anesth 12 (1), 40–47.
13. Brockwell, R.C., Andrews, J.J., 2007. Understanding your anesthesia workstation. In: Schwartz, A.J., Matjasko, M.J., Gross, J.B, (Eds.), ASA refresher courses in anesthesiology, vol. 35. Williams & Wilkins, Lippincott, Philadelphia.
14. Siegel E. New naming of Dräger medical anesthesia ventilation modes, Dräger (website): www.draeger.com. Accessed November 10, 2008.
15. OSHA. Anesthetic gases: guidelines for workplace exposures (website): http://www.osha.gov/dts/osta/anestheticgases/index.html#Appendix2. Accessed January 5, 2009.
16. ASA. 2008 recommendations for pre-anesthesia checkout procedures (website): http://www.asahq.org/clinical/fda.htm. Accessed January 8, 2009.

Chapter 6

Supraglottic Airway Devices

Jordan L. Newmark and Warren S. Sandberg

One of the most important interventions the anesthetist makes for his or her patient is to secure and maintain a patent airway. The anesthetist delivers therapeutic oxygen and maintains ventilation via this airway. This chapter will review a variety of devices used above the glottic opening to supply oxygen and other inhalational gases/agents and to maintain airway patency.

Supraglottic airway devices are simple to use and have qualitatively changed the practice of anesthesiology. However, a supraglottic airway device is commonly considered to be less secure because the larynx, trachea, and distal airways are not protected by the inflated cuff of an endotracheal device. Laryngospasm and active or passive aspiration of gastric contents are always possible when using the supraglottic devices discussed within this chapter.

Supraglottic airways have also changed the considerations when approaching unusual airway situations. For example, the prone position poses additional concerns about maintaining the supraglottic airway, yet these devices are easy to insert in the prone position. Supraglottic airway devices have a place in difficult airway management. Any patient with a known or suspected difficult airway requires the utmost diligence, planning, and back-up planning, and equipment and personnel readily available should an airway emergency occur. Part of this planning is to ensure that supraglottic devices are available. Moreover, the supraglottic airway is a first-line alternative when unrecognized airway problems are encountered.

A recent trend in supraglottic airway usage is to employ the devices in patients traditionally considered to have a full stomach, and hence to be at risk for regurgitation and aspiration. There exists debate whether or not cricoid pressure should be applied during the insertion of a supraglottic airway device in such a patient with full-stomach precautions.

Cricoid pressure impedes insertion of laryngeal mask airways and similar devices. Once inserted, these devices do not continue to protect the airway from gastric aspirate because they do not have endotracheal cuffs.

Supraglottic devices for oxygen delivery and airway maintenance are one area in anesthesiology where innovation and invention are rapidly changing practices. Thus this chapter serves as a starting point, but the reader is encouraged to follow the primary literature for the latest developments in practice.

Noninvasive Oxygen Delivery

Oxygen delivery systems are commonly divided into *variable* and *fixed* performance devices. The F_{IO_2} provided to the patient with variable performance devices can fluctuate and is sometimes difficult to predict. However, arterial blood gas sampling, along with oxygraphy[1] is a possible method for quantifying oxygen delivery to the patient when using any device. The delivered F_{IO_2} changes with a number of factors (Table 6–1), mainly those associated with equipment and the patient.

Understanding the interplay between these factors is key to understanding how variable performance devices function. Here, we will use a simple adult face mask as an example. A simple adult face mask holds a small volume of about 200 cc. The mask is continuously supplied with oxygen and fills when the patient is between inspiration and expiration. Oxygen can leak from the holes of the mask and from an imperfect seal at the face. As the patient inhales, the oxygen-rich air is first to enter the airway. As the patient continues to inhale, room air then enters the gas mixture through holes in the mask. This entrained room air reduces the delivered

Table 6–1 Factors Affecting Delivered F_{IO_2} in Variable Performance Devices

Equipment: Oxygen flow rate, mask reservoir volume, quality of fit, hole number, and size/area

Patient: Respiratory rate, tidal volume, peak inspiratory flow rate

Other: Presence of other gases (i.e., water vapor from humidification, rebreathed CO_2)

Adapted from Wheeler DW. Equipment for the inhalation of oxygen and other gases. In Davey AJ, Diba A, editors. *Ward's anaesthetic equipment*, ed 5, Philadelphia, Elsevier Saunders, 2005.[2]

Table 6–2 Variable Performance Devices Categorized by Reservoir Size

Reservoir Capacity	Volume (cc)	Example
Zero capacity	0 cc	Nasal cannulas
Low capacity	70-100 cc	Tracheostomy mask, pediatric face mask
Medium capacity	100-250 cc	Adult face mask
High capacity	250-1500 cc	Face mask with reservoir bag
Very high capacity	>1500 cc	Pediatric incubator, headbox, tent Oxygen bar/surgery bar under surgical drapes

Table 6–3 Pros and Cons of Nasal Cannulas for Oxygen Delivery

PROS

Less claustrophobic than face masks

Allow access to the face (i.e., for eating, speaking, brushing teeth, etc.)

Convenient for home usage

Improved patient compliance[4]

CONS

Very widely variable delivery[2] (i.e., volume of patient's nasopharynx, seating of prongs in patient's nose, patient's respiratory pattern, etc.)

Prong discomfort

Drying or damage to the nasal mucosa

Dilution of delivered F_{IO_2} by ambient air via nostrils and during mouth breathing[4]

Blocked nasal passages prevent oxygen from entering nasopharynx

Risk for surgical fire, especially if 100% F_{IO_2} delivered under surgical drapes[5]

Technically challenging to quantitate end tidal CO_2 during NC use, however, devices for this purpose are being studied and developed,[6] and some are commercially available

F_{IO_2}. Therefore, in this variable performance system, the F_{IO_2} delivered to the patient is increased when the mask is tightly fitted, and with high oxygen flow rates-in a patient with a low peak inspiratory flow rate, tidal volume and respiratory rate.[3] During this process, there is often some degree of CO_2 rebreathing.

The design of the variable performance device can be changed to increase the F_{IO_2} delivered to the patient, for example, by increasing the reservoir size. The above mentioned face mask used a 200 cc volume of oxygen—in other words, the reservoir size for oxygen was 200 cc. Variable performance devices are often categorized by their reservoir capacity (Table 6–2).

Nasal Cannulas and Simple Face Masks

Zero Capacity Variable Performance Devices—Nasal Cannulas

Nasal cannulas (NC) may be classified as a zero capacity device because there is no built-in oxygen reservoir. The "reservoir" is the volume of the patient's nasopharynx and is best used when the patient is not mouth breathing. However, there is some debate about this, as mouth breathing may still allow for inhalation of some oxygen from the nasopharyngeal reservoir. Specifically, "Mouth breathing causes inspiratory air flow. This produces a Venturi effect in the posterior pharynx entraining oxygen from the nose."[4]

NC consist of plastic tubing, two firm 1 cm plastic prongs which seat in the nose, and are held to the face by an adjustable

strap, which wraps around the patient's ears. Oxygen is usually not humidified when delivered by NC.

NC are typically used with an oxygen flow rate of 2 to 4 L/min to allow for an F_{IO_2} of about 0.26 to 0.36.[2,4] High flow rates are uncomfortable because they dry and irritate (or can even damage) the nasopharynx. Table 6–3 lists pros and cons of nasal cannulas.

A nasal sponge-tipped catheter (Figure 6–1) may be used to enhance the reservoir produced by NC oxygen delivery. The nasal catheter is a single lumen device that is placed into one nostril and held in place by a spongy foam cuff. The catheter is then taped to the patient's face—there are no straps. This device "should not be used when a nasal mucosal tear is suspected because of the risk of surgical emphysema."[4]

New zero capacity variable performance devices are being developed and tested to improve patient comfort and safety.[7] For example, the OxyArm, (Figure 6–2) which is shaped like a cellular phone headset, does not contact the patient's face and allows for greater comfort. It produces an "oxygen cloud" by the nose and mouth. At oxygen flow rates of 2 to 4 L/min, 0.28 to 0.35 F_{IO_2} can be administered.[8]

Medium Capacity Variable Performance Device—Simple Face Mask

Simple adult face masks (Figure 6–3) are considered medium capacity devices because they have a reservoir size of 100 to 250 cc, which covers the nose and mouth.

These masks are made of soft, clear plastic materials that are secured to the patient's face with an adjustable elastic strap, which fits around the head. Many of these masks include a bendable metal piece over the bridge of the nose,

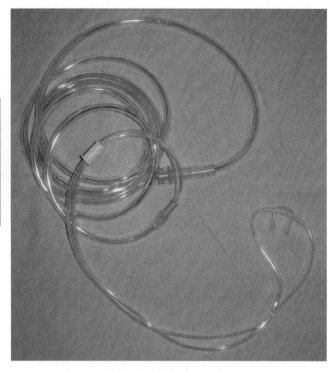

Figure 6–1   Nasal cannulas.

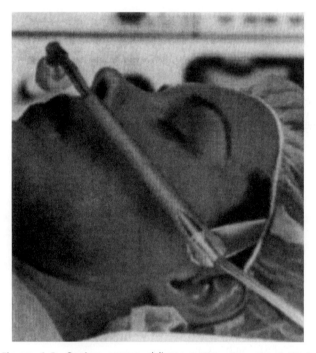

Figure 6–2   OxyArm oxygen delivery system. *(From Futrell JW Jr, Moore JL. The OxyArm: a supplemental oxygen delivery device. Anesth Analg 2006;102(2):491-494.)*[8]

which can be used to improve mask fit. The body of the mask contains an entry for oxygen supply tubing, and holes which help prevent mask collapse around the face during inspiration, and allow for exchange of ambient, exhaled, and excess gases.

Simple face masks deliver 2 to 6 L/min of oxygen, allowing for a widely variable F_{IO_2}. However, "a typical example of

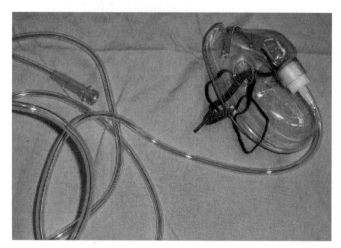

Figure 6–3   Simple adult face mask.

4 L/min of oxygen flow delivers an F_{IO_2} of about 0.35 to 0.40, providing there is a normal respiratory pattern."[9] Oxygen flow rates below 2 L/min (or a very high minute ventilation) makes for excessive rebreathing of CO_2; flow rates above 2 L/min help with ventilation of exhaled gas out of the reservoir through the holes of the mask, especially during respiratory pauses. The total dead space of the mask is about 100 cc, which is usually inconsequential. Large mask bodies and high resistance through the mask holes may increase CO_2 rebreathing.[9]

The F_{IO_2} supplied to the patient by these masks is affected by several factors, including the supplied oxygen flow rate, patient respiratory pattern, and mask fit. Increased oxygen flow rates and tight mask fit will increase the F_{IO_2}. For anxious pediatric patients who cannot tolerate wearing a mask, oxygen can be "wafted" by placing the mask within close proximity, although the F_{IO_2} supplied will decrease as a function of increasing distance.[10] Table 6–4 lists the functional properties and some of the pros and cons of simple face masks.

Similar to the simple face mask is the aerosol face tent (Figure 6–4). The face tent is also a variable performance, clear plastic device with adjustable face strap. The bottom is shaped to fit around the patient's chin, and the device is open at the top. This presumably produces less claustrophobia, easier phonation for the patient, and allows better access to the mouth for food, liquids, and suction. It is also useful in patients recovering from nasal surgery who cannot tolerate pressure on the nose. The oxygen reservoir is slightly larger than that of the simple face mask; however, more fresh gas is lost to the environment through the open top (see Figure 6–4).

High Capacity Variable Performance Devices—Partial Rebreather Masks

The above discussed medium capacity device, the simple face mask, may be converted to a high capacity device with the addition of a 600 to 1100 cc reservoir bag, increasing the F_{IO_2} delivered to the patient. The F_{IO_2} is increased by virtue of the oxygen supply flow rate and; reservoir oxygen, which is composed of exhaled and supplied oxygen as well as room air. These masks are sometimes referred to as partial rebreather masks, or nonrebreathing masks.

Table 6–4 Patient Factors Increasing F$_{IO_2}$ by Simple Face Mask

Lengthened duration of pause between inspiration and expiration → more time for reservoir filling with supplied oxygen

Low peak inspiratory flow rate → less room air entrained through mask holes

Decreased minute ventilation/low respiratory rate/hypoventilation → less CO_2 rebreathing

Patient inspiratory flow rate < oxygen supply rate

PROS

Low cost, convenient, easy usage

Patient comfort

CONS

Delivered F$_{IO_2}$ varies widely with oxygen flow rate, mask fit, patient respiration.

Small reservoir causes most adult patients to breathe ambient air through holes.

Vented masks allow for spread of infected respiratory droplets.[11,12]

Entrainment of ambient or exhaled gases.

In theory, patients who are dependent on hypoxia or hypercarbia for respiratory drive (i.e., patients with COPD) may lose respiratory drive when using this device.[9] An alternative explanation is that increased F$_{IO_2}$ deranges VQ matching, leading to worsened gas exchange.

CO_2 rebreathing (may be indicated by patient feeling warmth or humidity during respiration).[9]

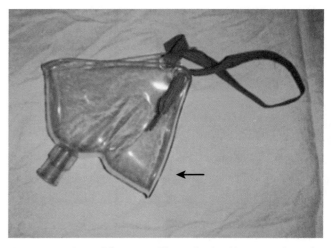

Figure 6–4 Aerosol face tent. The patient's chin seats where the arrow indicates, and the reservoir remains open, without contacting the patient's face.

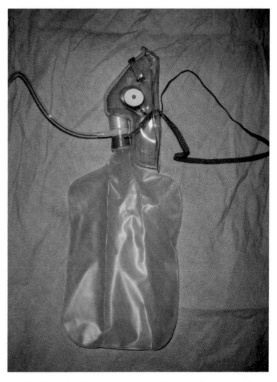

Figure 6–5 Partial rebreather mask. Note the large reservoir bag and white, one-way flap valves.

Simple face masks often waste supplied oxygen, especially when the patient's inspiratory flow rate is below that of the supplied oxygen flow rate and during patient expiration.[13] Nonrebreather masks help prevent this by filling with directly supplied and exhaled oxygen.

Reservoir bags are preferred to increasing mask size, which can increase CO_2 rebreathing, and require increased supplied oxygen flow rates to inefficient amounts (greater than 60 L/min) when attempting to provide an F$_{IO_2}$ near 100%.[13] Rather, these partial rebreather masks "probably deliver an F$_{IO_2}$ between 0.75 to 0.90 at oxygen flow rates of 12 to 15 L/min."[14]

CO_2 rebreathing is further decreased with partial rebreather masks with the addition of flap valves over the holes of the mask's body (Figure 6–5). These allow for vented gases to enter the environment and help to prevent entrance of these gases and ambient air into the system. Patients will preferentially breathe oxygen from the large reservoir bag. However, a poorly fitted mask allows ambient air to flow around the edges of the device to dilute the supplied oxygen.

Additional features sometimes associated with nonrebreather masks are one-way valves seated between the oxygen reservoir bag and the body of the mask itself. This valve decreases CO_2 rebreathing and allows the patient to preferably inhale oxygen from the reservoir bag. The addition of this valve requires a higher supplied oxygen flow rate because exhaled oxygen from the patient and oxygen from the mask body are vented into the environment.

Fixed Performance Oxygen Delivery Devices: Venturi Masks

Fixed performance devices provide a more consistent and predictable F$_{IO_2}$ to the patient. The most common such device is the venturi oxygen mask (Table 6–5).

Venturi masks consist of a clear plastic mask, similar to the simple adult face mask detailed in the prior section, and a plastic venturi device (Figure 6–6). The venturi device itself fits between the oxygen supply tubing and body of the mask (Figure 6–7). Each is color coded and has listed on it an oxygen flow rate that is needed to achieve a given F$_{IO_2}$. Each venturi device allows for a certain flow of air through open windows in the device and supplied oxygen through tubing.

Table 6–5 Examples of Indications for Fixed Performance Devices

Goal is to provide a known F_{IO_2} to the patient who is dependent on their hypoxic/hypercarbic drive (i.e., during a COPD exacerbation to preserve respiratory drive)

Calculation of the PaO_2/F_{IO_2} ratio to determine if a patient requires endotracheal intubation with mechanical ventilation to diagnose acute respiratory distress syndrome or respiratory failure

When prescribing an exact F_{IO_2} for oxygen therapy, rather than flow rate, to a hospitalized or critically ill patient

Providing a known F_{IO_2} in the setting of a patient with a varied or unstable respiratory pattern

Adapted from Wheeler DW. Equipment for the inhalation of oxygen and other gases. In Davey AJ, Diba A, editors. *Ward's anaesthetic equipment*, ed 5, Philadelphia, Elsevier Saunders, 2005.[15]

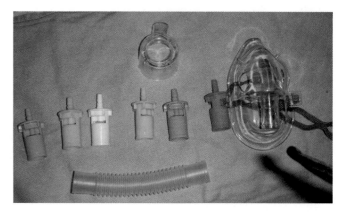

Figure 6–6 Venturi mask components.

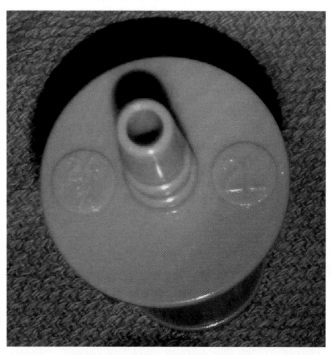

Figure 6–7 Venturi device. Note the flow rate indicated on the right (2 L in this example), and the associated F_{IO_2} that will be provided (24%).

It is important to understand how venturi devices work so they can be optimally used. These devices make use of the Bernoulli effect, which can be stated mathematically:

$$P + \tfrac{1}{2}(\rho v^2) = \kappa$$

where P = pressure, ρ = density, v = velocity, and κ = constant. Applying this principle to the venturi mask—as supplied oxygen flows through a fixed space within the device and into a larger chamber, velocity and kinetic energy of the oxygen increase distally. Because the total energy must be constant, the potential energy in the system simultaneously decreases. This creates a negative pressure gradient, causing room air to mix with the supplied oxygen in the venturi device in a predictable fashion. This allows for a fixed and constant F_{IO_2} to be delivered to the patient. Larger air entrainment windows are needed for more room air to mix, so that the delivered F_{IO_2} is decreased relative to venturis with smaller windows.

During the design and manufacturing of the venturi, these devices are calibrated such that a known oxygen flow rate and air entrainment window size will provide a known F_{IO_2}. Large oxygen and total gas flow rates are used in this system. No rebreathing can occur because both the supplied fresh gas flow rate exceeds the patient's peak inspiratory flow rate, and holes in the mask allow the fresh gas to displace expired CO_2 and other waste and ambient gases.

Most commonly, the clear masks are fitted with plastic conduits and venturi devices are packaged separately. The devices are manually assembled by linking together the venturi, conduit, and mask. This allows the F_{IO_2} to be changed by changing just the venturi. Alternatively, some vendors have designed single use masks with preattached venturi devices. These devices typically give overall flow rates of approximately 60 L/min, with each requiring a particular oxygen flow to give a fixed F_{IO_2} (usually 24%, 28%, 31%, 35%, 40%, and 60%).[16] See Table 6–6. Similar previously "calibrated variable venturi devices can be used to deliver the desired F_{IO_2}"[4] as well (Table 6–7).

Continuous Positive Airway Pressure (CPAP)

Continuous positive airway pressure (CPAP) and bilevel positive airway pressure (BiPAP) are both modes of noninvasive ventilation (i.e., not involving placement of an endotracheal tube and mechanical ventilation). They are used in several clinical situations, most commonly in the intensive care unit (ICU) for hospital applications. These include therapy for obstructive sleep apnea (OSA) both in hospital and at home, recovery from general anesthesia or ventilator weaning, acute respiratory failure, or other respiratory emergencies (i.e., COPD exacerbation, pulmonary edema, etc.).

As the name implies, CPAP provides a constant positive pressure to the airway in an effort to prevent airway collapse, and increasing the patient's functional residual capacity. CPAP valves deliver a set amount of positive pressure, regardless of respiratory cycle phase, in the range of 2.5 to 20 cm H_2O. On the other hand, BiPAP improves ventilation by decreasing the pressure provided during expiration, facilitating CO_2 release (Table 6–8). The anesthetist should check that the CPAP valve is continuously functioning during the entire respiratory cycle. "It is important to check that the

Table 6–6 Provided F$_{IO_2}$ and Associated Oxygen Flow Rates and Air Entrainment

F$_{IO_2}$ Provided	Oxygen Flow to Venturi	Air Entrained	Total Flow to Patient
(%)	(L/Min)	(L/Min)	(L/Min)
0.24	2	51	53
0.28	4	41	45
0.31	6	41	47
0.35	8	37	45
0.40	10	32	42
0.60	15	15	30

Adapted from Wheeler DW. Equipment for the inhalation of oxygen and other gases. In Davey AJ, Diba A, editors. *Ward's anaesthetic equipment*, ed 5, Philadelphia, Elsevier Saunders, 2005.[17]

Table 6–7 Pros and Cons of Fixed Performance Oxygen Masks

PROS

See indications table.

Low cost, disposable device.

Simple to use, robust to use-error.

CONS

Delivered F$_{IO_2}$ on average is 5% above desired F$_{IO_2}$.[18]

Highest F$_{IO_2}$ venturi device may underperform by 5%-10%.[16]

Most reliable when delivering low F$_{IO_2}$ with more air entrapment.[16]

Mask is cumbersome, noisy, and uncomfortable.

Table 6–8 Pros and Cons of CPAP/BiPAP Devices

PROS

Spares the patient invasive airway device and mechanical ventilation.

Can be used as temporizing measure to avoid intubation if the patient's primary problem is expected to improve.

Can be used at home for treatment of OSA.

Oxygen can be humidified for patient comfort.

CONS

CPAP/BiPAP may suffocate patient if fit and settings are inappropriate.

BiPAP must allow for ventilation of CO_2 via loose fit.

Exact mask fits difficult to achieve.

Patients often noncompliant because of comfort and noise, especially during sleep.

Water condensation in tubing may make nasal CPAP less reliable.[20]

Masks

Full Face Masks

Face masks, which seat over the patient's nose and mouth, are used to provide noninvasive positive pressure ventilation to the anesthetized patient. "The ability to hold the mask and to administer positive pressure ventilation is a basic skill that all anesthesia providers must master. In the past, the face mask was often used to administer an entire anesthetic."[21] The most commonly used face masks today are clear, disposable, and come in a variety of sizes to fit essentially any patient's anatomy equally well (i.e., not particularly well).

Face masks consist of a mount, body, and rim. The mount is standardized as a 22-mm female inlet for an anesthesia circuit or ventilator tubing, or an angle piece. The interface between the mount and body often contains a set of hooks, sometimes removable, used to secure a mask strap. The body of the mask seats between the mount and rim and is usually clear to visualize condensation or aspirates. The body volume and rim account for much of the mask's dead space, which has greater implication for the pediatric population. Therefore, Rendell-Baker masks were designed without rims to reduce dead space and allow a better fit in neonates and small children.

In standard masks, the rim itself is a soft, air-filled cushion, which is in direct contact with the face. Often the cushion contains a syringe inlet for addition or removal of air. Rims may be shaped anatomically, or generically as an oval. Masks come in a huge range of sizes, primarily to accommodate pediatric needs. Adult face masks typically come in three sizes in any vendor's product line: small, medium, and large. The medium size is inevitably the 90% solution, effectively fitting the vast majority of patients.

Most masks used today are made of plastics, mainly polyethylene and polyvinyl chlorides (PVCs) (Figure 6–8). This material is soft and clear, allowing for patient comfort and anesthetist convenience in observing the airway for condensation or emesis. Although these plastics are inexpensive, they cannot be autoclaved—plastic masks are made for single use (Figure 6–9, A and B). Allergic reactions are of no concern with these materials.

CPAP valve is being kept open by an adequate flow throughout the respiratory cycle."[19]

CPAP and BiPAP are delivered via a variety of face masks applied over the nose, mouth, or both. Masks range from simple nasal plugs, nasal masks, face masks over the nose and mouth, to full head helmets. A variety of shapes and sizes exist to allow for appropriate size and fitting. Straps and/or harnesses are used to secure the mask.

Wide bore tubing, similar to that used for anesthesia machine circuits, is connected to the CPAP/BiPAP machine and mask. The masks often contain a single female inlet, as do many anesthesia masks, to accommodate one limb tubing, or a "Y" piece for two limbs. Other masks may have two female inlets for both an oxygen delivery limb (from either wall oxygen or a mechanical ventilator) and a limb for direct CPAP valve application.

The oxygen and fresh gas flow delivered to the patient must overcome the patient's peak inspiratory flow rate so that positive pressure can be continuously provided. "Some systems incorporate a reservoir bag, otherwise a flow generator connected to piped high pressure oxygen outlet (wall CPAP) is used."[19] These flow generators are "high pressure oxygen driven Venturi injectors"[19]—these units and those similar can be very loud and bothersome to the patient.[19]

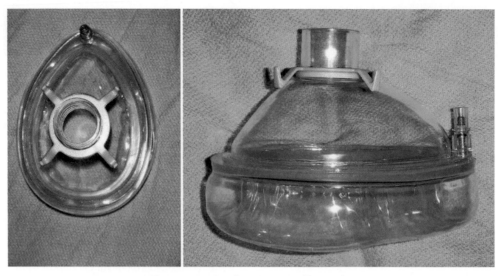

Figure 6–8   "Medium-Size" PVC face mask.

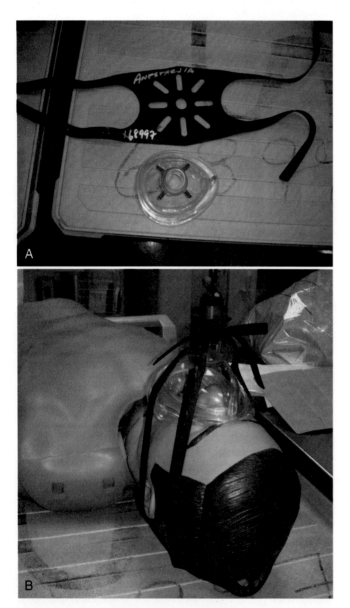

Figure 6–9   Face mask strap.

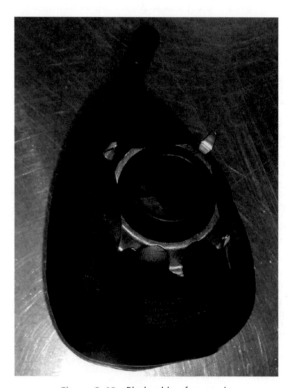

Figure 6–10   Black rubber face mask.

Some masks are made of inexpensive black rubber (Figure 6–10). Rubber, including natural latex rubber, comes from the bark sap of rubber plants, namely from the *Hevea brasiliensis* tree. Black rubber is made from the vulcanization of natural latex rubber, where extreme heat is used to destroy the allergic-causing plant proteins. Black rubber masks are reusable and may be autoclaved between patients. However, black rubber masks may be intimidating or anxiety provoking to patients, and do not allow the anesthetist to view the airway for condensation or secretions or emesis. The anesthetist may also want to avoid using these masks in latex sensitive, or latex allergic, patients (Tables 6–9 and 6–10).

Table 6–9 Natural Latex Rubber Reactions[22]

Type	Description	Treatment
Irritant contact dermatitis	Nonallergic reaction Local skin reaction consists of itching, scaling, edema, erythema	Avoid latex materials Topical antihistamines and/or topical steroids
Type IV, delayed hypersensitivity	T-cell mediated, local dermatitis Skin edema, erythema, itching hours after exposure, may persist and/or topical for days to weeks	Avoid latex materials Topical antihistamines and/or topical steroids PO antihistamines
Type I, immediate hypersensitivity	IgE-mediated, systemic allergic reaction Systemic urticaria, itching, wheezing, flushing, conjunctivitis, angioedema, rhinitis Anaphylaxis: hypotension, tachycardia, with above Type I symptoms	See Table 6–10

Table adapted from Vassallo SA. Latex allergy. In 37th Anesthesia review and update, Harvard Medical School, Boston, 2008.[22]

Table 6–10 Management of Latex Anaphylaxis[22,23]

Call for help.

Remove the antigenic stimulus. Identify and removal all latex products away from the patient.

Attention to the patient's airway. Ensure patent airway and ventilation, delivery 100% F_{IO_2}. Consider endotracheal intubation because angioedema may soon obstruct airway.

Support the patient's circulation with massive crystalloid resuscitation. Obtain large bore IV access.

Deliver 0.1 µg/kg of intravenous epinephrine (ACLS doses not indicated). Repeat as needed to obtain sufficient blood pressure, heart rate, and airway response.

Discontinue anesthetics if hypotension persists. However, volatile anesthetics may help combat bronchospasm.

Discontinue other potential antigens, such as antibiotics or blood products.

Discuss patient's condition with surgeons, remove any potential antigens from field. Plans may need to be made to halt surgery.

Deliver systemic steroids: dexamethasone, 0.2-2.5 mg/kg IV, methylprednisolone, 1 mg/kg IV.
Consider antihistamines: diphenhydramine, 0.5-1 mg/kg IV, ranitidine, 1 mg/kg IV.

Consider arrangements for ICU bed, anticipate further potential complications, such as loss of ability to oxygenate/ventilate, "pressor support" dependency, complete cardiovascular collapse, cardiac arrest, or hypertension/tachycardia from previously discussed treatments.

Table from Vassallo SA. Latex allergy. In 37th Anesthesia review and update, Boston, Harvard Medical School, 2008 and Gaba DM, Fish KJ, Howard SK, editors. *Crisis management in anesthesiology*, Philadelphia, Churchill Livingstone, 1994.[22,23]

Applying positive pressure ventilation via the mask may be achieved with the one-handed, "C-E" method of mask ventilation. In the anesthetist's left hand, an appropriately sized mask is applied to the face, such that the top of the mask seats over the bridge of the nose, and the bottom over the chin. The cheeks should fit within the edges of the mask's rim. Using the left hand, the thumb and index finger use downward force to seal the mask against the face. The third, fourth, and fifth fingers are placed on the patient's mandible—the fifth finger should be placed on the angle of the jaw. These fingers draw the patient's face up into the mask. With the fingers in correct position, the first two fingers create a letter "C" around the mask's mound, and remaining fingers form a letter "E" upon the patient's jaw (Figure 6–11). The aforementioned "downward force" applied by the thumb and index finger is actually a force meeting that is applied by the third through fifth fingers pulling the jaw up into the mask. Properly applied, many anesthetists can lift the patient's head with this mask-grip. The anesthetist's right hand is now free for positive pressure ventilation via a rebreathing bag or manual resuscitator. The patient's head is ideally at the level of the anesthetist's xiphoid, but a facile anesthetist can ventilate from virtually any position. With sufficient patient head tilt and jaw thrust during mask ventilation, the jaw may be moved anteriorly, and tongue maneuvered to relieve obstruction of the upper airway. Other mask ventilation techniques exist, including two-person mask ventilation, which are outside the scope of this chapter.

Insertion of an oropharyngeal or nasopharyngeal airway device (see next section) can facilitate mask ventilation. Use of mask straps allows for consistent mask seal and may free the hands of the anesthetist or offset user fatigue. Edentulous patients can be more difficult to mask ventilate, because their cheeks may not allow a secure seal against the mask. Leaving dentures in place, packing the buccal cavities with gauze, or using smaller masks partially subsiding into the mouth to ventilate the nose all may help improve mask effectiveness in edentulous patients.[24]

Nasal Masks

Similar to the previously mentioned face masks are nasal masks. These are often used in dental procedures to allow for easy access to the mouth, or with the use of CPAP or BiPAP machines. The Goldman and McKesson nasal inhalers are examples.[25] These masks come in various sizes to fit over the bridge of the nose, upper lip, and maxilla. These masks apply positive pressure ventilation to the nasopharynx alone. Nasal masks provide a pressure gradient between the nasopharynx and oropharynx to "overcome the effect of gravity on the soft palate and tongue, pushing forward and opening the upper airway."[26] Full-face masks do not generate such a gradient, allowing the tongue and soft palate to obstruct the posterior pharynx and gas flows (Table 6–11).[26] Some preliminary

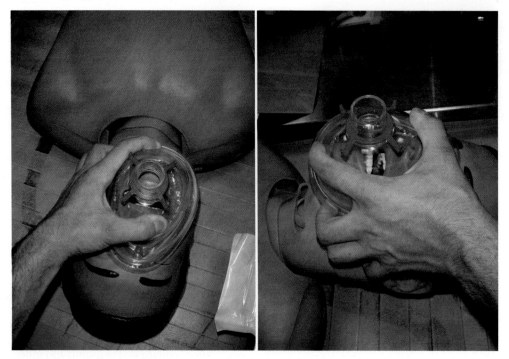

Figure 6–11   "C-E" method of face mask ventilation.

investigations using nasal masks during induction of anesthesia have suggested they are more effective than ventilation with full-face masks[26] (Figure 6–12). The mouth may remain open during nasal mask ventilation; however, simply closing the mouth would decrease any gas leak.

Similar to the nasal mask are nasal plugs—which seal onto the nares—used in CPAP. One study of neonatal resuscitation with bag-mask positive pressure ventilation showed using this "nasal cannula" plug mask may be more effective than traditional full-face mask bag ventilation.[27]

Oropharyngeal and Nasopharyngeal Airway

Oropharyngeal Airway

The oropharyngeal airway is a hard, rigid, plastic device curved to anatomically fit into the oropharynx to relieve upper airway obstruction caused by the tongue or epiglottis contacting the posterior pharyngeal wall. These pieces are designed with a flange which seats just outside the mouth to help prevent complete entrance into the mouth and airway. Just behind the flange is, a straightened area which serves as a bite block. The rest of the device is curved to situate over the tongue and into the oropharynx. The distal end is designed to settle deep at the base of the tongue, and superior to the epiglottis. The entire airway device is hollow to allow for airflow through a central channel. A diversity of shapes and sizes exist to fit neonates, children, and small and large adults. A standardized color coding and sizing system exists for these devices. For example, a large adult Guedel oropharyngeal airway would be a size number 10, or 100 mm, colored red. The most popular oropharyngeal airway is the Guedel airway (Figure 6–13).

Proper selection and insertion of any airway device are very important. To choose the appropriately sized airway for a given patient, "the distance from the flange to the distal tip of the airway should be about the same as from the patient's lips to the tragus of the ear."[28] Ideally the patient is anesthetized (or obtunded) enough to tolerate placement. These devices may be lubricated, although this is not essential. The patient's mouth should be opened wide and the head extended on the neck. Carefully place the airway to follow the anatomy and shape of palate and tongue. Sometimes the tongue perturbs placement because it may fold posterior as the airway is advanced. A tongue blade can aid in flattening the tongue and preventing its collapse.[29] Another method of placing an oropharyngeal device involves rotating the device 180 degrees, facing the opposite direction, such that the distal end is pointing toward the palate (Figure 6–14). Once advanced beyond the tongue, the device can be rotated to seat properly in the oropharynx.

Specially designed oropharyngeal airways have been developed to assist with intubations requiring the aid of a fiberoptic bronchoscope.[30] These airways act as both conduits for the bronchoscope to easily pass through secretions, and, once past the tongue, to approach the larynx. Bite blocks incorporated into these airways prevent damage to both the patient and fiberoptic equipment.[28] Several types of fiberoptic intubating oropharyngeal airways exist. The Optosafe has a large enough air passage to allow the bronchoscope, endotracheal tube, and all components to enter through the device. The Ovassapian or Berman airways are open and flexible, to allow the airway to be peeled around and away from the fiberoptic bronchoscope before deployment of an endotracheal tube over the scope (Figure 6–15). Lastly, the Williams Airway Intubator can be used for both fiberoptic intubations, blind intubations, or to relieve airway obstruction.[31]

Cuffed oropharyngeal airways (COPA) are of the Guedel variety and contain a distal inflatable cuff similar to that of endotracheal tubes, to allow for a more secure fit in the oropharynx. When the cuff is inflated, the tongue and epiglottis are displaced from the posterior pharynx, facilitating air flow

Table 6–11	Pros and Cons of Face Mask Ventilation for Administration of Anesthesia

PROS

Appropriate mask ventilation and/or oxygenation can be a lifesaving maneuver and may allow for denitrogenation of patient's airways during induction of anesthesia.

Inexpensive.

May be scented for patient comfort.

Clear mask bodies allow for detection of misting (implying ventilation) and blood and emesis.

Clear mask bodies may reduce claustrophobia compared with dark rubber masks.

Mask straps reduce anesthetist fatigue during mask ventilation.

Mask ventilation may allow patient to recover from anesthesia and/or neuromuscular-blocking drugs if endotracheal intubation cannot be achieved.

Mask ventilation may be used for dental surgery or for volatile or nitrous gas inductions in patients without intravenous access (pediatric patients or those with severe needle phobia).

CONS

Appropriate mask ventilation and/or oxygenation takes training to master.

Pressure injury to facial nerves, trigeminal nerves, etc.

Corneal abrasion, especially if mask is too large to seat over the eyes. Eye tape or coverings help prevent this.

Difficult to achieve airtight seal in large patients, edentulous patients, those with beards, and those with nasogastric tubes.

Claustrophobia.

Skin pressure sores or ulceration.

Improper use may lead to stomach inflation and increase risk of aspiration, especially if >20 cm H_2O is used during ventilation, because fresh gas may overcome lower esophageal sphincter pressure.

Increases dead space by up to 200 cc (adult masks).

During mask ventilation, patient's c-spine may be undesirably disturbed.

Patient may have jaw pain after mask ventilation.

User fatigue can occur, especially with ill-fitting masks or inexperienced anesthetists.

Multiple persons may be needed to achieve adequate fit and mask ventilate.

Gases, such as volatile anesthetic agents, may escape through the mask and pollute the operating room environment.

Allergic reaction to mask materials (i.e., latex allergy) if a rubber mask is used.

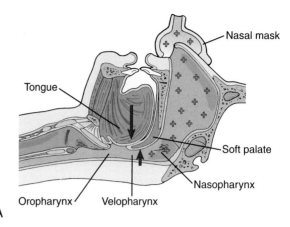

A

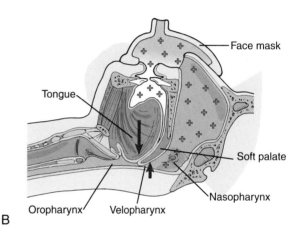

B

Figure 6–12   Nasal mask ventilation. *(From Liang Y, Kimball WR, Kacmarek RM, et al. Nasal ventilation is more effective than combined oral-nasal ventilation during induction of general anesthesia in adult subjects. Anesthesiology 2008;108:998-1003.)*[26]

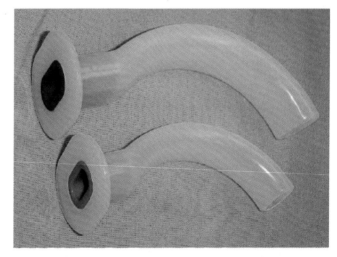

Figure 6–13   Guedel oropharyngeal airways. Size 10 is red, size 8 is green.

through the airway.[32] The COPA allows for attachment to the anesthesia machine breathing circuit with its distal connector. Several recent studies have emerged regarding the clinical use and safety concerns for the COPA (Table 6–12).

Nasopharyngeal Airway (Nasal Trumpets)

The nasopharyngeal airway is a curved, soft, flexible plastic tube, which comes in a variety of sizes, designed to anatomically fit through the curve of the nasopharynx (Figure 6–16).

The proximal end is splayed and thickened, and may contain a safety pin to remain outside the nares. The beveled distal end seats deep within the oropharynx, superior to the epiglottis. The beveled end, when lubricated, should pass easily through the nares and nasopharynx into proper position. It is important that this airway is sized properly, and long enough

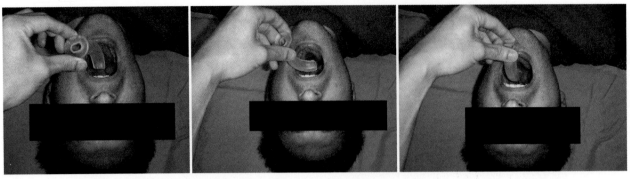

Figure 6–14   Insertion of oropharyngeal device with 180-degree rotation: sequence in this figure is from left to right.

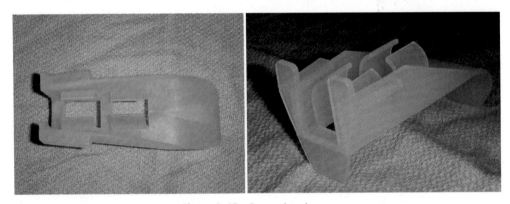

Figure 6–15   Ovassapian airway.

to bypass the tongue and/or the upper airway obstruction, even if the device is slightly uncomfortable. "The use of nasopharyngeal airways has almost disappeared from UK anesthetic practice, with the rising popularity of the LMA"[39] (Table 6–13).

Sizes are based upon both internal diameter in millimeters and size French. For example, a 7.0 mm nasopharyngeal airway would be a size 28 French.[40] Various shapes include cuffed/uncuffed, with or without balloons for inflation, or even binasal variants (two nasal trumpets attached with a connector) for positive pressure ventilation.[41]

The nasal trumpet should be inserted such that it "is inserted perpendicularly, in line with the nasal passage the airway held with the bevel against the septum and gently advanced posteriorly while being rotated back and forth."[42] If the airway does not seat well, or obstruction is not relieved, remove this device and try either the other nostril, or another size.

Laryngeal-Mask Airway (LMA)

The Laryngeal Mask Airway (LMA)

The LMA, first described in 1983 by Brain[49] and commercially available in 1989,[50] is a supraglottic airway device consisting of a curved lumen (or shaft, etc.) and a diamond/ovoid-shaped bowl (or cuff). This device, a hybrid of face mask and endotracheal tube, seats firmly within the posterior pharynx and over the laryngeal inlet to allow for gas exchange. The advent of the LMA has changed airway management in anesthetic practice, and that of other medical specialties, such as emergency medicine. The LMA is a key component of the ASA difficult

airway algorithm.[51] In 1984 Brain first described its potential use during emergencies.[52]

The LMA's lumen is made to fit with standard breathing circuits and resuscitation equipment. The distal end of the tube contains the bowl of the LMA. The rounded bowl, as described previously, is directly inflated with a pilot balloon, usually with 20 cc of air. The bowl is open to the lumen of the tube to allow for air passage. Protective bars are present on some LMA models at the junction between the lumen and bowl, which functions to shield the LMA lumen from the patient's epiglottis, which could potentially obstruct ventilation and gas flow. LMAs are available in neonate through adult sizes. Newer LMAs are made for one-time use and are disposable (Figures 6–17 and 6–20). Older models, such as the LMA-Classic (Figure 6–18) were made from silicone rubber and were autoclaved between uses.

Insertion of the LMA is best described by Brain in a correspondence to *Anesthesiology* in 1990 (Figure 6–19).[54] To insert the LMA, the patient should be anesthetized with an induction dose of a sedative-hypnotic, or receive local anesthesia to the airway to tolerate the procedure without airway reflexes, such as gag or cough. The bowl of the LMA should also be checked before insertion to ensure the bowl is not defective. For LMA size selection, see Table 6–14. Deflate the cuff and apply lubrication. Some anesthetists will inflate the cuff before insertion, although this is not recommended by most manufacturers.

Place the patient's head in a sniff position. An assistant may help open the mouth by placing traction on the jaw or lips. The anesthetist places his or her fingers within the bowl of the LMA, such that the concave side of the bowl will slide against the hard palate and into the oropharynx (Figure 6–21). At this point, the anesthetist may either continue to slide the LMA

Table 6–12 Clinical Uses and Safety of the COPA

Spontaneously ventilated patients[33]

For use during fiberoptic intubation[34]

Manual in-line stabilization[35]

Awake intracranial neurosurgery[36]

Lingual and glossopharyngeal nerve injury[37]

PROS

Relief of obstructed airway

Facilitate positive pressure ventilation with face mask

Variety of shapes and sizes for neonates to adults and for differing purposes

May be used as a conduit for instrumentation (i.e., suction, fiberoptic camera, etc.)

CONS

Trauma to teeth (especially if prior dental work such as caps or crowns), gums, lips, tongue, etc.

Further airway obstruction

Device aspiration[38]

Gagging, coughing, vomiting, laryngospasm, especially if airway reflexes not sufficiently suppressed by anesthetics or topical agents

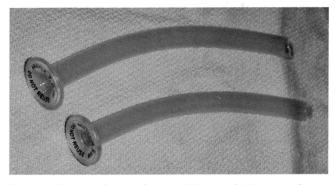

Figure 6–16 Nasopharyngeal airway. 7.0 mm and 6.5 mm are shown.

Table 6–13 Pros and Cons of Nasal Airways

PROS

Relatively noninvasive.

Although uncomfortable for some patients, can stimulate patients to breathe and is usually more comfortable than an oropharyngeal airway, which may not be practical for some patients (i.e., facial deformities, poor dentition, etc.).[39]

Can be used in patients who cannot open their mouth or have upper airway obstructions than cannot be otherwise relieved,[43] such as in the case of congenital facial anomalies.[44]

May act as a conduit for catheter suction, NG-tube placement, or other instrumentation.[42,43]

May facilitate noninvasive positive pressure ventilation with face mask or noninvasive mechanical ventilation. Can also maintain patent airway during dental procedures.[42] May also allow for continuous positive pressure ventilation (CPAP).[45]

CONS[40]

Patient discomfort or pain on insertion. Lubricant and/or vasoconstricting nasal spray helps reduce this pain.

Contraindicated in patients with anticoagulation, sepsis/DIC, pregnancy, other coagulopathies raising concern of bleeding. Epistaxis is always a possibility with this device.

Contraindicated in patients with abnormal nasopharyngeal anatomy, bleeding polyps, or suspected facial or skull fracture (i.e., trauma patient, cerebrospinal fluid rhinorrhea, etc.). Accidental intracranial placement may occur in this population.[46,47]

Pressure necrosis if left for prolonged amount of time.[48]

Potential for nasal or skull trauma if forced into airway.

Can migrate through nares into nasopharynx to oropharynx or larynx.

Further airway obstruction if not seated properly.

Gastric distention if device is too long, allowing air or gases to enter esophagus rather than into the airway.[48]

Can accidentally be placed into a false lumen[43] or through the cribriform plate and enter the sinus, skull, or frontal lobe of the brain.[46,47]

May stimulate the vagus nerve, causing vagal reflex (syncope, bradycardia).

Patients may gag/choke/aspirate.

Mucus plugging, however, some models have holes in the wall to bypass plugs.[39]

Rubber nasopharyngeal airways may cause allergy in latex sensitive patients. Latex free devices are available.

---

down into the supraglottic position until a "pop" or "snap" is felt, indicating the LMA is in the appropriate position for inflation. Others prefer to grip the shaft of the device like a pen, and advance the device downward through the pharynx. Once the "pop" or "snap" is felt, the pilot balloon is inflated with air through a syringe. See Table 6–14 to determine how much air is needed to inflate for a given LMA size.

It should be noted that there are many effective techniques for LMA insertion, reflecting the simplicity of the device and its robustness to user variation in practice.

To confirm proper seating of the LMA, which occurs in greater than 95% of insertions,[28] the patient can be allowed to breath spontaneously with normal chest rise and without signs of stridor or airleak.[28] In the apneic patient, positive pressure should be applied. Typical airway pressures are kept under or equal to 20 cm H_2O to minimize gastric distention. In practice, higher airway pressure may be needed, albeit rarely. Visible chest rise without hearing a leak or stridor, and no resistance to bag ventilation, suggests a patent airway with

the LMA. A bite block may now be placed, along with tape to the patient's face to secure the LMA.

The LMA may be removed inflated or deflated, although removing it inflated has the benefit of removing nasopharyngeal and oropharyngeal secretion from the airway. Convincing the patient to swallow at the moment of removal clears all secretions. Table 6–15 lists the pros and cons of LMAs for airway control.

The insertion and use of the LMA in the prone position is becoming popular in Europe. In one study in 2002, 73 healthy ambulatory surgery patients underwent LMA insertion while in the prone position and were ventilated prone during their procedures. Only minor complications were observed, although not infrequent, including four episodes of malposition, and one

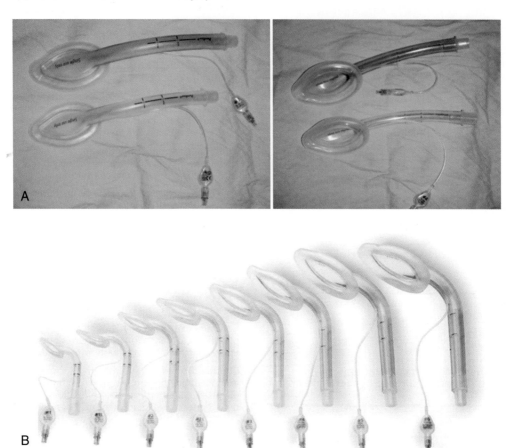

Figure 6–17 The basic LMA. Note this model does not contain epiglottis elevator bars. **A,** Sizes 4 and 5 are shown. **B,** All available sizes (1-6) for the AuraOnce basic LMA by Ambu. *(Shown with permission.)*

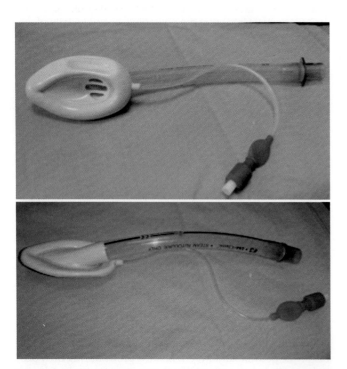

Figure 6–18 The LMA-Classic, size 3. This older model is reusable and has epiglottis elevator bars.

episode of laryngospasm.[55] In our own practice, we commonly insert LMAs after induction in the prone position for brief procedures. Mask ventilation and LMA insertion are inevitably easy. One recent case report describes the successful use of a prone LMA being inserted and used during a pediatric craniectomy and cervical laminectomy after accidental extubation.[56]

Since the LMA's development in 1983, a multitude of supraglottic airway devices have been invented and tested. For example, wire- reinforced, kink-resistant LMAs have been developed for use in head and neck surgeries, which can withstand the insertion of a throat pack (Figure 6–22).[59] Some others are listed next.

LMA with Esophageal Drains

Several LMAs have been developed that include an open conduit located at the distal portion of the LMA cuff, allowing drainage of oropharyngeal or esophageal contents. An oral-gastric tube may be introduced through this device as well. However, the ability of these LMAs to prevent aspiration has been questioned.[39]

The Pro-Seal LMA, for example, has a larger and softer cuff, esophageal drain, and an associated bite block. The Pro-Seal LMA claims to reduce rates of aspiration from gastric contents with at least a 10 cc inflation with air and optimal placement.[61] This device is designed for use during a "cannot intubate in a rapid sequence" induction situation for

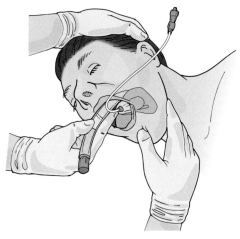

Figure 6–19 Proper insertion of the LMA. *(From Brain AIJ. Proper technique for insertion of the laryngeal mask. Anesthesiology 1990;73:1053.)*[54]

Table 6–14 Sizing of the LMA

LMA Size	Patient Weight (kg)	Max Cuff Volume (cc)
1	neonate 5	4
1.5	infant 5-10	7
2	child 10-20	10
2.5	child 20-30	14
3	adult 30-50, typically female	20
4	adult 50-70, most females	30
5	adult 70-100, most males	40
6	adult 100 (+), typically male	50

Adapted from Diba A. Airway management devices. In Davey AJ, Diba A, editors. *Ward's anaesthetic equipment*, ed 5, Philadelphia, Elsevier Saunders, 2005.[53]

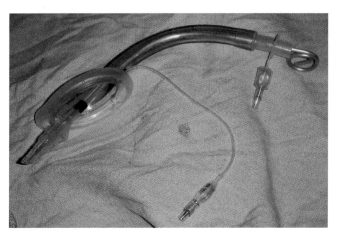

Figure 6–20 Size 5 disposable LMA with 7.0-mm endotracheal tube inserted through the lumen. Liberal use of lubrication is needed to allow for easy threading of the endotracheal tube through the LMA.

emergency surgery.[62] Another advantage is that it may allow for higher airway pressures during positive pressure ventilation.[63] A gastric drainage tube, such as a nasogastric tube, can be easily inserted through this device.[64] Cook et al in 2007[65] inserted a Pro-Seal LMA into 1000 consecutive patients and noted the following complications: development of partial obstruction, some necessitating reinsertion; visible blood-tinged secretions upon removal; minor gastric regurgitation without aspiration; and one case of hypoglossal nerve palsy after prolonged use—whether or not this was permanent was not mentioned.[65] Sore throat after use has also been reported as a common complication.[66] Cases of the gastric drain entering the trachea[67] and a case of mechanical vocal cord closure has also been described.[68]

LMA Supreme

This LMA device features a larger cuff, reinforcing tips, epiglottic fins, and a firm endotracheal tube, which contains a bite block and drainage tube (Figure 6–23). The LMA Supreme is less likely to fold or kink in the airway with the previously mentioned additions and can be used as an intubation

device[62] or for intubation via a fiberoptic scope. This device is disposable and comes in three adult sizes.

i-gel

This device uses "soft thermoplastic elastomer" materials as its noninflatable "cuff"[62] to allow for a patient specific fit. The stem of this device contains an associated bite-block and can be used for instrumentation with endotracheal tubes and fiberoptic cameras to obtain high Brimacombe scores,[69] which may allow it to be used in difficult airway situations (Figure 6–24). The i-gel also contains a "gastric channel" for drainage of stomach contents.[70] The i-gel is also disposable and comes in three adult sizes. It is now beginning to be studied in the pediatric population. Complications while using the i-gel have been reported, namely tongue trauma,[71] blood upon extubation and minor lip trauma,[72] and transient ulcerative pressure damage to the mental nerve.[73]

Intubating LMAs

A group of LMAs, such as the iLMA, or Fast-Trach-LMA, have been designed to facilitate blind endotracheal intubation through the LMA itself, by virtue of anatomic curves of the upper airway and intubation device. These devices play a very important role in the management of the anticipated, and unanticipated, difficult airway.[74,75] However, training and practice are required to obtain an appropriate skill level to use this device successfully (20 prior insertions are generally recommended).[74]

Intubating LMAs (or Fast-Trach-LMA) differ in structure from the classic LMA, seeking to and increase the chance for successful endotracheal intubation. The bowl and 15 mm LMA lumen, which can be used for ventilation, are made of rigid stainless steel. The bowl also contains a protective epiglottic lifting bar, as described previously with the classic LMA. A stainless steel handle bar is connected to the distal lumen to allow for external adjustments to the bowl for endotracheal intubation. The endotracheal tube itself, included with this device, is reinforced with metal wire to help prevent kinking during insertion. This endotracheal tube also contains a latex free, silicone rubber end, which allows for easier passage

Figure 6–21 Folding and kinking of the LMA. **A,** An example of infolding. **B,** An example of overfolding. **C,** An example of back folding. *(Adapted without permission from ISO. Anaesthetic and respiratory equipment-supralaryngeal airways and connectors, BSI, 2009.)*

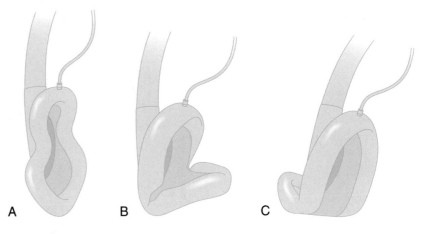

A   B   C

Table 6–15 **Pros and Cons of the LMA as a Primary Airway Device**
PRO
Easily placed, limited training needed.
Avoids intubation of the trachea and bag ventilation with a face mask (e.g., especially if patient is potentially difficult to bag mask, as in those with beards or without teeth).
Use in patients with potentially difficult airway or in airway emergencies. See ASA difficult airway algorithm.[51]
Use as a conduit for other instruments, such as fiberoptic camera, blind intubation with endotracheal tube, gum bougie wand.
Avoids the use of neuromuscular blocking drugs (NMBDs).
Use in short procedures in which the patient may spontaneously ventilate (i.e., 20-minute knee arthroscopy).
Insertion will not cause drastic changes in hemodynamics, bronchial tone, or intraocular/intracranial pressure.[57]
If removed with bowl inflated, secretions are removed with the LMA, avoiding instrumenting the airway with suction.
CON
Effective under 20 cm H_2O, or air leaks and gastric distention may occur. If high airway pressures are likely to be needed for ventilation, LMAs should be avoided.
Not a definitely secure airway—no protection from gastric aspirate or laryngospasm.
May not be safe in patients with gastroesophageal reflux disease (GERD), hiatal hernia, gastric neuropathy, or other "full-stomach" precaution.
Nitrous oxide may distend the cuff, increasing its pressure against the pharyngeal mucosal layers, leading to ischemia.
Obesity and abdominal insufflation with CO_2 during laparoscopic surgery may impede positive pressure ventilation.[57]
LMA can kink, fold, or dislodge during surgery, causing airway obstruction (see later figure).
Unclear how long the LMA can be used during surgery. By convention, it is commonplace to only use the LMA for less than 2 hr in the United States, whereas they will be used for much longer surgical cases in many European countries.
Insertion and use in prone cases still controversial, especially in the United States.
Anatomic defects or airway disease, such as epiglottitis, may limit its use.
Case reports of complications have included cranial nerve damage, paralysis, and temporary vocal cord paralysis.[58]

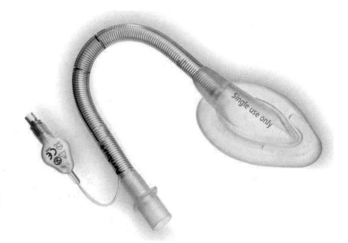

Figure 6–22 Wire-wound reinforced LMA. Shown here is the Auraflex LMA by Ambu. *(Shown with permission.)*

through the LMA lumen and larynx. However, conventional endotracheal tubes may also be used in conjunction with this device.[76] This LMA is limited to an 8 mm endotracheal tube. The intubating LMA is not manufactured for single usage, and should be preserved, cleaned, and sterilized between uses. Other features of the intubating LMA include an endotracheal tube "pusher" to allow the endotracheal tube to be advanced as the LMA itself is removed from the oropharynx. Lubrication of the LMA bowl and intubation components is recommended to increase successful placement. The Fast-Trach LMA may also be used to allow for endotracheal intubation with the aid of a fiberoptic bronchoscope; for example, during severe facial trauma[77] or in patients requiring manual in-line neck stabilization (Figure 6–25).[78]

As with all medical devices, several potential safety issues exist for the Fast-Trach LMA. For example, esophageal intubation occurs about 5% of the time,[74] the stainless steel material of this device is not MRI compatible,[79] and placement may put pressure on or cause movement of an injured cervical spine.[80]

The LMA Ctrach, similar to the iLMA, incorporates fiberoptic bundle technology, a camera within the LMA cuff, and a magnetically attached LCD display unit.[81] This allows for indirect laryngoscopy and view of the larynx during endotracheal tube placement. In patients with grade 3 views during direct laryngoscopy, this device can be used to obtain a view of the larynx and insertion of an endotracheal tube about 89% of the time.[82] This Ctrach LMA has also been described successfully for use in difficult or emergency airway situations.[82,83] This device as well comes in three adult sizes: 3, 4, and 5, and is reusable. As with all supraglottic airway devices, the risk of aspiration of gastric contents is always possible, and has been described in one morbidly obese patient while using the Ctrach during a difficult airway.[84]

Other Nonintubating Airways

Combitube

The Combitube is a disposable emergency airway management device consisting of two lumens and two inflation cuffs (Figure 6–26). Indications for this device are supraglottic obstruction or when personnel need an immediate airway, especially during a cannot ventilate or intubate scenario.[85] This device is lubricated and inserted blindly into the oropharynx until the tick marks on the tube reach the level of the teeth. A laryngoscope may also be used for insertion.[61] The Combitube enters the esophagus about 95% of the time, thus functioning as an esophageal obturator.[58] The proximal pharyngeal cuff fills with 100 cc of air, while the distal cuff is filled with 15 cc of air. Occasionally, this 100-cc cuff may block airflow into the distal airways, in which case the Combitube should be removed by 1 to 2 cm.[86] For each lumen, one opens beyond the inflation point of the 15-cc distal cuff (tube "2"), while the other (tube "1") opens in-between the cuffs via side holes. Once both cuffs are inflated, after insertion, tube 1 is ventilated first, and if ventilation is not possible, tube 2 is attempted next. Typically, tube 2 is used for gastric decompression, while the 15-cc inflated cuff seals off the esophagus for ventilation through the side holes in-between each cuff. This forces positive pressure ventilation/fresh gas into the airway—a concept similar to the esophageal obturator airway. An esophageal detector may be used in conjunction with the Combitube before test ventilation to prevent undesirable gastric distention (Figure 6–27).[86] If subsequent endotracheal intubation is attempted by direct laryngoscopy, the 100-cc oropharyngeal cuff must first be deflated. The 15-cc distal cuff should remain inflated to help protect the airway from gastric aspirate. One study even described using this device to help control severe oronasal bleeding during angiography in a facial trauma patient.[87]

The major safety concerns include gastric distention/inflation, therefore increasing the risk of regurgitation/aspiration, and esophageal rupture with the possibility of ensuing mediastinitis. The Combitube should only be left seated and inflated for several hours "to decrease the risk of ischemia of the tongue and subsequent edema formation."[32,88,89] Other safety issues include transient cranial nerve IX and XII dysfunction[90] and postoperative sore throat and/or hoarseness.[91] Only two adult sizes are currently available. Another disadvantage to the Combitube is its high monetary cost per unit.

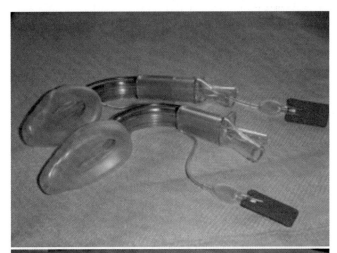

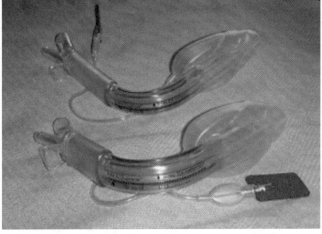

Figure 6–23   LMA Supreme, sizes 4 and 5. Note the bite block and esophageal drain associated with this LMA.

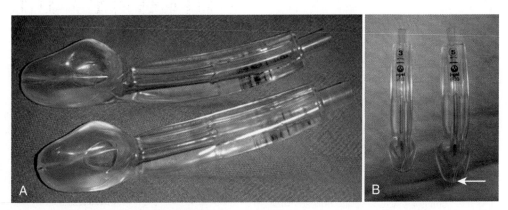

Figure 6–24   i-gel, sizes 3 and 5. Note this device's bite block, gastric drainage channel, and lack of an inflation tubing. The *arrow* denotes the proximal end of the gastric drainage channel.

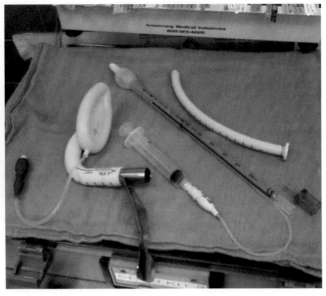

Figure 6–25 Fast-Trach LMA. Note the cuff of the endotracheal tube is inflated.

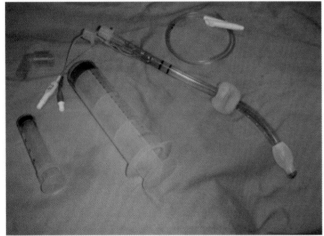

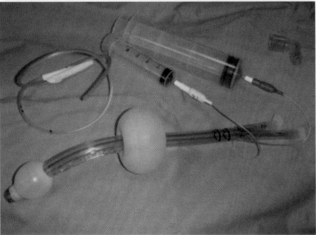

Figure 6–26 The Combitube. The 100-cc syringe connects to the blue tube (tube 1), which inflates the pharyngeal cuff, and the 15-cc syringe connects to the white tube (tube 2), which inflates (typically) within the esophagus. Included in the Combitube kit is a gastric drainage tube, seen in the upper right corner of this image. It is usually placed through tube 2.

Laryngeal Tube

Similar to the Combitube, the laryngeal tube is a shorter, single-lumen device with two cuffs. One cuff inflates within the oropharynx, the other within the esophagus. Ventilation and fresh gas then enters the airway by passing in-between the two cuffs. Some newer models also include an opening for gastric tube insertion. A fiberoptic scope can be introduced through the laryngeal tube, and tracheal intubation can be obtained nasally with the laryngeal tube in place.[92] These tubes are reusable and come in pediatric and adult sizes.[86] Sore throat and dysphagia after removal have been noted on occasion[93] and hoarseness.[94] A similar device, called the airway management device (AMD), has been developed in the United Kingdom; however, it has had mixed results.[86]

Pharyngeal Airway Xpress

An alternate supraglottic airway device, which uses a series of folded gill-like structures that sit in the hypopharynx/cricopharyngeus muscle and a pharyngeal cuff to allow ventilation. It is inserted blindly or with the aid of a light wand. An endotracheal tube may be introduced through this device to intubate the patient. The leak pressure was noted to be higher when compared with ventilation through an LMA (31 vs. 21 cm H_2O).[95] For 5 minutes after insertion, increases in systolic and diastolic blood pressure of about 20% were noted in one study,[96] and acute transient sialodenopathy.[97] A sore throat is not an uncommon complaint after placement,[95] as is mucosal trauma and/or blood-tinged secretions upon removal of this device.[98]

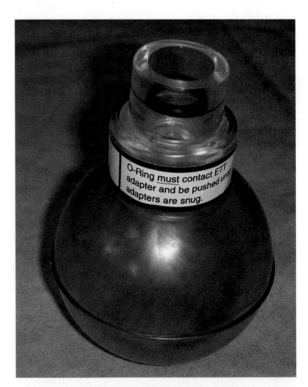

Figure 6–27 Esophageal detector bulb.

Glottic Aperture Seal (GAS) Airway[32]

This disposable airway device used a plastic epiglottic elevator, which is inserted during placement into the patient. It is secured in the airway with a spongy distal tip.

Conclusions

As surgery becomes less invasive and more efficient, office-based anesthesia and surgery is becoming increasingly prominent. This has allowed for the continued and expanded use of supraglottic airway devices, especially those within the LMA family, and development of new designs. Therefore the anesthetist must develop a complete understanding of these devices, how they work, their pitfalls, and how these may be avoided or overcome. These devices are now dominating airway management in Europe, are expanding in the United States, and are a key component of the ASA difficult airway algorithm.[51]

Suggested Reading

American Society of Anesthesiologists. 2003. Practice guidelines for management of the difficult airway: an updated report by the American Society of Anesthesiologists task force on management of the difficult airway. Anesthesiology 98, 1269–1277. *The American Society of Anesthesiologists difficult airway algorithm. The guidelines describe this fundamental algorithm and how supraglottic airway devices play a role in the management of the difficult airway.*

Hagberg, C.A., 2001. In: Schwartz, A.J. (Ed.), ASA refresher courses in anesthesiology, Current concepts in the management of the difficult airway, vol. 29 Lippincott Williams & Wilkins, Philadelphia. *A comprehensive review of many supraglottic and subglottic airway devices used to manage the difficult airway.*

Dorsch, J.A., Dorsch, S.E. 2007. Supraglottic airway devices. Understanding anesthesia equipment, ed 5. Lippincott Williams & Wilkins, Philadelphia. *A comprehensive and detailed chapter regarding the components, proper and alternate uses for, and safety issues regarding the LMA family of supraglottic airway devices.*

International Organization for Standardization. 2009. Anaesthetic and respiratory equipment-supralaryngeal airways and connectors, ed 1. BSI. *The first of its kind from the ISO, in this detailed document they provide technical standards for manufacturing and proper use for supraglottic airways and associated equipment. An important read for the anesthetist to ensure safe use of these devices.*

Brain, A.I.J. 1983. The laryngeal mask—a new concept in airway management. Br J Anaesth 55 (8), 801–806. *The article introducing the LMA into the world of anesthesia. An interesting and insightful read.*

Liang, Y., Kimball, W.R., Kacmarek, R.M., et al., 2008. Oral-nasal ventilation during induction of general anesthesia in adult subjects. Anesthesiology 108, 998–1003. *A thought-provoking article questioning some basic tenets of mask ventilation. Perhaps nasal masks will replace the oral-nasal/full-face mask in anesthetic practice.*

Davey, A.J., Diba, A. 2005. Manual resuscitators. Ward's anaesthetic equipment, ed 5. Elsevier Saunders, Philadelphia. *The current chapter excluded manual resuscitators from the discussion of supraglottic airway devices. However, manual resuscitators are important components of the anesthetist's airway equipment, and should be well understood. This chapter, and Chapter 5 in this text, provides an excellent review of these devices.*

References

1. Waldau, T., Larsen, V.H., Bonde, J., 1998. Evaluation of five oxygen delivery devices in spontaneously breathing subjects by oxygraphy. Anaesthesia 53 (3), 256–263.

2. Wheeler, D.W., 2005. Equipment for the inhalation of oxygen and other gases. In: Davey, A.J., Diba, A. (Eds.), Ward's anaesthetic equipment, ed 5. Elsevier Saunders, Philadelphia.

3. Wagstaff, T.A., Soni, N., 2007. Performance of six types of oxygen delivery devices at varying respiratory rates. Anaesthesia 62 (5), 492–503.

4. Al-Shaikh, B., Stacey, S. (Eds.), 2007. Essentials of anaesthetic equipment, ed 3. Churchill Livingstone, Philadelphia.

5. Lampotang, S., Gravenstein, N., Paulus, D.A., et al., 2005. Reducing the incidence of surgical fires: supplying nasal cannulae with sub-100% O_2 gas mixtures from anesthesia machines. Anesth Analg 101 (5), 1407–1412.

6. Yanagidate, F., Dohi, S., 2006. Modified nasal cannula for simultaneous oxygen delivery and end-tidal CO_2 monitoring during spontaneous breathing. Eur J Anaesthesiol 23 (3), 257–260.

7. Sasaki, H., Yamakage, M., Iwasaki, S., et al., 2003. Design of oxygen delivery systems influences both effectiveness and comfort in adult volunteers. Can J Anaesth 50 (10), 1052–1055.

8. Futrell J.W., Jr., Moore, J.L., 2006. The OxyArm: a supplemental oxygen delivery device. Anesth Analg 102 (2), 491–494.

9. Al-Shaikh, B., Stacey, S. (Eds.), 2007. Essentials of anaesthetic equipment, ed 3. Churchill Livingstone, Philadelphia.

10. Davies, P., Cheng, D., Fox, A., et al., 2002. The efficacy of noncontact oxygen delivery methods. Pediatrics 110 (5), 964–967.

11. Somogyi, R., Vesely, A., Azami, T., et al., 2004. Dispersal of respiratory droplets with open vs. closed oxygen delivery masks–implications for the transmission of severe acute respiratory syndrome. Chest 125, 1155–1157.

12. Hui, D., Hall, S., Chan, M., et al., 2007. Exhaled air dispersion during oxygen delivery via a simple oxygen mask. Chest 132, 540–546.

13. Wheeler, D.W., 2005. Equipment for the inhalation of oxygen and other gases. In: Davey, A.J., Diba, A. (Eds.), Ward's anaesthetic equipment, ed 5. Elsevier Saunders, Philadelphia.

14. Wheeler, D.W., 2005. Equipment for the inhalation of oxygen and other gases. In: Davey, A.J., Diba, A. (Eds.), Ward's anaesthetic equipment, ed 5. Elsevier Saunders, Philadelphia.

15. Wheeler, D.W., 2005. Equipment for the inhalation of oxygen and other gases. In: Davey, A.J., Diba, A. (Eds.), Ward's anaesthetic equipment, ed 5. Elsevier Saunders, Philadelphia.

16. Wheeler, D.W., 2005. Equipment for the inhalation of oxygen and other gases. In: Davey, A.J., Diba, A. (Eds.), Ward's anaesthetic equipment, ed 5. Elsevier Saunders, Philadelphia.

17. Wheeler, D.W., 2005. Equipment for the inhalation of oxygen and other gases. In: Davey, A.J., Diba, A. (Eds.), Ward's anaesthetic equipment, ed 5. Elsevier Saunders, Philadelphia.

18. Al-Shaikh, B., Stacey, S. (Eds.), 2007. Essentials of anaesthetic equipment, ed 3. Churchill Livingstone, Philadelphia.

19. Wheeler, D.W., 2005. Equipment for the inhalation of oxygen and other gases. In: Davey, A.J., Diba, A. (Eds.), Ward's anaesthetic equipment, ed 5. Elsevier Saunders, Philadelphia.

20. Bacon, J.P., Farney, R.J., Jensen, R.L., et al., 2000. Nasal continuous positive airway pressure devices do not maintain the set pressure dynamically when tested under simulated clinical conditions. Chest 118 (5), 1441–1449.

21. Dorsch, J.A., Dorsch, S.E., 2008. Understanding anesthesia equipment, ed 5. Wolters Kluwer-Lippincott Williams & Wilkins, Philadelphia.

22. Vassallo, S.A., 2008. Latex allergy. 37th Anesthesia review and update, Harvard Medical School, Boston.

23. Gaba, D.M., Fish, K.J., Howard, S.K. (Eds.), 1994. Crisis management in anesthesiology, Churchill Livingstone, Philadelphia.

24. Morgan, G.E., Mikhail, M.S., Murray, M.J. (Eds.), 2006. Clinical anesthesiology, ed 4. Lange Medical Books/McGraw-Hill, New York.

25. Bagshaw, O.N., Southee, R., Ruiz, K., 1997. A comparison of the nasal mask and the nasopharyngeal airway in paediatric chair dental anaesthesia. Anaesthesia 52 (8), 786–789.

26. Liang, Y., Kimball, W.R., Kacmarek, R.M., et al., 2008. Nasal ventilation is more effective than combined oral-nasal ventilation during induction of general anesthesia in adult subjects. Anesthesiology 108, 998–1003.

27. Capasso, L., Capasso, A., Raimondi, F., et al., 2005. A randomized trial comparing oxygen delivery on intermittent positive pressure with nasal cannulae versus facial mask in neonatal primary resuscitation. Acta Paediatr 94 (2), 197–200.

28. Diba, A., 2005. Airway management devices. In: Davey, A.J., Diba, A. (Eds.), Ward's anaesthetic equipment, ed 5. Elsevier Saunders, Philadelphia.

29. Dorsch, J.A., Dorsch, S.E., 2008. Understanding anesthesia equipment, ed 5. Wolters Kluwer-Lippincott Williams & Wilkins, Philadelphia.

30. Greenland, K., Irwin, M., 2004. The Williams Airway Intubator, the Ovassapian Airway and the Berman Airway as upper airway conduits for fiberoptic bronchoscopy in patients with difficult airways. Curr Opin Anaesthesiol 17, 505–510.

31. Dorsch, J.A., Dorsch, S.E., 2008. Understanding anesthesia equipment, ed 5. Wolters Kluwer-Lippincott Williams & Wilkins, Philadelphia.

32. Stoelting, R.K., Miller, R.D. (Eds.), 2006. Basics of anesthesia, ed 5. Churchill Livingstone, New York.

33. Brimacombe, J., Berry, A., 1998. The cuffed oropharyngeal airway for spontaneous ventilation anaesthesia. Clinical appraisal in 100 patients. Anaesthesia 53 (11), 1074–1079.

34. Ezri, T., Szmuk, P., Evron, S., et al., 2004. Nasal versus oral fiberoptic intubation via a cuffed oropharyngeal airway (COPA) during spontaneous ventilation. J Clin Anesth 16 (7), 503–507.

35. Koga, K., Sata, T., Kaku, M., et al., 2001. Comparison of no airway device, the Guedel-type airway and the cuffed oropharyngeal airway with mask ventilation during manual in-line stabilization. J Clin Anesth 13, 6–10.

36. Audu, P., Loomba, N., 2004. Use of cuffed oropharyngeal airway (COPA) for awake intracranial surgery. J Neurosurg Anesthesiol 16, 144–146.

37. Laffon, M., Ferrandiere, M., Mercier, C., et al., 2001. Transient lingual and glossopharyngeal nerve injury: a complication of cuffed oropharyngeal airway. Anesthesiology 94 (4), 719–720.

38. Lee, C.M., Song, K.S., Morgan, B.R., et al., 2001. Aspiration of an oropharyngeal airway during nasotracheal intubation. J Trauma 50 (5), 937–938.

39. Diba, A., 2005. Airway management devices. In: Davey, A.J., Diba, A. (Eds.), Ward's anaesthetic equipment, ed 5. Elsevier Saunders, Philadelphia.

40. Roberts, K., Whalley, H., Bleetman, A., 2005. The nasopharyngeal airway: dispelling myths and establishing the facts. Emerg Med J 22, 394–396.

41. Dorsch, J.A., Dorsch, S.E., 2008. Understanding anesthesia equipment, ed 5. Wolters Kluwer-Lippincott Williams & Wilkins, Philadelphia.

42. Dorsch, J.A., Dorsch, S.E., 2008. Understanding anesthesia equipment, ed 5. Wolters Kluwer-Lippincott Williams & Wilkins, Philadelphia.

43. Al-Shaikh, B., Stacey, S. (Eds.), 2007. Essentials of anaesthetic equipment, ed 3. Churchill Livingstone, Philadelphia.

44. Ahmed, J., Marucci, D., Cochrane, L., et al., 2008. The role of the nasopharyngeal airway for obstructive sleep apnea in syndromic craniosynostosis. J Craniofac Surg 19 (3), 659–663.

45. Ryan, D.W., Weldon, O.G., Kilner, A.J., 2002. Nasopharyngeal airway continuous positive airway pressure: a method to wean from or avoid mechanical ventilation in adults. Anaesthesia 57 (5), 475–457.

46. Schade, K., Borzotta, A., Michaels, A., 2000. Intracranial malposition of nasopharyngeal airway. J Trauma 49 (5), 967–968.

47. Steinbruner, D., Mahoney, P.F., 2007. Intracranial placement of a nasopharyngeal airway in a gun shot victim. Emerg Med J 24, 311.

48. Dorsch, J.A., Dorsch, S.E., 2008. Understanding anesthesia equipment, ed 5. Wolters Kluwer-Lippincott Williams & Wilkins, Philadelphia.

49. Brain, A.I.J., 1983. The laryngeal mask—a new concept in airway management. Br J Anaesth 55 (8), 801–806.

50. Dorsch, J.A., Dorsch, S.E., 2008. Understanding anesthesia equipment, ed 5. Wolters Kluwer-Lippincott Williams & Wilkins, Philadelphia.

51. ASA, 2003. Practice guidelines for management of the difficult airway. Anesthesiology 98, 1269–1277.

52. Brain, A.I.J., 1984. The laryngeal mask airway—a possible new solution to airway problems in the emergency situation. Arch Emerg Med 1, 229–232.

53. Diba, A., 2005. Airway management devices. In: Davey, A.J., Diba, A. (Eds.), Ward's anaesthetic equipment, ed 5. Elsevier Saunders, Philadelphia.

54. Brain, A.I.J., 1990. Proper technique for insertion of the laryngeal mask. Anesthesiology 73, 1053.

55. Ng, A., Raitt, D., Smith, G., 2002. Induction of anesthesia and insertion of a laryngeal mask airway in the prone position for minor surgery. Anesth Analg 94, 1194–1198.

56. Dingeman, R.S., Goumnerova, L.C., Goobie, S.M., 2005. The use of a laryngeal mask airway for emergent airway management in a prone child. Anesth Analg 100, 670–671.

57. Klock, P.A., Ovassapian, A., 2008. Airway management. In: Longnecker, D.E., Brown, D.L., Newman, M.F. (Eds.), Anesthesiology, ed 1. McGraw-Hill, New York.

58. Klock, P.A., Ovassapian, A., 2008. Airway management. In: Longnecker, D.E., Brown, D.L., Newman, M.F. (Eds.), Anesthesiology, ed 1. McGraw-Hill, New York.

59. Al-Shaikh, B., Stacey, S. (Eds.), 2007. Essentials of anaesthetic equipment, ed 3. Churchill Livingstone, Philadelphia.

60. ISO, 2009. Anaesthetic and respiratory equipment—supralaryngeal airways and connectors. BSI, .

61. Stoelting, R.K., Miller, R.D. (Eds.), 2006. Basics of anesthesia, ed 5. Churchill Livingstone, New York.

62. Popat, M. (Ed.), 2009. Difficult airway management, ed 1. Oxford University Press, New York.

63. Klock, P.A., Ovassapian, A., 2008. Airway management. In: Longnecker, D.E., Brown, D.L., Newman, M.F. (Eds.), Anesthesiology, ed 1. McGraw-Hill, New York.

64. Brain, A.I.J., Verghese, C., Strube, P.J., 2000. The LMA "ProSeal"—a larngeal mask with an oesophageal vent. Br J Anaesth 84 (5), 650–654.

65. Cook, T.M., Gibbison, B., 2007. Analysis of 1000 consecutive uses of the ProSeal laryngeal mask airway(TM) by one anaesthetist at a district general hospital. Br J Anaesth 99 (3), 436–439.

66. Evans, N.R., Garner, S.V., James, M.F.M., et al., 2002. The ProSeal laryngeal mask: results of a descriptive trial with experience of 300 cases. Br J Anaesth 88 (4), 534–539.

67. O'Connor, C.J., Stix, M.S., Valade, D.R., 2005. Glottic insertion of the ProSeal(TM) LMA occurs in 6% of cases: a review of 627 patients. Can J Anaesth 52 (2), 199–204.

68. Brimacombe, J., Richardson, C., Keller, C., et al., 2002. Mechanical closure of the vocal cords with the laryngeal mask airway Proseal(TM). Br J Anaesth 88 (2), 296–297.

69. Janakiraman, C., Chethan, D.B., Wilkes, A.R., et al., 2009. A randomized crossover trial comparing the i-gel supraglottic airway and classic laryngeal mask airway. Anaesthesia 64, 674–678.

70. Liew, G., John, B., Ahmed, S., 2008. Correspondence: aspiration recognition with an i-gel airway. Anaesthesia 68, 778–789.

71. Michalek, P., Donaldson, W.J., Hinds, J.D., 2009. Correspondence: tongue trauma associated with the i-gel supraglottic airway. Anaesthesia 64, 687–697.

72. Uppal, V., Fletcher, G., Kinsella, J., 2009. Comparison of the i-gel with the cuffed tracheal tube during pressure-controlled ventilation. Br J Anaesth 102 (2), 264–268.

73. Theron, A.D., Loyden, C., 2008. Correspondence: nerve damage following the use of an i-gel supraglottic airway device. Anaesthesia 63, 433–445.

74. Popat, M. (Ed.), 2009. Difficult airway management, ed 1. Oxford University Press, New York.

75. Ferson, D.Z., Rosenblatt, W.H., Johansen, M.J., et al., 2001. Use of the intubating LMA-Fastrach(TM) in 254 patients with difficult-to-manage airways. Anesthesiology 95, 1175–1181.

76. Lu, P., Yang, C., Ho, A.C.Y., et al., 2000. The intubating LMA: a comparison of insertion techniques with conventional tracheal tubes. Can J Anaesth 47 (9), 849–853.

77. Kannan, S., Chestnutt, N., McBride, G., 2000. Intubating LMA guided awake fiberoptic intubation in severe maxillofacial injury. Can J Anaesth 47 (10), 989–991.

78. Asai, T., Eguchi, Y., Murao, K., et al., 2000. Intubating laryngeal mask for fiberoptic intubation—particularly useful during neck stabilization. Can J Anaesth 47 (9), 843–848.

79. Dorsch, J.A., Dorsch, S.E., 2008. Understanding anesthesia equipment, ed 5. Wolters Kluwer-Lippincott Williams & Wilkins, Philadelphia.

80. Dorsch, J.A., Dorsch, S.E., 2008. Understanding anesthesia equipment, ed 5. Wolters Kluwer-Lippincott Williams & Wilkins, Philadelphia.

81. Popat, M. (Ed.), 2009. Difficult airway management, ed 1. Oxford University Press, New York.

82. Liu, E.H.C., Goy, R.W.L., Chen, F.G., 2006. The LMA CTrach (TM), a new laryngeal mask airway for endotracheal intubation under vision: evaluation in 100 patients. Br J Anaesth 96 (3), 396–400.

83. Goldman, A.J., Rosenblatt, W.H., 2006. The LMA CTrach (TM) in airway resuscitation: six case reports. Anaesthesia 61, 975–977.

84. Abdi, W., Ndoko, S., Amathieu, R., et al., 2008. Evidence of pulmonary aspiration during difficult airway management of a morbidly obese patient with the LMA CTrach (TM). Br J Anaesth 100 (2), 275–277.

85. Mort, T.C., 2006. Laryngeal mask airway and bougie intubation failures: the Combitube as a second rescue device for in-hospital emergency airway management. Anesth Analg 103, 1264–1266.

86. Diba, A., 2005. Airway management devices. In: Davey, A.J., Diba, A. (Eds.), Ward's anaesthetic equipment, ed 5. Elsevier Saunders, Philadelphia.

87. Morimoto, F., Yoshioka, T., Ikeuchi, H., et al., 2001. Use of esophageal tracheal Combitube to control severe oronasal bleeding associated with craniofacial injury: case report. J Trauma 51, 168–169.

88. Keller, C., Brimacombe, J., Boehler, M., et al., 2002. The influence of cuff volume and anatomic location on pharyngeal, esophageal, and tracheal mucosal pressures with the esophageal tracheal Combitube. Anesthesiology 96, 1074–1077.

89. McGlinch, B.P., Martin, D.P., Volcheck, G.W., et al., 2004. Tongue engorgement with prolonged use of the esophageal-tracheal Combitube. Ann Emerg Med 44, 320–322.

90. Zamora, J.E., Saha, T.K., 2008. Combitube rescue for cesarean delivery followed by ninth and twelfth cranial nerve dysfunction. Can J Anaesth 55 (11), 779–784.

91. Gaitini, L.A., Vaida, S.J., Mostafa, S., et al., 2001. The Combitube in elective surgery: a report of 200 cases. Anesthesiology 94, 79–82.

92. Asai, T., Shingu, K., 2005. The laryngeal tube. Br J Anaesth 95 (6), 729–736.

93. Yildiz, T.S., Solak, M., Toker, K., 2007. Comparison of laryngeal tube with laryngeal mask airway in anaesthetized and paralysed patients. Eur J Anaesthesiol 24, 620–625.

94. Zand, F., Amini, A., Sadeghi, S.E., et al., 2007. A comparison of the laryngeal tube-S (TM) and Proseal (TM) laryngeal mask during outpatient surgical procedures. Eur J Anaesthesiol 24, 847–851.

95. Casati, A., Vinciguerra, F., Spreafico, E., et al., 2004. The new PAXpress airway device during mechanical ventilation in anaesthetized patients: a prospective, randomized comparison with the laryngeal mask airway. Eur J Anaesthesiol 21, 663–672.

96. Casati, A., Vinciguerra, F., Spreafico, E., et al., 2004. Cardiovascular changes after extraglottic airway insertion: a prospective, randomized comparison between the laryngeal mask or new PAXpress. J Clin Anesth 16, 342–346.

97. Khan, R.M., Jafri, F., Huda, W., et al., 2002. Acute transient sialadenopathy after use of PAXpress (TM). Anesth Analg 95 (6), 1819–1820.

98. Ahmed, S.M., Khan, R.M., Maroof, M., et al., 2008. Assessment of manoeuvers required for successful blind tracheal intubation through the PAXpress (TM). Anaesthesia 63, 32–35.

Chapter 7

Intubation Equipment

Zhongcong Xie, Ali Diba, and Zhipeng Xu

Introduction

Visualization of the vocal cords for intubation was popularized by Sir Robert Macintosh and Sir Ivan Magill in the early 1940s. It was during the insertion of a Boyle-Davis gag that Macintosh conceived the idea of his laryngoscope, which is still the most popular design in use today and has spawned a wide variety of modifications. It consists of a blade that elevates the lower jaw and tongue, a light source near the tip of the blade to illuminate the larynx, and a handle to apply force to the blade. The handle also contains the power supply (battery) for the light source. The light comes on when the blade, which is hinged on the handle, is opened to the right angle position. Macintosh designed a slightly curved blade (Figure 7-1) with a small bulbous tip that was designed to be inserted anterior to the base of the epiglottis in an adult. The child and infant blades were not designed by him, and he criticized them as being anatomically wrong and unnecessary. Some blades for adults and many of those intended specifically for children or infants tend to be either straight or with a small shallow curve at the tip only. These are designed to be inserted deeper into the pharynx and posterior to the epiglottis and hence the blades are correspondingly longer.

In practice, the term "laryngoscope," when not further described, is still largely synonymous with the rigid retractor type and more specifically the Macintosh-designed laryngoscope.[1] The term "difficult laryngoscopy" therefore is largely used to describe any situation where only a suboptimal view

of the larynx can be obtained with these default devices.[2] For practical usefulness, given the variety of devices now routinely available, this term should always be further defined to describe the circumstances.

Intubation Devices

Intubation devices may be considered under two broad categories:

1. Retractor type, such as the Macintosh laryngoscope, reliant on retracting tissues to create an uninterrupted sight line between the operator and the objective. Fiberoptics may be used in the light source of these types.
2. Fiberoptic laryngoscopes, where a fiberoptic channel transmits the image from the tip of the device to an eyepiece or camera, thus allowing the observer to effectively view around an obstruction. Fiberoptic channels are hence also necessitated for light transmission to the objective.[3] Two types of fiberoptic laryngoscopes can be categorized:
   a. Rigid fiberoptic laryngoscopes, such as the Upsher and Bonfils, where the fiberoptic viewing channel is rigid and usually encased in metal. This type of device can also force tissues aside and act as a retractor. Accepted wisdom has it that such instruments require less dexterity and expertise to use than their

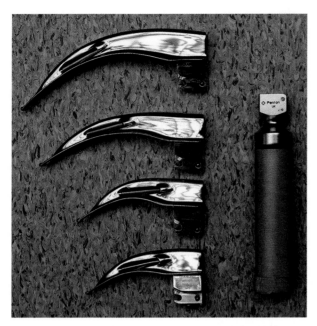

Figure 7–1   Macintosh laryngoscope with 4 sizes of interchangeable blade.

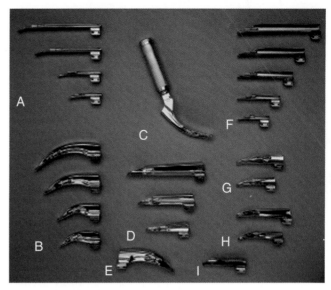

Figure 7–2   Laryngoscope blades. **A,** Miller pattern: 3 large; 2, adult; 1, infant; 0, premature. **B,** Macintosh pattern: 4, large; 3, adult; 2, child; 1, infant/neonate. **C,** Macintosh polio blade. **D,** Soper pattern: adult, child, infant. **E,** Macintosh pattern left-handed version. **F,** Wisconsin: large, adult, child, infant/neonate. **G,** Robertshaw's: infant and neonate. **H,** Seward: child and infant. **I,** Oxford: infant.

flexible counterparts. Other devices recently introduced include the Airtraq optical laryngoscope and the video laryngoscopes such as the GlideScope, Storz C-MAC, and the McGrath. Some of these are not truly fiberoptic devices—using mirrors or cameras and light sources at their tips instead—but they perform in fundamentally the same way.

    b. Flexible fiberoptic laryngoscopes. The viewing bundle (plus light transmission bundles and an optional instrument channel) is wrapped in a flexible casing. The instrument can thus be made to follow anatomical spaces and will bend as necessary to negotiate almost any route. The term "flexible fiberoptic bronchoscope" is synonymous in use.

Retractor-Type Laryngoscopes

Figure 7-2 shows some of the wide variety of blades currently available. The choice of blade for routine use is probably largely a matter of personal preference. One must keep in mind that the technique for laryngoscopy is different for the various designs of blade and differing designs may offer better views of the larynx in a given patient. Most blades are detachable from the handle for ease of cleaning and change of blade size where appropriate. The "hook on" connection for the blade, which allows easy detachment, is very convenient and was developed by Welch Allyn Ltd. in the early 1950s. Two new standards, ISO 7376/3 (green system) and ISO 7376/1 (red system) have been developed, which allow blades from different manufacturers to be interchangeable, but they have not been universally adopted. In both, the bulb is housed within the handle and light is transmitted through an optical "bundle" to the tip of the blade. Their difference lies in the dimensions of the hinges and the relative positions of the light sources. Prisms and mirrors are sometimes added to these devices to overcome the principal shortcoming of

this class of device, namely that the operator's eye and patient's larynx must be in a straight line with no interposed tissue. So far, such modifications have not proven popular or lasting.

Features of Modern Laryngoscopes

Figure 7-3 shows a typical instrument with a hook on type Macintosh blade. Some specific points are highlighted next:

- Detachable blade for interchangeable blade designs and ease of cleaning and sterilization.
- Light source sited within the handle. Much brighter xenon gas-filled bulbs are used to compensate for light loss during transmission.
- Light projection via a shaped bundle of glass fibers.[4] The bundle may be manufactured as an integral part of the blade, or may be detachable so that should it become damaged or opaque it may be replaced separately. Fiberoptic bundles are prone to degradation resulting in poor illumination and difficult laryngoscopy.
- Disposable single-use blades are gaining popularity as an alternative to the costly and damaging process of sterilization of laryngoscope blades. These may be of plastic or even metal design but must not be assumed to perform as well as traditional instruments.[5,6]

Laryngoscopy

Figure 7-4 shows how correct positioning of the patient's head with craniocervical extension and lower cervical flexion, the position known as "sniffing the morning air," allows the laryngoscope to retract the tongue and associated soft tissues into the elastic and distensible area of the floor of the mouth. Such positioning provides an uninterrupted sight line through

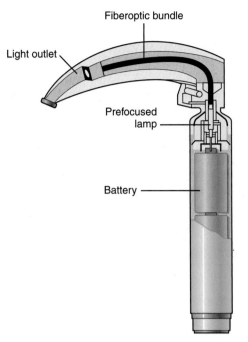

Fiberoptic bundle

Light outlet

Prefocused lamp

Battery

Figure 7–3 The Heine fiberoptic laryngoscope. Note that the lamp is within the handle, thus avoiding unreliable electrical contacts between the handle and the blade.

to the larynx.[7] Poor views of the larynx can be predicted from this model where there is:

- Inadequate craniocervical movement or jaw opening; reduction in volume of distensible area below floor of mouth as with small receding mandible or following scarring or distortion of the anatomy as from head and neck surgery or radiotherapy; tumors of tongue base or larynx; or swelling of the posterior pharyngeal wall.

The handle of the laryngoscope is used to lift (i.e., force is applied in the direction of the handle rather than using the handle as a lever). Curved blades are designed for the tip to be inserted into the vallecula with the standard Macintosh blade being inserted to the right of the tongue and hence forcing it to the left side, whereas the straight blade may be inserted posterior to the epiglottis and is particularly useful for small children and adults with a large floppy epiglottis. Different laryngoscope blades require different techniques for viewing the larynx, which must be learned to exploit that device. For example, the Henderson blade (Karl Storz, Germany), a modification of the Miller blade, is a long straight bladed design with a "C"-shaped cross section (Figure 7-5) and is intended to be inserted to the right of the tongue with the head turned aside in effectively a "retromolar" fashion. A poor view obtained with one design does not predict a poor view with a different design.

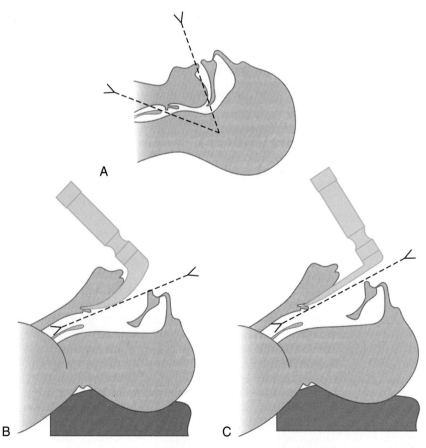

Figure 7–4 **A,** The "V" shape of the normal upper airway. The larynx cannot be seen from outside the mouth. **B,** With the neck extended at the upper cervical spine and the jaw protruded forward by the laryngoscope blade, the "V" extends into a straight line bringing the larynx into view. The curved blade fits between the base of the tongue and the epiglottis. **C,** The straight blade passes behind the epiglottis.

Laryngoscopes
Macintosh Blade

The Macintosh blade is probably the most commonly used blade in adults in the United States. The Macintosh blade is curved to better fit in the mouth and oropharyngeal cavity.[8] There is a small bulbous structure at the tip of the Macintosh blade designed to help lift the larynx (Figure 7-6). In the United

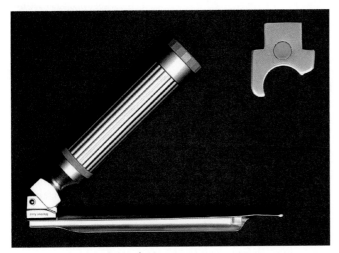

Figure 7–5 The Henderson blade attached to a laryngoscope handle (here in "ISO Green system" fitting). Inset shows the blade from the rear to demonstrate the profile in cross-section.

States, the Macintosh blade is available in the following sizes: large (Macintosh 4), adult (Macintosh 3½ and 3), child (Macintosh 2), infant (Macintosh 1), and premature (Macintosh 0).

During intubation, the Macintosh blade is traditionally inserted from the right side of the mouth. Then the tongue can be pushed over to the left side of mouth by the blade. The tip of the Macintosh blade is placed in the space between the base of the tongue and the pharyngeal surface of the epiglottis (compared with placement of the Miller blade beneath the laryngeal surface of epiglottis). The laryngoscope with Macintosh blade then can be lifted upwards, which will elevate the larynx and allow visualization of the vocal cords. The use of the Macintosh blade may cause less trauma to the teeth and allow more room for the passage of the endotracheal tube than other blades. The Macintosh blade may also cause less bruising of the epiglottis because the tip of Macintosh blade usually does not come in contact with it.

Even though the Macintosh blade is one of the most commonly used blades, it has some limitations. In the case of a difficult airway, the Macintosh blade may not be able to provide good exposure made possible by the lifting of the epiglottis that can be accomplished with the Miller blade. However, the choice of a laryngoscope is based on the operator's training and experience.

Miller Blade

The Miller blade is another of the most commonly used blades.[9] As can be seen in Figure 7-7, the tip of the Miller blade is straight. The size of the Miller blade can be large (Miller 4),

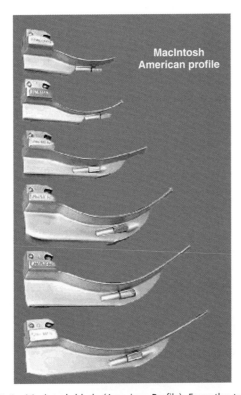

Figure 7–6 Macintosh blade (American Profile). From the *top to bottom*: Macintosh newborn size 0, Macintosh infant size 1, Macintosh child size 2, Macintosh medium adult size 3, Macintosh extended adult size 3½, Macintosh large adult size 4. *(From LaryngoscopeBlades. (website): http://www.laryngoscopeblades.com/photo-amer%20mac-5-5052-xx.htm.) Accessed 8-2-2010.*

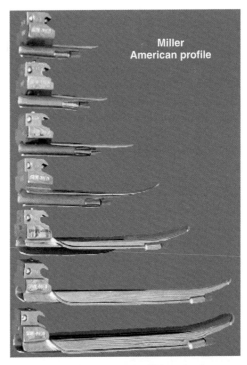

Figure 7–7 Miller blade (American Profile). From the *top to bottom*: Miller small premature size 00 light on left side, Miller premature size 0 light on left side, Miller infant size 1 light on left side, Miller small child size 1½ light on left side, Miller child size 2 light on right side, Miller medium adult size 3 light on right side, Miller large adult size 4 light on right side. *(From LaryngoscopeBlades. (website): http://www.laryngoscopeblades.com/photo-amer%20miller-5-5062-xx.htm.) Accessed 8-2-2010.*

adult (Miller 3), child (Miller 1½ and 2), infant (Miller 1), or premature infant (Miller 0 and 00).

Even though the Miller blade is commonly used, the choice of laryngoscope is based on personal preference and experience. Nevertheless, this blade is often used to intubate neonates and infants. The tip of the Miller blade is placed beneath the laryngeal surface of the epiglottis (versus in the space between the base of the tongue and pharyngeal surface of epiglottis if the Macintosh blade is used). Miller blade can potentially provide better exposure of the glottic opening and less frequent need for a stylette during intubation. The limitations of the Miller blade include the possibility of causing more trauma to the teeth and epiglottis than the Macintosh blade, and its insertion may result in less room for the passage of the endotracheal tube.

Macintosh Polio Blade

This variation alters the angle between the blade and the handle and is developed to allow the laryngoscope blade to be more easily inserted into the mouth in patients with abnormal anatomy. The polio blade is essentially a modification of the Macintosh blade. It is also a curved blade, but the angle between the polio blade and the handle is approximately 120 degrees (rather than 90 degrees in the Macintosh blade). This design allows the easier introduction of the blade into the mouth in specific groups of patients (Figure 7-8). The polio blade was originally designed to intubate patients housed in iron lungs. Now it can be used in patients who are using respirators or wearing body jackets, who are obese, have breast hypertrophy, or have restricted neck mobility. The polio blade can facilitate the introduction of the blade into the mouth of these patients. However, this blade does not have all the mechanical advantages of the Macintosh blade. For example, only a small amount of force can be applied when the polio blade is used. Alternatively, a regular Macintosh blade with a "stunted" handle may be used in the special patient populations discussed above. Another device, the Patil-Syracuse handle allows multiple locking positions for the blade attachment point.

Left-Handed Macintosh Blade

The "reversed" Macintosh blade has a flange on the right side in a mirror image of the traditional Macintosh blade. The right-sided flange can help move the tongue to the right side of the mouth when the blade is inserted from the left side of the mouth.[10,11] Although the reversed Macintosh is held in the right hand, manufacturers still named it a "left-handed" blade, referring to the hand which passes the endotracheal tube.

The left-handed Macintosh blade can be used by left-handed individuals. It can also be used for patients whose

anatomy (e.g., lesions on the right side of the tongue, mouth, or face) makes it difficult to insert the Macintosh blade from the right side of the mouth or for patients who need to be intubated while lying on their right side. The left-handed Macintosh blade is inserted from the left side of the mouth and then swept from left to right, creating a space on the left side of the mouth. The left-handed Macintosh blade comes in No. 3 size only. The use of the left-handed laryngoscope blade requires training and practice. A right-handed person (and most experienced left-handed anesthesiologists) would find the device most odd in use.

McCoy Blade

This blade is based on a standard Macintosh blade modified by the insertion of a hinge to give an adjustable tip that is operated by a lever on the handle (Figure 7-9). The blade is inserted in the normal way, and if the view is obscured, the tip can be flexed so that it further elevates the vallecula and epiglottis. Opinion is divided as to its usefulness: although the design has been commercially successful and it is included in many algorithms for airway management, there is little evidence to support its widespread use. The effect on laryngeal view is variable depending on whether the base of tongue and vallecula is already optimally elevated.[12] In difficult direct laryngoscopy, activation of the tip may improve the laryngeal view, where there is a grade 3 Cormack and Lehane view but is unlikely to do so where the epiglottis cannot be seen (grade 4 view).[13] Additionally, the incidence of grade 2 or worse views may be increased compared with a standard Macintosh blade even without activation of the tip.[14,15]

Soper Blade

The Soper blade is a straight blade that has a shallow vertical portion with a flange facing to the left (Figure 7-10). This blade comes in adult and pediatric sizes, it is generally used to intubate neonates and infants. This blade combines the "Z" section (outward flange) of the Macintosh design with the pattern common to Miller and other straight blades. The broad flat shape makes it easier to restrict the neonate and premature infant's tongue movement. The tip of Soper blade

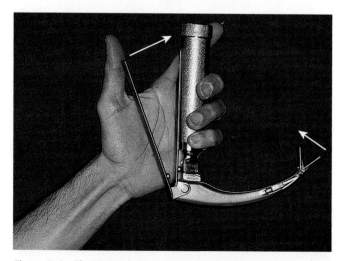

Figure 7–9   The McCoy laryngoscope with the lever deployed to show flexion of the tip.

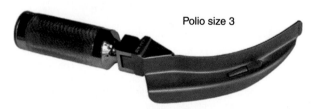

Polio size 3

Figure 7–8   Macintosh polio blade. *(Cited from LaryngoscopeBlades. (website): http://www.laryngoscopeblades.com/photo-polio-5-3077-53.htm.)* Accessed 8-2-2010.

is placed beneath the laryngeal surface of the epiglottis. Soper blades can be technically difficult to use and can lead to longer intubation times compared with straight blades.

Wisconsin Blade

The Wisconsin blade is a straight blade with a flange that is curved to form two thirds of a circle in cross section (Figure 7-11). The Wisconsin blade can extend slightly toward the distal portion of the blade, therefore increasing the visual field and reducing the possibility of trauma during intubation. Five sizes are available, and the Wisconsin blade is designed primarily for use in infants. After successful exposure of vocal cords by this blade, the endotracheal tube can then be inserted through the circle of the cross section or through the mouth for intubation. The space for the passage of the endotracheal tube can be too narrow when the Wisconsin blade is inserted.

Robertshaw Blade

The Robertshaw blade was originally designed for use in infants and children, but can be also used in adults. It is gently curved over the distal third and is designed to lift the epiglottis indirectly in the manner similar to the Macintosh blade (Figure 7-12). During intubation, the tip of the Robertshaw blade is placed in the space between the base of the tongue and the pharyngeal surface of the epiglottis. Usually, a size 0 Robertshaw blade is used for low-birth-weight babies because

the tapered tip of the blade makes it easier to navigate in a small pharynx. The Robertshaw blade allows binocular vision, and therefore the blade can potentially cause less trauma due to better visualization of the anatomy. The Robertshaw blade can be particularly useful in nasotracheal intubation because it provides a better view of the pharynx when Magill forceps are introduced into the mouth.[16,17]

Seward Blade

The Seward blade has a straight tongue with a curve near the tip, and a small reverse Z-shaped flange (Figure 7-13). The Seward blade is especially useful for nasotracheal intubation because the shape of the Seward blade allows Magill forceps to be introduced into the mouth with a minimum loss of view. It is intended for use in children younger than 5 years old.

Oxford Infant Blade

The Oxford infant blade has a straight tongue that curves up slightly at the tip. This blade has a "U shape" at the proximal end, and the distal part is open. It tapers from a maximum width at the proximal end to the smallest width at the tip (Figure 7-14). It is suitable for premature infants, babies, and children up to the age of 4. There is sufficient overhang on the open side, helping to prevent the lips from obscuring vision. The broad, flat lower surface is useful in a small child with a cleft palate. Similar to the Wisconsin blade, the space between the corner of the mouth and the Oxford infant blade can be

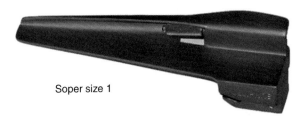

Soper size 1

Figure 7–10 Soper blade. *(From LaryngoscopeBlades. (website): http://www. laryngoscopeblades.com/photo-soper-5-5080-01.htm.) Accessed 8-2-2010.*

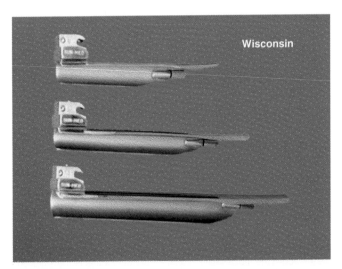

Wisconsin

Figure 7–11 Wisconsin blade. *(From LaryngoscopeBlades. (website): http:// www.laryngoscopeblades.com/photo-wisconsin-5-5057-xx.htm.) Accessed 8-2-2010.*

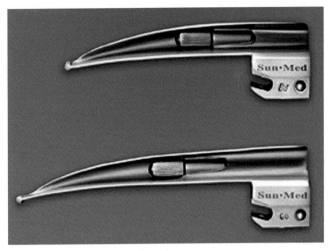

Figure 7–12 Robertshaw's blade. *(From LaryngoscopeBlades. (website): http://www.laryngoscopeblades.com/photo-robertshaw.htm.) Accessed 8-2-2010.*

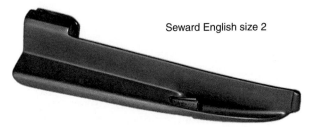

Seward English size 2

Figure 7–13 Seward blade. *(From LaryngoscopeBlades. (website): http:// www.laryngoscopeblades.com/photo-seward-5-5079-02.htm.) Accessed 8-2-2010.*

narrow, which could make it difficult to insert the endotracheal tube into the mouth.

Rigid Fiberoptic Laryngoscopes

Bullard Laryngoscope and UpsherScope

These two devices have a broadly similar curve to the blade and use fiberoptics to transmit the image from the tip to the eyepiece. They are designed to elevate the jaw without the need for neck extension and for use in patients with limited mouth opening. Physical alignment of the oral, pharyngeal, and laryngeal axes for direct visualization of the glottis is not required, unlike in direct laryngoscopy. Whereas the Bullard (Figure 7-15) uses a fixed stylet to carry the tracheal tube, the UpsherScope (Figure 7-16) has a "C"-shaped cross section, which will transmit a tube of the correct diameter to emerge in the field-of-view of the device.

Unlike the flexible fiberoptic bronchoscopes, which have become the "gold standard" for management of the difficult intubation, this class of device—in addition to "viewing around corners"—allows tissues to be retracted to create a view of the larynx. Intubation is, of course, limited to the oral route and applications are far more limited than for flexible fiberoptic intubation. However, there may be a particular

indication for these devices in the setting of difficult flexible fiberoptic intubation (where lack of intraoral space and collapsed overlying tissues are the cause of difficulty—as in patients with obstructive sleep apnea). It must be added this is usually only a problem in anesthetized patients, but awake intubation is not always possible, for example, in children. The utility of these devices is perhaps at best limited to patients with midline airways because they are dependent upon a largely normal supraglottic anatomy. In some studies of the Bullard scope, successful tube placement was achieved in at least 90% of patients and exceeded 80% on the first pass in patients deemed prospectively to have difficult airways.[18] To use the Bullard scope, lubricate the stylet that is attached to the device and insert it into the endotracheal tube until its tip extends out of the Murphy's eye. Held in the left hand, the scope is then advanced midline over the tongue into the pharynx. The device should be advanced as a single unit with the endotracheal tube held by the scope. With gentle elevation of the Bullard handle, the blade tip should retract the epiglottis to visualize the glottis. The endotracheal tube is then slid into the glottic opening, and the rest of the device is gently removed from the mouth.

The WuScope is a further example of this type. This class of device appears to enjoy greater popularity in the United States,[19] but its exact role is not obvious given its expense, the need for training and that it does not obviate the need for flexible fiberoptic intubation.[20, 21]

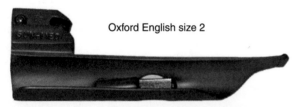

Oxford English size 2

Figure 7–14   Oxford infant blade. *(From LaryngoscopeBlades. (website): http://www.laryngoscopeblades.com/photo-oxford-5-5078-01.htm.) Accessed 8-2-2010.*

Bonfils Intubating Fiberscope

Recently, there has been a growing interest in a new type of device called an intubating fiberoptic stylette ("optical stylette") for the management of difficult airways. Several new optical stylette devices have been introduced in the last decade. These optical stylettes use fiberoptic imaging elements in an intubation stylette design. These devices offer an advantage of both the viewing capability of fiberoptics and the familiar handling of a stylette. Examples include the Shikani stylette, Bonfils fiberscope, and the Machida Portable Stylette Fiberscope.[22]

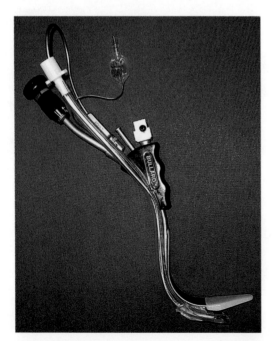

Figure 7–15   The Bullard laryngoscope (depicted with the light handle not connected).

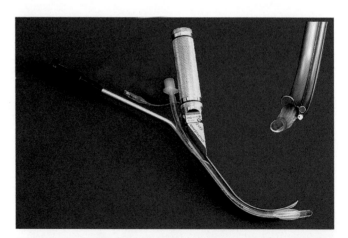

Figure 7–16   The UpsherScope. Figure shows the tip of the device with endotracheal tube emerging. The large light transmission fiberoptic bundle lies above the much smaller coherent bundle for image transmission. The size of the distal viewing lens explains why fiberoptic devices are so easily foiled by secretions.

The thin, stylettelike Bonfils (Figure 7-17), with a gentle anterior curve at its distal third, is designed to be introduced from the side of the mouth in a "retromolar approach" using the nondominant hand to elevate the jaw and tongue.[22] The preloaded tracheal tube is advanced off the device once it has been manipulated into the larynx. The design of this device and technique of intubation really dictate that a camera and monitor is used on the eyepiece. There exists limited published experience to advocate a role for this device.[23] It does, however, herald the arrival of a number of devices that may be seen as a crossover category of a "seeing stylette" falling between a laryngoscope and an intubation aid.[24]

Video Laryngoscopes

Video laryngoscopes have gained popularity as an alternative to conventional Macintosh and Miller blades because they can provide improved visualization of the glottic structures compared with direct laryngoscopy. These indirect-viewing video laryngoscopes use a video camera mounted on a scope used to provide access and view to the larynx for intubation and use fiberoptic imaging to improve the results. Currently, several video laryngoscopes are used in clinical practice, including the McGrath portable video laryngoscope, GlideScope, Storz C-MAC, Daiken Medical Coopdech C-scope vlp-100, Pentax AWS Scope, and Berci DCI (Figure 7-18).

The Storz C-MAC

The Storz C-MAC system consists of a TV camera that is incorporated into the handle of the laryngoscope, delivering an enlarged image of the laryngeal structures.[25] A short fiber light bundle exits from the handle and is inserted into a guide tube, recessed 40 mm from the tip of the blade to avoid interference during advancement of the endotracheal tube. A fiber light cord and a TV cable exit at the other end of the handle and connect to the light source and the camera control unit.[26] The image is enhanced using digital signal processing. The intubating blade is a modified Macintosh designed to accommodate the image light bundle. Thus after the blade is introduced into the mouth and into the vallecula in the same manner one would use the conventional Macintosh blade, the operator can observe the anatomy on the attached screen rather than alongside the blade. The blade is interchangeable and available in several sizes. It can be autoclaved for repeat use. The C-MAC blade offers an improved view of the glottic structures compared with the conventional laryngoscope likely due to the fact that the image fiber bundle tip is positioned close to the blade tip, thus changing the viewpoint from a straight line of sight that is required for conventional laryngoscopy.[26] The disadvantages of the Storz blade and other fiberoptic devices is that blood or secretions can quickly obscure the view. The Storz laryngoscope generally overcomes this by placing the lens about one third of the way back from the tip of the blade. However, the view can still become impaired in patients who have a lot of blood or secretions in the oropharynx. Fogging of the lens seems to be a particular problem with this device.

The Glidescope

The Glidescope Video Laryngoscope has an integrated high resolution camera and a 60-degree blade angulation designed to view the anterior glottis without the need for direct line of sight. This unique angulation of the blade provides access by reducing the need to remove the tongue from the line of sight to the larynx. The video camera in the Glidescope is placed back at the midpoint of the blade for protection from blood and secretions obscuring the view during intubation. The device has a heated lens and a wide camera viewing angle of 50 degrees. The GlideScope Cobalt is a single-use video laryngoscope and is available in four sizes; GlideScope Ranger is a reusable device and is available in two sizes. The GlideRite Rigid Stylet is used with the GlideScope Video Laryngoscope that has an ability to conform to the GlideRite blade shape, eliminating the need to manually shape the stylette to fit down the airway.

A recent study[27] compared the effectiveness of the three commonly used video laryngoscopes (GlideScope Ranger, Storz V-MAC, and McGrath VLS) in morbidly obese patients. This study showed that the Storz Video Laryngoscope had a better overall operator satisfaction score and shorter intubation time, fewer intubation attempts, and less need for additional intubation adjuncts compared with the other two devices.

Airtraq Laryngoscope
Description

The Airtraq laryngoscope (Figure 7-19) is a newly developed laryngoscope that provides a magnified wide-angle (panoramic) view without the need for an external monitor. Airtraq is a first disposable optical laryngoscope, and its visual guiding system can be used for both routine and complex airways. The high definition optical system provides a magnified view during laryngoscopic procedures. The Airtraq is an anatomically shaped laryngoscope with two separate channels: (1) the optical channel contains a high definition optical system, and (2) the guiding channel holds the endotracheal tube and guides it through the vocal cords.

The Airtraq has a built-in antifog system, and a low temperature light source at the tip of the blade (provides illumination up to 90 minutes), and can be used with any standard endotracheal tube. Available in several sizes, the Airtraq

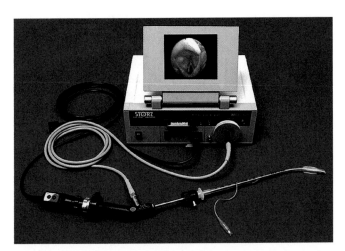

Figure 7–17 The Bonfils laryngoscope with endotracheal tube loaded and connected to a compact combination light source and image-processing unit. *(Both courtesy Karl Storz, Germany.)*

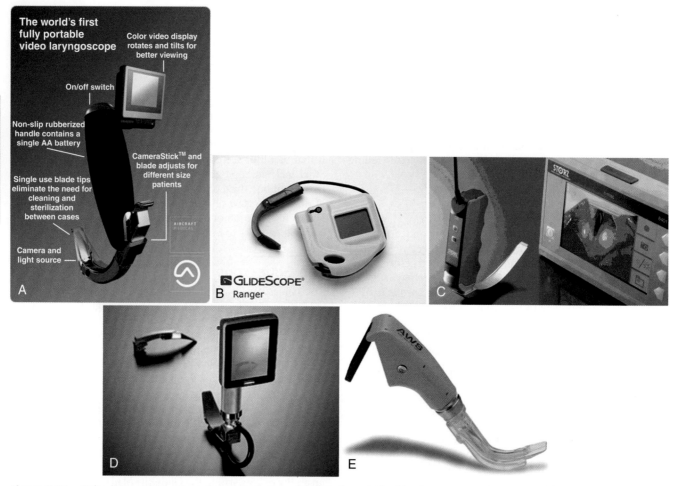

Figure 7–18   Video laryngoscopes. From the *top to bottom*: **A,** McGrath portable video laryngoscope series 5. **B,** GlideScope Ranger. **C,** Storz C-MAC. **D,** Coopdech Video Laryngoscope. **E,** Pentax Airway Scope AWS-S100 video laryngoscope. (**A,** *From LMA. (website): http://www.lmana.com/ mcgrath.php;* **B,** *from GlideScope Ranger, medGadget (serial online): http://medgadget.com/archives/2006/10/glidescope_rang.html;* **C,** *from Karl Storz. (website): http:// www.karlstorz.de/;* **D,** *from http://www.daiken-iki.co.jp/english/contents/products/main_an_9.html;* **E,** *from Clear and disposable: a new laryngoscope from Pentax, medGadget (serial online): http://medgadget.com/archives/2006/12/clear_and_dispo.html.) Accessed 8-2-2010.*

accommodates standard endotracheal tubes varying from an inner diameter size of 2.5 to 8.5 mm, and can be enhanced with a small, reusable clip-on video system to allow viewing on an external monitor. There are several sizes of Airtraq. Regular size (3, blue) is for size 7.0- to 8.5-mm endotracheal tube; small size (2, green) is for size 6.0- to 7.5-mm endotracheal tube; pediatric size (1, pink) is for size 3.5-to 5.5-mm endotracheal tube; and infant size (0, gray) is for size 2.5- to 3.5-mm endotracheal tube. The device requires a minimum mouth opening of 16 mm for a small size and 18 mm for the regular size, and 12.5 mm for a pediatric size. For nasal intubation, there are infant nasal (white) and nasal tracheal intubations (orange). Finally, there is one for double lumen endotracheal tubes (yellow).

The Airtraq allows visualization of the vocal cords without the need to hyperextend the patient's neck. Thus Airtraq can offer a view of the glottic opening without the need to align the laryngeal, pharyngeal, and oral axes, and can facilitate intubation in any position. This is potentially useful in patients with unstable cervical spine fractures, jaw immobility, anterior larynx, and trauma. The device is designed so that the image is transmitted to a proximal viewfinder through a combination of lenses and a prism, rather than fiber optics. This helps visualize the glottis, surrounding structures, and the tip of the tracheal tube.

The device provides a magnified angular view of the larynx and adjacent structures and has a short learning curve. Its uses, according to the manufacturer, include endotracheal tube placement or exchange and placement of other devices such as gastric tubes. A study by Maharaj et al[28] compared the Airtraq-assisted intubation with that using the conventional Macintosh laryngoscope. The Airtraq reduced the duration of intubation attempts, the need for additional maneuvers, and improved the intubation difficulty score. In addition, tracheal intubation using Airtraq reduced the degree of hemodynamic stimulation and minor trauma compared with the Macintosh laryngoscope. A recent study by Malin et al[29] examined the utility of the Airtraq laryngoscope after failed conventional tracheal intubation. The authors concluded that in patients with difficult airways, following failed conventional orotracheal intubation, Airtraq allows securing the airway in 80% of cases mainly by improving glottis view. However, the Airtraq does not guarantee successful intubation in all instances, especially in case of laryngeal and/or pharyngeal obstruction.

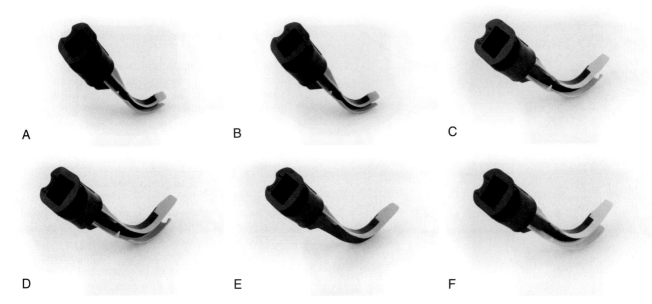

A B C

D E F

Figure 7–19 Airtraq laryngoscope. From the *top to bottom:* **A,** Airtraq for orotracheal intubation infant (gray, size 0, ET tube size 2.5-3.5). **B,** Airtraq for orotracheal intubation pediatric (pink, size 1, ET tube size 3.5-5.5). **C,** Airtraq for orotracheal intubation small (green, size 2, ET tube size 6.0-7.5). **D,** Airtraq for orotracheal intubation regular (blue, size 3, ET tube size 7.0-8.5). **E,** Airtraq for nasal tracheal intubation (orange). **F,** Airtraq for double lumen endobronchial tubes (yellow, for 35-41F standard and hooked). *(From AIRTRAQ. Airtraq sizes, (website): http://www.airtraq.com/airtraq/newmodel.list-prod.action?type=root&menuId=newmodel.)* Accessed 8-2-2010.

Before Airtraq is used, the LED (light emitting diode) light should be turned on and the endotracheal tube should be lubricated and placed into the channel. The antifogging system for the optics is activated by turning on the LED light, which must be turned on at least 30 seconds before use. After induction of general anesthesia, the patient head should be placed in the neutral position. The tip of the Airtraq device should also be lubricated and inserted in the mouth in the midline above the center of the tongue. Care should be taken not to push the tongue toward the larynx. If the surrounding structures (e.g., epiglottis) cannot be recognized, the operator should withdraw the Airtraq slightly and lift up. The tip of the Airtraq blade can be placed either in the vallecula (Macintosh style) and the epiglottis lifted by elevating the blade, or the blade can be placed under the epiglottis (Miller style). The Airtraq handle should be elevated straight up. Once the vocal cords are visualized, the endotracheal tube can be advanced slowly. After successful intubation, the device is slowly withdrawn from the mouth.

Flexible Fiberoptic Laryngoscopes (Bronchoscopes)

The first use of flexible fiberoptic technology in airway management can be credited to Dr. Peter Murphy[30] who in 1967 reported using the newly invented choledochoscope for intubation of the trachea.[31] Although initially ignored by fellow anesthesiologists, the approach now forms the mainstay of managing difficult intubations. The terms flexible intubating fiberscope, endoscope, scope, bronchoscope, laryngoscope, and even tracheoscope are used interchangeably with varying degrees of precision. For anesthetic purposes it is more important that the device has the correct length, insertion tube diameter, and operating channel for the intended task.

The flexibility of these devices means that they can be made to follow virtually any anatomic space to return an image of the objective. Because they presume no particular anatomic arrangement (i.e., unlike rigid devices there is no preshaped curve) and can work around most obstructions, the technique of flexible fiberoptic intubation has become a "gold standard" for management of the difficult laryngoscopy. This has tended to create the impression that the technique is the solution to all difficulties with the airway, but this is clearly not so. These devices are simply for seeing around corners. For example, where the tracheal additus, however small, can be seen directly by the naked eye (with a simple retractor type of laryngoscope), use of a fiberoptic scope can only make the situation more difficult. Additionally, the very small objective lens with its wide angle of view is easily obscured by blood and secretions.[32-34]

Principles and Design

The pathways through which the illumination and the image pass consist of thousands of very fine glass fibers, each typically of the order of 10 μm in diameter. Each fiber consists of a central glass core surrounded by a thin cladding of another type of glass with a different refractive index to that of the core glass. As a result of the difference in refractive indices at the interface of the two materials, light entering the glass fiber undergoes total internal reflection along the length of the fiber to emerge at the other end (Figure 7-20). For the purpose of transmitting illumination, the arrangement of the fibers is unimportant. For image transmission, however, the arrangement of the fibers relative to one another must be identical at either end of the bundle, as each fiber carries a tiny portion of the overall image (in the same way that many small dots make up the printed image in a newspaper). This is called a coherent bundle.

The fibers are so fine that they are easily flexible and they are lubricated so that they can move relative to each other.

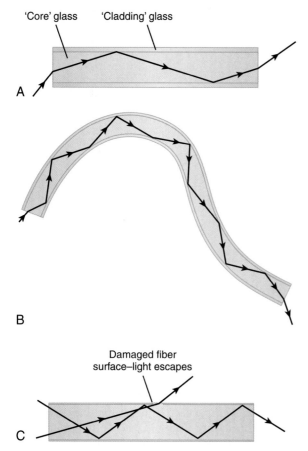

'Core' glass   'Cladding' glass

A

B

Damaged fiber
surface—light escapes

C

Figure 7–20 **A,** A single optical fiber. Note that the light ray is repeatedly internally reflected from the interface between the core and cladding glass. **B,** If the fiber is curved, the ray is still internally reflected within it. **C,** If the surface of the fiber is damaged, the light ray may not be totally internally reflected, and some light may escape from the bundle.

The whole bundle may therefore be flexed. The insertion tube of the typical flexible fiberoptic scope (Figure 7-21) carries:

- Two light bundles, running from the umbilical cord to the tip of the scope
- One image bundle, running from the eyepiece and its lens system to the objective lens at the tip of the scope
- One "working" or "biopsy" channel of a width dictated by the primary purpose of the endoscope
- Two angulation wires, which control the more flexible tip of the device

These then are held together with a stainless steel spiral wrap followed by a stainless steel braid before being covered in a waterproof material to give a rigid cross section while allowing overall flexibility (Figure 7-22). The fiberscope, while able to bend in any plane, is axially rigid to twisting forces, thus rotation of the control handle results in similar rotation of the tip of the device. This forms the basis for control of the tip, which can be rotated so that angulation of the tip, which occurs in only one plane relative to the scope, can be made to take place in any direction. The fiberscope uses a powerful external cold light source so that the tissues are not damaged by radiant heat. Modern scopes have a detachable light cable, which can be replaced by a miniature battery operated light source (Figure 7-23). These are not normally powerful enough for use with the video camera. The working channel is used to inject drugs or for suction via the valved port, which may be connected to an external high vacuum source.

Usage

Intubating fiberscopes are available with insertion tubes ranging in size from 2.5-mm external diameter for use in infants (this smallest size usually has no working channel) through to more than 6 mm with proportionately larger

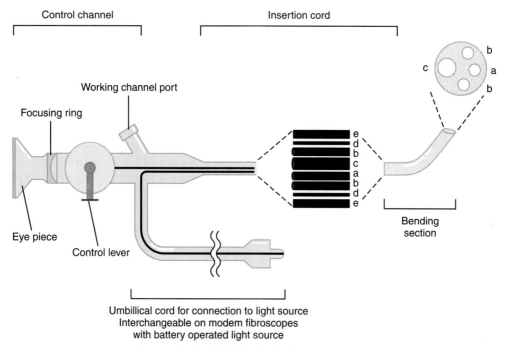

Control channel   Insertion cord

Working channel port

Focusing ring

Eye piece

Control lever

Bending
section

Umbillical cord for connection to light source
Interchangeable on modem fibroscopes
with battery operated light source

Figure 7–21 Schematic diagram of flexible intubating fiberscope. **A,** Coherent fiberoptic bundle for image transmission. **B,** Light transmission bundles for illumination. **C,** Working channel. **D,** Angulation wires. **E,** Outer casing with spiral wrap and flexible steel braid.

working channels. Only the channels on the largest sizes (primarily bronchoscopes with working channels of more than 2 mm) are wide enough for aspirating secretions or blood with any effectiveness; oropharyngeal secretions are best tackled with a handheld Yankauer sucker. A device with an external diameter of about 3.5 mm is optimal for use in adults (and nonspecialist pediatric practice) giving the best combination of:

- Stiffness for ease of insertion
- Bore, for access and endotracheal tube compatibility

The advent of the miniature video camera has revolutionized fiberoptic endoscopy. Without doubt, flexible fiberoptic endoscopes should be used with a video monitor rather than with the operator's eye at the eyepiece. The advantages in anesthetic practice are:

- Improvements in teaching techniques
- More useful assistance from the anesthetic team (e.g., jaw lift is better maintained by someone who can see the effect it has on the laryngeal view enjoyed by the endoscopist)
- More holistic view of patient's condition if not squinting through an eyepiece and hence less goal obsessed approach to endoscopy/intubation
- Facility to record images for review and documentation
- Operator comfort

Figure 7-24 shows the arrangement of components on a typical fiberoptic intubation cart (Figure 7-25). Ideally a

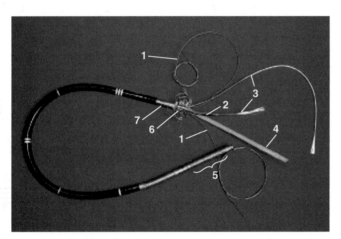

Figure 7–22 Cutaway photograph of Olympus intubating fiberscope to show constituent parts. *(1)* Angulation wire; *(2)* coherent bundle; *(3)* light transmission bundle; *(4)* working channel; *(5)* bending section; *(6)* spiral steel wrap; *(7)* flexible steel braid.

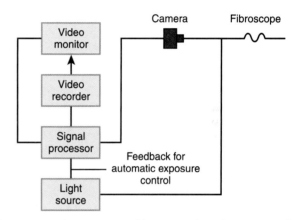

Figure 7–24 Arrangement and interconnection of components for a fiberoptic intubation trolley. The video monitor can toggle between a live image from the camera or playback recorded images.

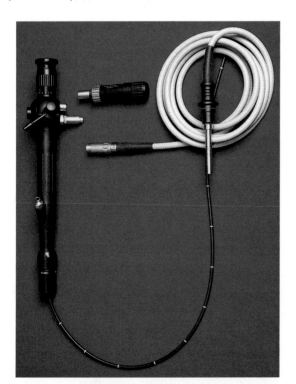

Figure 7–23 Storz "portable" flexible intubating fiberscope with choice of battery operated and remote light sources.

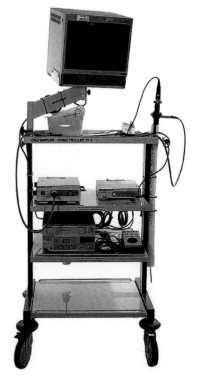

Figure 7–25 A fiberoptic intubation cart.

printer able to capture still images from the outputs of the signal processor or video recorder should also be incorporated.

The advent of the miniaturized CCD (charge-coupled device, effectively the "retina" of modern electronic cameras), has allowed a new generation of flexible fiberoptic endoscopes where the CCD is placed at the distal tip of the instrument and hence the image suffers no loss from transmission along a length of glass fibers while also dispensing with the expense of the coherent fiber image transmission bundle (Figure 7-26). Such instruments obviously do not have an eyepiece and must be used with a monitor. They are not yet commonplace for airway applications.

Care of the Fiberscope

The fiberscope must be cleaned and disinfected following use. Modern devices are fully immersible, this being denoted on Olympus equipment by a blue ring around the control handle (a red ring denotes an item such as the light cable which may be autoclaved). This is best done immediately following use by gentle scrubbing with a nailbrush and soapy water to remove adherent material followed by immersion in a proprietary sterilizing solution and final rinsing in sterile water. Automated machines exist that can even produce a printed paper trail to document completion of the process. The working channel also should be cleaned with a dedicated brush and subsequently flushed with appropriate solutions. Some manufacturers produce immersible and even autoclavable cameras.

Fiberoptic Intubation

Fiberoptic laryngoscopy via the oral or nasotracheal route may be performed on both the awake or asleep patient.[35] In a patient who is awake following suitable topical anesthesia or nerve block, the fiberscope may be inserted and advanced behind the tongue and into the larynx. Once in the trachea, a tracheal tube, which has been previously loaded onto the fiberscope, is advanced off the scope to lie within the trachea, and the fiberscope is then removed. The patient may be encouraged to protrude the tongue and or lower jaw to create

the space in the pharynx necessary for the fiberscope to be able to view, identify, and advance through the airway. Deep respiration assists the identification of the larynx, if needed. Intubation of the awake rather than anesthetized patient is often easier for these reasons. Sedation may be used for additional patient comfort but must not render the patient uncooperative or unconscious. For this reason "sedation" based on the titration of short-acting opiates is preferable in that the antitussive and analgesic properties are useful while the patient retains the ability to obey commands and pharmacological antagonism is easy in case of overdosage.

Training. Competent fiberoptic intubation requires a modicum of training and the maintenance of skills by regular deployment. "Hand-eye coordination" and the control of the fiberscope may be learned by most with only brief practice on an obstacle course, which may be made in minutes from items found in any anesthetic room. Thereafter, familiarization with airway anatomy as seen through the fiberscope is necessary. This is simplest and safest on the apneic, anesthetized, paralyzed, and preoxygenated patient.[36] If necessary, an assistant provides jaw thrust or tongue traction.

Associated Equipment

Endotracheal tubes. The ideal tube for intubation over a fiberscope would have a narrow kink-resistant wall with a blunt tapered tip that fits the fiberscope closely so that it may follow the scope easily without snagging on nasal or laryngeal structures,[37] although this, of course, would severely restrict the size of endotracheal tube orifice. Dedicated tubes are not yet available despite several prototype designs,[38] but Rüsch produces a centering aid designed to bridge the gap from scope to tube. Tubes with soft short bevels, such as the Portex Ivory and the Mallinckrodt reinforced ranges with an internal diameter of 6 to 7 mm, are generally preferred by specialists.

Bite blocks. For oral intubation, a dental prop or bite block (Figure 7-27) ensures that expensive fiberscopes are not inadvertently bitten and is comfortable for the patient.

Conduit airways aim to make oral intubation easier by centering the insertion point in the mouth and delivering the fiberscope closer to the larynx and acting as a supraglottic

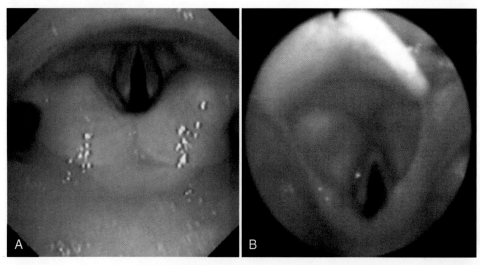

Figure 7–26   **A,** Image from an Olympus digital video intubating fiberscope. **B,** Image from optical system for comparison of image quality.

airway (Figure 7-28). A number of open or split designs are available that allow the fiberscope to be separated from the airway after tracheal insertion so as not to limit the size of the tracheal tube that may be used for intubation. They also function as a bite block; but they make tongue protrusion, which is a helpful maneuver, quite difficult. They are not necessary for awake intubation, and for the trainee endoscopist they remove too much of the learning that may be gained from an oral intubation. The laryngeal mask airway (LMA), as a conduit, is discussed separately later.

Tongue forceps with atraumatic broad-ridged rubber inserts at the tip (Figure 7-29) allow tongue retraction to create space in the pharynx for fiberoptic intubation and for injection of local anesthesia.

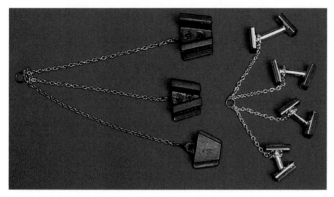

Figure 7–27 Dental props are ideal bite blocks for awake oral intubation because they allow tongue protrusion. The all rubber McKesson pattern on the left is more comfortable.

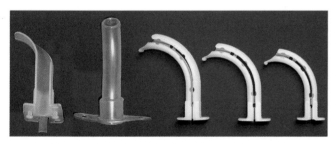

Figure 7–28 From *left to right*: VBM intubating airway and bite block, Optosafe airway, Bermann airways in 3 sizes.

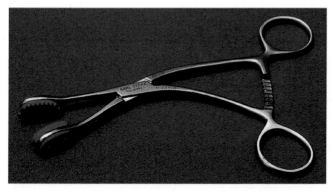

Figure 7–29 Tongue forceps, surprisingly tolerable.

Ventilation/intubation masks. Where anesthesia is maintained with an inhalational anesthetic, endoscopy may be performed through a mask or elbow with a silicone rubber diaphragm with an orifice that stretches to accommodate an endotracheal tube (Figure 7-30). Such arrangements are difficult to use.

Aintree intubation catheter (AIC) (Figure 7-31). Developed in Liverpool as "a ventilation-exchange bougie" and first described in 1996,[39] the AIC allows fiberoptic intubation through the LMA or other supraglottic airway. Produced as a single use device by Cook, it is a 56-cm-long hollow plastic catheter that will fit over fiberscopes of 4.0 mm or less in diameter, leaving the bending section of the scope free. The assembly is easily passed through the LMA and into the trachea (Figure 7-32). The fiberscope is then removed, followed by the LMA to leave the AIC in the trachea. Tracheal tubes of 7 mm or greater may then be railroaded into place over this. For rescue oxygenation, a 15-mm male ISO adapter and female Luer-Lok adapter are both supplied in the package. Great care must be taken if jetting through wide-bore catheters placed close to the carina, for which a much lower driving pressure should be used. The combination of LMA, AIC, and fiberscope constitutes a powerful technique for airway management because:

- The standard LMA is a familiar device with a proven track record for establishing an airway.
- The cuff of the LMA seals off the larynx from any blood or debris emanating from above, thus the conduit protects the fiberscope from its greatest adversaries.
- An absolute minimum of fiberoptic skills are needed to rapidly manipulate the scope into the trachea, the technique is thus within reach of almost all anesthesiologists.

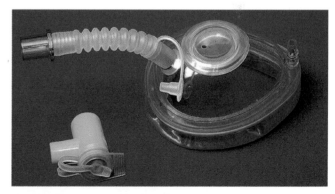

Figure 7–30 Face mask with perforated silicone membrane allowing fiberoptic intubation on the anesthetized patient; the tube can be forced through the membrane, which is replaceable. The same effect can be achieved using the Mainz Universal Adapter (pictured alongside) and an ordinary face mask.

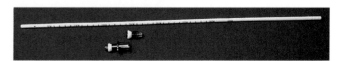

Figure 7–31 The Aintree Intubation Catheter, with Rapi-fit Luer-Lok and ISO 15-mm adaptors.

Aids for Intubation/Tube Exchange

Bougies and Stylettes

Occasionally during direct laryngoscopy, the larynx may be only partially visualized or may be hidden behind the epiglottis and beyond reach with the normal curvature of an endotracheal tube. Intubation may then possibly be accomplished by either:

- Altering the curvature of the endotracheal tube using a malleable plastic-coated metal stylette
- Initially inserting a long thin gum-elastic bougie (GEB) and using this as a guide over which the tube may be passed (railroaded) into the trachea (Figure 7-33, *A*)

Credited to Dr P. Hex Venn, the GEB with a coudé tip was designed in the 1970s as the Eschmann Tracheal Tube Introducer (now available from Portex Ltd).[40,41] It has been hugely successful due to the angled tip and the memory of the material for holding a curve. Latto, in his surveys of anesthetic practice, has found the preference for the GEB over other aids at difficult direct laryngoscopy to rise from 45% in 1984 to 100% in 1996.[42] Repeated autoclaving rapidly renders the material brittle. The new single-use versions of the device in plastic do not generally have the same characteristics in use,[43] and some are particularly unsatisfactory. On the other hand, the disposable version is sufficiently inexpensive to be deployed ubiquitously, requires little skill, and is quick to use. Cook has recently marketed the single use hollow

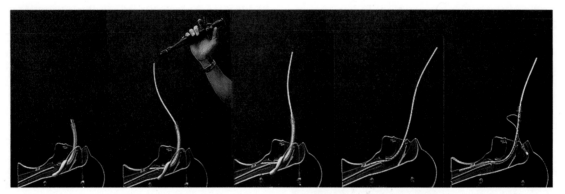

Figure 7–32   Photographic sequence to show fiberoptic intubation through the LMA using the Aintree Intubation Catheter.

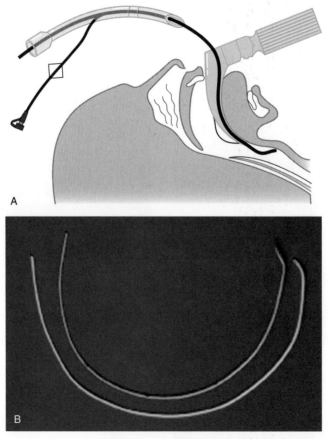

Figure 7–33   **A,** The endotracheal tube introducer with coudé tip. **B,** The Eschmann gum-elastic bougie and the blue single use Frova introducer from Cook.

Frova introducer (Figure 7-33, *B*), which has a comparable "memory" to the GEB, and is supplied with a Rapifit adapter in Luer-Lok and ISO 15 mm fittings to allow gas sampling or oxygenation.

Lightwand

A logical development from the stylette, is the lighted stylette, allowing transillumination of the neck tissues as a further aid to positioning of the tracheal tube (Figure 7-34).

Trachlight

The Trachlight (Laerdal Medical) develops the concept one stage further by aiming to allow intubation using only transillumination of the neck (without laryngoscopy). As such, the stylette is more rigid than the aforementioned aids to permit some tissue retraction. A reusable handle houses the battery to which are particularly bright disposable lighted stylettes of three different sizes attached. The tracheal tube is mounted on the stylette assembly and is held by the handle (Figure 7-35). The stylet is bent into an L-shape before insertion into the mouth. The nondominant hand grips and elevates the lower incisors and mandible and the Trachlight is rotated into place to transilluminate the thyroid cartilage in the midline. At this point the wire core of the stylette is held steady while the rest of the Trachlight and the tracheal tube are advanced into the trachea. The device is then disconnected from the tracheal tube and removed. Intubation in skilled hands appears simple and smooth enough for routine use, with some reporting only a 1% failure rate.[44,45] Sore throat and tracheal bleeding are reported,[45] and use in obese patients may not be straightforward.[46]

Airway Exchange Catheter

Endotracheal tubes can be more safely exchanged over a catheter or bougie that has been inserted through the tube into the trachea, the new tube then being simply railroaded into place over this. The Airway Exchange Catheter (AEC) by Cook (Figure 7-36) is long enough to allow comfortable removal of a nasal endotracheal tube without risk of losing hold of the catheter. Where there may be doubt as to the ability of a postoperative or sedated patient to maintain a patent airway following extubation, the AEC may be inserted first and extubation may be performed "over" this. It may then be removed some hours later or used to guide reintubation if needed. Because the plastic remolds at body temperature and the AEC is smaller than the tracheal tube it replaces, it is usually well tolerated[47] by patients. Oxygen insufflation or jetting is possible as with the Aintree Catheter (see previous discussion).

Retrograde Intubation

The larynx may be intubated in the following manner: A cannula is introduced diagonally through the cricothyroid membrane with its tip pointing cephalad. A flexible "J"-tipped guidewire is then passed via the cannula and the tip grasped in the mouth or as it emerges from the nose. A plastic catheter is passed over the J tip and back along the guidewire to provide a stiffer guide over which the endotracheal tube may be railroaded. An epidural catheter and other disparate items may be used where the dedicated kit (Figure 7-37) is not available. This "lo-tech" approach also has the advantage of being applicable where blood and secretions prevent use of the flexible fiberscope. The very high entry point of the wire into the trachea means that only a short length of tracheal tube can be inserted before it abuts the anterior tracheal wall, and the guidewire must be withdrawn (proximally). To ensure the ability to insert the tube further into the trachea before withdrawing the wire, a gum elastic bougie may be inserted through the endotracheal tube once it is within the trachea (Figure 7-38), or the emerging guidewire from the larynx may be introduced up the operating channel of a flexible fiberscope with a preloaded tracheal tube.

Magill Forceps

These are ergonomically designed forceps, the handles of which fit comfortably into the operator's right hand like a pair of scissors (Figure 7-39). The tips are spatulate and ridged for

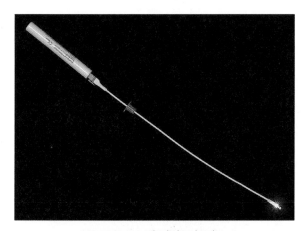

Figure 7–34   The lighted stylet.

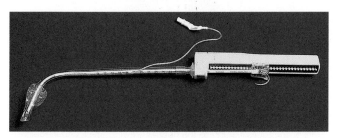

Figure 7–35   The Trachlight prepared for intubation.

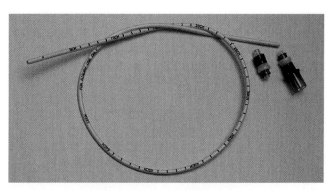

Figure 7–36   The Cook Airway Exchange Catheter with Rapi-Fit adaptors.

gripping the tip of an endotracheal tube so that it can be lifted from the back of the pharynx and into the larynx.

Drug Delivery Systems

Nebulizing sprays are used for the topical application of local anesthetic solutions (e.g., 4% lidocaine to the larynx and trachea). The principles of the Forrester spray are shown in Figure 7-40. When the reservoir bulb is compressed, air is blown into the chamber containing the solution. This forces the latter up and along a narrow bore delivery tube to the tip of the apparatus. The rest of the air from the bulb is directed to the tip where it mixes with and nebulizes the solution. These

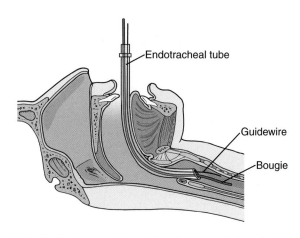

Figure 7–38   To assist in ensuring that the tracheal tube follows down the trachea after removal of the guidewire, a gum elastic bougie can be introduced through the tracheal tube first.

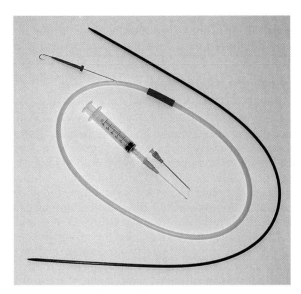

Figure 7–37   A retrograde intubation kit, the principal components of which are a stiff guidewire with a soft flexible J tip and an introducing cannula. A 70-cm 11F-Teflon catheter runs over the guidewire to give extra stiffness for railroading the endotracheal tube.

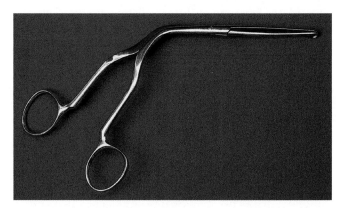

Figure 7–39   Magill's intubating forceps.

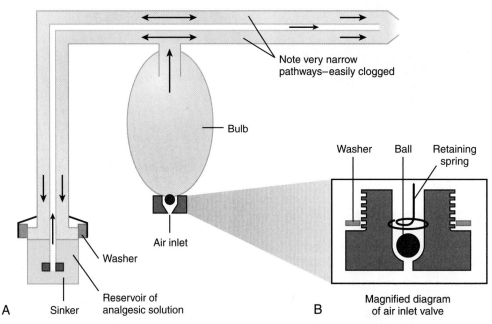

Figure 7–40   The Forrester spray. **A,** Working principles. Note that the diameters of the tubes leading to the nozzles are very small, and if analgesic solution is allowed to collect and crystallize out in this area, the spray will be blocked. **B,** The air inlet valve.

sprays tend to block if they are not cleaned shortly after use because the solution remaining at the nozzle dries out, leaving crystals that block the small orifice. This may be avoided by rinsing them out with distilled water or spirit, before cleaning and disinfecting for subsequent usage. The same principles are used in atomizers which utilize pressurized oxygen to drive the nebulization (Figure 7-41). For use through the fiberscope, single use dispensers are available with controlled dosing of drug from a small syringe using oxygen as the propellant. The Mucosal Atomization Device (Wolfe Tory Medical; Salt Lake City) (Figure 7-42) simply relies on forcing solution through a very narrow orifice for atomization. Lidocaine is available for topical use as a 4% solution or as a 10% solution in a multidose metered dispenser (Figure 7-43). Despite the small volume delivered (0.1 mL) because of the concentration of drug, care must be taken to prevent overdosage, particularly in children.

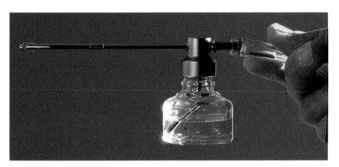

Figure 7–41   Oxygen powered atomizer.

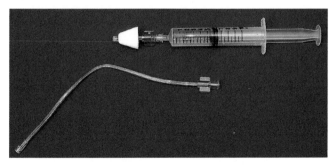

Figure 7–42   The Mucosal Atomization Device, *above* with syringe attached for intranasal application and *below* for intraoral and laryngeal use.

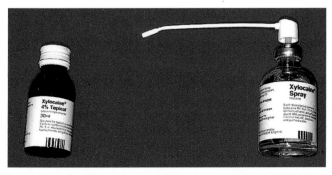

Figure 7–43   10% solution lidocaine in an oily base presented as a metered spray dispenser giving 10 mg lidocaine per spray (0.1 mL). The 4% solution is ideal for topical analgesia of the larynx and trachea.

References

1. Stoelting, R.K., Miller, R.D. (Eds.), 1994. Basics of anesthesia, ed 3. Churchill Livingstone, London.
2. Latto, I.P., Vaughan, R.S. (Eds.), 1997. Difficulties in tracheal intubation, ed 2. Elsevier Saunders, London.
3. Popat, M.T. (Ed.), 2001. Practical fibreoptic intubation, Butterworth-Heinemann, Boston.
4. Skilton, R.W.H., Parry, D., Arthurs, G.J., et al., 1996. A study of the brightness of laryngoscope light. Anaesthesia 51 (7), 667–672.
5. Twigg, S.J., McCormick, B., Cook, T.M., 2003. Randomized evaluation of the performance of single-use laryngoscopes in simulated easy and difficult intubation. Br J Anaesth 90 (1), 8–13.
6. Evans, A., Vaughan, R.S., Hall, J.E., et al., 2003. A comparison of the forces exerted during laryngoscopy using disposable and nondisposable laryngoscope blades. Anaesthesia 58 (9), 869–873.
7. Stoelting, R., Miller, R. (Eds.), 2006. Basics of anesthesia, ed 5. Churchill Livingstone, New York.
8. Stone, D.J., Gal, T.J., 2000. Airway management. In: Miller, R.D. (Ed.), Miller's anesthesia, ed 5. Churchill Livingstone, London.
9. Hagberg, C.A. (Ed.), 2007. Benumof's airway management, ed 2. Elsevier Mosby, Philadelphia.
10. Mace, S. (Ed.), 2008. Challenges and advances in airway management, an issue of emergency medicine clinics, Elsevier Saunders.
11. Hung, O., Murphy, M. (Eds.), 2007. Management of the difficult and failed airway, ed 1. McGraw-Hill Professional, New York.
12. Levitan, R.M., Ochroch, E.A., 1999. Explaining the variable effect on laryngeal view obtained with the McCoy laryngoscope. Anaesthesia 54 (6), 599–601.
13. Chisholm, D.G., Calder, I., 1997. Experience with the McCoy laryngoscope in difficult laryngoscopy. Anaesthesia 52 (9), 906–908.
14. Leon, O., Benhamou, D., 1998. Improvement of glottis visualization with a McCoy blade. Ann Fr Anesth Reanim 17 (1), 68–71.
15. Cook, T.M., Tuckey, J.P., 1996. A comparison between the Macintosh and the McCoy laryngoscope blades. Anaesthesia 51 (10), 977–980.
16. Orebaugh, S.L. (Ed.), 2006. Atlas of airway management: techniques and tools, ed 1. Lippincott Williams & Wilkins.
17. Finucane, B.T., Santora, A.H. (Eds.), 2003. Principles of airway management, ed 3. Springer, New York.
18. Pollack, C.V., Tiffany, B.R., Carty, J.P., et al., 1998. Teaching residents new airway management techniques: initial emergency department experience with the Bullard laryngoscope. Ann Emerg Med 32, S13.
19. Foley, L.J., Ochroch, E.A., 2000. Bridges to establish an emergency airway and alternate intubating techniques. Crit Care Clin 16 (3), 429–444.
20. Pearce, A.C., Shaw, S., Macklin, S., 1996. Evaluation of the UpsherScope. A new rigid fibrescope. Anaesthesia 51 (6), 561–564.
21. Fridrich, P., Frass, M., Krenn, C.G., et al., 1997. The UpsherScope in routine and difficult airway management: a randomized, controlled clinical trial. Anesth Analg 85 (6), 1377–1381.
22. Liem, E.B., Bjoraker, D.G., Gravenstein, D., 2003. New options for airway management: the intubating fiberoptic stylets. Br J Anaesth 91 (3), 408–418 (review).
22. Halligan, M., Charters, P., 2003. A clinical evaluation of the Bonfils intubation fibrescope. Anaesthesia 58 (11), 1087–1091.
23. Wong, P., Lawrence, C., Pearce, A., 2003. Intubation times for using the Bonfils intubation fibrescope. Br J Anaesth 91 (5), 757.
24. Liem, E.B., Bjoraker, D.G., Gravenstein, D., 2003. New options for airway management: intubating fiberoptic stylets. Br J Anaesth 91 (3), 408–418.
25. Kaplan, M.B., Ward, D.S., Berci, G., 2002. A new video laryngoscope - an aid to intubation and teaching. JCA 14, 620–626.
26. Kaplan, M.B., et al., 2006. Comparison of direct and video-assisted views of the larynx during routine intubation. JCA 18, 357–362.
27. Maassen, R., et al., 2009. A comparison of three videolaryngoscopes: the Macintosh laryngoscope blade reduces, but does not replace, routine stylet use for intubation in morbidly obese patients. Anesth Analg 109, 1560–1065.
28. Maharaj, C.H., 2008. Evaluation of the Airtraq and Macintosh laryngoscopes in patients at increased risk for difficult tracheal intubation. Anaesthesia 63 (2), 182–188.
29. Malin, E., et al., 2009. Performance of the Airtraq laryngoscope after failed conventional tracheal intubation: a case series. Acta Anaesthesiol Scand 53 (7), 858–863.
30. Calder, I., Pearce, A., Towey, R., 1996. Classic paper: a fibreoptic endoscope used for tracheal intubation. Anaesthesia 51 (6), 602.
31. Murphy, P., 1967. A fibreoptic endoscope used for tracheal intubation. Anaesthesia 22, 489–491.

32. Ronco, C., Bellomo, R., Kellum, J. (Eds.), 2009. Critical care nephrology, ed 2. Elsevier Saunders, Philadelphia.

33. Walls, R.M., Murphy, M.F., Luten, R.C. (Eds.), 2008. Manual of emergency airway management, ed 3. Lippincott Williams & Wilkins, Philadelphia.

34. Benger, J., Nolan, J., Clancy, M. (Eds.), 2008. Emergency airway management, ed 1. Cambridge University Press, Cambridge.

35. Gregg, Margolis (Ed.), 2003. Paramedic: airway management, ed 1. Jones & Bartlett, Sudbury, Mass.

36. Popat, M. (Ed.), 2001. Practical fibreoptic intubation, Butterworth-Heinemann, Oxford.

37. Jones, H.E., Pearce, A.C., Moore, P., 1993. Fibreoptic intubation. Influence of tracheal tube tip design. Anaesthesia 48 (8), 672–674.

38. Kristensen, M.S., 2003. The Parker Flex-Tip Tube versus a standard tube for fiberoptic orotracheal intubation: a randomized double-blind study. Anaesthesiology 98 (2), 354–358.

39. Atherton, D.P.L., O'Sullivan, E., Lowe, D., et al., 1996. A ventilation-exchange bougie for fibreoptic intubations with the laryngeal mask airway. Anaesthesia 51 (2), 1123–1126.

40. Venn, P.H., 1993. The gum elastic bougie. Anaesthesia 48, 274–275.

41. Henderson, J.J., 2003. Development of the "gum-elastic bougie." Anaesthesia 58 (1), 103–104.

42. Latto, I.P., Stacey, M., Mecklenburgh, J., et al., 2002. Survey of the use of the gum elastic bougie in clinical practice. Anaesthesia 57 (4), 379–384.

43. Hodzovic, I., Latto, I.P., Henderson, J.J., 2003. Bougie trauma—what trauma? Anaesthesia 58 (2), 192–193.

44. Hung, O.R., Pytka, M.D., Morris, I., et al., 1995. Clinical trial of a new light-wand device (Trachlight) to intubate the trachea. Anaesthesiology 83 (3), 509–514.

45. Tsutsui, T., Setoyama, K., 2002. A clinical evaluation of blind orotracheal intubation using Trachlight in 511 patients. Masui 50 (8), 854–858.

46. Nishiyama, T., Matsukawa, T., Hanaoka, K., 1999. Optimal length and angle of a new lightwand device (Trachlight). J Clin Anaesth 11 (4), 332–335.

47. Loudermilk, E.P., Hartmannsgruber, M., Stoltzfus, D.P., et al., 1997. A prospective study of the safety of tracheal extubation using a pediatric airway exchange catheter for patients with a known difficult airway. Chest 111 (6), 1660–1665.

Chapter 8

Endotracheal Airway Devices

Young K. Ahn and Warren S. Sandberg

Endotracheal airway devices provide a means of oxygenation and ventilation by directly accessing the trachea, allowing gas delivery and exchange to the lungs. Endotracheal tubes are endotracheal airway devices inserted orally or nasally, whereas tracheostomy tubes are placed surgically or percutaneously through the trachea. Additional types of subglottic airway devices, including those used for jet ventilation, can be used for short-term oxygenation requirements.

Endotracheal tubes and tracheostomy tubes, commonly with a tracheal cuff, are used when a patient's airway needs to be definitively secured from aspiration or when positive pressure ventilation is required. Indications for endotracheal intubation for invasive airway management take into account patient risk factors for aspiration. This includes unsatisfactory NPO status common in traumatic and emergent presentations. Pathophysiological states such as symptomatic gastric reflux, ileus, or bowel obstruction often require definitively securing the airway. Elevated risk of aspiration may also be present with anatomic variation due to a history of certain gastrointestinal operations (i.e., esophagectomy or gastrectomy). Additionally, patients who are morbidly obese or with primary lung disease should be strongly considered for endotracheal intubation, as effective ventilation with supraglottic airway devices may be difficult.

Situational factors warranting strong consideration of endotracheal airway management include the need for surgical access to the oropharynx, lengthy procedures, and positioning requirements limiting access to the airway. Postoperative intubation requirements also need to be factored into the decision to use an endotracheal tube (Table 8–1).

Tracheal Tubes (Endotracheal Tubes)

A properly positioned, cuffed endotracheal tube is currently the definitive method to secure an airway via the oropharynx or nasopharynx. It should be noted that uncuffed endotracheal tubes have traditionally been used for small children due to anatomic differences between children and adults. In adults, the narrowest part of the upper airway is the glottis whereas in children the cricoid cartilage is commonly believed to be the narrowest point in the airway.[1] Thus, cuffless tubes theoretically provide an adequate seal between the trachea and endotracheal tube while decreasing the risk of pressure injury and postintubation croup in children.[2] Studies have shown, however, that when endotracheal cuff pressures are properly monitored, the incidence of croup and other complications in full-term neonates and young children are not statistically different between cuffed and uncuffed endotracheal tubes[3] (Figure 8–1). Uncuffed endotracheal tubes may also need to be replaced with a larger sized tube if an adequate seal is not established, requiring reinstrumentation of the airway.

Endotracheal intubation provides the ability to ventilate with positive pressure while precisely titrating gas delivery. Intubation reduces the risk of aspirating native or foreign material in patients who cannot protect their own airway, which would include anyone under a general anesthetic. Finally, a properly secured endotracheal tube is intuitively less likely than a supraglottic device to be accidentally displaced during patient positioning and surgical manipulation.

Table 8–1 Considerations for Endotracheal Management of Airway

Patient Factors	Situational Factors
GENERAL RISK FACTORS FOR ASPIRATION • Trauma • Unsatisfactory NPO status	**PLAN OF CARE FOR PATIENT** • Intraoperative time • Postoperative intubation requirements (anticipated major fluid shifts)
ANATOMIC RISK FACTORS FOR ASPIRATION • History of gastrectomy • History of esophagectomy • Hiatal hernia • Tracheoesophageal fistula • Supraglottic airway obstruction	**SURGICAL CONCERNS** • Surgical site (oral/maxillary/facial, laryngeal procedures) • Surgical approach (thoracotomy, laparoscopic)
PHYSIOLOGIC RISK FACTORS FOR ASPIRATION • Symptomatic gastric reflux • Decreased state of consciousness • Decreased GI motility (ileus, gastroparesis, bowel obstruction)	**POSITIONING CONCERNS** • Limited access to airway intraoperatively • Prone positioning in certain cases • Frequent positioning change requirements
PULMONARY STATUS CONCERNS • Primary lung disease (COPD, restrictive lung disease) • Morbid obesity	
ANTICIPATED DIFFICULT AIRWAY	

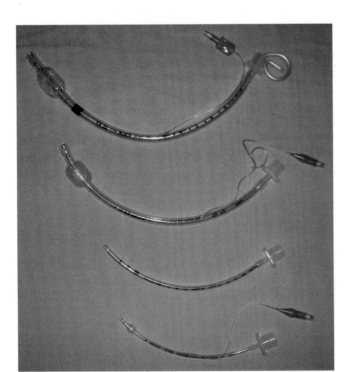

Figure 8–1 Variety of adult- and pediatric-sized endotracheal tubes, both cuffed and uncuffed.

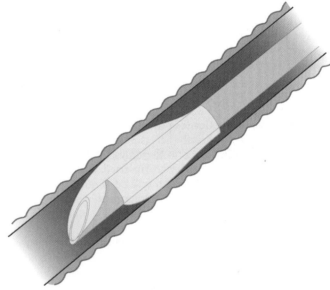

Figure 8–2 Rubber tube with kink and herniation of cuff. *(Image taken from Davey A, Diba A, editors.* Ward's anaesthetic equipment, *ed 5, Philadelphia, Elsevier Saunders, 2005.)*

Material

Endotracheal tubes were historically made of opaque rubber or soft latex. The elasticity of these materials and the low-profile cuff made insertion less traumatic, a particularly helpful characteristic for nasally inserted tubes. Although sterilization can be difficult to verify after each use, studies show that sterilization according to the Centers for Disease Control and Prevention guidelines results in properly sterilized reusable endotracheal tubes.[4]

Reports of foreign objects or dried mucus occluding the lumen of rubber or latex endotracheal tubes after sterilization are not uncommon. The integrity of the endotracheal tube and cuff can also become compromised over time and with repeated sterilization. This can result in easier kinking of the tube lumen and cuff herniation past the distal opening of the endotracheal tube (Figure 8–2). Additionally, these cuffs are at higher risk of transmitting pressures capable of causing tracheal mucosal ischemia due to the higher inflation pressures required. Finally, the use of natural rubber and latex poses a greater risk of irritation and allergic reactions in patients. For all these reasons, plastic endotracheal tubes made of polyvinyl chloride (PVC) and polyurethane have largely replaced rubber and latex endotracheal tubes.

Single use polyvinyl chloride (PVC) and polyurethane endotracheal tubes are often transparent, allowing easier visual inspection of the airway up to the point of entry to the body. They are reliably supplied sterilized from the manufacturer. Plastic endotracheal tubes can also be reproduced to more precise specifications than rubber or latex endotracheal tubes, which is especially important in endotracheal tubes with a very small inner diameter (ID). As noted, endotracheal tubes made with these newer materials are less allergenic and are ubiquitous in modern anesthesia practice.[5]

Recently, newer endotracheal tubes have been designed to address ventilator associated pneumonias (VAP) during prolonged intubation and ventilatory support. The incidence of VAP in the critical care setting was studied with silver-coated endotracheal tubes in multiple randomized controlled trials. Silver-coated endotracheal tubes were determined to reduce the bacterial burden and incidence of VAP while increasing the length of time to development of VAP, though long-term mortality was not affected.[6,7]

Design

Endotracheal tubes are shaped to follow the anatomic curve of the oropharynx (Figure 8–3, *A).* The distal end is beveled with the opening facing left of the laryngoscopist, allowing for visualization of the beveled tip as it passes between the vocal cords. Opposite the bevel may be a port referred to as a Murphy eye. If the beveled opening is obstructed by having its opening against the tracheal wall or becomes occluded by a foreign body, the Murphy eye theoretically enables some degree of oxygenation and ventilation (Figure 8–3, *C).* Endotracheal tubes without the Murphy eye are referred to as Magill endotracheal tubes.

At the distal end of the endotracheal tube is the tracheal cuff, providing occlusion of the space between the tracheal wall and endotracheal tube. Once the cuff is properly positioned and inflated, effective positive pressure ventilation can be delivered and the airway is considered "protected" against aspiration. The cuff is inflated via tubing that connects to a self-sealing valve and pilot balloon. The tubing is integrated closely to the endotracheal tube body.

Several notable markings are on the endotracheal tube. This includes the size of the endotracheal tube, which is a measure of the ID in millimeters, and the length of the endotracheal tube, marked by a radio-opaque line that can be visualized on a chest radiography. Numbers oriented to be easily read by the laryngoscopist, usually in intervals of 2 cm, show the length of the endotracheal tube from the distal end. Markings relating to certification that the plastic has been tested for tissue toxicity (i.e., I.T.Z. 79 or CE) are also printed on the endotracheal tube (Figure 8–3, *B).*

Size

Increasing the ID of an endotracheal tube exponentially decreases the resistance to gas flow through the tube, whereas decreasing the length linearly decreases the resistance. This relationship is given by the Poiseuille equation:

$$R = (8\eta)/(\Pi r^4)$$

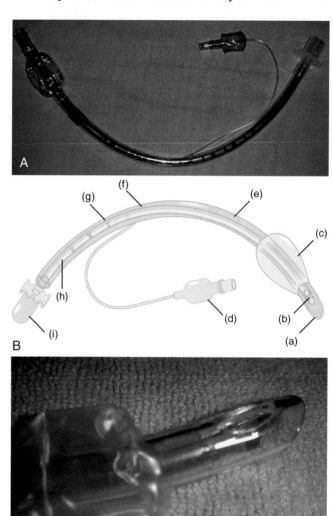

Figure 8–3 **A,** Normal curve of a standard, disposable endotracheal tube. **B,** Schematic drawing of PVC endotracheal tube. **C,** Close-up picture of the Murphy eye. *(B, from Davey A, Diba A, editors.* Ward's anaesthetic equipment, *ed 5, Philadelphia, Elsevier Saunders, 2005.)*

Resistance directly relates to the work a patient exerts to maintain sufficient ventilation through the narrow endotracheal tube. Thus, the largest ID endotracheal tube to pass through the narrowest part of the airway without trauma is typically chosen. Endotracheal tube size guidelines for adults and children based on this concept are shown in Table 8–2.

Routine use of larger diameter endotracheal tubes has come into question for brief procedures (such as operating room anesthetics) supported by mechanical ventilation. Positive pressure ventilation by the ventilator makes work of breathing by patients less relevant. Even with spontaneous ventilation modes, pressure support settings on most modern ventilators compensate for the increased resistance of endotracheal tubes.[8]

Although narrower endotracheal tubes do not effectively increase work of breathing for the ventilated patient, they do decrease trauma to the oropharynx and trachea. Endotracheal tubes size 7 mm ID and greater lead to an increased incidence of sore throats and vocal hoarseness, likely due to the increased area of contact between the tube and vocal cords and trachea.[9]

Table 8–2 Length/Internal Diameter of ETT

Internal diameter (mm)		Age (years)	Length (cm)	
Oral	Nasal		Oral	Nasal
2.5	2.5	PREMATURE	10.5	13.0
3.0	3.0	0-1	10.5	13.0
3.5	3.5		11.0	14.0
4.0	4.0	1-2	12.0	14.5
4.5	4.5		13.5	15.0
5.0	5.0	2-4	14.0	16.6
5.5	5.5		14.5	17.0
6.0	6.0	5-12	15.0	17.5
6.5	6.5		16.0	18.5
7.0	7.0	13-16	17.5	19.0
8.0	8.0		18.5	19.5
–	6.0	ADULTS — Small women Large men	–	24.0
–	6.5		–	24.0
7.0	7.0		–	24.0
7.5	7.5		–	25.0
8.0	8.0		23.0	26.0
8.5	–		24.0	–
9.0	–		25.0	–

However, narrower endotracheal tubes are associated with more kinking and difficulty in passing a suction catheter or bronchoscope. Larger endotracheal tubes are routinely used if fiberoptic bronchoscopy is to be performed through the tube.

The shortest length of endotracheal tube would ideally be used as well, but tubes are not routinely cut to minimize the length for each patient solely to decrease resistance. This is partly due to the safety and practical aspects of cutting each tube. There is risk with certain patient conditions such as edema after burns or prone positioning with large volume resuscitation, and patient positioning changes during surgery that can lead to displacement of shorter endotracheal tubes.

Special tubes preformed for oral or nasal intubation (i.e., RAE tubes) have a fixed length correlating to their internal diameters. It is more difficult to choose narrower internal diameters in these tubes because of considerations involving the height of the patient and the possibility of having an endotracheal tube that is too short or a cuff that is too small to achieve a satisfactory seal.

Endotracheal Tube Cuffs

Endotracheal tube cuffs can be categorized according to the pressure required to properly inflate the cuff.

High pressure (also referred to as low volume) cuffs are inflated in a spherical shape, allowing for minimal surface contact area between the tracheal mucosa and endotracheal cuff when properly inflated. The trachea tends to conform to the cuff shape, rather than the cuff conforming to the trachea. This design theoretically increases the chance of transmitting cuff pressure that exceeds the capillary perfusion pressure to the tracheal mucosa, which is about 25 to 34 cm H_2O in normotensive adults, and likely lower in children.[10] Conversely, overinflation of the cuff quickly leads to a significant amount of pressure transmission through the cuff and can lead to tracheal mucosal ischemia.

Medium pressure cuffs are made of more distensible material and need less pressure to properly inflate than high

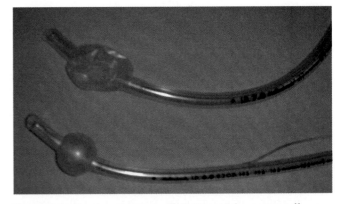

Figure 8–4 *Top,* Low pressure cuff. *Bottom,* High pressure cuff.

pressure cuffs. There is less risk of exceeding the transmucosal capillary perfusion pressure with inadvertent overinflation of the cuff. However, the cuffs are more susceptible to damage due to the compliant construction material (Figure 8–4).

Low pressure (also referred to as high volume) cuffs, are made from relatively inelastic material such as PVC. There is a large area that is in contact between the tracheal mucosa and cuff. A seal is formed between the cuff and trachea without compromising the capillary perfusion to the tracheal mucosa. The disadvantage is that multiple channels form due to the redundant folding of the large volume cuff when inflated, allowing passage of supraglottic material into the lungs (Figure 8–5).

Cuff size and shape thus involve a series of trade-offs. Currently, low pressure cuffs are the most commonly used in general practice because of their lower likelihood of causing tracheal injury and the low likelihood of injury from passage of material past the cuff during brief intubations (i.e., elective procedures).[11]

During prolonged intubation, neither high pressure nor low pressure cuffs have been shown to satisfactorily prevent ventilator-associated pneumonias. However, some authorities have attributed the decline in iatrogenic tracheal stenosis to the turn away from high pressure cuff designs. Newer low

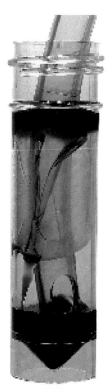

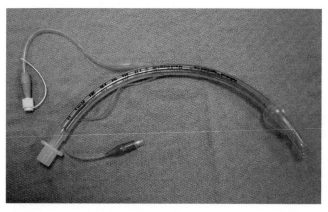

Figure 8–6 Endotracheal tube with additional suction channel to remove material that might otherwise migrate past the cuff into the trachea.

Figure 8–5 Low pressure cuff model, showing passage of dye material past redundant folds of the endotracheal tube cuff. *(From Davey A, Diba A, editors.* Ward's anaesthetic equipment, *ed 5, Philadelphia, Elsevier Saunders, 2005.)*

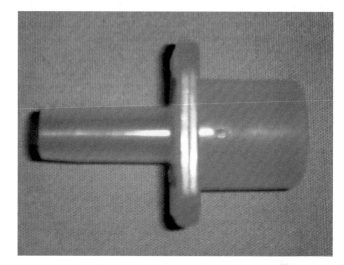

Figure 8–7 15-mm ISO connector.

pressure (high volume) designs use thin polyurethane cuffs that may be superior to the low pressure polyvinylchloride cuffs, by virtue of reducing redundant folds. Initial data seem to support a reduced incidence of early and late onset ventilator-associated pneumonia, though more clinical studies are required.[12] This is an area of active product development by vendors, seeking a competitive advantage by adding features. For example, Figure 8–6 illustrates an endotracheal tube with a thin cuff intended to minimize translocation of material past the cuff and a special channel designed to allow frequent suctioning of the area above the cuff to minimize the load of potentially aspirated material.

The endotracheal tube cuff is usually connected to a pilot balloon with a self-sealing valve by thin tubing incorporated into the body of the endotracheal tube. The pilot balloon can be used to gauge the degree of inflation pressure in the endotracheal cuff, at least in a crude way. It is important to remember that the cuff should only be inflated enough to prevent leaks with positive pressure ventilation, and this inflation criterion can be readily assessed by listening for air leaks during positive pressure inspiration. This goal-directed cuff pressure management not only lessens the chance of ischemic injury to the tracheal mucosa, but it allows for a "safety leak" if airway pressure becomes too high.

Connectors/Catheter Mounts/ Tracheal Tube Adaptors

The proximal end of the endotracheal tube is connected to the remainder of the breathing circuit via a 15-mm International Organization for Standardization (ISO) connector

(Figure 8–7). The distal male end of the ISO connector securely fits into the proximal end of the endotracheal tube. It is important to note that the ISO connector and endotracheal tube is connected loosely when shipped because the seal is hard to break once firmly secured. The 15-mm proximal male end of the ISO connector is inserted firmly into the 15-mm female end of the breathing circuit or catheter mount.

The proximal end of the 15-mm ISO connector can also insert into a variety of special purpose connectors, enabling swiveling or increased flexibility to reduce torsion and positioning away from surgical sites, and ports for bronchoscopy or suction catheters (Figure 8–8). One such adaptor that provides both flexibility and a port for suction catheters is a catheter mount, also known as a tracheal tube adaptor.

Common Problems with Endotracheal Tubes and Safety Considerations

Many common problems encountered with use of endotracheal tubes are easily correctable if recognized quickly. We will review some common issues one may expect to encounter during placement of the endotracheal tube.

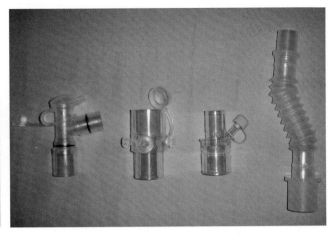

Figure 8–8 *From left to right,* Elbow connector with suction/bronch port, straight connector with MDI port, straight connector with gas sampler port, and straight expandable connector.

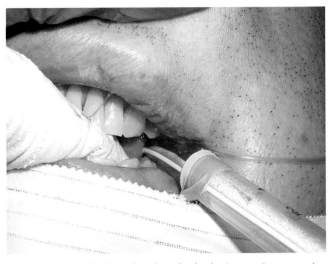

Figure 8–9 Bite block and endotracheal tube in a patient emerging from anesthesia. The patient has compressed the bite block to the point that the tube is partially collapsed, and head movement has led the softened tube to kink.

Issues may arise with the initial placement of the endotracheal tube, such as esophageal intubation or advancement of the tube into a mainstem bronchus (usually the right main bronchus). Database searches show that dislodgment of the endotracheal tube is by far the most common issue with placement and ensuing complications.[13]

Failure to obtain a sufficient endotracheal cuff seal can be due to an improper size of the endotracheal tube, improper placement of the endotracheal tube, or problems with the cuff. Issues with the endotracheal cuff can range from insufficient inflation, progressive deflation, or damage to the cuff. Endotracheal cuffs can be damaged from overinflation (unlikely), by teeth during passage through the oropharynx (likely), or from defects in the manufacturing process (unlikely).

Difficulty in achieving ventilation with appropriate airway pressures can be the result of obstruction at any point along the length of the endotracheal tube or breathing circuit. The warm oropharynx and nasopharynx can soften the endotracheal tube and make it susceptible to kinking. Specially designed and reinforced tubes address this, but most modern PVC tubes are not as susceptible to the kinking as softer plastics and rubber tubes were. The tube can also become kinked at points where torsion is applied throughout the breathing circuit, especially with changes in patient positioning.

The patient may also bite and obstruct the endotracheal tube. There have been reports of patients biting through the tube completely, resulting in the loss of an airway and highlighting the need for a properly placed bite block in orally intubated patients who have not been administered muscle relaxants. Figure 8–9 illustrates kinking and insufficiency of a bite block, highlighting the fact that problems with endotracheal tube patency can happen in concert. Apart from the obvious visible evidence of tube obstruction, the capnogram would almost certainly also demonstrate an obstructed pattern.

An obstructive ventilatory pattern can also be observed if the distal end of the endotracheal tube rests against the trachea or carina. This can occur when the endotracheal tube is advanced too far or with changes in positioning after initial proper placement of the endotracheal tube, particularly flexion or rotation at the neck.

Native and foreign bodies, most commonly mucus plugs, but even teeth, dental caps, plastic packaging, needles, and various objects able to fit through an endotracheal tube have been found obstructing the lumen. Careful attention while initially placing the endotracheal tube is key to preventing such problems, but promptly recognizing the cause of an endotracheal tube obstruction is equally essential.

Finally, when using positive pressure ventilation, barotrauma and pneumothorax must always be considered as possible causes of difficult oxygenation and/or ventilation. Clinical examination, including breath sounds, chest wall movement, and all available vitals signs and monitors, as well as communication with the surgical team are essential in prompt recognition, prevention, and treatment of life-threatening airway compromise.

Although endotracheal tubes protect the airway, they also bring nonintuitive risks. For example, the high concentrations of oxygen and nitrous oxide delivered by an endotracheal tube create risk for ignition and explosion, particularly during laser surgeries. Endotracheal tubes designed to address this safety issue will be described in a following section.

Guidelines have been published to improve patient safety, especially during prolonged intubations, as seen in intensive care units. These include the use of capnography, availability of emergency equipment such as bag-valve-mask systems near the patient, and drills to quickly act on damaged or blocked tubes. In addition, skin damage and ulcerations should be evaluated by using standard descriptive terms to enhance communication and accurate documentation of progression of any lesions.[13]

Nitrous Oxide and the Endotracheal Tube

Special discussion regarding nitrous oxide is needed because it is commonly used as an anesthetic agent. Nitrous oxide diffuses readily into the endotracheal tube cuff, and this agent commonly replaces nitrogen in the anesthetic gas mixture.

One would expect the cuff volume and pressure to remain constant as nitrogen and nitrous oxide exchange over the course of an anesthetic. However, nitrous oxide diffuses across surfaces more quickly than nitrogen, and this kinetic imbalance can lead to problems. The rate of nitrous oxide diffusion is directly affected by the following three factors[14]:

- The permeability and compliance of the cuff determined by the construction material. High pressure cuffs usually have low compliance and high permeability (i.e., rubber cuffs). They are more susceptible to early rises in pressure from diffusion of nitrous oxide. Low pressure cuffs have more volume to expand with the initial diffusion of nitrous oxide leading to only a minimal increase in pressure. However, once the cuff is fully expanded, the low compliance of the cuff causes significant and abrupt increases in cuff pressures that can also lead to tracheal mucosa damage.
- The surface area of the cuff exposed to diffusion of nitrous oxide. The more surface area available, the quicker the diffusion of nitrous oxide into the cuff.
- The partial pressure of nitrous oxide in the delivered concentration of inhaled agents. The higher partial pressure of nitrous oxide inhaled, the quicker and more significant the diffusion of nitrous oxide.

The simplest way to prevent progressively increasing cuff pressure is to monitor the pilot balloon regularly when nitrous oxide is being administered and remove appropriate volume from the cuff as needed to maintain a sufficient seal. Other methods of preventing increasing cuff pressure includes filling the cuff with sterile saline or a concentration of gases with the same composition as that which will be administered.

Commercial devices have been developed that address the changes in endotracheal cuff pressure intraoperatively. These include devices that address the extra volume diffusing into the cuff by providing a reservoir for the extra gas in the pilot balloon, such as the Mallinckrodt Brandt and Mallinckrodt Lanz devices. Another product, the Portex Soft Seal cuff, reduces the permeability of the cuff to nitrous oxide by 80% and has been shown to mainly decrease cuff pressure by increasing compliance.[15] Finally, the Bivona "Fome-Cuf" uses foam to inflate the cuff while leaving the pilot balloon open, preventing a closed system, which diffused nitrous oxide could pressurize (Figure 8–10).

Specially Designed Tracheal Tubes

Preformed Tubes

The most common type of preformed tubes are the orotracheal and nasotracheal RAE (Ring, Adair, Elwin) tubes (Figure 8–11). The orotracheal RAE tube has a preformed bend at the mouth to angle the tube and connector down across the chin and away from the face. This is especially useful in procedures requiring facial exposure. Orotracheal tubes can be inserted with direct laryngoscopy as one would do with conventional endotracheal tubes. They can also be placed with the assistance of McGill forceps or with fiberoptic guidance.

In patients with coagulopathies or sinus abnormalities and children under the age of 10 who naturally have prominent adenoids, there is an increased risk of bleeding with nasal intubation and it is avoided if possible.[16] However, nasal

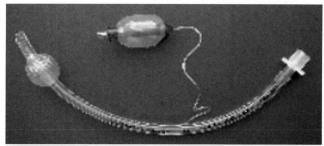
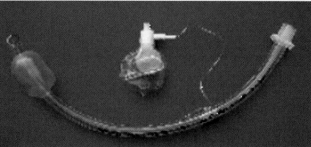
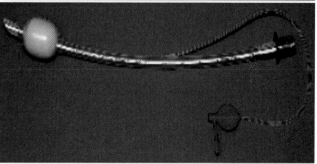
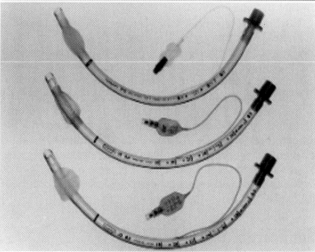

Figure 8–10 Commercial devices addressing nitrous oxide diffusion into ETT cuffs. *From top to bottom,* Mallinckrodt Brandt, Mallinckrodt Lanz, Bivona Fome Cuff, and the Portex Soft Seal, which is the bottommost of three endotracheal tubes placed for comparison. *Top three panels from Davey A, Diba A, editors.* Ward's anaesthetic equipment, *ed 5, Philadelphia, Elsevier Saunders, 2005. Bottom panel from Karasawa F, Mori T, Okuda T, et al. Profile soft-seal cuff, a new endotracheal tube, effectively inhibits an increase in the cuff pressure through high compliance rather than low diffusion of nitrous oxide. Anesth Analg 2001;92:140-144.)*

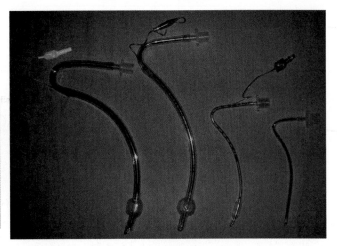

Figure 8–11 Nasal RAE endotracheal tubes. *From left to right,* Two standard adult cuffs, then a pediatric-sized cuff, and finally a pediatric uncuffed nasal RAE tube.

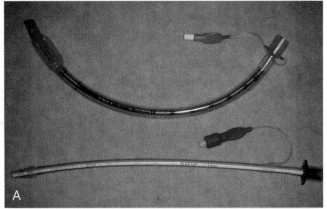

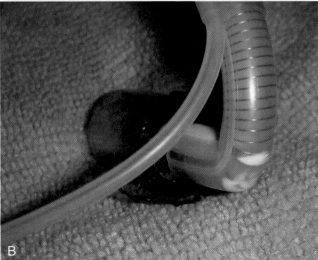

Figure 8–12 **A,** Two different reinforced endotracheal tubes. Stylets are necessary because of the flexibility of the reinforced tubes. **B,** Close-up of reinforcing wire and unreinforced vulnerable point between 15-mm ISO connector and ETT tube.

intubation is required during certain oral and maxillary surgeries for surgical exposure. The nasotracheal RAE tube has a preformed bend designed to angle the tube and connector up and over the forehead, away from the lower face and oropharynx. The nasopharyngeal RAE tube is inserted using fiberoptic guidance or direct laryngoscopy aided by head positioning or with McGill forceps. Because placement of the nasal RAE tube is more involved than the usual orotracheal intubation, and because the tube is inaccessible during surgery, it is often sutured in place by the surgical team at the nasal septum to prevent dislodgement.

The Portex Ivory Polar tube also has a preformed bend at the nares, which brings the tube up and over the forehead, away from the lower face and oropharynx. An advantage of the Polar tube is the soft plastic material, allowing for less nasopharyngeal trauma during intubation.

Both the nasal and oral RAE tubes have a fixed length distal to the preformed bend. This fixed nasopharyngeal and oropharyngeal length is proportional to the inner diameter of the tube. As previously discussed, consideration must be given to a patient's height when determining the proper size RAE tube. Thus tall people with small noses can present a challenge to the anesthesiologist trying to insert the large diameter nasal RAE tube dictated by the patient's height.

Reinforced Tubes

Reinforced tubes can be constructed from softer latex or rubber because of a reinforcing spiral of nylon or steel running the length of the tube (Figure 8–12, *A*). Due to the softness and inability of reinforced tubes to hold their shape during intubation, they are usually inserted over a malleable stylet or over a bougie catheter that has already been passed into the trachea. The benefit of having this flexible, yet reinforced tube is its resistance to kinking during positioning and surgical manipulation. However, with newer PVC endotracheal tubes, which decrease kinking issues, this concern is less of an absolute indication for usage of reinforced endotracheal tubes.

Disadvantages of reinforced tracheal tubes are a by-product of the advantages they offer. The reinforced tubing is thicker

in total outer diameter for a given inner diameter. Additionally, they are usually longer for a given inner diameter than traditional endotracheal tubes and due to the reinforcement cannot be cut shorter according to patient height. Thus extra care must be given to prevent mainstem bronchial intubation. Finally, there is a short length of the endotracheal tube that is not reinforced where the ISO connector is attached. This portion is susceptible to kinking, especially in reusable reinforced tracheal tubes, where the integrity of the soft rubber may be compromised (Figure 8–12, *B*).

Microlaryngeal Tubes

Microlaryngeal tubes are typically used during surgery of the larynx. They have a smaller outer diameter and can be inserted orally or nasally to allow relatively unobstructed surgical access to the larynx. McGill forceps are used to guide proper placement if the microlaryngeal tube is too narrow to accommodate a bougie or stylet. The cuff is usually standard size as needed to properly secure an airway, and can be brightly colored for easy visibility. Due to the small diameter of microlaryngeal tubes, mechanical ventilation to overcome high tube resistance is necessary (Figure 8–13).

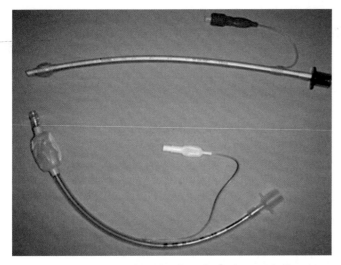

Figure 8–13　Two types of oral/nasal microlaryngeal tubes.

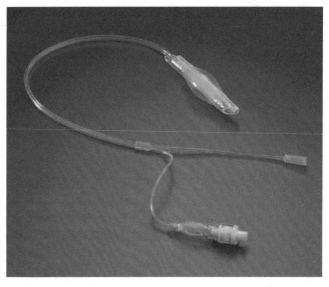

Figure 8–14　Carden tube. *From Smiths Medical. (website):* http://www. smiths-medical.com/catalog/tracheal-tubes/silicone-cuffed-endotracheal-tubes/bivona-tts-carden-laryngoscopy.htm *Accessed August 14, 2010.*

Carden Tubes

The Carden tube was designed for jet ventilation with minimal surgical field obstruction during microlaryngeal surgery. It consists of a small outer diameter tube except the distal end, which resembles the distal end of a regular endotracheal tube (Figure 8–14).

McGill forceps are commonly used to insert the Carden tube into its proper subglottic position. Alternatively, anesthesiologists have found different ways to insert the Carden tube. One method describes threading the smaller diameter portion of the Carden tube and stylet into a standard endotracheal tube. Under direct laryngoscopy, the Carden tube and distal end of the standard endotracheal tube are advanced into the proper subglottic position and the Carden tube's cuff is inflated. The standard endotracheal tube and stylet can be removed for surgical access, allowing for jet ventilation.

Laser Surgery Tubes

Laryngeal surgeries commonly employ various lasers, such as carbon dioxide, Nd-YAG, Holmium-YAG, argon, and KTP beams. Conventional endotracheal tubes in the presence of high concentrations of oxygen or nitrous oxide are extremely flammable and ignition can result in serious injury to the upper airway and oropharynx. Deflected laser beams can also cause significant damage to the surrounding soft tissue. Examples of commercially available endotracheal tubes that are more resistant to ignition from laser beams are described below.

Mallinckrodt Laser-Flex endotracheal tubes are disposable tubes with laser resistant construction. The tube is constructed of a metal helix with a surface that deflects laser beams with dispersed energy to minimize tissue damage. There are two sequential endotracheal tube cuffs at the distal end (Figure 8–15, *A*). Both cuffs are inflated with saline, with the proximal cuff protecting the distal cuff. Addition of dye to the saline allows visualization of a leak if the integrity of either cuff is breached. Pilot cuffs are connected via tubing that is run through the lumen of the tube. The lumen of the Laser Flex tube is also narrow in diameter, necessitating mechanical ventilation, and adequate expiratory time to prevent lung

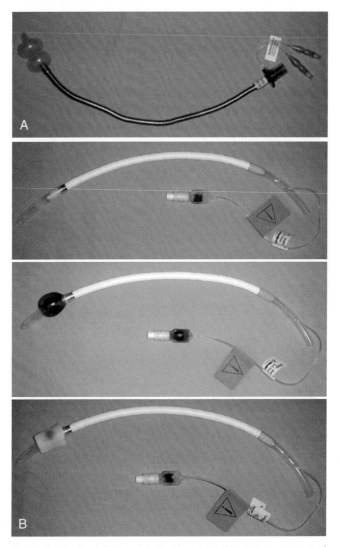

Figure 8–15　**A,** Mallinckrodt Laser-Flex. **B,** Medtronic Laser ETT out of package, with normal saline and methylene blue in cuff and with leak on gauze.

hyperinflation. Medtronic produces a Laser-Shield II endotracheal tube that is similarly wrapped with material to deflect and disperse laser beams. The pilot cuff is manufactured with methylene blue dye, which fills the cuff when inflated with normal saline as suggested by the manufacturer. The manufacturer also suggests wrapping the endotracheal tube cuff with a normal saline-soaked gauze to act as a heat sink and allow for visualization of methylene blue leakage (Figure 8–15, B).

Other commercially and independently prepared endotracheal tubes have been wrapped in foil and then wrapped in saline-soaked foam or gauze to make the endotracheal tube more laser resistant with good results. Clearly, the method of careful preparation of the endotracheal tube and filling of the cuff with an inert substance, in combination with judicious surgical use of the laser, is paramount to safe laser surgery.

Hunsaker Tubes

Hunsaker tubes are double lumen tubes, with one lumen for jet ventilation and the adjacent, narrower lumen for airway pressure monitoring and gas sampling (Figure 8–16, A). The tube is constructed of laser resistant plastic. A stainless steel wire is incorporated into the tubing to prevent loose fragments in the event a portion of the endotracheal tube breaks off after extended damage from high energy laser beams. A thin stylet allows for placement of the Hunsaker tube under direct laryngoscopy, and placement of the distal end approximately 7.5 cm distal to the vocal cords. The distal end of the Hunsaker tube incorporates a dispersive cage to direct the jet ventilation air flow (Figure 8–16, B). Fiberoptic confirmation of proper placement is recommended, and care must be taken to prevent kinking throughout the length of the thin tube lumen.

Laryngectomy Tubes

Laryngectomies necessitate the establishment of a transtracheal airway intraoperatively with a tracheotomy. Laryngectomy tubes are also preformed with a "U" shape that addresses the issues of stability, kinking, and interference with the surgical site. The distal end to the cuff is usually shortened like a tracheostomy tube to reduce mainstem bronchial intubation. The "U" shape reduces excessive movement compared with a standard endotracheal tube inserted through the tracheotomy, while the rest of the tube is oriented caudally, away from the surgical field (Figure 8–17).

Other Endotracheal Tube Variations

Other endotracheal tubes are designed to have special functions to assist in a variety of situations. Pulling on a wire attached to the distal end of the Endotrol endotracheal tube increases the curvature of the tube from the neutral position, allowing for greater manipulation of the endotracheal tube during intubation.

Endotracheal tubes also can have extra lumens incorporated into the body. Uses for the extra lumen include delivery of medications, such as topical anesthetics, jet ventilation, and monitoring of tracheal pressure.

Secretions above the endotracheal cuff are always of concern, particularly with low pressure cuffs during prolonged intubations. Endotracheal tubes with dedicated suction channels used to clear subglottic secretions above the endotracheal tube cuff are available, but results on the clinical significance in the prevention or delay of ventilator-associated pneumonia remain uncertain.[18]

Tracheostomy Tracheal Tubes

A cuffed tracheostomy tracheal tube is the definitive method of transtracheal airway management, just as the endotracheal tube is the definitive method of oropharyngeal or nasopharyngeal airway management. A tracheostomy tube is most often inserted due to long-term need for mechanical ventilation or airway protection. An inability to orally intubate due to various reasons, and certain procedures such as laryngectomies, are also common reasons for tracheostomies to be performed and tracheostomy tubes used.

Tracheostomy tubes are made of similar materials as endotracheal tubes, namely PVC, polyurethane, and newer plastics. However, because many tracheostomy tracheal tubes are

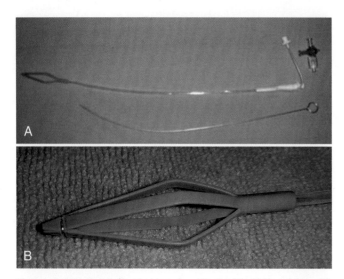

Figure 8–16 **A,** Medtronic Hunsaker MonJet Ventilation tube with stylet and 3-way stopcock. **B,** Medtronic Hunsaker MonJet Ventilation tube's distal end dispersive cage.

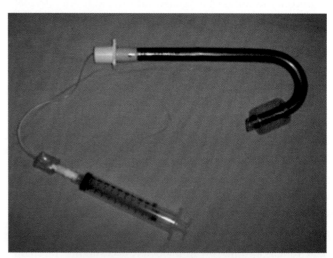

Figure 8–17   Reusable laryngectomy tube.

anticipated to remain for prolonged periods, materials such as silicone for ease of secretion clearance, silastic for comfort and flexibility, and armoured tubes for durability and preventing kinks are available.[19] The needs of patients requiring tracheostomy tubes are highly variable and certain manufacturers take special orders for custom tracheostomy tubes (Figure 8–18).

Tracheostomy tubes can be placed in the operating room or percutaneously at the bedside in many patients. Bedside percutaneous tracheostomy is advantageous in that it requires fewer resources, with no operating room involvement, avoids the hazards of transporting an intubated patient, and is a less involved surgical procedure. Elective percutaneous insertion of tracheostomy tubes is usually done with the aid of a fiberoptic bronchoscope to ensure the posterior tracheal wall is not breached and the positioning of the tracheostomy tube is optimal.[20]

The variations between tracheostomy tracheal tubes are many. Tracheostomy tubes can be cuffed or uncuffed depending on whether positive pressure ventilation or airway protection from aspiration is required. Cuffed tracheostomy tubes lead to the same issues of overinflation and tracheal mucosal ischemia as orotracheal endotracheal tubes. Foam cuffs and devices that deal with nitrous diffusion into the cuff are also available to counteract cuff overinflation.

Also available are tracheostomy tubes with suction catheters that end directly above the cuff, a common area for secretions to pool in the larynx. Another tracheostomy design allows for expiration supraglottically, around an inflated cuff, which allows for vocalization even with positive pressure ventilation.

Fenestrated tracheostomy tubes also allow for some degree of vocalization as patients can exhale through the glottis. If positive pressure ventilation is intermittently required, a nonfenestrated inner cannula can be inserted to preserve adequate pressure and tidal volumes. It is important that the fenestrated portion of the tube always be placed correctly in the trachea.

In patients with significant anatomic abnormalities, a tracheostomy tube that is too short is of great concern. One method to overcome this challenge is making longer tubes. Typically the side flanges in these tubes are of more significance than usual in preventing mainstem bronchial advancement. Many times, armoured tubes are used in conjunction with longer tubes to prevent kinking in situ.

Inner tubes can be used to further adapt the tracheal tube to patient needs. As discussed above, they can be used to "block" fenestrated tubes or used for easier maintenance and cleaning of tracheal tubes in situ. The clear downside is the reduction

of the tracheal lumen diameter and the risk of displacing an established airway.

Passy-Muir valves, or speaking valves, are essentially caps with a one-way valve that allows inspiration normally through the tracheostomy tube, but directs expiration supraglottically for vocalization (Figure 8–19).

Common Issues with Tracheostomy Tubes and Safety Issues

The major differences between endotracheal tubes and tracheostomy tracheal tubes are due to anatomic considerations. Additionally, issues with tracheostomy tubes must be quickly identified and resolved because of underlying pulmonary pathology and poor respiratory reserve in many of these patients. The tracheostomy tube enters the trachea through the anterior tracheal wall, with the distance between the cricoid and carina ranging from 10 to 20 cm in patients 8 years and older and approximately 5 to 6 cm in children up to 1 year of age. Thus tracheostomy tubes have a higher risk of tracheal mainstem intubation due to the short length between the tracheal cuff and the carina, in addition to the obtuse angle between the trachea and right mainstem bronchus. This is why tracheostomy tubes have a shorter length of tube distal to the tracheal cuff.[21]

Due to the acute angle of entry when entering transtracheally, occlusion against the tracheal wall is also of concern. The tip of the tracheostomy tube is not beveled and is formed at a right angle on entry to decrease occlusion against the posterior tracheal wall. Swelling of the posterior tracheal wall up to a week after placement, in addition to formation of granulation tissue can also lead to obstruction of the tracheal lumen, occurrences that must be on the differential diagnosis for obstructive ventilation presentations. The initial placement of tracheostomy tubes involves risks including tracheal ring fractures, subcutaneous emphysema (1.4%), pneumothorax (0.8%), and massive hemorrhage from tracheoarterial fistulas (less than 1%).[22]

Recommendations to improve patient safety with the placement of tracheostomy tubes include having emergency airway equipment and personnel qualified to deal with airway issues during the placement and immediately after placement

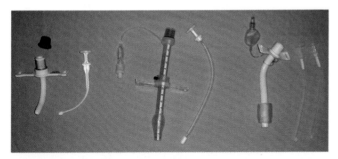

Figure 8–18 Multiple tracheostomy types. *Left,* Uncuffed, pictured with button cover; *middle,* cuffed with adjustable flange; *right,* cuffed with flange.

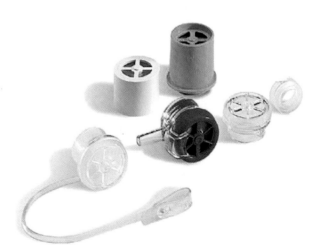

Figure 8–19 Passy-Muir valve. *(From Passy-Muir (website): http://www. passy-muir.com/products/.) Accessed* August 13, 2010.

of the tracheostomy, use of variable flange tubes in patients with abnormal tracheal anatomy, and use of tubes with inner sleeves when appropriate.[13]

Minitracheostomy and Other Emergency Cricothyrotomy Tubes

When insertion of an orally or nasally inserted airway device is not possible when managing an airway, emergency transtracheal airway access may be necessary. Anesthesiologists will likely be responsible for establishing an airway in these patients when faced with a "cannot intubate, cannot ventilate" situation.

One can establish transtracheal access emergently as follows: As always, the patient should be positioned optimally as their clinical condition allows. Ideally, the patient is positioned supine with the head slightly extended and the neck midline. The cricothyroid membrane is located, and either a 12-gauge or 14-gauge IV, which has been attached to a 10-cc syringe half filled with saline, is inserted perpendicular to the cricothyroid membrane. The entire time the IV is being advanced, one should aspirate on the syringe. Confirmation of entry into the trachea is made by a definitive aspiration of bubbles. At this point, the IV should be inserted slightly further, just enough for the catheter to enter the tracheal lumen, and the catheter should be threaded caudally into the trachea and the introducing needle and syringe removed. The catheter is attached to a 3cc syringe barrel, which can then be attached to a 15-mm ISO connector from a standard endotracheal tube.

Due to the small diameter of the catheter inserted during emergency cricothyrotomy procedures, conventional methods of oxygen delivery (Ambu bag or wall source) cannot generate high enough pressures to sufficiently oxygenate and ventilate the patient. A high pressured system capable of delivering 25 to 30 psi of oxygen (i.e., the auxiliary oxygen flow meter of the anesthesia machine) can be used at a rate of 12 times per minute, for a duration of 1.5 seconds per insufflation. This allows time for passive expiration through the larynx, and decreases the chance of barotraumas from continuous high pressure insufflation.

Clearly, an emergency situation does not lend itself well to an improvised method of establishing percutaneous transtracheal access and obtaining a high pressure oxygen source. Commercial products are available, such as the Ravussin Jet Ventilation catheter, which consists of a 13-G kink resistant catheter for adults, 14-G catheter for children, and 18-G catheter for babies. A 15-mm ISO connector is integrated into the proximal end of the catheter, allowing for transtracheal jet ventilation on insertion (Figure 8–20). A high pressured oxygen source and a commercially prepared emergency percutaneous tracheostomy kit should be available wherever the anesthesiologist will be managing an airway because this is one of the last lines of establishing an emergency airway.

Double Lumen Endobronchial Tubes

Intrathoracic operations often require deflating one lung to improve surgical access. This can be achieved with one-lung ventilation (OLV) using a double lumen endobronchial tube

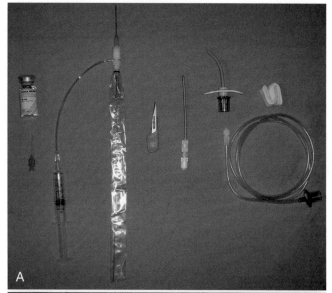
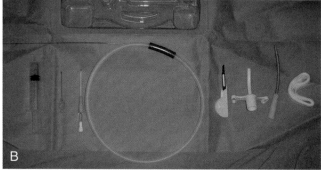

Figure 8–20   Two different emergency cricothyrotomy commercial kits.

to secure and control ventilation of both lungs independently. There are absolute indications to control ventilation of one lung, such as bronchopleural fistulae, extreme hypoxia from a unilateral pulmonary process, or surgical or traumatic opening of a major conducting airway. Additionally, there are absolute indications to isolate one lung from the other while maintaining ventilation, including unilateral pulmonary hemorrhage or infection at risk of contaminating the unaffected lung.

Double lumen tubes essentially consist of two different length endotracheal tubes fused together, each tube with its own cuff and pilot balloon (Figure 8–21, A and B). The bronchial cuff and pilot balloon are blue, whereas the tracheal cuff and pilot balloon are clear. Because the two lumens are semilunar, the inner diameter is not used to describe double lumen tube sizes. Instead an estimation of the circumference is made in units of French, with typical sizes being 28, 35, 37, 39, and 41 Fr. These sizes may be too large for use in some pediatric cases, but a range of estimates based on height and age are detailed below (Table 8–3). Historically, some double lumen tubes had a small, soft hook that settles on the carina a few centimeters from the distal end of the tube, assisting in confirmation of tube placement.[23] Modern single use tubes do not have this feature and are instead positioned with the assistance of fiberoptic bronchoscopy.

Double lumen tubes have two points of curvature and have a left bronchial or right bronchial design. The first curve is

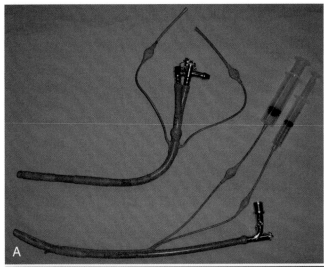
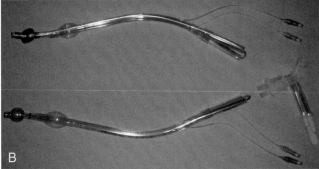

Figure 8–21 **A,** Reusable rubber double lumen tubes, Rubber tubes are now mostly of historical interest. **B,** Disposable PVC double lumen tubes.

Table 8–3 Estimating the Size of Double Lumen Endotracheal Tubes

Patient Factors	Double Lumen Tube Size (French)
Height 4' 6"–5' 5" Height 5' 6"–5' 10" Height 5' 11"–6' 4"	35-37 37-39 39-41
Age 8 Age 10 Age 12 Age 13-14	Consider 26 Consider 28 Consider 32 (manufactured as left-sided tube only) Consider 35 (manufactured as left-sided tube only)

Adapted from Miller RD, editor. Miller's anesthesia, Philadelphia, Elsevier, 2005.

Table 8–4 Clinically Confirming Proper Double Lumen Tube Placement

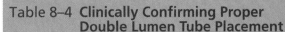
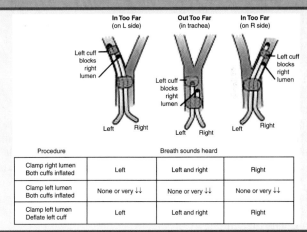

Procedure	Breath sounds heard		
Clamp right lumen Both cuffs inflated	Left	Left and right	Right
Clamp left lumen Both cuffs inflated	None or very ↓↓	None or very ↓↓	None or very ↓↓
Clamp left lumen Deflate left cuff	Left	Left and right	Right

for passage through the oropharyngeal pathway, much like a standard endotracheal tube. The second curve depends on left or right bronchial intubation. Under direct laryngoscopy the double lumen tube is inserted with the endobronchial lumen facing up. After passage through the trachea, the double lumen tube is rotated counterclockwise toward the left main stem bronchus or clockwise toward the right main stem bronchus. The connectors on the double lumen tube are then attached to the remainder of the breathing circuit with twin tube adaptors.

Proper placement requires the tracheal cuff to be inflated at the level of the trachea and the bronchial cuff to be inflated at the level of the bronchus, which can be verified by auscultation. Inflation of the tracheal cuff should lead to bilateral breath sounds with both lumens ventilating. The tracheal lumen is then occluded, leading to ventilation through the bronchial lumen, with breath sounds on the side of bronchial intubation, but decreased breaths sounds on the side opposite of bronchial intubation. The bronchial cuff is then carefully inflated until breath sounds are absent on the side opposite of bronchial intubation, indicating proper seal of the double lumen cuffs. The tracheal lumen is then unclamped, enabling effective one-lung ventilation.

A variety of maneuvers involving sequential cuff inflation, deflation, and auscultation are described in Table 8–4 to assist in confirming proper double lumen tube placement. However, a smaller diameter fiberoptic bronchoscope is usually used to definitively confirm placement of the tube in addition to auscultation of breath sounds. Proper confirmation is especially important in right-sided double lumen tubes due to the short length of the right main bronchus from the carina before steeply giving a branch off into the right upper lobe. There is a greater risk of inserting the double lumen tube too deeply and completely intubating the right main bronchus or just occluding the right upper lobe branch. A port (Murphy eye) at the level of the bronchial cuff on the right-sided tube assists in ventilation of the right upper lobe in this case (Figure 8–22). There is also a risk of incomplete isolation of either lung, but again more common with right-sided tubes that have not been advanced far enough.

Endobronchial Tubes

Endobronchial tubes are long tubes with a cuff at the distal end. They are usually guided fiberoptically to the left main bronchus where the cuff is isolated and the left lung can be ventilated. The right lung will then collapse and allow for better procedural access or isolation. Although either lung can be isolated in this manner, the short length between the carina and the takeoff of the right upper lobe bronchus makes it prone to obstruction by the cuff.

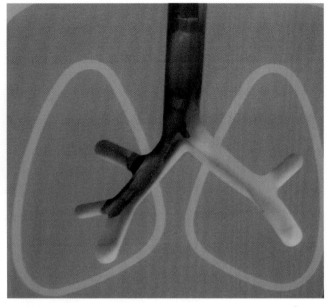

Figure 8–22 Murphy eye providing ventilation to RUL after advancing too far with right sided DLT in airway model.

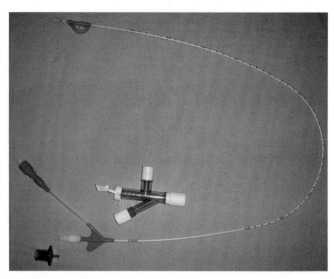

Figure 8–23 Endobronchial blocker with adaptor for connection to circuit to endotracheal tube, insertion of blocker, and insertion of fiberoptic bronchoscope.

Endobronchial Blocker

Endobronchial blockers can be incorporated into special endotracheal tubes or standard endotracheal tubes (Figure 8–23). In fact, it was not uncommon to carefully use a Foley or Fogarty catheter with a normal endotracheal tube to create a bronchial blocker. The endobronchial blocker is advanced through the tube and further distally, usually with the aid of a fiberoptic bronchoscope, and inflated at the proper location to isolate the lung.

Endobronchial blockers may be preferred in certain cases where a standard endotracheal tube is already in place or if there are concerns about transitioning from a double lumen tube to a standard endotracheal tube, particularly for long cases. They are particularly advantageous when selective lobar blockade (SLB) is desired (see Figure 8–24 for example), which has been shown to improve oxygenation intraoperatively, with or without the use of concomitant CPAP. Patients who have had previous lung resection or have comorbidities, such as COPD that makes one-lung ventilation difficult, can also benefit from the improved oxygenation of SLB. In addition, commercially produced independent bronchial blockers and variations—such as the Fuji Uniblocker, Arndt wire-guided endobronchial blocker, and the Flexitip endobronchial Cohen blocker—have hollow suction channels to facilitate lobar collapse.[24]

Other Subglottic Airway Devices

The airway exchange catheter can be categorized as a subglottic airway device because it is used to maintain access to the airway while exchanging endotracheal tubes (Figure 8–25). This device has an inner diameter large enough to provide temporary oxygenation and ventilation if the patient cannot be easily reintubated. It has been demonstrated that patients with known or presumed difficult intubations who

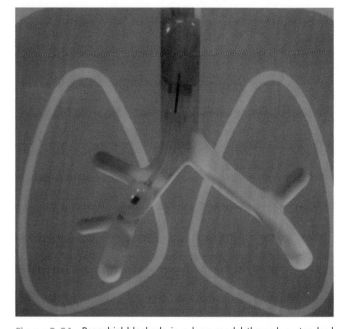

Figure 8–24 Bronchial blockade in a lung model through a standard endotracheal tube. This would selectively collapse the right middle and lower lobes.

were reintubated over an airway exchange catheter were reintubated over the AIC almost every time when properly used.[25] Nevertheless, the device is not a failsafe. There have been instances of dislodging the airway exchange catheter and unintentionally removing it from the trachea while exchanging endotracheal tubes, or advancing the device too far and causing a pneumothorax. Additionally, it is important to remember jet ventilation or a high flow oxygen source is mandatory for temporary oxygenation through this long, thin tube, and an outflow path from the lungs is also needed for ventilation of the gases.

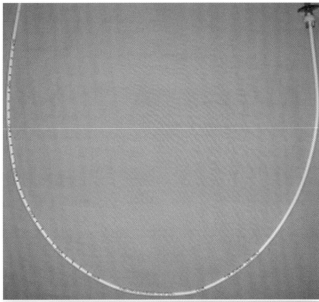
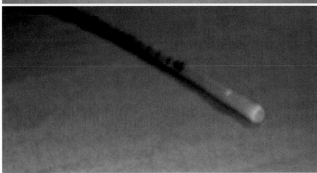

Figure 8–25 *Top,* Airway exchange catheter. *Bottom,* AEC tip with openings for jet ventilation.

Conclusion

An anesthesiologist's responsibility is wide ranging, but the most recognized and perhaps the most essential in the first few moments of an acute medical crisis is to secure and ensure an appropriate airway for the patient. Additionally, when establishing an elective anesthetic plan, appropriate airway management consideration is paramount. Intimate knowledge of the airway devices available is important in effectively and safely managing an airway. New devices continually appear and existing devices are regularly improved, but the fundamental issues of airway management remain constant.

Further Reading

The following textbook and journal articles are important in demonstrating that the clinical context and practice of striving for patient care and safety are what drive new innovations in anesthesia equipment, particularly subglottic airways. In the anesthesia or critical care setting, these airway devices are not only just temporary breathing devices, but also an essential part of the long-term airway management plan that should be used with the ultimate medical goals of the patient in mind.

1. Diba, A. 2005. Airway management devices. In: Davey, A., Diba, A. (Eds.), Ward's anaesthetic equipment, ed 5. Elsevier Saunders, Philadelphia. *This textbook provides a concise review of endotracheal tubes, tracheostomies, and other subglottic airway devices. This textbook served as an important reference for this chapter.*

2. Dorsch, J., Dorsch, S. 2008. Tracheal tubes and associated equipment. Understanding anesthesia equipment, ed 5. Lippincott Williams & Wilkins, Philadelphia. *This textbook provides a thorough review of endotracheal tubes and subglottic airway devices. It is recommended for more in-depth reading.*

3. Kollef, M., Afessa, B., Anzueto, A., et al., 2008. Silver-coated endotracheal tubes and incidence of ventilator-associated pneumonia: the NASCENT randomized trial. JAMA 300, 805–813. *This primary journal article is important for recognizing the morbidity and mortality of VAP. Although these significant findings did not show long-term decreases in morbidity and mortality, it is important in that researchers and clinicians recognized addressing VAP not only from a medical standpoint, but also from a technological and equipment standpoint.*

4. Pneumatikos, I., Dragoumanis, C., Bouros, D. 2009. Ventilator-associated pneumonia or endotracheal tube-associated pneumonia? An approach to the pathogenesis and preventive strategies emphasizing the importance of endotracheal tube. Anesthesiology 110, 673–680. *This journal article emphasizes the clinical significance of VAP and recognizing not only the ventilator as the source of infection, but also the actual endotracheal tube. Just as important is the approach to address endotracheal tubes as a possible source of infection.*

5. Polderman, K., Spijkstra, J., de Bree, R., et al., 2003. Percutaneous dilatational tracheostomy in the ICU: optimal organization, low complication rates, and description of a new complication. Chest 123, 1595–1602. *An example of the many recent reports that support the use of bedside tracheostomy in the ICU, which in the bigger picture, logistically safely supports the practice of early tracheostomy versus late tracheostomy in the ICU.*

6. Mort, T. 2007. Continuous airway access for the difficult extubation: the efficacy of the airway exchange catheter. Anesth Analg 105, 1357–1362. *This journal article highlights the importance of the anesthesiologist's responsibility in airway management—preparing for the worst case scenario. In this case, the worst case scenario is illustrated by failure to reintubate for whatever reason—but having not only a tube exchanger in place, but one that is also capable of oxygenating.*

References

1. Klock, P.A., Ovassapian, A. 2008. Airway management. In: Longnecker, D.E. (Ed.), Anesthesiology, McGraw-Hill Medical, New York.

2. Larson, C. 2006. Airway management. In: Morgan, G., Mikhail, M., Murray, M. (Eds.), Clinical Anesthesiology, ed 4. Lange Medical Books/McGraw-Hill, New York.

3. Khine, H., Corddry, D., Kettrick, R., et al., 1997. Comparison of cuffed and uncuffed endotracheal tubes in young children during general anesthesia. Anesthesiology 86, 627–631.

4. Yoon, S., Jeon, Y., Kim, Y., et al., 2007. The safety of reused endotracheal tubes sterilized according to Centers for Disease Control and Prevention guidelines. J Clin Anesth 19, 360–364.

5. Diba, A. 2005. Airway management devices. In: Davey, A., Diba, A. (Eds.), Ward's anaesthetic equipment, ed 5. Elsevier Saunders, Philadelphia.

6. Kollef, M., Afessa, B., Anzueto, A., et al., 2008. Silver-coated endotracheal tubes and incidence of ventilator-associated pneumonia: the NASCENT randomized trial. JAMA 300, 805–813.

7. Rello, J., Kollef, M., Diaz, E., et al., 2006. Reduced burden of bacterial airway colonization with a novel silver-coated endotracheal tube in a randomized multiple-center feasibility study. Crit Care Med 34, 2766–2772.

8. Koh, K., Hare, J., Calder, I. 1998. Small tubes revisited. Anaesthesia 53, 46–50.

9. Stout, D., Bishop, M., Dwersteg, J., et al., 1987. Correlation of endotracheal tube size with sore throat and hoarseness following general anaesthesia. Anaesthesiology 67, 419–421.

10. Dorsch, J., Dorsch, S. 2008. Tracheal tubes and associated equipment. In: Understanding anesthesia equipment, ed 5. Lippincott Williams & Wilkins, Philadelphia.

11. Diba, A. 2005. Airway management devices. In: Davey, A., Diba, A. (Eds.), Ward's anaesthetic equipment, ed 5. Elsevier Saunders, Philadelphia.

12. Pneumatikos, I., Dragoumanis, C., Bouros, D. 2009. Ventilator-associated pneumonia or endotracheal tube-associated pneumonia? An approach to the pathogenesis and preventive strategies emphasizing the importance of endotracheal tubes. Anesthesiology 110, 673–680.

13. Thomas, A., McGrath, B. 2009. Patient safety incidents associated with airway devices in critical care: a review of reports to the UK National Patient Safety Agency. Anaesthesia 64, 358–365.

14. Diba, A. 2005. Airway management devices. In: Davey, A., Diba, A. (Eds.), Ward's anaesthetic equipment, ed 5. Elsevier Saunders, Philadelphia.

15. Karasawa, F., Mori, T., Okuda, T., et al., 2001. Profile soft-seal cuff, a new endotracheal tube, effectively inhibits an increase in the cuff pressure through high compliance rather than low diffusion of nitrous oxide. Anesth Analg 92, 140–144.

16. Al-Shaikh, B., Stacey, S. 2007. Tracheal and tracheostomy tubes and airways, Essentials of anaesthetic equipment, ed 3. Elsevier, Philadelphia, Churchill Livingstone.

18 Dorsch, J., Dorsch, S. 2008. Tracheal tubes and associated equipment. Understanding anesthesia equipment, ed 5. Lippincott Williams & Wilkins, Philadelphia.

19. Russell, C. 2004. Tracheostomy tubes. In: Russell, C., Basil, M. (Eds.), Tracheostomy: a multi-professional handbook, Greenwich Medical Media Limited, London.

20. Polderman, K., Spijkstra, J., de Bree, R., et al., 2003. Percutaneous dilatational tracheostomy in the ICU: optimal organization, low complication rates, and description of a new complication. Chest 123, 1595–1602.

21. Klock, P.A., Ovassapian, A. 2008. Airway management. In: Longnecker, D.E. (Ed.), Anesthesiology, McGraw-Hill Medical, New York.

22. Bauman B, Hyzy R. Overview of tracheostomy, UpToDate (website): www.uptodate.com.

23. Diba, A. 2005. Airway management devices. In: Davey, A., Diba, A. (Eds.), Ward's anaesthetic equipment, ed 5. Elsevier Saunders, Philadelphia.

24. Campos, J. 2009. Update on selective lobar blockade during pulmonary resections. Curr Opin Anaesthesiol 22, 18–22.

25. Mort, T. 2007. Continuous airway access for the difficult extubation: the efficacy of the airway exchange catheter. Anesth Analg 105, 1357–1362.

Chapter 9

Noninvasive Physiological Monitors

Jordan L. Newmark and Warren S. Sandberg

Introduction

The hallmark of anesthesiology is providing patients with pain relief, comfort, and safety during unpleasant diagnostic studies, treatments, and surgery. Imparting safety to anesthetized patients requires vigilance, and continuous observation and monitoring of the patient. This forms the basis of the American Society of Anesthesiologists (ASA) seal, which depicts a watchtower and the word "vigilance" (Figure 9-1). Historically, and at present, stress of medical interventions and from anesthetics themselves causes physiological derangements in anesthetized patients, manifesting as erratic and unstable vital signs sensed by monitors. Monitors are the topic of this chapter.

The work of Joseph T. Clover, MD (1825–1882), renowned British anesthetist, was paramount in the development of monitoring for anesthetized patients. In Clover's time chloroform and nitrous oxide formed the basis of surgical anesthesia. He was a strong advocate of palpating the patient's pulse during anesthesia, and can be seen doing so in photographs (Figure 9-2) and depictions of him providing anesthesia care.[1]

The American Society of Anesthesiologists (ASA) House of Delegates approved on October 21, 1986, and last amended on October 25, 2005, a set of standards outlining basic anesthesia monitoring (otherwise known as the "ASA Standard Monitors"), to be followed whenever general, regional, or monitored anesthesia care (MAC) anesthesia is provided.[2] These vital monitors and their associated equipment/technology are noninvasive and will be discussed in this chapter.

The ASA Standard Monitors[2] include measures of patient oxygenation, ventilation, circulation, and, if necessary, the ability to monitor body temperature. Why did the ASA choose these patient variables and not others? The reason is because it is the responsibility of the anesthetist to provide adequate oxygenation and respiration to the organs of the patient at the tissue level to prevent cellular damage or cellular death. The ideal monitor would provide information regarding cell oxygenation and respiration safely, noninvasively, accurately, reliably, consistently, and in real time. This monitor should also require little to no maintenance, no calibration and should be monetarily inexpensive. Unfortunately, there is no single monitor in existence that can provide this information to the anesthetist. Therefore, surrogate measures must be obtained: inspired oxygen analysis, end-tidal CO_2 analysis, electrocardiography, blood pressure, and pulse oximetry. It is the task of the anesthetist to synthesize and interpret the data from these indirect monitors in order to infer adequacy of tissue oxygenation and respiration.

Assessment of oxygenation must include an oxygen analyzer to measure the amount of inspired oxygen within a breathing circuit, and a measurement of blood oxygenation (usually via pulse oximetry). Ventilation, in addition to clinical observation, may be detected by measuring carbon dioxide in the patient's exhaled gas. Capnography, capnometry, or mass or Raman spectrometry are used to quantify expired carbon dioxide. Appropriate monitoring of circulation requires a continuous electrocardiogram and perfusion assessment, in addition to measurement of blood pressure and heart rate at least every 5 minutes. Lastly, temperature, if deemed necessary by the anesthesiologist, can be measured with a thermistor or thermocouple probe. Each monitor is prone to error, so all of the above monitors are best used when the data are pooled together, in conjunction with clinical data from direct patient observation, physical examination, and assessment, such as chest auscultation or direct palpation of pulses, to fully gauge the well-being of the patient under anesthesia.[3]

The anesthetized patient often needs additional noninvasive monitors, such as inhalational agent concentration analyzers,

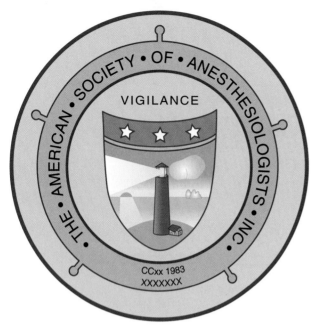

Figure 9–1   ASA seal. *(From ASA. (website): www.asahq.org.) Accessed* August 30, 2010.

peripheral nerve stimulation for neuromuscular blockade, or central nervous system monitoring. These adjunct monitors will also be discussed.

Monitors Connected to the Patient

Cardiovascular System

Electrocardiogram (ECG)

The ECG monitors the conduction of electrical impulses through the heart. These yield potentials of 0.5 to 2.0 mV at the patient's skin, to produce PQRST waveforms. This monitor is used to determine the heart rate and to detect and diagnose arrhythmias, myocardial ischemia, structural defects, pacemaker function, and electrolyte abnormalities. Note that the presence of an ECG signal does not guarantee adequate cardiac contraction or output (e.g., pulseless electrical activity).

Mechanism of Monitoring

Electrode pads containing a silver/silver chloride electrode bound to adhesive material and a conductive gel, which decreases the electrical resistance of the skin surface, are applied to the patient's skin (Figure 9-3). ECG electrodes measure a small electrical signal (about 1 mV), which is amplified and broadcasted over a 0.01- to 250-Hz bandwidth. This allows for the filtration of "noise."[4,5] The ECG is prone to electrical interference from outside sources, and requires proper electrode application to clean, dry skin, ideally free of hair. Severely burned patients or those with certain dermatological conditions may require sterile subcutaneous needle electrodes rather than electrode pads.[6] In normal patients, the injury risk from ECG monitor application is essentially zero. However, ECG skin electrodes can cause skin irritation if left on for a prolonged duration of time without being changed,

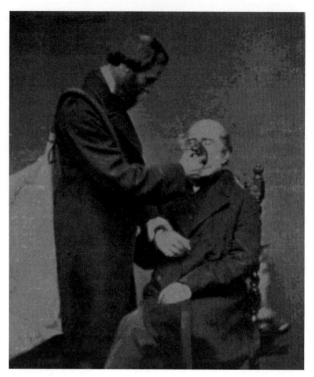

Figure 9–2   Joseph Clover, MD, administering chloroform and palpating the radial pulse.

as is often the case for intensive care unit (ICU) patients (Table 9-1).[7]

ECG skin electrodes, and peripheral nerve electrode pads, should be placed upon skin which is cleaned to remove dead skin, decrease signal impedance and allow for more accurate signal measurement.[8]

Appropriate electrode placement and location is an important component of proper ECG monitoring. To effectively detect arrhythmias and ischemia, the pads must be placed in consistent locations on the patient (Figure 9-4). Limb leads must be placed on, or near, their appropriate limbs and the precordial lead (V_5) at the fifth intercostal space, anterior axillary line. Note that lead RL is a "ground" lead, or earth reference.[5] Therefore, placement of RL anywhere on the patient is acceptable (Figure 9-5).

MODES AND OPTIONS FOR ECG MONITORING

The ECG monitor has several choices for the filtering of noise, most commonly called "diagnostic" and "monitor" modes. The monitor mode filters out noise by using a narrowed band pass (0.5 to 40 Hz), while the diagnostic mode filters less signal and noise by using a wider band pass (0.05 to 100 Hz).

Rate Detection

The ECG is an excellent measure of heart rate (Figure 9-6). Visual or audible alarms alert the anesthetist to bradycardia and tachycardia.

Rhythm Detection

It is important to monitor and ensure the anesthetized patient maintains a normal sinus rhythm—a P wave before each QRS complex. P waves are best seen in lead II.

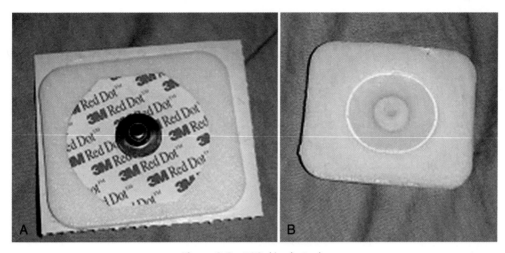

Figure 9–3   ECG skin electrode.

Ischemia Detection

This diagnostic mode should be used when monitoring for ischemia. Automatic trending of ST segment changes is often available and useful for monitoring the development of ischemia over time. Continuous monitoring of leads II and V_5 simultaneously allows for detection of ischemia anywhere in a large area of the myocardium. Lead II monitors the inferior portion of the heart, supplied by the right coronary artery. Lead V_5 monitors the bulk of the left ventricle, supplied by the left anterior descending artery. Lead I may be monitored for patients in whom the left circumflex artery is at risk. Visual and/or audible alarms may be configured to provide the anesthetist a warning of possible ischemic changes.

Impedance Pneumography and Apnea Detection

Many ECG monitors have the ability to measure a patient's respiratory rate through impedance pneumography (Figure 9-7). Impedance pneumography works by measuring the electrical impedance of the thoracic cavity. The baseline thoracic impedance is often represented as "Z." As air enters the thoracic cavity, lung volume increases, thus increasing the thoracic impedance. During expiration, lung volume decreases, and the impedance of the thoracic cavity goes down. These changes in Z are sometimes called ΔZ. These data are processed and displayed in waveforms representing inspiration and expiration, allowing the anesthetist to observe respiratory rate and depth of breathing. ECG lead I allows for monitoring of the upper chest breaths, while ECG lead II gives data from the lower chest and diaphragmatic area. Impedance pneumography is most commonly used by the anesthetist within the postanesthesia care unit (PACU) or intensive care unit in spontaneously ventilating patients. Cessation in impedance, or when ΔZ becomes equal to Z, will activate an apnea alarm, alerting the anesthetist that the patient may have stopped making respiratory effort.

Implantable Cardiac Rhythm Management Devices

The ECG is capable of monitoring cardiac pacemakers by displaying pacing spikes while the device is functioning (Figure 9-8). If the patient's heart rate is higher than the device's programmed rate, no pacer spikes will be seen because the

Table 9–1   Sources of ECG Error/Interference

- Electrocautery (especially monopolar) causes (i) ECG artifacts (ii) malposition of electrocautery plate in relation to ECG skin electrodes can leave burns at the electrode sites.[4] (See Figure 9-7 for image of electrocautery artifact)

- Movement of the patient or OR table/stretcher or excessive muscle tone.[11] This affect can be reduced by placing electrodes over bony prominences and by using low-pass filters.[4]

- Inadequate adhesion of electrodes to skin (see Figure 9-10).

- Incorrect lead placement (see image).

- Electrical interference.

- Obesity will decrease wave amplitude, whereas patients with thin walled chests will show amplification of the ECG waves. The displayed waveform appearance may be amplified on many ECG monitors to allow for closer inspection.

device is not firing (or not needed). Pacer spikes occur at a constant rate. Patients who are atrial-chamber paced will reveal pacer spikes before each P wave, while patients who are ventricular-chamber paced will have pacer spikes before each QRS complex and QRS widening. Lastly, pacers that are dual atrial and ventricular paced will display pacer spikes before each P wave and each QRS complex (Figure 9-9). If the patient has an implanted cardioverter-defibrillator (ICD), an ECG (and the capability to deliver an external defibrillating shock) should be monitored during surgery and transport (Figure 9-10). This is because ICDs are often programmed perioperatively to "no response," and to respond to external magnet placement.[10]

Noninvasive Blood Pressure Monitoring

The circulatory system is responsible for perfusing organs with blood. Oxygen delivery to, and removal of waste products from, organs must be maintained at all times to sustain life, including during anesthesia.

Blood flow to organs is directly related to pressure gradients and inversely related to vascular resistance. Flow = Pressure/Resistance. Therefore, even if pressure is high, flow may be reduced in the face of elevated resistance. Pressure gradients can be estimated by the difference between mean

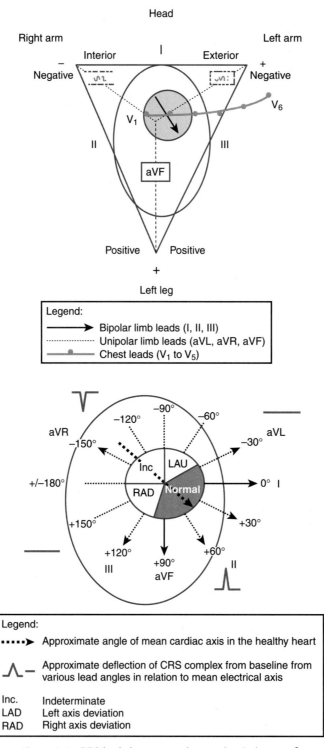

Figure 9–4 ECG lead placement and mean electrical vectors.[9]

arterial pressure (MAP) and venous pressure, or, in the case of increased intracerebral pressure (ICP), the difference between MAP and ICP.

The arterial blood pressure is used as a surrogate measure of blood flow and organ perfusion and is comprised of resistance and flow. Thus blood supply to an organ may be low despite adequate blood pressure because of high resistance. Individual organs manifest various degrees of autoregulation, which allows for local changes in resistance to maintain a constant blood flow.

Systolic and diastolic blood pressures are measured by a variety of methods. The pressure created by a contracting heart corresponds to the systolic blood pressure, while the pressure during relaxation corresponds to the diastolic blood pressure. Mean arterial blood pressure is the average arterial blood pressure during systole and diastole; MAP is approximately

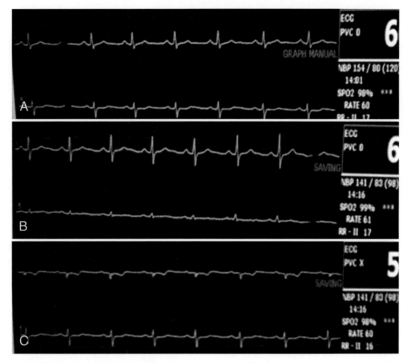

Figure 9–5   ECG displaying II on *top column* and V5 on *bottom column*. **A,** Correct lead placement, displaying II and V5. **B,** V5 and left leg limb leads switched. **C,** LA and RA leads switched.

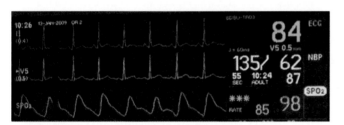

Figure 9–6   Normal ECG waveform with associated Spo₂ plethysmograph.

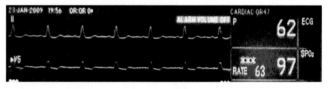

Figure 9–9   V-paced ECG. Same patient with the DDD pacer, now V-paced. Note widened QRS. V-pacer spikes buried under QRS complex and cannot be appreciated.

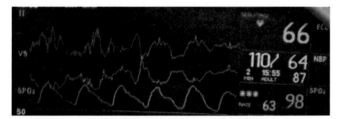

Figure 9–7   Electrocautery artifact and ECG waveform. Note the associated plethysmographic wave from the pulse oximeter is regular and appropriate in morphology. This can be used to reassure the anesthetist that the patient has not developed a dangerous arrhythmia.

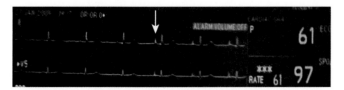

Figure 9–8   A-pacer spikes. Patient with DDD pacer, programmed to A-pace at 60 beats per minute. The letter *P* next to the heart rate indicates pacer detection is on.

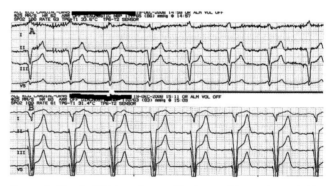

Figure 9–10   **A,** ECG impedance artifact caused by uncleansed skin. **B,** Same patient and ECG lead placement after skin was cleaned with NuPrep (Weaver and Company, CO)[12] gel, which is an abrasive gel that removes dead skin to decrease the electrical resistance of the skin to ECG signal transmission. *(Image and caption courtesy of Scott Streckenbach, MD, Dept. of Anesthesia and Critical Care, Massachusetts General Hospital, Harvard Medical School, Boston.)*

Table 9–2 Selection of an Appropriate Blood Pressure Cuff[13]

- Width of the inflatable bladder of the cuff should be ~40% of upper arm circumference (about 12-14 cm in the average adult).
- Length of inflatable bladder should be ~80% of upper arm circumference (practically enough length to encompass the arm).
- If an aneroid manometer is used, recalibrate periodically before use.
- Ideally, for lower extremity blood pressure measurements, use a wide, long thigh cuff that has a bladder size 18 × 42 cm and apply to the midthigh with it centered over the popliteal artery.

Table 9–3 Limitations, Precautions, and Additional Considerations for Auscultatory Blood Pressure Measurement

- Cuff size may give incorrect values; a cuff that is too small may result in falsely high blood pressures, whereas a cuff that is too large may result in falsely low blood pressures. The cuff width should cover two thirds of the upper arm or thigh.
- Requires active operator participation; labor intensive.
- Prone to operator error and subjective interpretation.
- Vasoconstriction, low blood pressure, and operating room noise may make auscultation difficult.
- Rapid deflation may give low pressure readings.
- Clothing or other objects trapped between the bladder and patient's skin may interfere with auscultation and/or blood pressure measurements.
- Palpate the artery of interest before initial measurement of blood pressure. Ensure the limb is free of clothing, lesions, lymphedema, arteriovenous fistulas, etc.[14]
- Auscultated vessel should be at the level of the heart. Vessels auscultated above the level of the heart are measured to be falsely low and vice versa.[14,6]
- Auscultatory gaps are periods of silence during the auscultation of systolic through diastolic blood pressures. These can be prevented by estimating the systolic blood pressure. Palpate a major distal artery and inflate the cuff until the pulse is no longer palpable and occluded—note the pressure. Deflate the cuff, wait 15-30 sec, and raise the cuff again above the occlusion pressure.[15]

equal to (2DBP + SBP)/3. It may be either directly measured or calculated from the systolic and diastolic values.

Manual Blood Pressure

Manual blood pressure directly measures the systolic and diastolic blood pressure by auscultation of Korotkoff sounds. The occlusive cuff contains a bladder attached to a tube through which air is entrained with an inflation bulb until a desired pressure is produced. The pressure is often measured with an aneroid manometer. A stethoscope is placed over the occluded artery. The occlusive cuff is inflated above the systolic blood pressure and is slowly deflated (3 to 5 mm Hg/sec) while auscultating for blood flow. The first sound of blood flow corresponds to the systolic blood pressure, while the point at which the sounds diminish reveals the diastolic blood pressure. Auscultation using a stethoscope will detect these Korotkoff sounds. Right- and left-sided, and upper and lower extremity blood pressures should be approximately the same. Both single and twin hose cuffs are available (see below under automated noninvasive blood pressure monitoring) (Table 9-2).

Automated Noninvasive Blood Pressure (NIBP)

Automated noninvasive blood pressure is the most common method of noninvasive blood pressure monitoring during anesthesia (Table 9-3). The blood pressure cuff is inflated initially to a preset point (150 mm Hg, or 40 mm Hg above prior measurement) and then incrementally decreased while the transducer senses the pressure oscillation in the cuff with an accuracy of +/− 2%.[4] This method directly measures the mean arterial blood pressure, which correlates to the point of maximum oscillation amplitude, and the systolic and diastolic pressures are estimated by an algorithm (roughly: MAP = (2DBP + SPB)/3. More specifically, the systolic blood pressure is interpreted as the initial detection of rising oscillation, while the diastolic blood pressure is interpreted as the initial detection of falling oscillations (Table 9-4). The automated cuff allows passive participation by the operator and limits operator interpretation by programming the cuff to measure the blood pressure at preset increments of time (e.g., every 5 minutes). NIBP cuffs and/or monitors may contain a single or twin hose system. These systems can be successfully mixed

Table 9–4 Limitations of Oscillometric Blood Pressure Monitoring

- Motion artifact may result in erroneous values or not give any values at all, resulting in a delay in accurate measurements (e.g., a shivering patient).
- Venous congestion, bruising at the site of cuff application, and limb ischemia may result from frequent blood pressure measurements during rapid or large blood pressure fluctuations. This can be prevented with a fast inflation and slow deflation time.
- Nerve damage.
- Intravenous or arterial line occlusion during cuff inflation.
- If placed proximal to a pulse oximeter or invasive blood pressure monitor, false decrease in Spo_2 and/or dampening of invasive blood pressure trace.
- Dysrhythmias may make values difficult to interpret or increase cycle time.
- Very low or high blood pressures may not correlate with intraarterial measurements; noninvasive blood pressure often overestimates low blood pressure (e.g., systolic blood pressure below 80 mm Hg).
- Different manufacturers of NIBP monitors may record differing blood pressures because each make uses a nonstandardized algorithm in estimating NIBP from the oscillometric waveform to derive SBP, DBP, and MAP.[15]
- See limitations of manual auscultation.

Table 9–5 Limitations of Doppler and Palpation Blood Pressure Measurement

- Only SBP can be measured.
- Palpation underestimates SBP.
- Doppler ultrasound is more sensitive than direct palpation in the obese, pediatric patients, or patients in shock.
- Misplacement of Doppler probe away from the artery prevents appreciation of the blood pressure and may lead to false diagnosis of severe hypotension.
- Inadequate amounts of ultrasound gel causing interference.

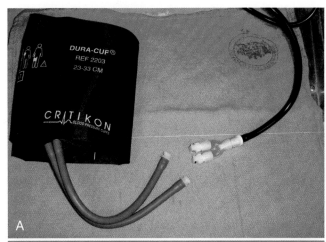

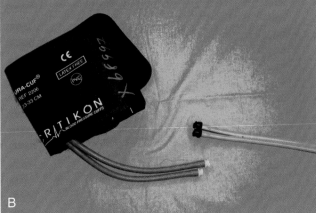

Figure 9–11 NIBP cuff with **(A)** single and **(B)** twin hosing systems.

in the case of a mismatched cuff and monitor, as long as a Y-piece adapter is used.[14] Table 9-5 denotes some common problems with automated NIBP monitors. Commonly, the cuff will keep cycling to try and obtain a blood pressure under some of the circumstances listed in Table 9-5 (Figure 9-11). If a blood pressure cannot be determined, error messages may be displayed, such as "pump time-out."

Doppler Ultrasound and Direct Palpation to Estimate Blood Pressure

Doppler or palpation uses ultrasound or touch, respectively, in conjunction with an inflatable cuff respectively, to estimate the blood pressure. The systolic pressure correlates to the point during cuff deflation at which first pulse is palpated or Korotkoff sounds are heard. Therefore, these methods entail placing a blood pressure cuff proximal to the artery of interest, and inflating the cuff until the pulse is occluded. The cuff is then gradually deflated until the pulse is appreciated once again. Palpation may also be used to determine approximate systolic blood pressure based on whether the pulse may be palpated at key points: radial artery (~80 mm Hg), femoral artery (~60 mm Hg), or carotid artery (~50 mm Hg). This method provides estimates when the blood pressure is very low. Note that these methods cannot determine diastolic or mean blood pressure, and has the same limitations as the auscultation method.

The Doppler probe works by transmitting ultrasonic waves through the underlying tissue into the flowing blood within the artery, which is then reflected back to the probe. The movement of blood creates a frequency shift, which is also transduced by the probe and can be aurally appreciated. This change between the transmitted and reflected frequencies produces the audible sounds of pulsation. Coupling gel must be placed between the probe and skin to minimize interference from air.

Arterial Tonometry

Arterial tonometry measures beat-to-beat blood pressure in a noninvasive fashion and produces a waveform similar to that of an invasive arterial blood pressure monitor (Table 9-6). Arterial tonometry works by placing numerous independent pressure transducers on the skin over a superficial artery, which overlays bony support, such as the temporal, radial, or dorsalis pedis arteries.[16,17] The tonometer flattens the artery against the bone without occluding flow (Figure 9-12). Wall tension from the tonometer then acts perpendicular to the blood pressure,

such that force measured by transducers at the skin surface reflect the patient's blood pressure within that artery.[16]

Respiratory System

The respiratory system is responsible for oxygen uptake and carbon dioxide removal, and provides a conduit for delivery of anesthetic agents. Mandatory respiratory monitors during general anesthesia include pulse oximetry, capnography, an inspired oxygen analyzer, and a disconnect alarm. In addition, direct visualization of the chest and a precordial or esophageal stethoscope may provide additional clinical information, such as detection of airway obstruction. During regional anesthesia, respiration may be monitored with direct visualization, oximetry, or capnography.

Oxygenation is most easily measured by pulse oximetry. Other methods include qualitative assessment of skin color, transcutaneous oximetry, and arterial blood gas sampling.

Pulse Oximetry

The advent of pulse oximetry in medicine has revolutionized the monitoring of patients, especially that of the anesthetized and critically ill patient (Figure 9-13). It is an extremely important monitor that allows for the continuous measurement of arterial hemoglobin oxygenation (Table 9-7). Oxygenated and deoxygenated hemoglobin absorb light differently at most wavelengths, including the wavelengths of

Table 9–6 Limitations of Arterial Tonometry

- Need for frequent calibration.[6]
- Motion artifact.
- Need for optimal placement directly over an artery, which can change with changes in blood pressure and arterial tone.[17]
- Tonometry apparatus can be cumbersome or uncomfortable for the patient.

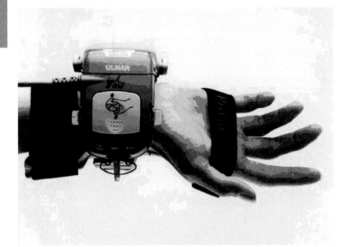

A

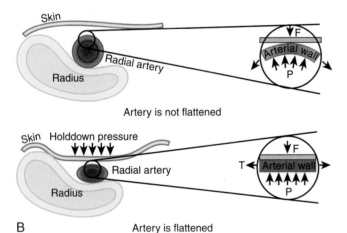

B

Figure 9–12 Arterial tonometry. (*From Tensys Medical (website):* www.tensysmedical.com[18] *and Kemmotsu O, Ueda M, Otsuka H, et al. Arterial tonometry for noninvasive, continuous blood pressure monitoring during anesthesia. Anesthesiology 1991;75(2):333-34.*[16])

660 nm (red light) and 960 nm (infrared light) examined by most devices. The Beer-Lambert law allows the concentration of each species to be calculated from the absorption of light at those wavelengths. The ratio of absorption is processed to give the percentage of hemoglobin saturated by oxygen, or the fractional saturation. The sensor has at least two light emitting diodes (960 nm and 660 nm) and a light detector. This sensor may be applied to fingers, toes, earlobes, tongue, or, with a special probe, the nose.

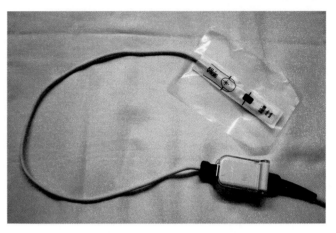

Figure 9–13 Pulse oximeter probe.

Table 9–7 Limitations of Pulse Oximetry

- Oximetry is a late reporter of inadequate gas exchange. Modern oximeters impose a ~10-sec delay between physiological changes and the displayed SpO_2 on the monitor.
- Oxyhemoglobin dissociation curve shifts may change the patient's PaO_2 without changes to the SpO_2.[20]
- Carboxyhemoglobin produced by carbon monoxide poisoning or cigarette smoking absorbs light similarly to oxygenated hemoglobin at 660 nm and will provide falsely elevated readings, although it does not contribute to O_2 delivery.
- Methemoglobin absorbs light at both 660 nm and 940 nm, resulting in a saturation of 85%, which does not correlate with the true saturation. Methemoglobinemia may often be treated with methylene blue.
- Methylene blue, indocyanine green, indigo carmine, and isosulfan blue injections transiently result in falsely low saturation readings.
- SpO_2 tends to be falsely overestimated at low saturations (below 80%).
- Malpositioned sensors affect results. For example, the *penumbra effect*[5,22] occurs because the path length of the 660-nm red light and 940-nm infrared light markedly differ. Therefore if the pulse oximeter does not appropriately fit on the patient's finger, which can be seen in pediatric patients, a falsely high SpO_2 is observed if the SaO_2 is <85%, and a falsely low SpO_2 is seen if the SaO_2 is >85% because light is shunted from the LED to the photodetector (optical shunting).
- Low perfusion (e.g., from a proximal blood pressure cuff, cardiac arrest, increased systemic vascular resistance).
- Cold or ischemic measured extremity.
- Ambient light.
- Motion.
- Hypotension/hypovolemia.
- Nail polish.
- Severe anemia with hematocrit <25%, SpO_2 is less reliable when the SpO_2 is decreased. With a hematocrit <10%, SpO_2 is less reliable at all SpO_2 levels.[20]
- Electromagnetic interference from bipolar electrocautery or cellular phones.[5]
- Skin pigmentation may or may not falsely underestimate SpO_2.[4,5,20]
- Rarely, burns, pressure sores, or pressure necrosis from the light emitting diode of the sensor.

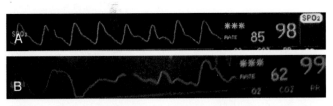

Figure 9–14 **A,** Normal plethysmographic waveform. Note the three asterisks indicating that the signal strength is optimized. **B,** Abnormal/ unreliable plethysmographic waveform.

Normal arterial oxygen saturation, or pulse oximetry (SpO_2) ranges in a healthy adult is 96% to 99%, while values above 88% may be acceptable in patients with lung disease. The percentages are associated with audible pitches, which allow the anesthetist to know the patient's relative level of oxygenation without seeing the monitor. The monitor also provides alarms when saturation falls below a level selected by the user. A high SpO_2 generally indicates that oxygen is available in the lungs from the environment or breathing circuit, taken up in the blood, and delivered to distal tissues. A low SpO_2 implies a problem along the above pathway, or an error in monitoring.

Certain hemoglobinopathies, most notably the presence of carboxyhemoglobin or methemoglobin, can falsely raise or lower the SpO_2, respectively. This is because carboxyhemoglobin appears like oxyhemoglobin at 660 nm, thus raising the apparent percent of total hemoglobin which is oxygenated. By extension, methemoglobin appears like deoxyhemoglobin at 660 nm, thereby lowering the apparent fraction of deoxyhemoglobin. Co-oximeters exist with a sensor using four or more wavelengths, which can separate a variety of hemoglobin species to calculate a more accurate fractional saturation.[4,19]

The pulse oximeter detects a pulse plethysmographic waveform (Figure 9-14). Without a clear waveform, the accuracy of the detected SpO_2 should be questioned. The characteristics of this waveform itself may reveal important clinical information, especially when used in conjunction with other monitors. For instance, electrocautery may cause ECG interference, which could be confused with a dangerous cardiac arrhythmia. However, a consistent plethysmographic waveform can easily rule this out. There have been case reports of the plethysmograph diagnosing the degree of airway trapping in obstructive airway disease with pulsus paradoxus, and degree of waveform respiratory oscillations predicting fluid responsiveness in the operating room and ICU.[20]

Some pulse oximetry systems include a signal strength indicator, which can be used to help analyze waveform quality, and therefore assess the validity of the signal and SpO_2 value. For example, the General Electric (GE)/Masimo SET system displays either one, two, or three asterisks, or three dashes, in the display screen to convey the quality/validity of the SpO_2 signal.

End-Tidal CO₂ Monitors

Ventilation is assessed by end-tidal carbon dioxide ($PetCO_2$) measurements and spirometry. Capnometry and capnography are often used as synonyms, as both analyze and record carbon dioxide (CO_2), with the latter including a waveform. Capnography not only evaluates respiration, but also confirms endotracheal intubation, and is diagnostic for certain pathological conditions. Lastly, mass spectrometry or Raman spectrometry may be employed as a technology to quantify $PetCO_2$, assuming a sidestream capnometer, rather than a mainstream capnometer, is used.

METHOD

The measurement of CO_2, due to its molecular structure, is frequently based on infrared light absorption. $PetCO_2$ can be measured continuously, in real time, to produce waveforms, which will be discussed below. With absorption infrared CO_2 analyzers (a commonly used analyzer), $PetCO_2$ is measured by diverting a gas sample from the patient into a sample chamber. Infrared light is shined through two chambers (a reference/control chamber and a testing chamber), and is sensed by a photodetector. CO_2 absorbs infrared light optimally of a wavelength between roughly 4.2 μm and 4.3 μm. Thus radiation of this wavelength is used. As CO_2 enters the sample chamber, it absorbs the infrared light. With higher concentrations of CO_2, absorption increases and less infrared radiation reaches the photodetector. With this information, and that from the control chamber, $PetCO_2$ can be calculated by the CO_2 analyzer.

Other than absorption infrared based CO_2 analyzers, photo-acoustic spectroscopy may be used. This device uses a microphone to detect sound produced by the contraction and expansion of the gas sample when it is exposed to pulsatile infrared radiation of an appropriate wavelength. Photoacoustic spectroscopy allows for less frequent calibration and is faster to detect $PetCO_2$ changes when compared with absorption infrared CO_2 analyzers.

Carbon dioxide may be measured either at the breathing circuit (mainstream capnograph), or via aspiration of gas samples by the capnograph (sidestream capnograph) at a constant rate (from 50 to 250 mL/min), facilitated by a pump, by the above listed CO_2 analyzers. See Tables 9-10 and 9-11 for advantages and disadvantages of each sampling method.

Mass spectroscopy is considered the gold standard expired gas monitor. It determines the amount of a large variety of gases within a sample by firing electrons through it. This imparts a charge (usually positive) onto the sampled gases, and the charged gas moves toward a negatively charged acceleration plate. As the gases travel, they exit through a small hole in the system called a molecular leak, after which the gases are exposed to a magnetic field. This field deflects the path of the gases, whereby gases of lower molecular weight become separated from gases of higher molecular weight. The gases soon reach a photovoltaic detector at different locations, depending on the particle mass, allowing for the identification and calculation of the partial pressure of each gas in the sample.[19] The limitation of this technology is that it must be used with a sidestream sample line, it must be within close proximity of the patient for real-time analysis, and water vapor can collect in their sample line.[19] These machines are also rather expensive, which also limits its practical use.[21]

Raman spectroscopy uses an argon laser with a wavelength of 485 nm, which is fired into the gas sample of the patient. As the gases are exposed to this radiation, they undergo an energy change and frequency shift, which is unique for each gas. Based upon the frequency shift wave number, the spectroscope can calculate the concentration of each gas in the sample in real-time, including volatile anesthetic agents, nitrous oxide, and molecular oxygen. This device requires a sidestream sample line, and consumes a large amount of electrical power. This machine is also very noisy.[19,21]

Table 9–8 Components of the Time-Based Capnogram Waveform

- The normal end-tidal CO_2 ($Petco_2$) waveform contains the expiratory portion (phases I, II, III, and occasionally IV) and inspiratory portion (phase 0).

- Two angles, the α-angle (between phase II and III) and the β-angle (between phase III and 0), also aide in interpretation (Figure 9-14).

- Phase 0 is the inspiratory segment.

- Phase I shows CO_2-free gas that is not involved in gas exchange (dead space).

- Phase II is the rapid upswing and includes both alveolar gas and dead space gas.

- Phase III is a plateau that involves alveolar gas and has a small positive slope.

- $Petco_2$ is measured at the end of phase III.

- Phase IV is a terminal upswing seen in obese and pregnant patients with reduced thoracic compliance.

- The α-angle is between phases II and III and is related to the V/Q matching of the lung. The β-angle is between phases III and 0 and usually about 90°and may be used to assess rebreathing.

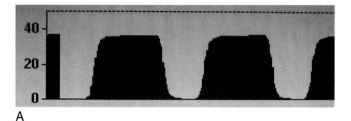

A

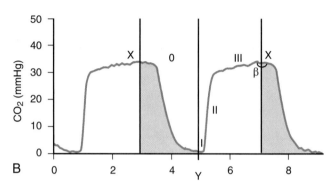

B

Figure 9–15 **A,** Capnogram waveforms. **B,** Phases of the capnogram. See Table 9-8 for definitions. *(From Bhavani-Shankar K, Philip JH. Defining segments and phases of a time capnogram. Anesth Analg 2000;91:973-977.)*

Time-Based Versus Volume-Based Capnography

Time-based capnograms are the most commonly used waveforms in the operating room and intensive care unit (Table 9-8). They plot $Petco_2$ on the y-axis and time on the x-axis (Figure 9-15). A detailed discussion of their interpretation will follow below. It is important to note that volume-based curves may be used and differ from time-based capnograms in several key ways, which allows for the calculation of cardiac output, anatomic dead space volume, physiological dead space fraction, the exhaled CO_2 volume, and even the patient's metabolic rate if CO_2 is known.[20] Volume-based capnography plots Pco_2 on the y-axis and volume on the x-axis.[20]

Range and Analysis

Normally, $Petco_2$ is approximately 2 to 5 mm Hg lower than $Paco_2$ due to dead space in the patient and breathing system. Therefore the ideal range for end-tidal carbon dioxide during general anesthesia is 30 to 40 mm Hg. Due to swallowed gas, esophageal intubation may result in carbon dioxide return similar to that of endotracheal intubation, except that $Petco_2$ diminishes to zero within a few breaths.

An early sign of malignant hyperthermia is a rapidly rising end-tidal carbon dioxide, especially if it is unresponsive to hyperventilation.

During a period of apnea or prolonged expiration, the measured $Petco_2$ becomes zero, even though $Paco_2$ is likely elevated. Providing a breath to the patient will produce another waveform. Sometimes cardiogenic oscillations may be seen on the $Petco_2$ waveform in this context (Figure 9-16). These are the result of the heart beating and displacing gas from the lungs, which leads to very small amounts of CO_2 being expelled into the sample line. In pressure support ventilation, these oscillations may be mistaken for an attempted patient breath, thus unintentionally triggering the ventilator to provide a breath.[23] These unintentional triggers may be avoided

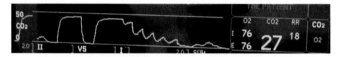

Figure 9–16 Cardiogenic oscillations.

by increasing the threshold for breath delivery, for example, by increasing the degree of negative inspiratory flow required to allow for the delivery of a breath by the ventilator (e.g., from 3 L/min to 4 L/min).

Widening of the β-angle with an elevation of both phase 0/I and III is a sign of inspiratory valve failure. Elevation of both phase 0/I and phase III is a sign of expiratory valve failure or absorbent malfunction. Inspired CO_2 will also rise in the face of absorbent exhaustion.

Alarms may be configured to warn the anesthetist of high or low $Petco_2$ measurements during inspiration or expiration (Table 9-9). The apnea alarm can also be based on capnography (Tables 9-10 and 9-11) (Figure 9-17).

Miscellaneous Monitors

The following monitors are required to be available, but need not be used at all times, according to the ASA standards for basic monitoring of the anesthetized patient. This does not detract from the importance of the following devices, which are very important for the safety and well-being of patients under anesthesia.

Temperature Monitoring

Temperature may be measured intermittently or continuously. The limitation of more external methods of temperature determination is that they may not reflect changes in the core body temperature, especially in the presence of vasoconstriction.

Table 9–9 Causes of High and Low End-Tidal CO₂

HIGH PETco₂[20]

Increased CO₂ delivery/production

Malignant hyperthermia, fever, sepsis, seizures, increased metabolic rate or skeletal muscle activity, bicarbonate administration/medication side effect, laparoscopic surgery, clamp/tourniquet release

Hypoventilation

COPD, neuromuscular paralysis or dysfunction, CNS depression, metabolic alkalosis (if spontaneously breathing), medication side effect

Equipment problems

CO₂ absorbent exhaustion, ventilator leak, rebreathing, malfunctioning inspiratory or expiratory valve

LOW PETco₂

Decreased CO₂ delivery/production

Hypothermia, hypometabolism, pulmonary hypoperfusion, low cardiac output or arrest, pulmonary artery embolism, hemorrhage, hypotension, hypovolemia, V/Q mismatch or shunt, auto-PEEP, medication side effect

Hyperventilation

Pain/anxiety, awareness/"light" anesthesia, metabolic acidosis (if spontaneously breathing), medication side effect

Equipment problems

Ventilator disconnection, esophageal intubation, bronchial intubation, complete airway obstruction or apnea, sample line problems (kinks), endotracheal tube or laryngeal mask airway leaks

Table 9–11 Limitations of Mainstream Versus Sidestream Capnometers[4,6,20]

MAINSTREAM

- Sensor plugging with secretions or humidity
- Sensor is heated and cumbersome, could burn or place traction on the endotracheal tube, respectively
- Cannot measure nitrous oxide
- Impractical for spontaneously respiring patients
- Sensor damage in some models[4]
- Sensors must be reused and sterilized
- Older models cannot determine inspired CO₂[6]
- Do not expose patient or healthcare personnel to gas exhaust as a matter of infection control[7]

SIDESTREAM

- Sensor plugging with secretions
- Sample tubing is delicate and easily kinked/damaged/leakage
- Water trap required
- Lag time from patient to analyzer
- Small tidal volumes (e.g., in pediatric patients) with high aspiration rates dilute the Petco₂ measurement with fresh gas. Low aspiration rates during hyperventilation may also underestimate Petco₂
- Older models must be calibrated
- Do not expose patient or healthcare personnel to gas exhaust as a matter of infection control[7]

Table 9–10 Advantages of Mainstream Versus Sidestream Capnometers[4,6,20]

MAINSTREAM

Sensor location is close to the airway

- Fast response/real time tracing
- No sample flow to reduce tidal volume
- Heater stops the accumulation of water vapor condensation

SIDESTREAM

- Less cumbersome equipment
- Safety (less potential to burn the patient with radiant heat)
- Disposable sample line
- Use with patients who are spontaneously respiring
- Allows for other gas measurements (e.g., nitrous oxide, volatile agents)
- Can be connected to a mass or Raman spectrometer and a portable Petco₂ analyzer for patient transport

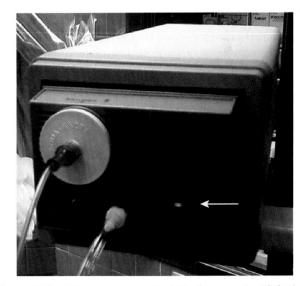

Figure 9–17 Sidestream capnometer. Note the green "on" light, indicating the pump is active.

INDICATIONS

Although temperature need not be measured during all anesthetics, it is important to note that the anesthetized patient is prone to temperature perturbations. This results from surgical site exposure, cold operating rooms, long surgical durations, vasodilation, and hypothalamic thermoregulatory inhibition from anesthetics, mechanical ventilation, and high gas flows through the endotracheal tube. Processes including evaporation, radiation, convection, and conduction draw heat away from the patient over time.

Temperature monitoring is indicated in several circumstances, and will be discussed below. It is desirable to measure temperature when the need to control it arises, such as during induced hypothermia and rewarming (e.g., during cardiopulmonary bypass or vascular neurosurgery), or when warming devices are used prophylactically. Infants and small children are prone to thermal liability due to their high surface area to volume ratio and will require temperature measurement. Adults who are subjected to large evaporative losses or low ambient temperatures (as occurs with exposed body cavities, large volume transfusion of unwarmed fluids, or burns) are prone to hypothermia. Febrile patients need to be monitored because of the risk of hyperthermia or hypothermia. Patients with autonomic dysfunction are unable to autoregulate their body temperature. Trauma patients, especially those exposed to the elements for long amounts of time, need temperature measurements. Lastly, malignant hyperthermia is a rare, but always possible pharmacogenetic complication. Therefore, temperature monitoring must be always readily available.

MONITORING SITES AND PROBE OPTIONS

Several types of temperature probes exist and can be classified into thermistors and thermocouples. Both are available as disposable sensors. A thermistor is a semiconductor that undergoes a linear and predictable decrease in resistance with increasing temperature. The nasopharyngeal probe is a thermistor. A thermocouple uses the *Seebeck effect* to monitor the patient. The device made of two dissimilar metals. The two are connected to one another, with one end maintained at a constant/reference temperature and the other exposed to the patient. When the two metals are at different temperatures, a potential difference is produced, which is mathematically correlated in a nonlinear fashion and allows the probe to function.[5,6] The technology involved in tympanic thermometers includes infrared radiation and thermocoupling. Infrared radiation from the eardrum is sensed by thermocouples within the thermometer, producing a potential difference as described above. This potential difference is correlated, again in a nonlinear way, to the eardrum temperature.[5]

Skin temperature, as measured on the forehead with a color changing liquid crystal strip, is normally 3° F to 4° F below core temperature, and this gradient may increase with further cooling. This is a poor temperature measure and cannot be used on patients with facial burns and can easily lose its adhesive ability, especially if a patient becomes diaphoretic (e.g., due to fever or light anesthesia). Lastly, this monitor is slow to display changes in temperature and may be influenced by the operative room environment (e.g., gusts of air from heating or cooling vents).[5]

The axilla is a common site for noninvasive temperature determination, and is usually 1° below body temperature. A nasopharyngeal (or similar) probe can be placed at the axillary artery with the arm adducted. This site is prone to measurement error, such as when the probe becomes dislodged.

Tympanic membrane temperature correlates well with core temperature by measuring near the eardrum. Intervening cerumen may enlarge the gradient with respect to core temperature. It is possible to perforate the tympanic membrane with this probe.

Rectal temperature changes lag behind those of core body temperature. This phenomenon is often noted during rewarming after hypothermia and indicates the slower peripheral, or "shell," rewarming. Accidental placement of the probe into stool will increase the lag time of this monitor. Rectal perforation is a rare complication.

Nasopharyngeal temperature probes monitor temperature at the posterior nasopharynx, and reflect the brain temperature. This measurement is performed by measuring the distance from the external meatus of the ear to the external nares, and inserting the temperature probe to that distance. This method may be associated with epistaxis in coagulopathic or pregnant patients, or result in skin necrosis if the probe is allowed to press on the nares during longer procedures. This method is discouraged with patients with head trauma or cerebrospinal fluid rhinorrhea.

Esophageal temperature monitoring reflects the core temperature well. The probe should be located at the lower third of the esophagus behind the level of the heart. It is rarely misplaced into the airway.

Blood and bladder temperature measurements may be obtained using the thermistor of a pulmonary artery catheter, or a bladder probe, respectively. However, these will be discussed further in the invasive monitoring chapter.

Although not typically used in the operating room, traditional mercury filled glass thermometers, which are placed in the mouth, axilla, or rectum, are sometimes used in postanesthesia recovery units (PACU). PACUs may also use newer temporal artery "swipe" thermometers, which are passed along the skin above the temporal artery and use infrared technology to determine the patient's temperature. However, these devices may be inaccurate, especially in the adult population, which Suleman et al speculate could be related to underlying temporal artery arthrosclerosis.[24,25] A more recent study comparing a variety of noninvasive temperature devices in a PACU revealed "oral, deep forehead, and temporal artery temperatures correlated best with [invasive] bladder temperature.[25]" These authors concluded more studies are needed to fully evaluate the utility of temporal artery "swipe" thermometers.[25]

Neuromuscular Junction Monitoring

To facilitate endotracheal intubation, optimize surgical field conditions, or protect the patient from injury due to unwanted movement, it is often necessary to administer direct neuromuscular blocking agents. These agents, in addition to the CNS depression achieved with hypnotics, represent an important class of drugs managed by anesthetists. The need to assess and monitor the level of neuromuscular blockade has led to the creation of several devices and technologies that allow the anesthetist to monitor the skeletal muscle relaxation, and titrate neuromuscular blocking drugs (NMBDs) to effect and monitor efficacy of reversal agents. Another important use of these monitors is to help locate peripheral nerves to be blocked by regional anesthetics.

METHODS AND MECHANISMS OF MONITORING NEUROMUSCULAR BLOCKADE

Peripheral nerve stimulators consist of a battery-powered direct current pulse generator connected to two electrodes. One electrode is positive, the other negative. For proper use of the device, the negative electrode should be placed over the distal portion of the nerve, while the positive electrode placed over the proximal aspect of the nerve. This prevents direct muscle stimulation.[4]

Several electrode types exist: skin surface (pregelled) electrode pads, ball electrodes, and subcutaneous needle electrodes. Skin electrode pads are similar to ECG pads

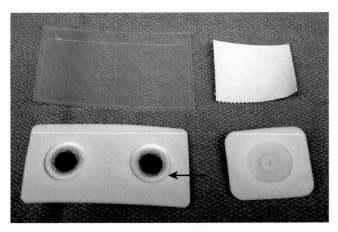

Figure 9–18 PNS skin electrode *(left)*. Note the green 10% chloride wet gel on adhesive side of pad, which is absent on the ECG skin electrode *(right)*.

(Figure 9-18). They contain a silver/silver chloride electrode attached to adhesive material and a conductive gel, which decreases the electrical resistance of the skin surface. Ideally, a supramaximal response is obtained with these pads during nerve testing. Therefore the smallest surface area possible should be contacted by the pads, so the current density may be increased.[19] If alligator clips are used in association with the electrode pads, one must ensure the clips do not touch each other during nerve testing, or the output from the unit can be shorted.[26] Stainless steel surface ball electrodes allow for more precise location of nerves and may be particularly useful in patients with edema or obesity (Figure 9-19).[27] These electrodes, most commonly used in the ICU setting, may be less reliable than adhesive pad electrodes. Sterile needle electrodes are best for burned patients or certain dermatological disorders.

It is commonplace in many institutions to connect peripheral nerve stimulators to ECG pads, rather than peripheral nerve stimulator (PNS) pads designed for the peripheral nerve stimulator itself. PNS pads contain a 10% chloride wet gel that adheres to the patient's skin, allowing for improved electrical conduction during nerve stimulation. The practice of substituting PNS pads with ECG pads may lead to an increase in impedance and less testing or reliable results.[8]

Nerve stimulators themselves are small, portable battery-powered units that deliver a constant current of 10 to 70 mA through the electrodes, through a variable tissue resistance, usually less than 2.5 kΩ. Greater tissue impedance seen in certain patients will not allow for supramaximal stimulation,[5] and therefore a greater current may need to be applied (e.g., in the obese). The nerve stimulators are capable of delivering train-of-four twitches at a frequency of 2 Hz, or tetany at a 50 Hz frequency (Figure 9-20). These stimuli depolarize the peripheral nerve of interest and the associated muscle group responds in less than 0.2 to 0.3 ms. Measures of neuromuscular function are described below. If using this device to locate nerves in an awake patient for regional anesthesia, much lower currents, below 5.0 mA, with short stimulation times, below 40 ms will maintain the patient's comfort (Figure 9-21).[4] In practice, most nerve stimulators used for neuromuscular blockade monitoring are not well suited for nerve location and vice versa (Table 9-12). Please see Chapter 14 for more details regarding nerve stimulation for regional anesthesia.

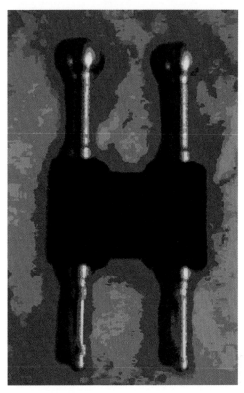

Figure 9–19 Stainless steel diagnostic bipolar probe/ball electrode. *(Courtesy of Richard Pino, MD, PhD, Dept. of Anesthesia and Critical Care, Massachusetts General Hospital, Harvard Medical School, Boston.)*

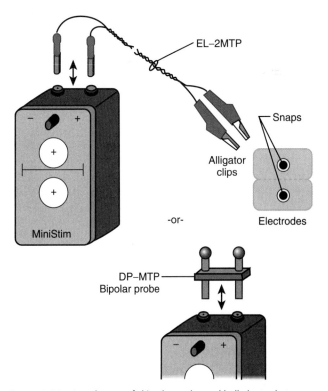

Figure 9–20 Attachment of skin electrodes and ball electrode to nerve stimulator.[26]

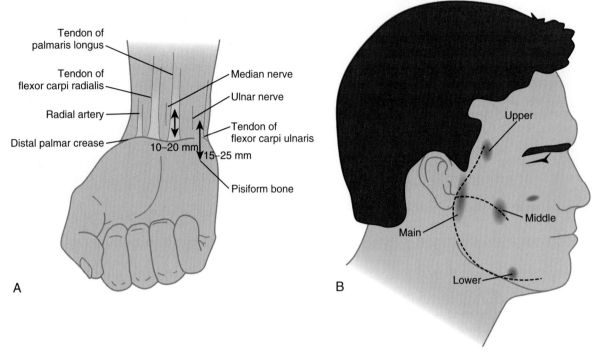

Figure 9–21 Wrist and facial motor points for nerve stimulation. **A,** Ulnar nerve. **B,** Facial nerve.[28]

Table 9–12 Testing Sites for Neuromuscular Blockade Monitoring
• Ulnar nerve/adductor pollicis brevis muscle
• Facial nerve/orbicularis oculi muscle
• Tibial nerve
• Posterior tibial nerve
• Common peroneal nerve
• Deep peroneal nerve

Table 9–13 Management of the TOF Ratio[29]
• 90% suppression of the first twitch; only one twitch observed. This is likely adequate for upper abdominal surgery.[4]
• 80% suppression of the first twitch; only two twitches observed.
• 75% suppression of the first twitch; only three twitches observed.
• TOF ratio = 0.75%; 5 sec–head lift, 15–20 mL/kg vital capacity, –25 cm H_2O inspiratory force, effective cough. In some settings, this would indicate adequate reversal to allow for extubation. Some anesthetists have found that a TOF ratio >90% is required to maintain a patent airway and keep oral secretions out of the trachea.
• At least one twitch must be present for NMBD antagonists to be administered, and large doses will be required.

Single Twitch Stimulation

Short duration twitches are applied over 0.1 to 0.2 ms at a 0.1 Hz frequency. The current applied is slowly increased in increments until the *supramaximal stimulus* is obtained (which is a slightly higher current needed to achieve a maximum twitch). This serves as the control twitch, to which future twitches will be compared once a muscle relaxant is given to the patient. Without the control twitch, this method is of little use.[29]

Train-of-Four (TOF) Stimulation

This is the most commonly used method to assess the degree of neuromuscular blockade. Four twitches are applied over a 2-second interval at a frequency of 2 Hz. This is repeated every 10 to 12 seconds. The strength of the fourth twitch is then compared with that of the first, otherwise known as the TOF ratio (TOF ratio = Fourth Twitch/First Twitch). When the neuromuscular junction is free of NMBDs, all four twitches will be of equal (or increasing) magnitude. When an NMBD is administered, the first twitch will be

the strongest, and each subsequent twitch will be of a lesser strength. This is because the motor nerve releases acetylcholine (Ach) during the first twitch, which in turn allows the NMBD to compete for binding at the neuromuscular junction. As the second, third and fourth stimulus is applied to the nerve, successively more receptors are blocked by the NMBD, and twitch fade is observed. The ratio of the fourth twitch needs to be compared with the strength of the first to determine the degree of neuromuscular blockade. Determining the degree of neuromuscular blockade via the TOF ratio requires a subjective assessment by the anesthetist, which some studies have shown that even experienced clinicians may not be able to reliably detect accurately.[30] See Table 9-13.

Sustained Tetany and Post-tetanic Potentiation

Tetanic stimulation involves applying a 50-Hz stimulus for 5 seconds to the nerve, which is in turn transmitted to the neuromuscular junction. The associated skeletal muscle will contract, releasing large amounts of Ach into the neuromuscular junction. If the contraction remains unchanged for the 5 seconds, this is a reasonable indicator that NMBD antagonists have achieved blockade reversal, or that the NMBD has been eliminated.

After applying tetanus to a peripheral nerve, the TOF twitch count will increase in number and strength for 20 to 45 minutes. This is called the post-tetanic potentiation, and it is due to the high concentration of Ach at the neuromuscular junction after tetanus. If TOF stimulation is absent before and after tetany, NMBD antagonists will not effectively reverse the relaxant.[29] However, with an unresponsive TOF, the observation of post-tetanic potentiation can assure the anesthetist that relaxation will soon lessen, and allow for NMBD antagonist administration.

Double Burst Suppression

Three 50-Hz pulses of 0.2 ms are applied to the selected peripheral nerve, and another three are applied 750 ms later. The anesthetist will either visualize or palpate a single muscle contraction associated with each of the two "bursts." If the second contraction is less than that of the first, muscle relaxation is still present. This method may be more accurate than monitoring the TOF ratio.[4,29]

Mechanomyography

A transducer measures the contraction force generated by a given muscle upon a known tension. As NMBDs are administered and the muscle becomes paralyzed, the force generated decreases.

Acceleromyography

A piezoelectric, ceramic wafer transducer is used to measure the acceleration of a muscle across a joint when stimulated. The degree of acceleration is assumed to correlate with contraction force (see Mechanomyography section). Unlike the TOF ratio palpated by hand, which requires the anesthetist to subjectively detect the degree of neuromuscular blockade, acceleromyography offers an objective, quantitative measure of neuromuscular transmission. Acceleromyography is therefore more sensitive than qualitative measures of the degree of blockade.[30] However, the measured accelerations may be prone to inconsistencies.[29]

Figure 9-22 illustrates the accelerometer and stimulating electrode properly applied with an ideal hand position. In practice, it is often desirable to tuck the arms during surgery, which complicates measuring TOF by palpation. However, acceleromyography can be used with tucked extremities (see Figure 9-23 for an example of how the hand can be positioned) and gives a quantitative assessment of neuromuscular blockade without needing to touch the patient. Figure 9-24 illustrates the typical output of the device. Before paralysis (and during recovery) the TOF ratio is displayed as a percentage of the first twitch strength. In normal patients, the TOF ratio before paralysis is greater than 100% (Figure 9-24, left panel). At high levels of paralysis, a twitch count is displayed (4, 3, 2, 1 or 0), as illustrated in Figure 9-24, right panel.

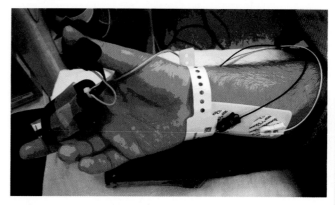

Figure 9–22 Acceleromyographic neuromuscular monitoring; ideal hand and monitor placement.

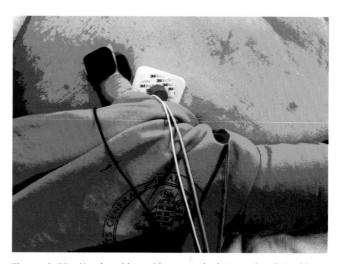

Figure 9–23 Hand position with arm tucked. Note thumb is able to move freely.

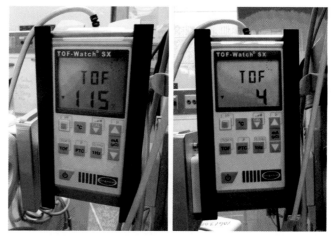

Figure 9–24 Acceleromyography output (examples).

Electromyography (EMG)

EMG measures the action potentials associated with a measured muscle group. Two sensing electrodes and two stimulus electrodes are placed over the muscle of interest. A ground lead is needed in-between. The amplitude of

Table 9–14	Limitations of Peripheral Nerve Stimulation for NMB Monitoring

- Hypothermia of a muscle (reduce twitch tension by 6%/° C)[6]
- Nerve damage/skin irritation at electrode site
- False-negative testing results because different muscle groups relax and return from blockade at rates times
- Skin impedance/poor adherence to skin

these signals allows the EMG to calculate how many action potentials are occurring during exposure to NMBDs— NMBDs decrease the number of action potentials. Action potentials occur within a few milliseconds and at very high frequencies after EMG stimulation (bandwidth of DC-10,000 Hz).[5,29] This technique is not widely used for routine NMB monitoring.

Clinical Measures: Visualization, Palpation, and Petco2

It is important to note that certain muscles regain their function after exposure to NMBDs at varying rates. For example, diagrammatic and laryngeal muscle function both relaxes and recovers from NMBDs before the adductor pollicis brevis. This is also true of the orbicularis oculi and rectus abdominis. Therefore the absence of peripheral nerve response to the above monitoring technologies does not generalize to all muscles of the anesthetized patient. Petco$_2$ fluctuations, coughing or wincing, or a "tight" surgical field, for example, can imply recovery from NMBDs of these central muscle groups even in the face of negative neuromuscular monitoring results for the adductor pollicis or other clinically monitored sites.

Lastly, to fully maximize the utility of the above mentioned monitors, a baseline measure of the peripheral nerve activity should be tested before any relaxants are administered. By extension, a repeat measure should be obtained before more agents are given to ensure accurate and appropriate management of NMBDs (Table 9-14). And, as described earlier in this section, these nonobjective measures are prone to clinician error.[30]

Neurological System Monitors
Bispectral Index (BIS) Monitor

This technology uses electroencephalography (EEG) and electromyography (EMG) to calculate the level of conciseness and sedation of the anesthetized patient (Figure 9-25). BIS monitors are used to titrate anesthetics to decrease the likelihood of intraoperative awareness.[31] See Chapter 11, level of consciousness monitoring, of this text for a more detailed discussion.

Cerebral Oximetry

Cerebral oximetry is a noninvasive monitor used to measure regional blood hemoglobin oxygenation saturation (rSO2) via near-infrared optical spectroscopy (NIRS). This technology is similar to that of the pulse oximetry and can be used for patients at risk for stroke (neurosurgical patients, cardiac or vascular surgery patients, patients with history of stroke, etc.).

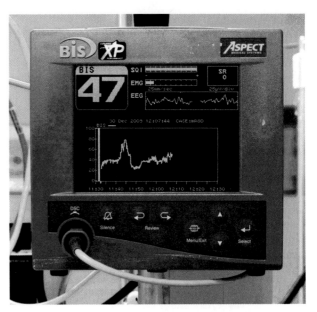

Figure 9–25   Display front of BIS monitor.

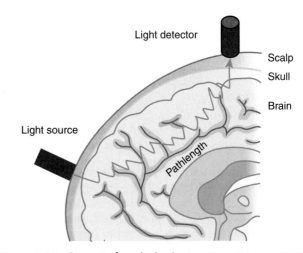

Figure 9–26   Concept of cerebral oximetry. *(From Watzman HM, Kurth CD, Montenegro LM, et al. Arterial and venous contributions to near-infrared cerebral oximetry. Anesthesiology 2000;93(4):947-953.)*[33]

The only commercially available monitor is manufactured by Somanetics; In-Vivo Optical Spectroscopy (INVOS).

The monitor is used by placing a noninvasive sensor on the left, right, or (ideally) both frontal-temporal regions of the patient—over the forehead away from the scalp and hair (Figure 9-26). This sensor emits low intensity light of two wavelengths, 730 and 805 nm (near infrared wavelength) through two light-emitting diodes, which are alternately illuminated.[34] This light penetrates the skin, skull, dura, and CSF, into the blood of the cerebral cortex. The light is then reflected back to the skin sensor and an rSO$_2$ is calculated based on light intensity changes as it passes through the brain (Table 9-15). Cerebral O$_2$ saturation is related to light intensity at the source, the detector, and light path-length through the tissue according to the Beer law.[33] An rSO$_2$ of 70% is normal because this percentage includes both arterial, capillary, and venous blood. A change greater than 20% to 30%, or an index value less than 50 is associated with neurological change.[32]

Table 9–15 Causes of rSO₂ Desaturation

- Hypoxia
- Embolic stroke/ischemia
- Unilateral or bilateral cerebral atherosclerosis
- Patient position (Trendelenburg leads to venous congestion in the cerebral circulation)
- Blood steal syndromes
- Hypothermia
- Left-shifted curve can lead to false positives
- Cardiac arrest
- Some patients have baseline low values and normal neurological function[34]
- IV indigo carmine administration[36]
- The scalp/hair follicles/hair can interfere with the measurement

Table 9–16 Indications for Monitoring Evoked Potentials[6,21,35]

- Spinal fusion/deformity surgery (e.g., tethered cord surgery, scoliosis repair, meningomyelocele surgery)
- Spinal instrumentation or hardware placement (e.g., pedicle screws, rods)
- Spinal tumor resection
- Spinal trauma/fracture repair
- Spinal vascular surgery
- Plexus surgery
- Peripheral nerve surgery
- Thoracoabdominal aortic aneurysm surgery
- Epilepsy surgery
- Brainstem or posterior fossa surgery
- Aneurysm repair
- Aortic cross clamping
- Carotid endarterectomy
- Cerebral tumor resection
- Cortical mapping and/or regional cortical function
- Probe localization during stereotactic neurosurgery[6]
- Facial nerve monitoring during acoustic neuroma resection[35]

According to Watzman et al, "the intensity of the [cerebral oximetry] light source is oscillated at high frequency. After the light passes through the tissue, the detected intensity is amplitude demodulated and phase shifted. Cerebral O₂ saturation is related to amplitude and phase, corresponding to intensity and path-length in the Beer law."[35]

Evoked Potentials

The nervous system reacts to somatosensory, motor, and auditory stimuli by generating electrical signals, called evoked potentials (EPs). Somatosensory evoked potentials (SSEPs), motor evoked potentials (MEPs), or brainstem auditory evoked responses (BAERs) may be monitored during surgery which puts the brain, spinal cord, or certain peripheral nerves at risk for damage or injury, namely from ischemia. See Table 9-16 for indications for evoked potential monitoring. Use of EPs requires adequate exposure to certain areas of the patient, equipment with a computer, and involvement of a trained technician.

SSEP monitors the function of the posterior spinal cord/sensory tracts and entails placing skin electrodes or needle electrodes over the distal portion of a peripheral nerve and delivering stimulation, to induce an SSEP. Common sites of measurement are the median nerve or ulnar nerve at the wrist, along with the posterior tibial nerve at the ankle, or peroneal nerve near the head of the fibula. During peripheral nerve stimulation with a square wave signal of 0.2 to 2 msec, electroencephalogram (EEG) activity is measured with recording electrodes on the scalp or areas near the spinal cord, or with cortical surface electrodes during neurosurgery. Spontaneous EEG activity within the brain is typically in the 50 to 100 mV range, while a single SSEP is of a much lower amplitude—1 to 2 mV. Repeated SSEPs are delivered to the upper and lower extremity nerves, and the EP waves are isolated and monitored from rest of the EEG pattern, often on the contralateral side away from the stimulus. EP waveforms are averaged and plotted as voltage versus time and contain a certain amplitude, latency, and morphology. Three positive peaks and three negative peaks (P1, P2, P3 and N1, N2, and N3, respectively) are also typically seen within the wave. The

Table 9–17 Anatomy and Physiology of Evoked Potentials

- Anterior spinal artery, supply to anterior cord, motor function.
- Posterior spinal artery, supply to posterior cord, sensory function. The majority of the measured SSEPs are created by the posterior column spinal pathways.
- Perforating branches of basilar and vertebral artery, brainstem.
- MCA, upper extremity SSEPs.
- ACA, lower extremity SSEPs.
- Decreases in cerebral perfusion to 18 cc/min/100 g brain tissue will decrease the electrical activity of the brain and the SSEP. A perfusion of 15 cc/min/100 g brain tissue will not allow for the measurement of SSEPs. Perfusions below this can lead to permanent electrical changes in the brain.[35]

latency is a measure of time between the applied stimulus and the associated EP.

There is no set standard or consensus on what constitutes a clinically significant change in SSEPs. However, a 50% or greater decrease in the peak amplitude of the positive peaks or loss of one or more of the negative peaks, or both, or a 10% increase in the latency, likely indicates damage to a peripheral nerve, the spinal cord, or a false positive test result from anesthesia or hypothermia. This monitor is very sensitive but not particularly specific, and it is not uncommon to observe false-positive SSEP changes. Therefore, it is important to obtain baseline measures before anesthesia, and before surgery has begun. Lastly, the site of stimulus and change is important and can help locate potential damage to a more specific area (Table 9-17).

Many anesthetic agents will affect EEG and SSEPs. The largest depressant affect is seen at the level of the cortex, versus a small depressant affect at spinal or subcortical levels of the brain. The anesthetic must be tailored appropriately to minimize changes to this monitor. Essentially, according to Banoub et al,[35] all potent inhaled agents prolong SSEP latency and diminish SSEP amplitude in a dose dependent fashion. Also, "sole use of 60% nitrous oxide decreases SSEP amplitude but does not affect latency," while "additive use of nitrous oxide with a potent inhalational agent further decreases SSEP amplitude but does not increase latency more than that seen with the potent agent alone."[35] Banoub et al[35] also note that intravenous anesthetics generally affect SSEPs less than volatile agents; etomidate and ketamine increase SSEP amplitude, while propofol, midazolam, and barbiturates have a mild to moderate depressant effect on SSEP amplitude. Opioids have a minuscule affect upon the SSEP amplitude.

At the level of the medullary nuclei, general anesthetics will not influence the ascending SSEPs. Measurements of SSEPs here imply the monitor is working, and to serve to measure the effect of anesthetics on the monitor. It should not be used to diagnose damage to the spinal cord because these signals reflect spinal cord white matter activity, and not spinal cord gray matter activity.[35]

BAERs are monitored during brainstem surgery, posterior fossa surgery, and surgery including the eighth cranial nerve (CN-VIII) (e.g., acoustic neuroma removal surgery, facial nerve decompression, etc.). BAERs are induced by placing earphones on the patient and sending clicking sounds to the tympanic membrane, repeatedly. These sounds evoke a response through CN-VIII, brainstem, and auditory cortex. BAER waves are produced and measured along with EEG activity through electrodes placed on the vertex and earlobe. They are processed and evaluated in a similar fashion described for the SSEPs at the level of the synapses between CN-VIII through to the auditory cortex.

MEPs are measured to assess the well-being of the anterior spinal cord/motor tracts, brainstem/cranial nerves VII/IX/X/XII, and corticospinal tract during the prior mentioned surgeries. MEPs are monitored by stimulating, often with multiple techniques in repetition, the motor cortex, anterior (cervical) spinal cord, or peripheral nerve with either electrical or transcranial magnetic signals. Stimulating needle electrodes are placed on the scalp, and recording electrodes put on contracting muscle. In response to this stimulation, a myogenic (muscle) or neurogenic (motor nerve) MEP is produced. Volatile anesthetics may depress motor neuron and cortical function, so intravenous anesthetic agents may be best used while monitoring MEPs. Neuromuscular blocking drugs (NMBDs) obviously will also affect MEPs. The level of neuromuscular relaxation resulting from NMBD administration should be monitored in conjunction with MEPs.

Electromyography (EMG) may be used in conjunction with MEPs to assess peripheral motor nerve or cranial nerve motor function during anesthesia and surgery. Surface electrodes or needle electrodes are placed upon muscles of interest to measure compound muscle action potentials (CMAPs), in response to either passive or active stimuli. Passive stimuli entail the observation of unwanted CMAPs during surgical stimulation. This monitor will then alarm the surgical team that a peripheral nerve may be in jeopardy and should be avoided. Active stimulation is just the opposite and allows the surgical team to figure out which muscle is innervated by a specific peripheral or cranial nerve.

As with any electrode, skin damage, pressure ischemia, and burns are possible at placement sites. MEPs are contraindicated in patients with retained intracranial metal, skull defects, postictal states, and after a major cerebral insult.[6]

Monitors Connected to the Anesthesia Machine

Oxygen Concentration Analyzers

Measuring the oxygen concentration within the gases administered to the anesthetized patient is necessary and is considered an ASA standard monitor. Oxygen concentration analyzers measure the partial pressure of oxygen delivered to the patient (fraction of inspired oxygen, or F_{IO_2}) and compute a percentage. Three methods are most commonly used for monitoring the F_{IO_2}: galvanic, polarographic, and paramagnetic.

Galvanic (fuel) cells contain a noble metal (gold) cathode and lead anode submerged in a solution of electrolytes, namely potassium and chloride. The cathode is exposed to and measures inspired or exhaled oxygen from the breathing circuit, which is filtered through a membrane, to isolate the oxygen from the other gases in the circuit. The oxygen enters through a sensing membrane into the potassium chloride solution and gold cathode. A current potential is produced, which is proportional to the F_{IO_2}. The current flow is dependent on the presence of oxygen, thus acting like a battery which requires oxygen.[4] The following equations describe this reaction:

$$O_2 + 4e^- + 2H_2O \rightarrow 4(OH)^-$$

$$Pb + 2(OH)^- \rightarrow PbO + H_2O + 2e^-$$

This monitor must be calibrated against room air oxygen and 100% oxygen, and the cell's life is limited to about 1 year of usage. There is a delay of about 20 seconds and an accuracy of +/− 3% associated with this monitor.[4]

Polarographic (Clark Electrode) oxygen analyzers measure oxygen in a similar fashion to that of galvanic cells. Polarographic analyzers use a platinum cathode and silver anode within electrolyte solution. A power source of 600 to 800 mV is used to polarize the electrodes. Oxygen samples from the breathing circuit pass through a Teflon membrane and create an electrical current—the cathode donates electrons to the anode. Each oxygen molecule causes the cathode to donate 4 electrons. This relationship allows this monitor to calculate the partial pressure of oxygen within the sample. This calculation is an average of the inspired and expired O_2.[4] The equation below illustrates reactions at the cathode and anode, respectively:

$$O_2 + 2H_2O + 4e^- \rightarrow 4OH^-$$

$$4Ag \rightarrow 4Ag^+ + 4e^-$$

$$4Ag^+ + 4Cl^- \rightarrow 4AgCl$$

Polarographic analyzers must also be regularly calibrated and the device has a 20 to 30 second delay. It has the same accuracy of a galvanic cell. The Teflon membrane breaks down over the course of 3 years, requiring replacement of the monitor.

Paramagnetic (Pauling) oxygen analyzers sample room air (reference sample) and gases administered to the patient simultaneously in two separate chambers, separated by a very sensitive, differential pressure transducer. The two chambers join together within an electromagnetic field, which is turned on/off at high frequency (100 to 110 Hz), which produces an oscillating pressure of 20 to 50 μbar in the chambers. Molecular oxygen is attracted to the field because it is paramagnetic—it has two electrons in unpaired orbits. The other anesthetic gases are diamagnetic and are repelled by the magnetic field. As the oxygen within each chamber interacts with the magnetic field, the transducer senses oxygen pressure fluctuations on either side (a pressure difference). More specifically, the magnetic field "causes an intermittent differential reduction in pressure upstream in the tubes that is detected and measured by [the] pressure transducer." This pressure difference is proportional to the oxygen partial pressure difference between each chamber.[4] The oxygen partial pressure is then calculated and conveyed to the anesthetist as a volume percent. This monitor is very accurate and continuously measures the volume percent of oxygen, breath-by-breath, essentially in real-time. High and low volume percent alarms can be arranged to alert the anesthetist of critical values. A similar technology involves magneto-acoustic spectroscopy, which converts the on/off oscillating pressures into sounds of various amplitudes, from which oxygen concentration can be calculated and displayed.

Older paramagnetic oxygen monitors work somewhat differently. These units contain a magnetic field. This magnetic field is occupied by a weakly diamagnetic gas—namely nitrogen. Within the poles of the field, two glass spheres are supported by threads, in a dumbbell-shaped position. Gas samples of oxygen are introduced into the system. Oxygen is attracted to the field, resulting in glass sphere movement. The amount of oxygen within the sample can be calculated based upon the degree of sphere movement (or similarly, the amount of current needed to place the spheres back into their original position). This type of oxygen monitoring is very accurate, within 0.1% O_2. The caveat is its slow response time, up to 60 seconds, and measurement errors associated with water vapor, high fresh gas flows, pressurization, and vibration.[19]

Volatile Agent and Nitrous Oxide Analyzers
Infrared Technology

It is desirable for the anesthetist to know the amount (or "dose") of inhalational anesthetics that are being inspired and expired by the patient. Infrared technology is employed to monitor, breath by breath, volatile agent concentration in the breathing circuit (Table 9-18). Circuit gas is brought through sampling tubing into a chamber where exposure to infrared radiation occurs. Sample gases absorb the infrared radiation at specific wavelengths, thereby preventing this radiation from reaching the photodetector. Unique absorption spectra produced by each volatile agent create an electrical signal, which is related to agent concentration and allows the monitor to perform its analysis.[4] The amplitude of the spectrum

Table 9-18 **Monitors Used for Gas Analysis**[4]				
Technology	O_2	CO_2	N_2O	Volatile agents
Infrared	No	Yes	Yes	Yes
Paramagnetic	Yes	No	No	No
Polarography	Yes	No	No	No
Fuel cell	Yes	No	No	No
Mass spectrometry	Yes	Yes	Yes	Yes
Raman spectrometry	Yes	Yes	Yes	Yes
Piezoelectric resonance	No	No	No	Yes

Adopted from Al-Shaikh B, Stacey S. Non-invasive monitoring. In *Essentials of anaesthetic equipment*, ed 3, Edinburgh, Churchill Livingstone, 2007.

is inversely related to the amount of agent present.[4] Various agents absorb best at different wavelengths. Therefore optical filters are used to ensure light of appropriate wavelength is exposed to sample gas. This technology uses infrared light of a 4.6-μm wavelength for nitrous oxide, and 7 μm and 13 μm for volatile agents. Multiple agents can be detected and analyzed simultaneously as a result.

Piezoelectric Quartz Crystal Oscillation

This technology uses two piezoelectric quartz crystals, one of which is covered in a lipophilic silicone oil to measure the concentration of volatile agent. The crystals are connected to a power source and allowed to oscillate at their natural frequencies. When the oil-covered crystal is exposed to a lipid soluble agent, its natural frequency changes proportionally to the amount of inhalational agent absorbed into the oil. This allows this monitor to calculate agent concentration. However, manual identification is required by the anesthetist or user.[19]

Raman spectroscopy may also be used to monitor inhalational anesthetic concentrations. Please see previous discussion under End-Tidal CO_2 Monitors.

Respirometer and Pneumotachograph

The most commonly used respirometer (or respiratory volume monitor) is the Wright respirometer, which is used to measure the tidal volume and minute volume of gas flow in a given direction (unidirectional). This monitor works by allowing gas to enter through an inlet, inside of which sits a rotating vane with slits. Slits are arranged such that incoming gas will rotate the vane at a rate of 150 revolutions per liter of flowing gas. A pointer on the face display of the respirometer moves as the vane turns. The main face has markings at 100 mL divisions, and a smaller inner face front displays 1 L per marking. A minimum flow of 2 L/min is needed for accurate measurements, as this monitor functions optimally with 4 to 24 L/min flow +/− 5% to 10%.[4] This meter displays falsely low volumes at low flows and falsely high volumes at high flows. Water vapor/condensation and friction decrease its accuracy. For optimal function, the

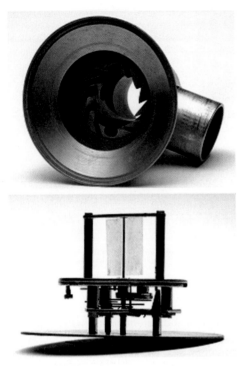

Figure 9–27   Wright respirometer. *(From Sheffield Museum of Anaesthesia. (website):* http://www.soa.group.shef.ac.uk/museum/wrights_respirometer.htm.)[36]

meter should be placed as close to the patient's airway as possible, and connected to the expiratory side of the circuit to minimize loss of volume from leaks and tube expansion. The pointer can be re-zeroed between usages. Improved versions of the Wright respirometer measure tidal volume with either light reflection or semiconductive components within a magnetic field, which are not prone to the above sources of inaccuracies (Figure 9-27).

Hot-wire anemometers are gas flow sensors, which are used by GE and Drager anesthesia machines. These devices contain a heated wire, which is cooled by gases flowing past the wire. The degree of cooling is directly related to the amount of fresh gas flow, which this monitor is able to determine. To make this determination, however, the density of the fresh gas must be known. This information is inputted to the hot-wire anemometer by the above-mentioned gas analyzers. The advantage of these monitors is that they are unaffected by water vapor or other sources of friction because none of the components physically moves.[37]

The pneumotachograph is another monitor that is used to measure gas flow and calculate gas volume in a bidirectional fashion (during inspiration and expiration). The pneumotachograph consists of an inlet and outlet, between which sits fixed resistors (often a bundle of parallel tubes) and a heating coil. Pressure transducers sit on either side of the resistors. Gas flow is laminar through the resistors, and the pressure change is measured. Flow rate of the gas is calculated because it is proportional to the pressure change across the resistance. Minute volume can be extrapolated. The heating coil minimizes condensation within the resistors, which can cause gas flow to become turbulent rather than laminar.[4]

The pneumotachograph can be connected to a Pitot tube to allow for increased accuracy, and measurement of a patient's

compliance, airway pressure, gas flow, and volume/pressure and flow/volume loops. The Pitot tube contains two ports connected to a pressure transducer. One port faces the gas flow, the other is perpendicular. This arrangement measures unidirectional flow, although this arrangement can be changed to allow for the measurement of bidirectional flow. This monitor calculates flow by the following:[4]

Pressure Difference Between Ports =
Square Root of Flow Rate

Uninterrupted evaluation of gas composition through a sampling tube can offset the density and viscosity of the flowing gases, which can make this monitor less accurate.[4]

Conclusion and Future Directions in Noninvasive Monitoring

The use of noninvasive monitors is paramount in appropriately caring for the anesthetized patient. As medical device and information technology continue to expand, more and more noninvasive monitors will be developed and brought to the bedside. It is important to remember that one of the fundamental goals of monitoring is to assure adequate tissue oxygenation and respiration. Future developments in monitoring that move towards this goal by replacing the current indirect measurements with more direct ones would be very welcome.

Author's note: Before the advent of photography, and even well into the twentieth century, the scientific discourse in medicine was frequently informed by the observations of individual clinicians, and particularly by their ability to capture their observations visually, mostly by drawing. Photography produced better, more realistic and faithful images, supplanting drawing, but it was not as widely available to the observing clinician as paper and pencil had been. Illustration as a regular skill died out, but photography remained esoteric until the advent of the digital point and shoot camera, which allowed on-camera review of the image and reshooting until the desired illustration had been captured. Eventually, such cameras became ubiquitous, mounted in cellular telephones. And thus illustration as a pool for exposition and communication was returned to the hand of the conscientious clinician. In a living expression of this fact, many of the images in this chapter were captured on the cell phone camera of one of the authors.

The message? The tools that record medical phenomena are now with us always.

Suggestions for Further Reading

ASA Committee on Standards and Practice Parameters. Standards for basic anesthetic monitoring, ASA (website): http://www.asahq.org/publications AndServices/standards/02.pdf. Accessed August 30, 2010. *This document puts forth the basic, minimum standard for monitoring the anesthetized patient as per the ASA.*

Dunn, P.F., Alston, T.A., Baker, K.H., et al., 2007. Monitoring. In: Clinical anesthesia procedures of the Massachusetts General Hospital, ed 7. Lippincott Williams & Wilkins, Philadelphia. *A very practical and easily read chapter regarding the use of noninvasive and invasive physiologic monitor usage at the Massachusetts General Hospital for anesthetized and intensive care unit patients.*

GE Medical Systems Information Technologies, 2005. Critical care monitoring clinical reference and troubleshooting guide. Compact Disc, Milwaukee, General Electric. *A comprehensive resource and user manual describing the technical details, proper usage, and troubleshooting of clinical monitors in the operating room and ICU.*

Barash, P.G., Cullen, B.F., Stoelting, R.K. (Eds.), 2005. Clinical anesthesia, ed 5. Lippincott Williams & Wilkins, Philadelphia. *Includes detailed information regarding pacemaker monitoring and management and tracings for common arrhythmias and data tables on limb placement and coronary anatomy.*

Bickley, L.S., Szilagyi, P.G., 2003. Beginning the physical examination: general survey and vital signs. In: Bate's guide to physical examination and history taking, ed 8. Lippincott Williams & Wilkins, Philadelphia. *Provides the fundamentals of clinically assessing the patient by "look, listen, feel." This chapter describes how to properly observe, auscultate, palpate, and use equipment such as the stethoscope and blood pressure cuff.*

Magee, P.T., 2005. Physiological monitoring: principles and non-invasive monitoring. In: Davey, A.J., Diba, A. (Eds.), Ward's anaesthetic equipment, ed 5. Elsevier Saunders, Philadelphia. *Classifies various noninvasive monitors by transducer and outlines the basics of signal and information transduction. Also provides important information regarding electrical impendence.*

Kemmotsu, O., Ueda, M., Otsuka, H., 1991. Arterial tonometry for noninvasive, continuous blood pressure monitoring during anesthesia. Anesthesiology 75, 333–340. *One of the first papers regarding the theory and development of arterial tonometry and noninvasive, beat-to-beat blood pressure monitoring.*

Keifer, J.C., Borel, C.O., 2008. Intraoperative neurologic monitoring. In: Longnecker, D.E., Brown, D.L., Newman, M.F., et al., (Eds.), Anesthesiology, ed 1. McGraw-Hill, New York. *A detailed comprehensive discussion of the basic science and clinical utility of evoked potentials.*

Pino, R.M., Ali, H., et al., 2008. Monitoring and managing neuromuscular blockade. In: Longnecker, D.E., Brown, D.L., Newman, M.F., et al.,(Eds.), Anesthesiology, ed 1. McGraw-Hill, New York. *An outstanding review of neuromuscular blockade monitoring.*

Avidan, M.S., et al., 2008. Anesthesia awareness and the bispectral index. N Engl J Med 358 (11), 1097–1108. *One of the largest clinical trials studying the use of BIS monitoring to prevent awareness during anesthesia.*

Watzman, H.M., et al., 2000. Arterial and venous contributions to near-infrared cerebral oximetry. Anesthesiology 93, 947–953. *An early research study regarding the use and development of cerebral oximetry in humans. Provides an excellent overview and conceptualization of this technology.*

References

1. Bar-Yosef, S., Schroeder, R.A., Mark, J.B., 2008. Hemodynamic monitoring. In: Longnecker, D.E., Brown, D.L., Newman, M.F. (Eds.), Anesthesiology, McGraw-Hill Medical, New York.

2. ASA Committee on Standards and Practice Parameters. Standards for basic anesthetic monitoring, ASA (website): http://www.asahq.org/publications AndServices/standards/02.pdf. Accessed August 30, 2010.

3. Webb, R.K., van der Walt, J.H., Runciman, W.B., et al., 1993. The Australian incident monitoring study. Which monitor? An analysis of 2000 incident reports. Anaesth Intensive Care 21 (5), 529–542.

4. Al-Shaikh, B., Stacey, S., 2007. Non-invasive monitoring. In: Essentials of anaesthetic equipment, ed 3. Churchill Livingstone, Edinburgh.

5. Magee, P.T., 2005. Physiological monitoring: principles and non-invasive monitoring. In: Davey, A.J., Diba, A. (Eds.), Ward's anaesthetic equipment, ed 5. Elsevier Saunders, Philadelphia.

6. Morgan, G.E., Mikhail, M.S., Murray, M.J. (Eds.), 2006. Clinical anesthesiology, ed 4. Lange Medical Books/McGraw-Hill, New York.

7. GE Medical Systems Information Technologies, 2005. Critical care monitoring clinical reference and troubleshooting guide, Compact Disc, Milwaukee, General Electric.

8. Yasuda, A., Pino, R.M., 2008. Impedance of ECG and peripheral nerve stimulation electrodes used to monitor neuromuscular blockade. Anesthesiology v109, A359.

9. Kuhn, L., Rose, L., 2008. ECG interpretation part 1: understanding mean electrical axis. J Emerg Nurs 34, 530–534.

10. Barash, P.G., Cullen, B.F., Stoelting, R.K. (Eds.), 2005. Clinical anesthesia, ed 5. Lippincott Williams & Wilkins, Philadelphia.

11. Magee, P.T., 2005. Physiological monitoring: principles and non-invasive monitoring. In: Davey, A.J., Diba, A. (Eds.), Ward's anaesthetic equipment, ed 5. Elsevier Saunders, Philadelphia.

12. Weaver and Company. (website): http://www.doweaver.com/Nuprep.html. Accessed August 30, 2010.

13. Bickley, L.S. (Ed.), 2003. Bate's guide to physical examination and history taking, ed 8. Lippincott Williams & Wilkins, Philadelphia.

14. Amoore, J.N., Scott, D.H., 1993. Noninvasive blood pressure measurements with single and twin-hose systems—do mixtures matter? Anaesthesia 48 (9), 799–802.

15. Amoore, J.N., Geake, W.B., Scott, D.H.T., 1997. Oscillometric non-invasive blood pressure measurements: the influence of the make of instrument on readings? Med Biol Eng Comput 35, 131–134.

16. Kemmotsu, O., Ueda, M., Otsuka, H., et al., 1991. Arterial tonometry for noninvasive, continuous blood pressure monitoring during anesthesia. Anesthesiology 75 (2), 333–340.

17. Janelle, G.M., Gravenstein, N., 2006. An accuracy evaluation of the T-Line Tensymeter (continuous noninvasive blood pressure management device) versus conventional invasive radial artery monitoring in surgical patients. Anesth Analg 102 (2), 484–490.

18. Tensys Medical. (website): www.tensysmedical.com. Accessed August 30, 2010.

19. Magee, P.T., 2005. Physiological monitoring: gases. In: Davey, A.J., Diba, A. (Eds.), Ward's anaesthetic equipment, ed 5. Elsevier Saunders, Philadelphia.

20. Hess, D.R., Kacmarek, R.M., 2008. Monitoring respiratory function. In: Longnecker, D.E., Brown, D.L., Newman, M.F., et al., (Eds.), Anesthesiology, ed 1. McGraw-Hill, New York.

21. Stoelting, R.K., Milller, R.D. (Eds.), 2007. Basics of anesthesia, ed 5. Churchill Livingstone, Philadelphia.

22. Bhavani-Shankar, K., Philip, J.H., 2000. Defining segments and phases of a time capnogram. Anesth Analg 91, 973–977.

23. Sheikh, E., Maguire, D.P., Gratch, D., 2009. Autotriggering during pressure support ventilation due to cardiogenic oscillations. Anesth Analg 109, 470–472.

24. Suleman, M., Doufas, A., Akca, O., et al., 2002. Insufficiency in a new temporal-artery thermometer for adult and pediatric patients. Anesth Analg 95, 67–71.

25. Langham, G., Maheshwari, A., Contrera, K., et al., 2009. Noninvasive temperature monitoring in postanesthesia care units. Anesthesiology 111 (1), 90–96.

26. Life-Tech, 2003. Ministim instruction manual. Stafford, Tex, Life-Tech.

27. Wilson, W.C., Grande, C.M., Hoyt, D.B. (Eds.), 2007. Trauma: critical care, vol. 2, Informa Healthcare, New York.

28. Life-Tech. EZ-Stim II dual purpose peripheral nerve stimulator brochure, (website): http://www.life-tech.com/documents/ezstimbrochure.pdf. Accessed August 30, 2010.

29. Pino, R.M., Ali, H.H., et al., 2008. Monitoring and managing neuromuscular blockade. In: Longnecker, D.E., Brown, D.L., Newman, M.F., et al., (Eds.), Anesthesiology, ed 1. McGraw-Hill, New York.

30. Capron, F., Fortier, L., Racine, S., et al., 2006. Tactile fade detection with hand or wrist stimulation using train-of-four, double-burst stimulation, 50-hertz tetanus, 100-hertz tetanus, and acceleromyography. Anesth Analg 102, 1578–1584.

31. Avidan, M.S., Zhang, L., Burnside, B.A., et al., 2008. Anesthesia awareness and the bispectral index. N Engl J Med 358 (11), 1097–1108.

32. Somanetics. Our technology FAQs (website): http://somanetics.com/Our-Technology-FAQs.asp. Accessed August 30, 2010.

33. Watzman, H.M., Kurth, C.D., Montenegro, L.M., et al., 2000. Arterial and venous contributions to near-infrared cerebral oximetry. Anesthesiology 93 (4), 947–953.

34. McDonagh, D.L., McDaniel, M.R., Monk, T.G., 2007. The effect of intravenous indigo carmine on near-infrared cerebral oximetry. Anesth Analg 105 (3), 704–706.

35. Keifer, J.C., Borel, C.O., 2008. Intraoperative neurologic monitoring. In: Longnecker, D.E., Brown, D.L., Newman, M.F., et al., (Eds.), Anesthesiology, ed 1. McGraw-Hill, New York.

36. Sheffield Museum of Anaesthesia, (website): http://www.soa.group.shef.ac.uk/museum/wrights_respirometer.htm. Accessed August 30, 2010.

37. Olympio, M.A., 2008. How do flow sensors work? In response. APSF Newsl 28, 10.

Chapter 10

Invasive Hemodynamic Monitoring

Beverly J. Newhouse and Rafael Montecino

The goals of hemodynamic monitoring in the operating room are to maintain optimal perfusion and oxygen delivery to tissues, ensure rapid detection of changes in clinical status, and monitor for response to surgery, anesthesia, resuscitation, and therapies. Although noninvasive monitors (such as a blood pressure cuff) are associated with less risks and complications, it is often necessary to use invasive monitoring techniques to achieve these goals, particularly in high-risk patients.[1] The necessity for invasive monitoring may be driven by patient condition or by the surgical procedure. In general, invasive hemodynamic monitoring is indicated if significant physiological disturbances are anticipated based on patient comorbidities or the surgical procedure. Examples of patient comorbidities that may warrant invasive monitoring include previous cardiopulmonary illness, multiple trauma, age greater than 70 years and/or limited reserve, septicemia or other form of shock, respiratory failure, acute renal failure, and vascular disease.

Invasive Arterial Blood Pressure Monitoring

Invasive arterial monitoring is the "gold standard" blood pressure device. In addition to being the most accurate form of blood pressure monitoring, arterial cannulation allows continuous beat-to-beat monitoring. It also serves as a site for obtaining serial lab measurements of oxygenation, ventilation, pH, lactate, base deficit, electrolytes, and hematological data.

General Indications for Arterial Blood Pressure Monitoring[2]

- Hemodynamic instability or predicted hemodynamic instability.
- Surgical procedures that will be prolonged, involve major fluid shifts, or significant blood loss.
- Monitoring the safety of certain anesthetic techniques, such as deliberate hypotension, cardiopulmonary bypass, or major vascular surgery involving arterial clamping.
- Monitoring the response to vasoactive drugs.
- Frequent blood gas measurements.
- Frequent blood sampling needed in patients without central venous access.
- Patients who are severely obese, have burned extremities, or are in shock (where noninvasive blood pressure monitoring may not be feasible).

Sites for Arterial Catheterization

The most common sites for arterial cannulation are radial or femoral arteries, but other arteries including the brachial, axillary, and dorsalis pedis can also be used. Axillary or brachial arterial catheterization, though feasible, may be associated with increased risk of extremity ischemia because they are end-arteries. Choice of artery is dependent on the ability to palpate a pulse or to locate it by Doppler ultrasonography. It may be prudent to assess the collateral circulation if cannulating the smaller arteries such as the radial or dorsalis pedis arteries. However, the commonly used Allen's test has not been shown to be a reliable way of evaluating collateral circulation in the hand. The extremity distal to the catheter should be assessed frequently both before and after insertion, and the catheter should be removed immediately if there is evidence of ischemia. The risk of clinically significant arterial thrombosis is decreased if the catheter is continuously flushed.

Options for Arterial Catheterization

The *radial artery* can be palpated on the distal portion of the forearm between the radius and the tendon of the flexor carpi radialis.

The *brachial artery* can be palpated as it courses medial to the biceps muscle and tendon into the antecubital fossa, with the arm extended and the palm facing up.

The *axillary artery* may be best palpated in the axillary space, with the arm abducted and externally rotated.

The *femoral artery* may be best palpated below the inguinal ligament, midway between the anterior superior iliac spine and the symphysis pubis.

The *dorsalis pedis* artery may be palpated on the arch of the foot, between the first and second metatarsals.

Figure 10–1 shows the normal waveforms associated with pressures of the aortic root, brachial artery, radial artery, and femoral artery. Systolic pressure increases with progression away from the aorta due to a counterreflection phenomenon in which the forward-traveling wave generated by left ventricular ejection meets a later-arriving reflected wave from the periphery. In patients with significant peripheral arterial disease (and calcified vessels), this phenomenon is more pronounced. However, the mean arterial pressure (MAP) should be equivalent at all arterial sites.

Insertion of an Arterial Catheter[3]

The most common method for gaining access into any desired vessel is the Seldinger technique, which was initially described by Sven-Ivar Seldinger in 1953. The technique begins by locating the artery with an introducer needle or catheter. Next a guidewire is passed through the lumen of the introducer needle/catheter and the introducer is removed leaving only the guidewire in the vessel. A soft dilator may be passed over the guidewire and then removed to dilate the skin and soft tissues leading to the artery. Finally, the arterial catheter is passed over the wire into the artery and the wire is removed. Special arterial catheterization kits are available in which the guidewire and arterial catheter are attached to the introducer needle, reducing the number of steps necessary and minimizing blood loss during the procedure. Figure 10–2, *A*, shows the Seldinger technique (without the dilator step) and Figure 10–2, *B*, shows the modified technique with use of a specialized arterial catheter.

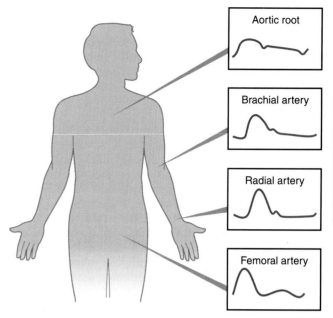

Figure 10–1 Normal pressure waveforms of the aortic root, brachial artery, radial artery, and femoral artery.

Contraindications to Arterial Cannulation

Absolute contraindications to cannulation include localized infection at the site of insertion, preexisting ischemia, nerve damage, Raynaud phenomenon, or traumatic injury proximal to the site of insertion. It is usually possible to identify another artery that is amenable to cannulation. Relative contraindications include failure to demonstrate collateral flow in small vessels (e.g., by Doppler ultrasonography), presence of an arteriovenous fistula in the same limb, and history of surgery disrupting the lymphatics of the same limb (e.g., axillary lymphadenectomy). If there are no other arterial sites that can be used, these relative contraindications may be outweighed by other considerations.

Complications

Complications of invasive arterial blood pressure monitoring may be related to the placement of the catheter, care of the indwelling catheter, length of time the catheter is in place, or patient characteristics. Table 10-1 lists the complications associated with arterial cannulation[4,5] and precautions to decrease these risks.

Other Considerations

As with all invasive pressure monitors, the transducer height should be level with the right atrium. An exception to this rule is when monitoring cerebral perfusion pressure, in which case the transducer height should be level with the tragus of the earlobe. If the patient's head is elevated, the manometer will therefore be higher than the heart.

Volume status can be indirectly assessed by evaluating the arterial pressure height during controlled mechanical ventilation. Positive pressure ventilation will lead to greater systolic variation (>10 mm Hg) of the blood pressure in patients who are hypovolemic (Figure 10–3).

Cardiac Output

Global oxygen delivery to the tissues is dependent on the oxygen content of blood (CaO_2) and cardiac output (CO). Cardiac output is equal to the product of heart rate (HR) and stroke volume (SV):

$$CO = HR \times SV$$

The variables that affect stroke volume include preload, afterload, and contractility. Preload is an estimate of left ventricular volume at the end of diastole. The Frank-Starling curve shows the relationship between preload and stroke volume (Figure 10–4). In general, increases in preload lead to greater stroke volume. However, a point on the Frank-Starling curve is eventually reached where further increases in preload do not increase stroke volume and may instead lead to decreased stroke volume (as in congestive heart failure). Because it is difficult to measure ventricular volume, ventricular pressure is commonly used to estimate volume and thus preload. Use of a central venous catheter enables monitoring of right atrial pressure or central venous pressure (CVP), which is an estimate of right ventricular preload. In a patient without significant pulmonary hypertension or valvular disease, it can be assumed that right ventricular preload correlates with left ventricular preload because the same blood volume that enters the right heart will traverse the pulmonary circulation to enter the left heart. By way of this assumption, CVP is often used as an estimate of left ventricular preload.

Afterload refers to the myocardial wall tension that is required to overcome the opposing resistance to blood ejection. Right ventricular afterload is indirectly represented by the pulmonary vascular resistance (PVR) and left ventricular afterload is indirectly represented by the systemic vascular resistance (SVR). SVR may be calculated from the following equation if cardiac output has been measured:

$$SVR = [(MAP - CVP/CO)] \times 80$$

where MAP = mean arterial pressure.

Contractility refers to the ability of the myocardium to contract and eject blood from the ventricle. Contractility depends on preload and afterload, so these variables should be optimized first to improve contractility. Contractility can be directly measured with the use of echocardiography to estimate ejection fraction. However, once preload and afterload are optimized, contractility is often indirectly represented by cardiac output. If cardiac output remains low despite improvements in preload and afterload, the use of inotropic pharmacological agents may be initiated to improve contractility.

Central Venous Pressure Monitoring

As described above, invasive central venous pressure (CVP) monitoring[6] allows continuous measurement of right heart pressures, which can be used to reflect volume status. The catheter also provides venous access for rapid infusion of fluids or drugs. Normal CVP during positive pressure ventilation ranges from 6 to 12 mm Hg. A low CVP with hypotension and tachycardia usually corresponds to hypovolemia. Persistent hypotension following a fluid challenge and higher than normal CVP usually indicates cardiac congestion (as can occur with cardiac tamponade, tension pneumothorax, or myocardial ischemia). In addition to monitoring of pressures, central venous catheterization enables collection of blood from the superior vena cava (central venous blood) for measurement of central venous blood oxygenation that can be used as an indirect marker of global tissue perfusion and oxygenation.

Indications for Central Venous Catheterization

- Assessment of volume status
- Inability to obtain adequate peripheral intravenous access

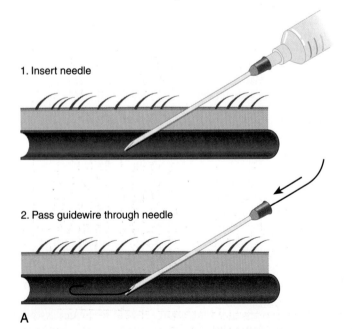

1. Insert needle

2. Pass guidewire through needle

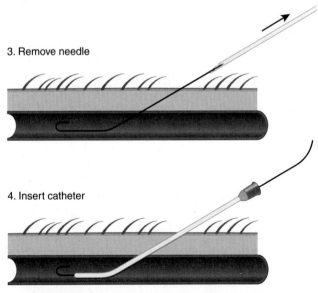

3. Remove needle

4. Insert catheter

A

Figure 10–2 Arterial cannulation via two different techniques: **(A)** Seldinger technique.

(Continued)

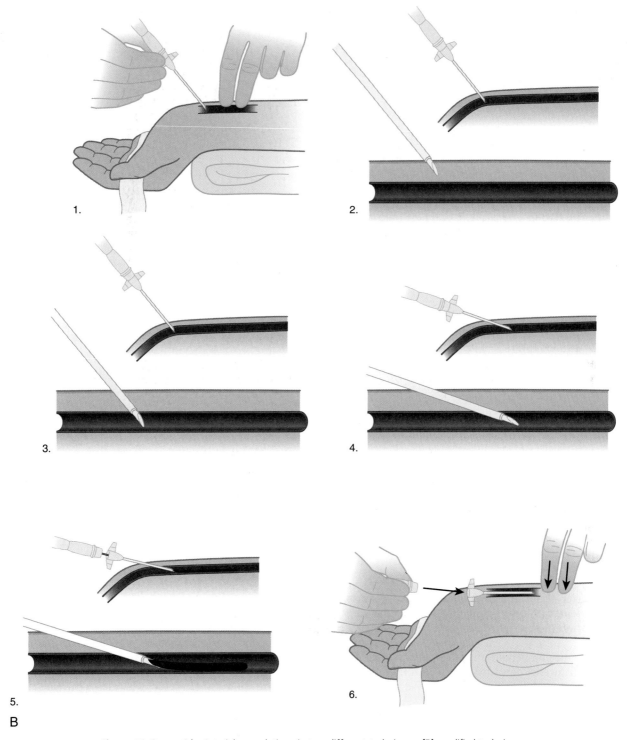

Figure 10–2, cont'd   Arterial cannulation via two different techniques: **(B)** modified technique.

- Rapid infusion of fluids through a large cannula (e.g., trauma patients, surgery with significant blood loss)
- Administration of drugs that may be toxic to peripheral veins (e.g., concentrated vasoactive drugs, hyperalimentation, certain antibiotics)
- Aspiration of venous air emboli (e.g., sitting craniotomy or other surgery with high-risk of venous air embolism)
- Blood sampling for frequent laboratory measurements

- Transvenous cardiac pacing
- Temporary hemodialysis
- Introducer for pulmonary artery catheterization

Sites for Central Venous Catheterization

Cannulation sites for CVP placement include subclavian, internal jugular, and femoral veins. Occasionally the external jugular vein may be used if it is large enough. Long-arm CVP

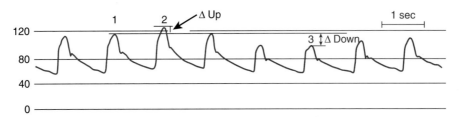

Figure 10–3 Arterial blood pressure tracing showing systolic pressure variation during mechanical ventilation. *(1)* represents end-expiration, *(2)* represents positive pressure inspiration in which systolic pressure increases slightly, *(3)* represents the large (>10 mm Hg) decrease after inspiration consistent with hypovolemia.

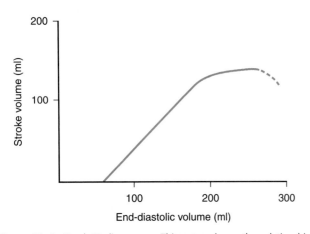

Figure 10–4 Frank-Starling curve. This curve shows the relationship between end-diastolic volume (preload) and stroke volume. Increases in end-diastolic volume lead to increased stroke volume until a point is reached where further increases in end-diastolic volume lead to congestive heart failure.

catheters can also be passed from the brachial or cephalic vein into the central circulation.

Insertion of a Central Venous Catheter

The Seldinger technique is commonly used to insert a central venous catheter. Figure 10–5 shows the steps to catheterization of the right internal jugular vein with this technique.

To reduce the number of cannulation attempts and the risk of inadvertent arterial puncture, a portable ultrasound vessel-imaging device is often used to visualize the vascular structures as shown in Figure 10–6.

There are several different kinds of catheters that can be inserted centrally, including single-lumen catheters, multilumen catheters, and introducer sheaths. Often a multilumen catheter will be inserted if the catheter is primarily intended for administration of medications and/or CVP monitoring. Introducer sheaths are used when there is the need for a larger catheter, such as for rapid volume administration or for the insertion of a pulmonary artery catheter. When placing an introducer sheath, the use of a tapered-tip, stiff dilator should be placed into the introducer to facilitate passage of this large cannula over the guidewire from the skin, through the subcutaneous tissues, and into the vein. Figure 10–7 shows examples of a multilumen catheter and an introducer catheter.

Complications of Central Venous Catheterization

Contraindications to central venous catheterization include trauma at the site or localized infection. Complications associated with placement of a central line[7-9] are presented in Table 10–2. To decrease the risk of infection, strict sterile technique should be used. In emergency situations when lines are inserted without adherence to sterile technique, they should be replaced as soon as it is feasible (i.e., when surgery is over and the patient is stable [usually within 12 to 24 hours]).

Central Venous Pressure Waveforms

There are many useful parameters that can be analyzed from the central venous pressure waveform. Table 10–3 lists the components of the CVP waveform and their corresponding phase of the cardiac cycle. Figure 10–8 shows the normal waveform and its components in association with an EKG and arterial pressure waveform. There are also certain physiological abnormalities that are associated with specific changes in the CVP waveform components. Table 10–4 and Figure 10–9 review some of the more common abnormalities and how the CVP waveform is affected.

Pulmonary Artery Catheter[10]

Indications for Pulmonary Artery Catheterization

As described earlier, left heart pressures may be estimated from right heart pressures in most circumstances and CVP may be used to approximate pulmonary capillary wedge pressure (PCWP). However, when left ventricular function is impaired, or significant valvular disease or pulmonary hypertension is present, the use of a pulmonary artery catheter (PAC) may be indicated for more accurate estimations of left heart pressures. Other possible indications for the use of a PAC include severe coronary artery disease, shock, massive trauma, severe lung disease, severe renal disease, and the need to place a temporary ventricular pacing wire via the PAC. Use of a PAC allows continuous monitoring of pulmonary artery pressures, intermittent monitoring of PCWP, and thermodilution for estimation of cardiac output and calculation of systemic vascular resistance. PCWP is used as the best estimation of left ventricular end-diastolic volume (preload), analogous to CVP estimation for the right ventricle.

The PAC can also be used to obtain blood samples for mixed venous oxygen saturation for evaluating the body's oxygen

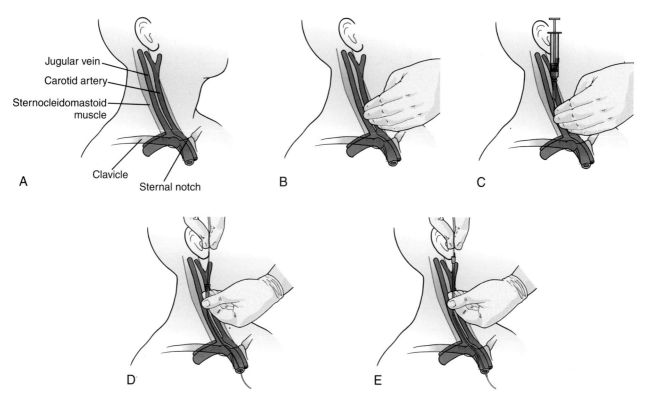

Figure 10–5   Catheterization of the right internal jugular vein.

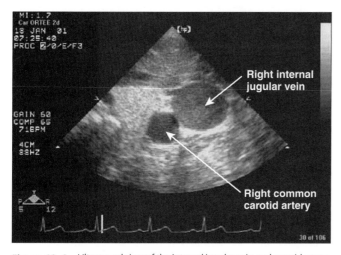

Figure 10–6   Ultrasound view of the internal jugular vein and carotid artery.

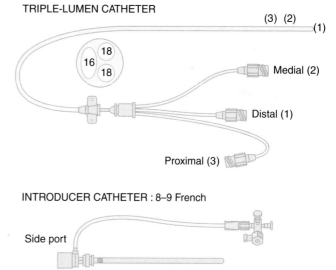

Figure 10–7   Examples of a multilumen catheter and an introducer catheter.

balance (by calculating oxygen consumption and delivery). Specialized PACs can be used that enable continuous Svo_2 monitoring.

Complications Associated with Pulmonary Artery Catheterization

Risks associated with PAC placement include those associated with central line placement and additional anatomic and functional disturbances (also see Table 10–2). The risk of complication increases with the duration of catheterization even when optimally placed; therefore, in general a PAC should not persist beyond 72 to 96 hours.

Standard PAC balloons contain latex and there have been reports of severe anaphylactic reactions attributed to the latex. Therefore, latex allergy or sensitivity is a contraindication to the use of a PAC, unless a special nonlatex catheter is used.

It should be noted that the use of a PAC has not been shown to improve survival. In addition, the value of the PAC is dependent on attainment of accurate measurements and the user's ability to appropriately interpret these measurements.

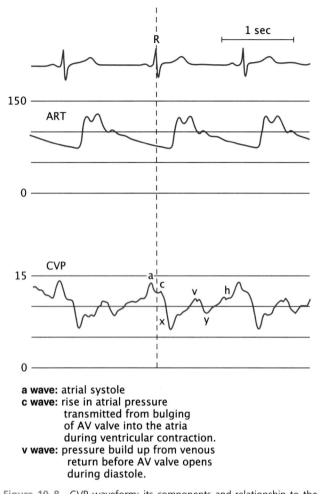

a wave: atrial systole
c wave: rise in atrial pressure
transmitted from bulging
of AV valve into the atria
during ventricular contraction.
v wave: pressure build up from venous
return before AV valve opens
during diastole.

Figure 10–8 CVP waveform: its components and relationship to the ECG tracing and arterial pressure waveform.

Insertion of Pulmonary Artery Catheter

The PAC can be placed into any of the central venous cannulation sites that have been described. The procedure begins with the same steps as described above using the Seldinger technique to place a large-bore (7.5 to 9.0 French) introducer sheath into a central vein. This introducer has a hemostasis valve at its outer end, through which the PAC will be inserted, and a sidearm extension that allows continuous central venous access for fluid and drug administration. The final steps in placing a PAC require the aid of a skilled assistant to help prepare the catheter and attach it properly to pressure monitoring transducers. The assistant attaches the distal and proximal port hubs to the pressure monitoring system that will allow waveforms to be displayed on the bedside monitor. All ports should be flushed to remove air from the catheter lumens. The balloon should be tested to make sure there is no leak and that it inflates symmetrically. The balloon should only be inflated with air, not with liquid.

The PAC is inserted through the hemostasis valve of the introducer to a depth of 20 cm, or approximately 5 cm beyond the tip of the introducer sheath. A characteristic CVP waveform must be identified to confirm that the PAC tip is in the vena cava or right atrium. The gentle curvature of the PAC (Figure 10–10 A) should be oriented to point just leftward

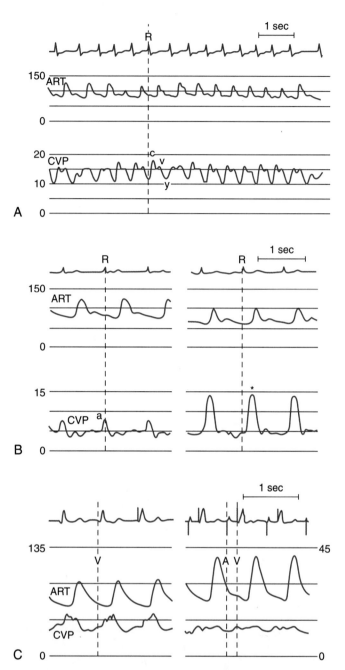

Figure 10–9 Central venous pressure (CVP) changes caused by cardiac arrhythmias. **A,** Atrial fibrillation. Note the absence of the a wave, a prominent c wave, and a preserved v wave and y descent. This arrhythmia also causes variation in the electrocardiographic (ECG) R-R interval and left ventricular stroke volume, which can be seen in the ECG and arterial pressure (ART) traces. **B,** Isorhythmic atrioventricular dissociation. In contrast to the normal end-diastolic a wave in the CVP trace *(left panel)*, an early systolic cannon wave is inscribed *(asterisk, right panel)*. The reduced ventricular filling accompanying this arrhythmia causes decreased arterial blood pressure. **C,** Ventricular pacing. Systolic cannon waves are evident in the CVP trace during ventricular pacing *(left panel)*. Atrioventricular sequential pacing restores the normal venous waveform and increases arterial blood pressure *(right panel)*. The ART scale is shown on the *left*, the CVP scale on the *right*. (Redrawn from Mark JB. *Atlas of cardiovascular monitoring*, New York, Churchill Livingstone, 1998.)

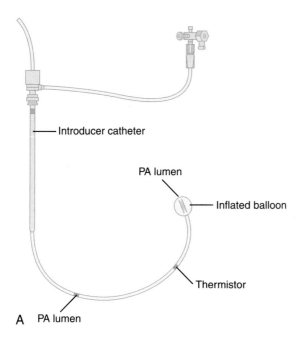

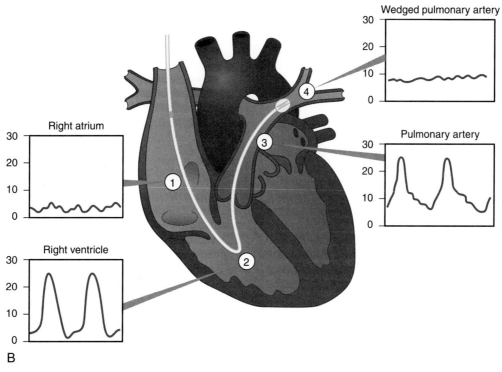

Figure 10–10   **A,** A pulmonary artery catheter showing the natural curvature of the device. **B,** Characteristic pressure tracings along the path of PAC insertion.

of the sagittal plane (the 11-o'clock position as viewed from the patient's head). This orientation will facilitate catheter passage through the anteromedially located tricuspid valve. Before further insertion of the catheter, the balloon should be inflated, and then the catheter is advanced into the right atrium, through the tricuspid valve into the right ventricle, through the pulmonic valve into the pulmonary artery, and finally into the pulmonary capillary wedge position. Characteristic waveforms from each of these locations confirm

proper catheter passage and placement. After the pulmonary capillary wedge pressure is measured, the balloon should be deflated, and the pulmonary artery waveform should reappear for continuous monitoring. PCWP may be obtained periodically as needed by reinflating the balloon with 1.5 mL of air to allow the catheter to float distally until the pulmonary artery occlusion again occurs. Figure 10–10 B shows the characteristic pressure tracings along the path of PAC insertion.

Determination of Cardiac Output Using the Pulmonary Artery Catheter
Cardiac Output by Thermodilution

Cardiac output measurement using a pulmonary artery catheter is based on the principle of thermodilution, in which a known volume of cold fluid is injected into the catheter at a proximal point and the temperature change (cooling effect) is measured in the blood at a downstream point by a thermistor. The temperature change in blood caused by the cold injectate flowing past the thermistor is measured and plotted against time. The shape of the resulting curve is determined by the cardiac output. When cardiac output is low, there will be a larger temperature change because there is a longer delay from the time of injection until the blood reaches the thermistor (more time for cooling effect to occur).

The theory and calculation of cardiac output by thermodilution depend on proper representation of the volume and temperature of the injectate fluid, the thermodynamic properties of blood and injectate solution, and the integral of the temperature-time curve. Both patient and injectate factors can affect the accuracy of thermodilution. Patient factors that can lead to inaccuracy include the presence of tricuspid regurgitation, intracardiac shunts, dysrhythmias, or abnormal respiratory patterns. Injectate factors include errors in injectate volume, rate of injection, and injectate temperature.

Cardiac Output by the Fick Principle

Determination of cardiac output can also be based on the Fick principle, which states that in steady state conditions, the amount of oxygen consumed per unit of time is equal to the arterial oxygen content minus the venous oxygen content multiplied by the blood flow (cardiac output).

In equation form, the Fick principle can be represented by the following equation:

$$\dot{V}O_2 = (CaO_2 - CvO_2) \times CO$$

where $\dot{V}O_2$ = oxygen consumption; CaO_2 = arterial oxygen content; and CvO_2 = venous oxygen content.

Solving this equation for cardiac output yields:

$$CO = \dot{V}O_2 / (CaO_2 - CvO_2)$$

Oxygen consumption ($\dot{V}O_2$) can be measured by indirect calorimetry while arterial and venous oxygen concentrations can be calculated using the following formulas after arterial and venous oxygen saturations and hemoglobin levels are measured:

$$CaO_2 = (1.39 \times Hb \times SaO_2) + (PaO_2 \times 0.003)$$

$$CvO_2 = (1.39 \times Hb \times SvO_2) + (PvO_2 \times 0.003)$$

Once the variables are measured or calculated, they can be substituted back into the Fick equation to determine the cardiac output.

Limitations in Using the Pulmonary Artery Catheter

Use of the PAC for measurement and calculation of hemodynamic variables is based on several assumptions, which in certain clinical conditions, do not hold true. Recall that PCWP

is an estimation of left ventricular end-diastolic pressure (LVEDP). This estimation is based on the assumption that when a static column of fluid is created (by inflation of the PAC balloon into the wedged position) there will be equalization of diastolic pressures in the cardiac chambers such that:

$$PCWP = LAP_d = LVEDP$$

where LAP_d = left atrial diastolic pressure.

The following clinical conditions can make this relationship inaccurate:

a. Mitral stenosis or regurgitation—left atrial pressure (and thus PCWP) will be greater than LVEDP because there is obstruction to flow across the mitral valve (mitral stenosis) or the regurgitant blood flow raises left atrial pressure (mitral regurgitation).

b. Aortic regurgitation—LVEDP will be greater than left atrial diastolic pressure (and PCWP) because the mitral valve closes before end diastole.

Recall, also, that LVEDP is used as a surrogate for left ventricular end-diastolic volume (LVEDV, or preload) such that:

$$PCWP = LAP_d = LVEDP \approx LVEDV$$

The following clinical conditions can make this assumption false:

a. Decreased compliance of the LV (diastolic dysfunction)—if LV compliance is reduced, then LVEDP (and PCWP) will overestimate LVEDV.

b. Increased intrathoracic pressure—if intrathoracic pressures are increased by positive pressure ventilation, positive end-expiratory pressure, or increased intraabdominal pressure, this may be transmitted to intravascular pressures and cause LVEDP (and PCWP) to overestimate LVEDV.

c. Ventricular interdependence—if the right ventricle is dilated, it can cause the interventricular septum to move leftward and decrease LV compliance, leading to overestimation of LVEDV by LVEDP.

Less Invasive Monitors for Cardiac Output

Esophageal Doppler

The esophageal Doppler technique is based on the concept that flow in a cylinder is equal to the cross-sectional area of the cylinder multiplied by the velocity of the fluid flowing through the cylinder. With the placement of a thin ultrasound probe (Figure 10–11) into the esophagus, sound waves are transmitted toward the descending aorta. As blood flows through the aorta, the frequency of the sound waves changes by the Doppler effect. The Doppler effect states that the frequency of sound waves emitted by a moving object (blood) is altered proportionately to the relative velocity between the object (blood) and the observer (probe). Since the change in frequency (Doppler shift) is proportional to the velocity of blood flow, aortic blood flow velocity can be calculated and a nomogram is then used to estimate stroke volume and cardiac output.

Advantages of the esophageal Doppler method include its relative noninvasiveness and its ability to provide continuous monitoring of cardiac output once the probe is placed into

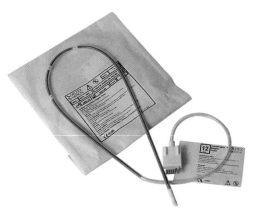

Figure 10–11 Doppler probe (CardioQ). Note the flexible probe shaft, three depth markers, and patient interface connector.

the esophagus and patient variables have been entered into the algorithm.

However, there are also several limitations of the esophageal Doppler method including the following:

a. Estimated cardiac output is based only on blood flow in the descending thoracic aorta, which does not include the portion of cardiac output to the upper part of the body and may not be an accurate representation of total cardiac output.

b. Blood flow velocity measurements may not be accurate when aortic blood flow is turbulent (such as with tachycardia or aortic stenosis).

c. Probe placement is contraindicated in patients with esophageal disease or severe coagulopathy.

d. Probe placement may be poorly tolerated in awake, nonintubated patients.

Indirect Fick Partial Rebreathing Method

The Noninvasive Cardiac Output (NICO, Novametrix Medical Systems, Wallingford, Conn.) monitor measures pulmonary blood flow by applying the Fick equation to the lungs, substituting Vco_2 for Vo_2 such that:

$$\text{Pulmonary Blood Flow} = Vco_2 / (CVco_2 - CaCo_2)$$

where Vco_2 = elimination of CO_2; $Cvco_2$ = mixed venous content of CO_2; and $CaCO_2$ = arterial content of CO_2.

Since the blood pumped out of the heart (cardiac output) travels through the lungs, measurement of pulmonary blood flow is a measurement of cardiac output. The NICO uses a partial CO_2 rebreathing technique and employs algorithms to calculate pulmonary blood flow based on changes in Vco_2 and $Caco_2$ without directly measuring $Cvco_2$ (because this is technically more difficult to do). Advantages of this method include its noninvasiveness (except that the patient must be intubated), the ability to obtain continuous measurements of cardiac output, and that it requires minimal operator experience. The algorithms used to calculate cardiac output are based on assumptions that hold true under stable conditions, but may not be true during the rapidly changing conditions of patients undergoing anesthesia and surgery. For example, changes in CO_2 production during periods of ischemia and reperfusion (e.g., tourniquet use, arterial clamping) may

lead to inaccurate measurements. Other limitations of the NICO are that it can only be used in intubated patients, the use of partial CO_2 rebreathing adds dead space, changes in mechanical ventilator settings can produce alterations in cardiac output measurements, and that accuracy may be limited in patients who do not have normal alveolar gas exchange or who have floridly abnormal cardiac outputs.

Transpulmonary Thermodilution

Transpulmonary (or transthoracic) thermodilution uses arterial thermodilution from a near-central artery (in contrast to the pulmonary artery) for the measurement of stroke volume and cardiac output. Because it is necessary to have a central venous catheter and a near-centrally placed (femoral, axillary, or brachial) arterial catheter, this method is still relatively invasive, although less so than the PAC. Cold indicator fluid is injected into the central venous catheter and temperature of the blood mixed with the cold indicator is measured at the arterial catheter (which has a thermistor at its tip). Although several studies have shown comparable validity and reliability of the transpulmonary thermodilution technique to pulmonary artery thermodilution, changes in systemic arterial compliance in response to changing hemodynamic conditions may lead to inaccurate measurements of cardiac output. In addition, because there is no measurement of pulmonary artery pressures or pulmonary capillary wedge pressure, transpulmonary thermodilution cannot aid in the discrimination between left and right heart function.

Lithium Dilution Cardiac Output

The Lithium Dilution Cardiac Output (LiDCO Ltd, Cambridge, UK) monitor uses lithium dilution instead of thermodilution to measure cardiac output. A bolus of lithium indicator solution is injected intravenously, mixes with the patient's blood, and the resulting lithium concentration-time curve is recorded by a sensor connected to the patient's arterial catheter. The sensor is outside the artery and requires withdrawal of a blood sample with each measurement. Analysis of the lithium dilution curve enables calculation of cardiac output. An advantage of this technique is that a central venous catheter is not necessary, nor is a near-central arterial catheter; thus this technique is less invasive than both pulmonary arterial catheterization and transpulmonary thermodilution, but still shows good correlation of cardiac output values. Limitations of the LiDCO include inaccuracy in patients receiving lithium therapy or receiving muscle relaxants. Also, because it does not require central catheterization, use of central pressures to directly estimate cardiac preload cannot be obtained unless a separate central catheter is placed.

Arterial Pulse Contour Analysis

During systole, blood pressure increases due to ejection of blood from the ventricles, as can be seen on an arterial blood pressure tracing. Pulse contour analysis is based on the assumption that the systolic part of the arterial pressure waveform is proportional to stroke volume. Beat-to-beat analysis of this waveform (or the pulse contour) is therefore used to estimate stroke volume and cardiac output. It is important to recognize that stroke volume at any given time is also influenced by the impedance or compliance of the aorta. To compensate for the effect of aortic impedance on stroke volume, cardiac output must be determined by another method first and used for calibration of the pulse contour analysis. Available monitors for continuous pulse contour analysis include the PiCCO (Pulsion Medical Systems, Munich, Germany), the LiDCO, and the Vigileo (Edwards Lifesciences, Irvine, Calif.). Both PiCCO and LiDCO require external calibration by manual injection of an indicator. PiCCO uses transpulmonary thermodilution for calibration while LiDCO uses the lithium dilution technique. The Vigileo has a special blood flow sensor (called the FloTrac™) that connects to the patient's arterial catheter to enable its use without external calibration. In addition to cardiac output monitoring, pulse contour analysis enables dynamic continuous measurement of stroke volume variation. Stroke volume variation can be used as a predictor of fluid responsiveness in the same way that arterial systolic pressure variation can be used (see Figure 10–3), and may be a better predictor of fluid responsiveness. Limitations of pulse contour analysis include inaccuracy whenever the arterial waveform is distorted, such as with mechanical occlusion or kinking of the cannula, overdampening of the waveform, and in patients with severe vasoconstriction or dysrhythmias.

Monitors for Pulse Contour Analysis

a. FloTrac/Vigileo—stroke volume is calculated using arterial pulsatility and then cardiac output is calculated from the equation $CO = HR \times SV$. Although there is no requirement for external calibration, which makes the Vigileo easier to use, rapid changes in vascular tone may lead to problems with accurate cardiac output monitoring.
b. PiCCO—cardiac output is first obtained by transpulmonary thermodilution, and this is used as the reference for obtaining continuous pulse contour-derived cardiac output measurements. Accuracy has been shown to be sufficient if frequent recalibration is performed, particularly after significant changes in arterial compliance or hemodynamics. However, this need for frequent recalibration is a major limiting factor of the PiCCO monitor. One advantage of the PiCCO monitor is the ability to monitor additional parameters, including global end-diastolic volume (GEDV), intrathoracic blood volume (ITBV), and extravascular lung water (EVLW). ITBV can be used as a surrogate for cardiac preload and EVLW can be used as a surrogate for pulmonary edema. However further studies are needed to validate these indices.
c. LiDCO—the pulse contour analysis is calibrated with cardiac output obtained by lithium dilution. Again, the need for frequent recalibration is a limitation of the LiDCO monitor.

Bioimpedance Cardiography

Thoracic bioimpedance is the electrical resistance of the thorax to high-frequency, low-magnitude current. Changes in bioimpedance are related to cardiac events and blood flow in the thorax such that as the amount of thoracic fluid increases, the thoracic bioimpedance decreases. Changes in bioimpedance are used to estimate changes in stroke volume and cardiac output. Six electrodes are placed on the patient's thorax to detect changes in bioimpedance. The individual determinants of overall thoracic fluid include tissue fluid volume, pulmonary

and venous blood volume, and aortic blood volume produced by myocardial contractility. Therefore, changes in tissue fluid content (such as pulmonary edema, pleural effusions, or chest wall edema) will alter bioimpedance readings and lead to errors in measurement of cardiac output. Patients in the operating room often have significant intrathoracic fluid shifts, which limits the utility of bioimpedance cardiography.

Echocardiography (see also Chapter 11)

a. Transthoracic echocardiography (TTE) is the least invasive way of imaging cardiac structures because it simply requires the placement of an ultrasound probe over the chest. However, access to the chest may be limited by the surgical field and TTE may result in inadequate images in patients who are obese or who are being mechanically ventilated.
b. Transesophageal echocardiography (TEE) requires placement of the ultrasound probe into the esophagus or stomach so it is more invasive than TTE, but still less invasive than many other monitors of cardiac function (including the PAC). TEE enables direct visualization of cardiac structures and evaluation of ventricular function, and it is an excellent means of assessing hemodynamics in the operating room. The factors that interact to affect systolic cardiac function (heart rate, preload, afterload, and contractility) can all be evaluated in real time with 2-dimensional and Doppler imaging via TEE. TEE measurements of cardiac output have been found to correlate well with thermodilution measurements. Thus the advantages of TEE include its minimal invasiveness with a low incidence of procedure-related complications, the ability to observe frequent changes in cardiac status immediately in real time, and its accuracy in detection of hypovolemia, left ventricular dysfunction, and ischemia. Contraindications to TEE include esophageal rupture, stricture, diverticulum, tumor, or recent esophageal or gastric surgery. Another limitation of TEE is that it is not applicable during induction or once patients are awake and extubated.

References

1. Ingelmo, P., Barone, M., Fumagalli, R., 2002. Importance of monitoring in high risk surgical patients. Minerva Anestesiol 68 (4), 226–230.
2. Bigatello, L.M., Schmidt, U., 2003. Arterial blood pressure monitoring. Minerva Anestesiol 69 (4), 201–209.
3. Franklin, C., 1995. The technique of radial artery cannulation. Tips for maximizing results while minimizing the risk of complications. J Crit Illn 10 (6), 424–432.
4. Frezza, E.E., Mezghebe, H., 1998. Indications and complications of arterial catheter use in surgical or medical intensive care units: analysis of 4932 patients. Am Surg 64 (2), 127–131.
5. Scheer, B., Perel, A., Pfeiffer, U.J., 2002. Clinical review: complications and risk factors of peripheral arterial catheters used for haemodynamic monitoring in anaesthesia and intensive care medicine. Crit Care 6 (3), 199–204.
6. Magder, S., 2006. Central venous pressure monitoring. Curr Opin Crit Care 12, 219.
7. Bowdle, T.A., 2002. Complications of invasive monitoring. Anesthesiol Clin North America 20 (3), 571–588.
8. Domino, K.B., Bowdle, T.A., Posner, K.L., et al., 2004. Injuries and liability related to central vascular catheters: a closed claims analysis. Anesthesiology 100 (6), 1411–1418.
9. McGee, D.C., Gould, M.K., 2003. Preventing complications of central venous catheterization. N Engl J Med 348 (12), 1123–1133.
10. Vincent, J.L., Pinsky, M.R., Sprung, C.L., et al., 2008. The pulmonary artery catheter: in medio virtus. Crit Care Med 36 (11), 3093–3096.

Further Reading

1. Hadian, M., Pinsky, M.R., 2006. Evidence-based review of the use of the pulmonary artery catheter: impact data and complications. Crit Care 10 (suppl 3), S8.

2. Hofer, C.K., Senn, A., Weibel, L., et al., 2008. Assessment of stroke volume variation for prediction of fluid responsiveness using the modified FloTrac™ and PiCCOplus™ system. Crit Care 12 (3), R82.

3. Mathews, L., Singh, R.K., 2008. Cardiac output monitoring. Ann Card Anaesth 11 (1), 56–68.

4. Morgan, P., Al-Subaie, N., Rhodes, A., 2008. Minimally invasive cardiac output monitoring. Curr Opin Crit Care 14 (3), 322–326.

5. Polanco, P.M., Pinsky, M.R., 2007. Principles of hemodynamic monitoring. Contrib Nephrol 156, 133–157.

Chapter 11

Transesophageal Echocardiography

Jacob Kaczmarski and Sugantha Sundar

Transesophageal echocardiography (TEE) is now frequently used as a monitor and diagnostic tool in the operating room and it is becoming increasingly important that anesthesiologists learn to acquire and interpret basic images.[1-4] The diagnosis of certain life-threatening conditions, such as cardiac tamponade, aortic dissection, hypovolemia, and severe left ventricular dysfunction, can be made with even limited training.[5,6] A competent echocardiographer needs to have a working knowledge of certain theoretical and practical aspects of TEE for it to be of use clinically.[7] These include the basic physics of ultrasound, navigating the computer workstation, important safety issues, and general maintenance of equipment.

A basic TEE machine requires a system for ultrasound beam generation, a system capable of receiving the returning ultrasound beams, a system to process these received signals and last, but not least, a way to display these images so the human eye and brain can appreciate it.

Basic Physics

TEE uses ultrasound (sound above the audible frequency in humans), to formulate images of cardiovascular structures. A transducer at the tip of the TEE probe transmits and receives ultrasonic waves, which are then computer processed and displayed in real time on a monitor. Sound waves typically demonstrate a sinusoidal pattern (Figure 11–1). The *wavelength* (λ) is the distance between successive peaks (or troughs) of the wave, and the *frequency* (F) is the number of wavelengths per unit of time measured in hertz (cycles per second). When used in medical ultrasound, the wavelength is related to the resolution of the displayed images and the frequency influences the depth of penetration. The maximum depth of penetration is usually about 200 to 400 times the wavelength. Typically, ultrasound waves with frequencies between 2.5 and 7.5 MHz with wavelengths of 0.2 to 0.6 mm are used in TEE. This correlates to a resolution of 0.4 to 1.2 mm and a depth of penetration of up to 24 cm.

The speed or *propagation velocity* (C) of sound is determined by the medium in which it travels and is approximately 1540 m/s in heart tissue. The mathematical relationship of frequency, wavelength, and propagation velocity is as follows:

$$C = \lambda \times F$$

Since the speed of sound in cardiac tissue is constant, frequency and wavelength are inversely proportional. Thus improved resolution at higher frequencies is obtained at the expense of decreased tissue penetration, and vice versa. Also, the distance of a structure of interest from the transducer may be determined by calculating the time a transmitted wave takes to return to the probe.

When an ultrasound wave reaches an interface of two substances with differing *acoustic impedances*, or densities, part of it is reflected back toward the transducer and part is transmitted through. The degree to which a wave is reflected is directly proportional to the size of the difference in acoustic impedance. An example of this is when air bubbles enter the heart. Blood and air differ significantly in density, so air bubbles reflect the vast majority of the ultrasound and are seen as very bright white specks. The type of reflection a sound wave undergoes is classified as either specular or scattered (Figure 11–2). *Specular* reflection occurs when a wave hits an object

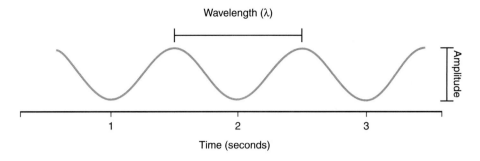

period = time of one cycle (wavelength)
above: one second from crest to crest

frequency = number of cycles/second
above: 1 cycle/sec = 1Hertz (Hz)

Figure 11–1   A sound wave.

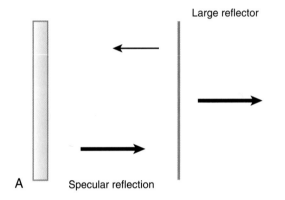

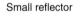

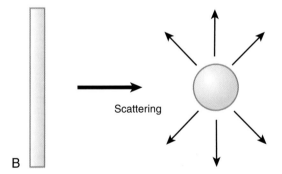

Figure 11–2   **A,** Specular reflection. **B,** Scattering.

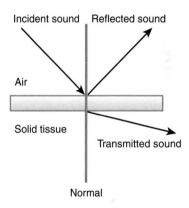

Figure 11–3   Fate of incident sound.

the screen as a result. Both specular and scattering reflection play a role in the acquisition of images in TEE. Probe position and multiplane angle should be directed in such a way as to obtain optimal visualization of the structure of interest.

The concept of *refraction* deals with the portion of ultrasound that is transmitted through at the interface of two different substances and is involved in the production of artifacts. The TEE machine assumes that the transmitted beam will continue to travel linearly throughout its course. However, the direction of the beam is actually altered as it passes from one medium to the next. The magnitude of the change is proportional to the difference in density of the two media, and the acuity of the angle of incidence (Figure 11–3). Visualization of the pulmonary artery catheter in the aorta is a frequent occurrence and is an example of artifact secondary to refraction.

Attenuation refers to the progressive loss in amplitude of an ultrasound signal as a function of the distance traveled within a certain medium, usually due to the processes of *absorption* and *scattering*. Absorption is the conversion of sound energy into heat, and scattering refers to the progressive divergence of sound waves from their original course as they travel further away from their source. The intensity of an attenuated ultrasound signal can be augmented by increasing the *gain* controls on the TEE machine. Images on the screen will appear brighter as the gain is increased and certain structures may

with a large, smooth surface. It will be strongly reflected at an angle equal and opposite to the angle of incidence. The greatest degree of reflection occurs when the angle of incidence is 90 degrees. Therefore, manipulating the TEE probe to align the ultrasound beam perpendicular to a structure of interest will aid in visualization.

Scattering reflection occurs with substances that possess uneven surfaces. Only a portion of the ultrasound waves return to the receiver and the remainder are reflected in diverging directions. These structures will appear darker on

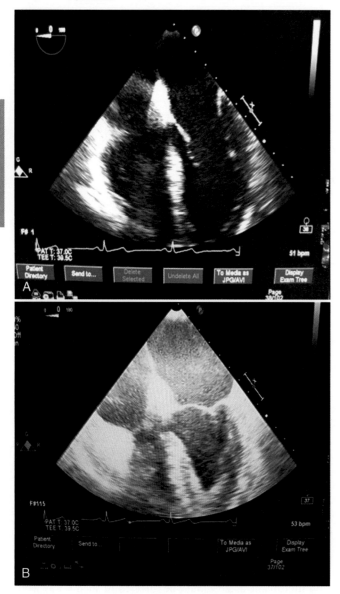

Figure 11–4   Gain settings.

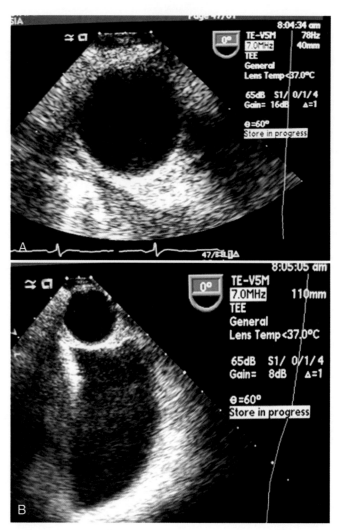

Figure 11–5   **A,** Depth, 4 cm—good for measuring the size of the aorta and looking for atheroma. **B,** Depth, 11 cm—left pleural effusion is now visible.

be easier to visualize. However, the amount of noise will also be amplified and the borders of other structures may appear fuzzy and difficult to differentiate (Figure 11–4, *A* and *B*).

Depth controls the distance at which objects are visualized on the TEE monitor. Increasing the depth will result in a decrease in size and resolution of the displayed images, but potentially more structures will be able to be seen. Normally a depth of approximately 15 cm is an adequate starting point at which to begin an examination. A greater depth is appropriate in certain circumstances such as an assessment of a pericardial or pleural effusion, whereas it is best to perform planimetry or caliper functions of a structure with the view as close as possible (Figure 11–5).

A *focus* function is available that enables the echocardiographer to concentrate the area of highest resolution on a structure of particular interest, such as on the mitral valve in the midesophageal four chamber views. The image of this area appears as slightly higher quality than that of the surrounding structures. The TEE machine performs this automatically

by manipulating certain dimensions of the transmitted ultrasound beam. It is important to be cognizant of the location of the focus sector when evaluating any ultrasound image.

Two-dimensional echocardiography is excellent for visualizing the structure and motion of the heart but is unable to provide information about blood flow within the cardiovascular system. Doppler echocardiography was developed for this purpose and is an integral part of a comprehensive TEE examination.[8] It is useful to assess intracardiac velocities and in the gradation of valvular stenosis and regurgitation. The direction and speed of blood flow are determined by the changes in frequency and wavelength of an ultrasound wave as it is reflected off of moving red blood cells, with the transducer serving as the reference point. The *Doppler shift* describes the changes in frequency of an ultrasonic wave as it is reflected off moving targets (Figure 11–6). It is mathematically expressed as follows:

$$\Delta F = V \times \cos \theta \times 2F_t / C$$

where *V* is the velocity of the target, θ is the angle of incidence, and F_t is the transmitted frequency. Since the frequency of the transmitted wave and the speed of sound in

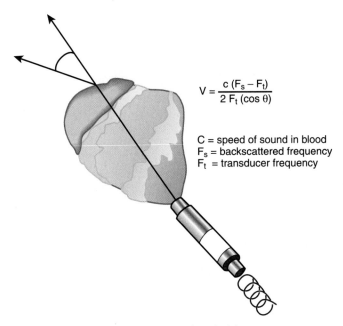

$$V = \frac{c\,(F_s - F_t)}{2\,F_t\,(\cos\theta)}$$

C = speed of sound in blood
F_s = backscattered frequency
F_t = transducer frequency

Figure 11–6   Doppler principle.

heart tissue (C) are constant, the detected change in frequency is directly proportional to the velocity of blood flow and the cosine of the angle of incidence. The estimation of the blood flow velocity is truest when the angle of incidence is 0 degrees (Cos 0 is 1) so it is most important that every effort be made to align the ultrasound beam properly. The underestimation of Doppler shift remains clinically irrelevant until the angle of incidence of the ultrasound beam is greater than 30 degrees. Particular images are better suited for this task, such as the deep transgastric view for determining blood flow velocity through the aortic valve.

All ultrasound systems have the ability to present an audiologic display of the beat-to-beat Doppler information obtained along with the acquisition and spectral display. The system is programmed such that the stronger the Doppler signal, the louder it is. This property in turn can be used to accurately position and align the transducer probe with the direction of flow to obtain the maximal velocity.

The quantitative Doppler data obtained is spectrally displayed after a series of preprocessing and postprocessing functions such as demodulation, fast Fourier transformation, and Chirp-Z transformation have been applied. The isolated frequency is displayed as clean envelopes (velocity over time) on the display monitor. Most machines also have a built-in software system that calculates velocity and peak gradient using the modified Bernoulli equation as depicted below:

$$\text{Pressure gradient} = 4 \times \text{Velocity}^2$$

Imaging Modalities

One-Dimensional Echocardiography—A-, B-, and M-Mode Echocardiography

Single dimensional echocardiographic imaging assesses the distance between the transducer and the interface and the intensity of the reflected ultrasound beam. A and B modes differ in the manner in which the imaging is displayed on the monitor. In the A mode, the display is in the form of vertical

lines on the oscilloscope, with the height corresponding to the intensity of the returning signal. In B mode the display is in the form of bright spots based on the intensity of the signal. In M mode there is the added component of time to the display, which is helpful in determining the motion of the structures evaluated (Figure 11–7).

Two-Dimensional Echocardiography

Two-dimensional imaging is an extension of B mode echocardiography. There is a phased array transducer that emits ultrasound waves in a sequential manner predetermined by the electrical signals received. The transmission and receiving of these ultrasound beams occur at the rate of 60 to 100 times per minute. This information is then processed by the computer and converted to images of the structures interrogated.

Doppler Echocardiography

The Doppler principle is used in this imaging modality.

Pulsed wave Doppler (PWD) uses a single transducer to both transmit and receive ultrasound waves and possesses the ability to analyze the velocity of blood flow at any specific point along the path of the ultrasound beam (Figure 11–8). This process, known as *time gating*, processes only ultrasound signals received after a certain period of time has elapsed since transmission. The amount of time is determined by the distance to the area of interest, or *"sample volume,"* which is chosen by the echocardiographer. The *pulse repetition frequency* (PRF) is the rate at which the transducer transmits ultrasonic waves. The PRF will be lower with sample volumes farther from the transducer as more time is necessary to allow for the return of the transmitted signals. A limitation of PWD is the inability to analyze objects with very high velocities caused by the presence of *aliasing*. Aliasing occurs when the Doppler frequency shift generated by the sample volume is greater than one half the PRF (called the *Nyquist limit*). In this case, the velocity flow profiles are ambiguous and appear to "wrap around" the baseline on the monitor. Nyquist limit refers to the maximum velocity that can be analyzed by PWD. Analysis of the maximum recordable velocities is related to the transducer frequency. A low frequency transducer can record higher velocities at a given depth. PWD is frequently used to interrogate velocities in the pulmonary veins, the left atrial appendage, and the left ventricular outflow tract (LVOT).

Continuous wave Doppler (CWD) uses two separate crystals for analyzing blood flow velocity: one for transmitting and the other for receiving ultrasonic signals. It is able to constantly analyze returning sound waves, and there in no Nyquist limit when using this technique. CWD is best for determining the area of highest velocity along the course of the ultrasound beam, which in most situations lies at the level of the valve orifice (Figure 11–9). There is also no operator selected sample volume and multiple velocities from various points may be present in a single spectral profile. These will often appear as different shades within the envelope.

Color flow Doppler uses PWD information to provide a color visualization of blood flow that is superimposed onto real-time 2-D images (Figure 11–10). The echocardiographer is able to select the height, width, and location of the sample to be analyzed by controlling a box displayed on the computer

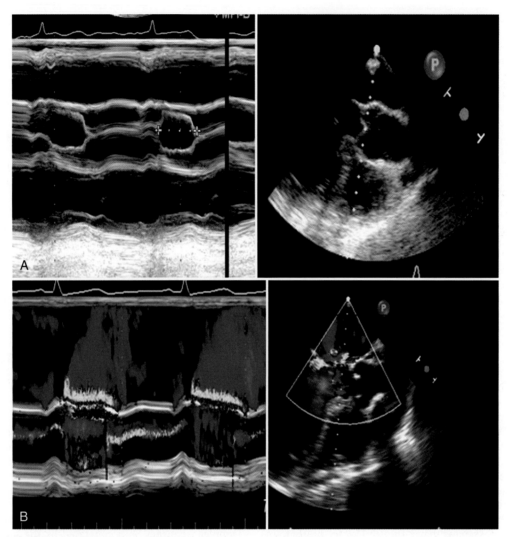

Figure 11–7   **A,** M- Mode. **B,** Color M- Mode.

screen. A color-coding system provides information about the velocity and direction of blood flow within the sample. Many echo cardiographers use color flow Doppler as a starting point to look for regurgitant or stenotic valvular lesions. For example, the relative size and direction of an eccentric mitral valve regurgitant jet are easily detected with color flow Doppler. These abnormalities can then be characterized further with continuous and PWD methods.

Doppler tissue imaging is directed at detecting velocities from myocardial tissue rather than blood (Figure 11–11). The modern TEE machines are equipped to measure myocardial velocities in the range of 0.2 to 0.4 cm/sec and detect amplitudes greater than 20 decibels. The signals obtained are displayed spectrally on the monitor. Tissue Doppler imaging has been used mostly to evaluate diastolic dysfunction.[9]

Three-Dimensional Echocardiography

Recent advances in technology have enabled three-dimensional (3-D) imaging of cardiac structures.[10,11] Two-dimensional images that are obtained in a sequential manner are recorded aligned and reconstructed to 3-D data. Images are collected using a multiplane probe over a 180-degree rotation at periodically set intervals. These images are gated to electrocardiography and respiration to minimize artifacts. Hence presence of arrhythmias can make it challenging. It takes 1 to 5 minutes to acquire the entire data set. The image quality of the 3-D reconstruction depends on the quality of the 2-D images obtained, the number of 2-D images used to reconstruct the 3-D image, ability to minimize motion artifacts, and ability to adequately gate all the beats. This methodology requires offline data analysis using customized or commercially available software depending on the machine used, making it somewhat cumbersome to use efficiently in an intraoperative setting (Figure 11–12). However, real-time 3-D (RT3D) imaging technology has revolutionized the intraoperative management of patients undergoing cardiac surgical procedures. RT3D uses a matrix array transducer that has more than 3000 imaging elements thereby offering better quality images. Images can be obtained real time, with zoom and using a wide angle. Having acquired the data set it has to be sliced or cropped using the crop functions to visualize the structures of interest (Figure 11–13).

It is important to remember to optimize the gain settings before acquiring the images. The American Society of Echocardiography position paper reviews the protocols that have

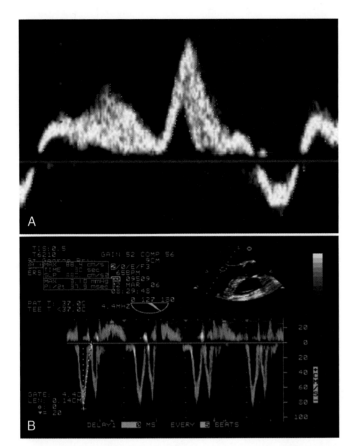

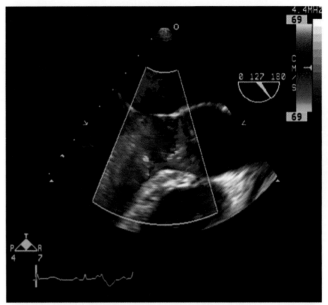

Figure 11–10 Color Doppler.

Figure 11–8 **A,** Pulsed- wave Doppler—pulmonary vein. **B,** Pulsed- wave Doppler—transmitral inflow.

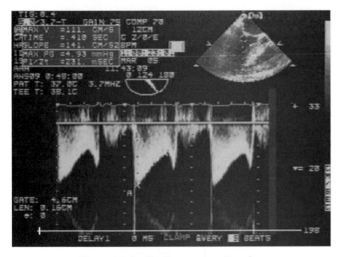

Figure 11–9 Continuous wave Doppler.

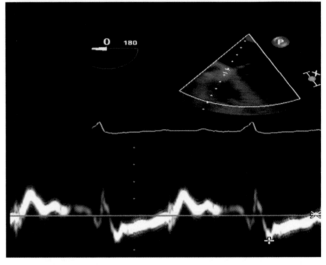

Figure 11–11 Tissue Doppler.

to be followed for transthoracic imaging.[12] Currently no such protocol exists for 3-D transesophageal echocardiographic imaging.

Workstation and the Probe

The two main components of a typical TEE machine are the computer workstation and the probe. The size, specifications, and portability of the unit vary according to the model and the

manufacturer. The TEE probe is a long, thin, flexible structure approximately 60 cm long (Figure 11–14). It is important to be careful when using the probe because it is relatively fragile and quite expensive to purchase and repair. The distal end contains the transducer, which is responsible for sending and receiving ultrasonic signals, and the proximal end is the handle. The handle contains several structures that allow the sonographer to manipulate the transducer and precisely control the direction of the ultrasound beam. Standardized terminology exists to describe these movements. The large wheel allows for *anteflexion* and *retroflexion* in an anterior-posterior direction, while the smaller wheel is used to *flex* the probe to the right or left. The large wheel is frequently useful in obtaining the midesophageal ascending aorta short axis view and the deep transgastric long axis view. The probe may be *advanced* into the stomach or *withdrawn* to the upper esophagus. The transgastric short axis view of the left ventricle is seen from the stomach, while the aortic arch is viewed from the upper

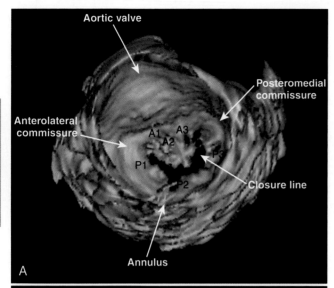

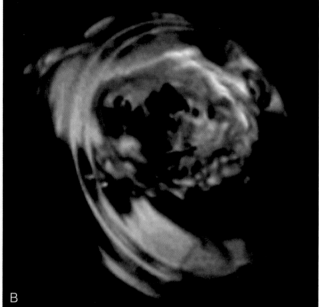

Figure 11–12 **A,** Reconstructed 3D image of mitral valve. **B,** Reconstructed 3-D image of mitral valve with color Doppler.

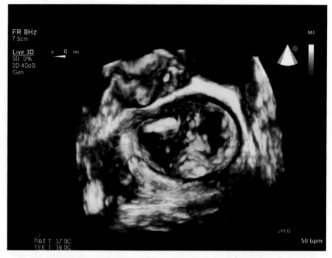

Figure 11–13 Live 3D imaging of mitral valve.

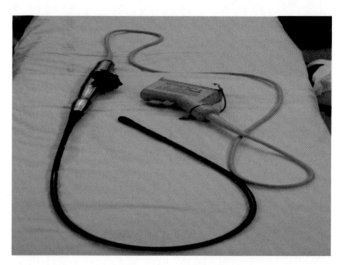

Figure 11–14 TEE probe.

esophagus. The probe may also be rotated in a clockwise and counterclockwise fashion. This is referred to as *turning to the right and to the left*, respectively, and is of use when developing the bicaval view from the midesophagus or the descending aorta short axis view from the stomach. An additional button is used to control a motor, which rotates the transducer at an angle from 0 to 180 degrees. The cardiac structures viewed at 90 degrees will appear distinctly different than those viewed at 0 degrees at the same level of the esophagus. This angle is displayed on the monitor. A mechanism also exists for locking the transducer head into a desired position. It is important that the probe not be manipulated while the head is locked to prevent damaging the esophagus. The TEE probe is detachable from the remainder of the machine so that it can be sterilized and stored separately. The American Society of Echocardiography and the Society of Cardiovascular Anesthesiologists have published a combined paper that offers guidelines

for performing a complete intraoperative TEE examination, and discusses the various echocardiographic views in greater detail. Due to variations in cardiac and thoracic anatomy, the exact angle and esophageal depth at which the standard views are acquired will differ. Adequate windows can almost always be obtained by using the aforementioned techniques to situate the TEE probe and transducer into a satisfactory position.

The computer workstation contains the monitor and a panel with various controls for image optimization, acquisition, and storage (Figure 11–15). A *keyboard* is usually present for entering patient information and annotating particular images, such as those that are "postcardiopulmonary bypass (CPB)." A *roller ball* controls among other things, an onscreen cursor, the location of the color flow Doppler box, and the direction of the CWD and PWD signals. *Caliper* and *trace* functions are available for tasks as measurement of the ascending aorta and outlining of blood flow velocity profiles through the valves of the heart (Figure 11–16). *Clip store*, *image store*, and *review* buttons allow recording of the images for viewing and reading at a later time. Images and clips can also be "*frozen*" for measurements and scrolled through for a frame-by-frame assessment.

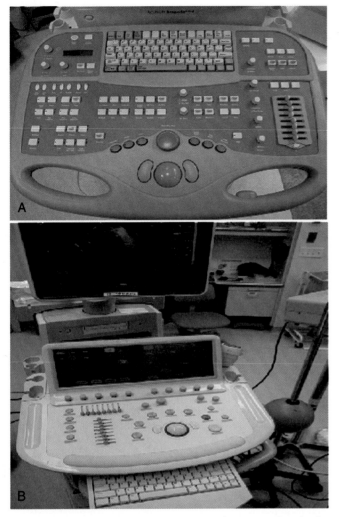

Figure 11–15   A, Workstation for Siemens machine. **B,** Workstation for Philips machine.

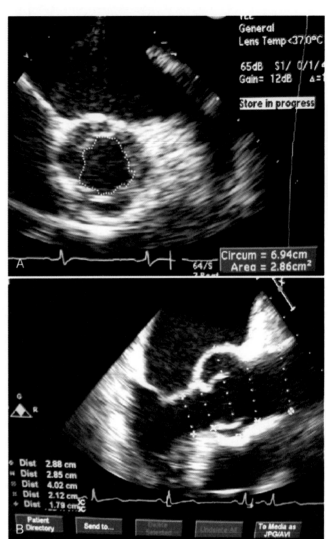

Figure 11–16   A, Calipers for trace function. **B,** Calipers for measure function.

The transducer at the head of the TEE probe transmits and receives ultrasonic waves (Figure 11–17). Although it fulfills both functions, the overwhelming majority of the time is spent receiving. It is composed of several complementary structures designed to generate optimum images of cardiovascular anatomy. The centerpiece of the transducer is a *piezoelectric crystal* that is composed of tightly packed polarized molecules. Piezoelectricity refers to the ability of some materials to generate an electric potential in response to an applied force, and vice versa. The force in TEE is sound waves. A pair of *electrodes* is placed adjacent to the crystal. When they generate an electrical current, the positive and negative charges within the molecules of the crystal align themselves in accordance with the electric field. This movement creates vibrations and the formation of ultrasound. When the sound waves reflected from the heart strike the crystal, the force induces tiny movements in the individual dipoles. This movement creates an electrical signal that is sensed by the electrodes. Thus the crystal converts electrical energy into acoustic energy during transmission and acoustic energy into electrical energy upon reception. These piezoelectric crystals are arranged in arrays (linear, annular, or convex). The rate of firing of these crystals can happen all together at once as in the switched array probes or be programmed with time delays as in the modern phased array probes. The duration of the vibration is limited by the addition of *damping material*. It is important that the vibration be brief because shorter pulse lengths improve the longitudinal resolution of the image. An *acoustic lens* helps to focus the ultrasound beam. A *faceplate* or *impedance matching layer* lies in between the crystal and the esophagus. This structure is designed to have impedance similar to the esophagus to limit the amount of ultrasound that is initially reflected back by the esophagus. A plastic or metal coating surrounds the elements of the transducer.

The accuracy with which a transducer is able to image is called resolution. Spatial resolution refers to the distance two objects have to be separated to identify them as two separate objects. Longitudinal resolution or axial resolution is the ability of the system to identify two objects as separate parallel to the direction of the ultrasound beam whereas lateral resolution is the ability of the system to identify two objects as separate perpendicular to the direction of the ultrasound beam. This translates to the fact that the higher the frequency of the transducer, the greater the resolution.

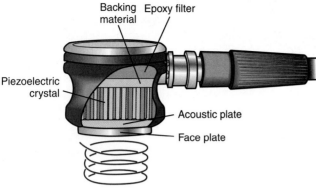

Figure 11–17 Transducer design.

However, the downside to this is the depth of penetration of the ultrasound beam is compromised. Temporal resolution refers to resolution in relation to time. This translates to the ability of the ultrasound system to accurately locate structures in transit at a given time. This is determined largely by the number of frames per second (frame rate) of the ultrasound beam.

Preprocessing Functions

Preprocessing refers to signal modification before it is displayed on the monitor. Filtering of noise from returning echoes is the first step in this process. The process of demodulation converts the echo voltages to video format displaying only the positive components. The process of differentiating accentuates the leading edge. Dynamic range manipulation allows excessively strong and excessively weak signals to be excluded, thereby keeping only the signals within the preferred dynamic range of the system. Hence image quality is much improved. The compression function reduces the dynamic range, further producing a higher contrast image.

Postprocessing Functions

Once the image has been stored into memory, the signals can be processed to provide better quality images. B color improves contrast by distinguishing subtle differences in echo density between adjacent tissues. Read zoom is yet another postprocessing function that is available.

Image Optimization

The quality of the images obtained depends on setting the machine functions appropriately. The depth should be adjusted to include the entire structure of interest and centered on the screen. The gain and the compressions should be set so that the blood appears black and distinct from the shades of gray of the surrounding tissue. The time gain controls (TGC) should be set so that there is uniform brightness in the near and the far fields. Some machines also allow setting the transducer frequency based on the depth of the image to be interrogated. The higher the frequency, the better it is to image nearer structures.

Artifacts

The ability to recognize the *artifacts* encountered during TEE is an essential skill to be developed as misinterpretations can lead to incorrect diagnoses and clinical decision making.[13-16] Problems attributed to artifacts can be minimized by ensuring proper machine control settings and by understanding the aforementioned principles of ultrasound physics. The apparent appearance of a Swan-Ganz catheter in the aorta and the "wrap around" effect seen with PWD are two previously mentioned examples. Another common artifact in the operating room is due to the interference caused by electrocautery (Figure 11–18). The screen becomes filled with multiple dots and speckles, which makes viewing of both 2-D and color flow images quite difficult. Therefore, it is helpful to acquire the most important echocardiographic information before incision if possible. The presence of synthetic (especially mechanical) or heavily calcified heart valves creates artifacts because of *acoustic shadowing*. Their acoustic impedance is dramatically different from surrounding tissues, and the vast majority of ultrasound waves are reflected back to the transducer before being able to reach more distal tissues. These areas simply appear dark. *Reverberation* artifacts may lead to the apparent "doubling" of certain objects. In these cases, returning echoes are reflected off of the transducer and the structure a second time before being displayed onto the monitor. The artifact resembles the true structure, but is twice the distance from the transducer (Figure 11–18). This is frequently seen during imaging of the descending thoracic aorta, and one must be careful not to interpret the duplicated aorta as an intimal tear or dissection. Strong differences in density at the lung-tissue interface, or severe aortic atherosclerosis, are often to blame. *Side lobe* artifacts result in the placement of objects outside the path of the main ultrasound beam within the image displayed that is on the monitor. They are due to the computer misplacing returning echoes from outlying ultrasound waves alongside those that have come from the main beam. This occurs most often with strong reflectors, such as a pulmonary artery catheter. Several other pieces of normal anatomy are frequent sources of confusion for novice echocardiographers. These include *Lambl excrescences, moderator band, Coumadin ridge,* and *eustachian valve.* Lambl excrescences are thin, stringlike cords that project from the aortic valve leaflets and can mimic vegetations. The moderator band is a muscular cord that traverses from the ventricular septum to the right ventricular free wall. The Coumadin ridge, aptly named for imitating a left atrial clot or thrombus, lies between the left atrial appendage and left upper pulmonary vein. The eustachian valve is an embryological remnant seen in the distal inferior vena cava in the bicaval view. Physicians should familiarize themselves with the appearance of these to correctly identify them in the intraoperative setting.

Maintenance of Equipment

Although the initial cost of purchasing equipment is significant, maintenance of the TEE equipment is also just as important. The TEE probe is at significant risk of damage due to the significant number of personnel that handle the equipment. There is also a space constraint in the operating room that leads to increased susceptibility to damage. Ideally all probes

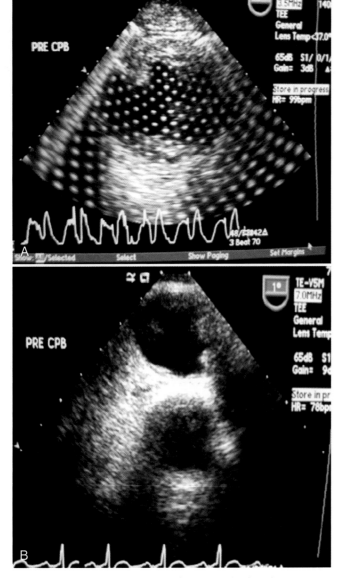

Figure 11–18   **A,** Cautery artifact. **B,** Double barrel aorta.

cavitation. The thermal effects are due to an increase in temperature because of absorption and scattering of ultrasound beams by the tissue. This is more of an issue with the live 3-D probes. Hence the 3-D probes have thermistors at their tip that automatically shut off the transmitting power once the probe tip has reached a certain temperature. The recommended spatial peak and temporal average intensity (SPTA) are 100 milliwatts/cm^2 for unfocused beams and 1 watt/m^2 for focused beams. The effects of cavitation are related to the interaction of the ultrasound beam with the microscopic gas bubbles, which causes them to contract and expand leading to bubble rupture and release of energy.

Cleaning and Disinfection

It is not uncommon to transmit organisms from one patient to another due to contaminated TEE probes. Hence meticulous attention should be paid to proper disinfection of TEE probes. Although no standardized protocol exists, most clinicians that perform TEE use the guidelines published by the gastroenterologists to disinfect endoscopes.[17,18] There should be a dedicated space outside the operating rooms for disinfecting the TEE probes. Glutaraldehyde-based solutions are used to disinfect the probes. Personnel involved in this process should be given a thorough in-service and be provided with protective gear, including eyewear and heavy duty gloves. All probes should be precleaned to remove blood and other particulate matter. Soap and water or isopropyl alcohol could be used for this purpose. Once the probe is precleaned, it should be placed immediately in glutaraldehyde-based solutions approved by the FDA. It is important to remember to immerse the probe only up to the last depth mark on the TEE probe as total immersion can lead to damage to the probe. At least 20 minutes of immersion in glutaraldehyde should be followed by 30 minutes of rinse in water to get rid of any residual glutaraldehyde solution. Use of autoclaving, dry heat sterilization, ultraviolet sterilization, and gas sterilization is not recommended. Iodine-based solutions should also be avoided. The work station should also be wiped down with isopropyl alcohol between cases. At the end of the day, the machine should be shut down properly and a cover inserted over it.

Antibiotic endocarditis prophylaxis is not recommended by the American Heart Association for TEE in the perioperative setting since the incidence of bacteremia associated with upper gastrointestinal endoscopy is very low.

Conclusion

TEE is increasingly becoming a well sought after diagnostic and monitoring tool, not only in the cardiac operating rooms but also in the noncardiac surgical setting. Understanding the basic functioning of this technology allows its safe and efficient use in the operating room. With the new certification process that is being developed by the American Society of Anesthesiologists and the National Board of Echocardiography for noncardiac anesthesiologists, we will see a significant rise in the use of this modality of monitoring. The equipment is also becoming increasingly portable and less expensive, making its use even more attractive. Digitally acquired data can be stored

should be housed in protective cases until ready for use. Consideration should be given to the use of wall-mounted TEE probe holders in the operating room. This will minimize tension on the cable connections and hence cause less damage to the probe. Probe damage can lead to transducer malfunction and pose an infection risk to patients if there are cracks in the transducer. There is also the potential for electrical safety to be compromised in the setting of a damaged TEE probe. Hence periodic maintenance checks are vital for safe use of this technology.

Ultrasound Safety

Safe use of the ultrasound technology warrants an understanding of the contraindications to TEE and knowledge of the bioeffects of the ultrasound. Bioeffects of ultrasound includes thermal and mechanical damage and the effects of effortlessly in fast access storage media for immediate retrieval and for long-term storage of older studies.[19] Recent advances in computer technology have enabled echocardiographic data to be connected to hospital information systems for purposes of billing as well. Most echocardiography laboratories have gone digital and the huge advantage with this system is the remote access capability. However, the increasing use of intraoperative TEE by anesthesiologists does not seem to be related to the availability of reimbursement from Medicare.[20] Availability of TEE has certainly revolutionized decision making in the cardiac operating room and changed the role of the anesthesiologist in the operating room.[21]

References

1. Perrino, A.C., Reeves, S.T. (Eds.), 2007. A practical approach to transesophageal echocardiography, Lippincott Williams & Wilkins, Philadelphia.
2. Otto, C., 2004. Textbook of clinical echocardiography, ed 3. Saunders, Philadelphia.
3. Savage, R.M., Solomon, A. (Eds.), 2005. Comprehensive textbook of intraoperative transesophageal echocardiography, Lippincott Williams & Wilkins, Philadelphia.
4. Matthew, J., Ayoub, C. (Eds.), 2005. Clinical manual and review of transesophageal echocardiography, McGraw-Hill, New York.
5. Suriani, R.J., Neustein, S., Shore-Lesserson, L., et al., 1998. Intraoperative transesophageal echocardiography during noncardiac surgery. J Cardiothorac Vasc Anesth 12 (3), 274–280.
6. Denault, A.Y., Couture, P., McKenty, S., et al., 2002. Perioperative use of transesophageal echocardiography by anesthesiologists: impact in noncardiac surgery and in the intensive care unit. Can J Anaesth 49 (3), 287–293.
7. Edelman, S., 2005. Ultrasound physics and instrumentation. ESP.
8. Quinones, M.A., Otto, C.M., Stoddard, M., et al., 2002. Recommendations for quantification of Doppler echocardiography: a report from the Doppler quantification task force of the nomenclature and standards committee of the American Society of Echocardiography. J Am Soc Echocardiogr 15 (2), 167–184.
9. Skubas, N.J., 2009. Two-dimensional, non-Doppler strain imaging during anesthesia and cardiac surgery. Echocardiography 26 (3), 345–353.
10. Garcia-Orta, R., Moreno, E., Vidal, M., et al., 2007. Three-dimensional versus two-dimensional transesophageal echocardiography in mitral valve repair. J Am Soc Echocardiogr 20 (1), 4–12.
11. Sugeng, L., Shernan, S.K., Salgo, I.S., et al., 2008. Live 3-dimensional transesophageal echocardiography initial experience using the fully-sampled matrix array probe. J Am Coll Cardiol 52 (6), 446–449.
12. Shanewise, J.S., Cheung, A.T., Aronson, S., et al., 1999. ASE/SCA guidelines for performing a comprehensive intraoperative multiplane transesophageal echocardiographic examination: recommendations of the American Society of Echocardiography council for intraoperative echocardiography and the Society of Cardiovascular Anesthesiologists task force for certification in perioperative transesophageal echocardiography. Anesth Analg 89, 870–884.
13. Piercy, M., McNicol, L., Dinh, D.T., et al., 2009. Major complications related to the use of transesophageal echocardiography in cardiac surgery. J Cardiothorac Vasc Anesth 23 (1), 62–65.
14. Cote, G., Denault, A., 2008. Transesophageal echocardiography-related complications. Can J Anaesth 55 (9), 622–647.
15. Vignon, P., Lang, R.M., 1999. Use of transesophageal echocardiography for the assessment of traumatic aortic injuries. Echocardiography 16 (2), 207–219.
16. Vignon, P., Spencer, K.T., Rambaud, G., et al., 2001. Differential transesophageal echocardiographic diagnosis between linear artifacts and intraluminal flap of aortic dissection or disruption. Chest 119 (6), 1778–1790.
17. Mentec, H., Vignon, P., Terre, S., et al., 1995. Frequency of bacteremia associated with transesophageal echocardiography in intensive care unit patients: a prospective study of 139 patients. Crit Care Med 23 (7), 1194–1199.
18. Banerjee, S., Shen, B., Nelson, D.B., et al., 2008. Infection control during GI endoscopy. Gastrointest Endosc 67 (6), 781–790.
19. Lambert, A.S., Miller, J.P., Foster, E., et al., 1999. The diagnostic validity of digitally captured intraoperative transesophageal echocardiography examinations compared with analog recordings: a pilot study. J Am Soc Echocardiogr 12 (11), 974–980.
20. Morewood, G.H., Gallagher, M.E., Gaughan, J.P., 2002. Does the reimbursement of anesthesiologists for intraoperative transesophageal echocardiography promote increased utilization? J Cardiothorac Vasc Anesth 16 (3), 300–303.
21. Kneeshaw, J.D., 2006. Transesophageal echocardiography (TOE) in the operating room. Br J Anaesth 97 (1), 77–84.

Further Reading

1. Armstrong, W.F., Ryan, T., 2009. Feigenbaum's echocardiography, ed 7. Lippincott Williams & Wilkins, Philadelphia. *Provides a more in-depth understanding of echocardiography for the interested reader.*
2. Denault, A.Y., Couture, P., McKenty, S., et al., 2002. Perioperative use of transesophageal echocardiography by anesthesiologists: impact in noncardiac surgery and in the intensive care unit. Can J Anaesth 49 (3), 287–293. *Excellent article discussing the role of TEE in the noncardiac surgery and intensive care setting.*
3. Mahmood, F., Christie, A., Matyal, R., 2008. Transesophageal echocardiography and noncardiac surgery. Semin Cardiothorac Vasc Anesth 12 (4), 265–289. *A comprehensive review of the role of TEE in noncardiac surgery.*

Chapter 12

Depth of Anesthesia Monitors: Principles and Applications

Roy Esaki and George Mashour

Why Monitor Depth of Anesthesia?

The problem of awareness during general anesthesia has become an increasingly prominent issue for both the anesthesiology community and the lay public. The Joint Commission issued a Sentinel Alert regarding awareness in 2004,[1] and the American Society of Anesthesiologists (ASA) subsequently established a Task Force on Intraoperative Awareness that published a practice advisory regarding the use of brain function monitoring.[2] This attention reflects the clinical significance of awareness because patients distressed by the recall of intraoperative events may develop severe psychological sequelae, including PTSD.[3,4]

To address this problem, various devices have been developed to help assess the depth of anesthesia. It is worth noting that estimates of the incidence of awareness have ranged from 0.0068% in a study by Pollard et al[5] to 1.0% in a study

by Errando et al,[6] making the identification of patients at risk for awareness and the reduction of this rare event a challenging task. There is a possibility that depth of anesthesia (DoA) monitors may also help anesthesia providers titrate medications, and help prevent oversedation, which may result in decreased morbidity and mortality.[7] Regardless of the motivation for monitoring brain function, the anesthesia provider should consider the evidence regarding the clinical utility of the device with respect to the outcome of interest.

Currently Available Depth of Anesthesia Monitors

This chapter will discuss the following devices:
- Bispectral index monitors (Aspect Medical Systems)
- S/5 Entropy module (GE Healthcare)
- Narcotrend monitor (MonitorTechnik)

- Cerebral state monitor (Danmeter)
- SEDLine/patient state analyzer (Hospira)
- SNAP II monitor (Stryker)
- AEP Monitor/2 (Danmeter)

We will focus on these monitors because they represent the main devices that are currently used and researched and were the devices mentioned in the ASA Practice Advisory for Intraoperative Awareness and Brain Function Monitoring.[2] Bowdle,[8] Bruhn,[9] and Jameson and Sloan[10] have written reviews outlining the basic principles behind EEG monitoring and discuss the devices as they existed in 2006.

The Ideal Monitor

The ideal DoA monitor would (1) detect whether the patient is too lightly anesthetized and is at risk of awareness; (2) detect whether the patient is unnecessarily deeply anesthetized, and thus at risk for prolonged recovery; (3) work similarly across different patients; and (4) work similarly regardless of anesthetic modality and medications.[1] Bruhn[9] discusses the principles of validity and reliability of DoA monitors. The first two criteria relate to the concept of validity, which is the "accuracy" of the monitor in correctly determining the anesthetic depth. The latter two criteria relate to the concept of reliability, or "consistency" of the monitor in reporting the same result for a given depth of anesthesia.

The clinical utility of the device depends on how well it meets these criteria. By being accurate and consistent, a device should theoretically be able to demonstrate improvements in certain clinical end points, such as decreased awareness events or recovery times.

Assessment and Comparison of Awareness Monitors

This chapter will demonstrate the underlying computational approach of key monitors and examine the available evidence regarding the clinical utility of the devices. The intention is not to compare technologies with each other to determine the "best" equipment to use. Algorithms and technologies are continually updated, and there is much heterogeneity in studies in terms of patient populations and clinical end points. Generalizations made across various studies are thus often misleading, if not invalid. Sources purporting to provide product comparisons should be examined judiciously for both accuracy and bias. For example, an online "distributive evidence database" (*brainmonitor.doctorevidence.com*) offers to objectively synthesize and compare the outcome-oriented evidence for DoA monitors, but is funded by Aspect Medical Systems.

To discuss the merits of each DoA monitor, it is useful to have an easily communicated metric to describe the accuracy and reliability of the device. Sensitivity/specificity analyses or the comparison of likelihood ratios are two possible approaches. An alternate approach, adopted by the ASA Practice Advisory for Intraoperative Awareness and Brain Function Monitoring along with the majority of publications on DoA monitors, is to compare prediction probabilities.

Smith et al[11] explains the concept of prediction probability (Pk) as applied to DoA monitors. Conceptually, Pk represents

a measure of how well an index value (such as the BIS index) provided by the device can differentiate between different clinical states (e.g., response vs. no response to command, or levels of a graded sedation scale).[2] If an index value were perfectly associated with the clinical state (i.e., a higher index value always represents a higher clinical level of arousal), the Pk value would be 1. If the index value were no better than chance in predicting a higher or lower clinical state, the Pk value would be 0.5.

The Pk is independent of scale, and does not make assumptions about the underlying distribution. It is thus commonly used for evaluating and comparing different monitors. The Pk essentially represents "criterion validity" (which is the agreement of the monitor with another instrument). However, the range of Pk values produced by various studies performed across different patients and anesthetic regimens are sometimes used as a measure of the *reliability* of the monitoring device.

Pk values are best used to compare devices in the same study. Comparisons between different studies may be confounded by differences in patient populations and anesthetic regimens. Pk values are also dependent on the clinical scale and assessment method used for comparison. For example, the Pk value for the prediction of loss of response to verbal command may be different from the Pk value for the prediction of loss of response to painful stimulus. The order of events is also important due to potential physiological hysteresis (i.e., loss of response during induction is not necessarily the reverse process of regaining response during emergence).

For purposes of evaluating a device's ability to detect and prevent impending awareness, it may be best to use Pk values that assess some measure of response to stimulus upon emergence. It is also very important to note that Pk depends on the coarseness of the scale.[12] A Pk value calculated using an "awake" versus "not awake" dichotomization would tend to have a higher value compared with a Pk calculated using multiple ordinal categories such as a 1 to 10 scale. This underscores the need to compare Pk values very cautiously.

In addition, Pks can be misleading if they are used as an indicator of the "believability" of a particular DoA monitor in predicting awareness in a given patient. Pks represent how well the monitor can predict a particular state across multiple patients; it does not offer direct information about the significance of a particular index value in a given patient. Index values must always be used as one piece of information that helps modify the individual pretest probability of awareness as determined by the clinician.

Basic Principles of EEG Analysis

In 1937, Gibbs et al[13] published a study on the relationship between electroencephalography (EEG) patterns and drug-induced changes in neuronal activity. The authors presciently recognized the potential application of EEG technology as a monitoring device, commenting:

"a practical application … might be the use of the electroencephalogram as a measure of the depth of anesthesia during surgical operations. The anesthetist and surgeon could have before them on tape or screen a continuous record of the electrical activity of both heart and brain."

The regular adoption of EEG as a monitoring technology can be facilitated by the development of computerized EEG processing systems to analyze complex waveform patterns. Most current awareness monitors similarly collect EEG information with frontal electrodes, but they differ significantly in how these EEG signals are processed to yield an index value representing the depth of anesthesia. Processing techniques unique to certain devices will be discussed in the device-specific section of this chapter. Rampil[14] provides an excellent technical primer on the physiology of EEG physiology and monitoring, while Sigl and Chamoun[15] provide a very clear explanation of the basic mathematics behind EEG signal analysis.

EEG Activity and Anesthetic Depth

Synaptic activity of cells in the cortex results in voltage changes that can be detected by electrodes placed on the scalp. There are various waveform patterns within certain frequency ranges, which correspond to various neurophysiological processes. These patterns are grouped into frequency bands called, in order of increasing frequency, δ-, θ-, α-, β-, and γ-waves. Each band exhibits certain changes under the influence of anesthetic agents. A review by Jameson et al[10] provides a detailed description of these neurophysiological and EEG effects.

Delta waves (<3 Hz) have the slowest frequencies of the various frequency bands and are seen in deep sleep; they may result from extreme thalamic depression. Θ-waves (4 to 7 Hz) may similarly arise from the inhibition of thalamic pacemaker cells. Theta waves are readily seen in young children and become less prominent with age, although they are normally seen during sleep at any age. Δ- and θ-waves are often referred to as "slow waves." α-Waves (8 to 12 Hz) are prominently seen in awake patients and are prominent over the vertex in a relaxed or sedated state. They are thought to reflect the cyclical activity of thalamic pacemaker cells when anesthetics decrease the inhibition of the thalamus by the nucleus reticularis. The pyramidal area of alpha wave prominence tends to move to more frontal regions with increased depth of anesthesia in a process called "anteriorization" or "frontal predominance."

Beta waves (12 to 24 Hz) are present in the prefrontal regions, and presumably reflect thalamocortical pathways with higher frequencies than α-waves due to desynchronization of the thalamus by sensory stimuli. Beta waves are normally present during alert states and can increase during initial central nervous system depression due to disinhibitory effects. This "β-activation" can be seen in Figure 12–1. β activity is most prominent in the frontal regions and tends to move posteriorly with increased depth of anesthesia.

Gamma waves, also known as β₂-bands, are of a higher frequency range (25 to 50 Hz) and may play a role in sensory processing and perception. Recent evidence suggests that organized γ activity may be essential for consciousness and interrupted during anesthesia.[16] The EEG of an alert individual mostly consists of higher frequency α- and β-waves. With the addition of anesthetic agents, the overall amplitude of the EEG waveform initially increases as the EEG is synchronized in the 8 to 10 Hz range, and subsequently decreases with increased anesthetic depth.[10] Similarly, the predominant frequencies initially increase during the early stages of anesthesia, after which the EEG shifts to lower frequency θ- and δ-waves.[17]

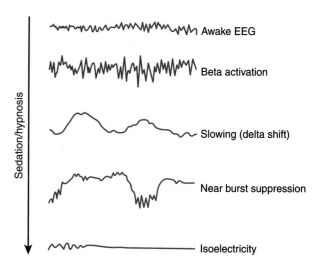

Figure 12–1   EEGs showing the progression of characteristic changes associated with increased anesthetic depth. *(Image from Tonner PH, Bein B. Classic electroencephalographic parameters: median frequency, spectral edge frequency etc. Best Pract Res Clin Anaesthesiol 2006;20:147-159.)*[18]

With sufficiently deep anesthetic states (often minimal alveolar concentration [MAC] values of 1.5 or higher[10]), the EEG demonstrates a bilateral pattern of slow and mixed waves. A pattern of high amplitude activity (bursts) upon a flat baseline (suppression) is called "burst suppression." A burst suppression ratio, comparing the percent duration of suppression, is often calculated. Burst suppression can also be seen with brain-injured conditions, such as postischemic states. Further deepening of the anesthetic state results in no discernable voltage changes (isoelectricity) (Figure 12–1).

Electromyography (EMG) Component of Surface Voltages

Electrodes placed on the forehead may pick up voltage changes resulting from frontal facial muscle activity. This electromyographic (EMG) component can have a significant influence on the EEG recordings and may be either treated as an artifact or as a useful signal, depending on the particular DoA monitor. The band from 35 to 127 Hz, which may reflect muscle activity, was found in one study to provide the best performance for detecting awareness,[19] but there is no clear agreement about the overall benefit of including EMG activity in EEG algorithms.

EEG Processing Techniques

The EEG can be analyzed in either the time domain or the frequency domain. Many of the improvements in DoA monitoring have resulted from the ability to process the EEG in the frequency domain. In the time domain, voltage changes in the EEG are plotted against time. Burst suppression is identified in the time domain. There are other time-domain techniques, such as the calculation of zero crossing frequency (ZXF), which is the number of times the EEG crosses the baseline, or a periodic analysis, which calculates the time between two consecutive minima of the waveform. Although these metrics are useful parameters in limited circumstances, complex signals cannot be fully analyzed by solely using time domain-based methods.[18]

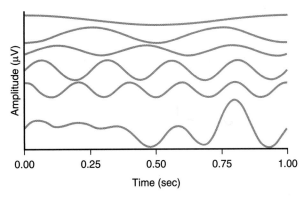

Figure 12–2 The five *upper* waveforms (with frequencies of 1, 2, 3, 4, and 5 Hz and amplitudes of 1, 1.5, 1, 2, and 1.5, respectively) combine to yield the waveform on the *bottom*. A Fourier transformation allows the combined waveform to be deconstructed into the five constituent sinusoids. *(Image from Sigl JC, Chamoun NG. An introduction to bispectral analysis for the electroencephalogram. J Clin Monit 1994;10:392-404.)*[15]

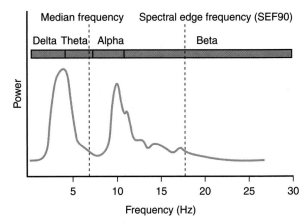

Figure 12–3 A schematic of the power spectrum. The horizontal axis represents the frequency of the component wave, and the vertical axis represents the power, or the degree to which the frequency is represented. Here, 90% of the power exists below the spectral edge frequency. *(From Tonner PH, Bein B. Classic electroencephalographic parameters: median frequency, spectral edge frequency etc. Best Pract Res Clin Anaesthesiol 2006;20:147-159.)*[18]

The advancement of microprocessing over the past few decades enabled fast calculations of Fourier transformations, which enable analysis of the frequency domain, wherein the frequencies of component signals present in the EEG are compared with the degree to which these frequencies are present. The general premise of EEG-based DoA monitors is that changes in EEG patterns can be detected, through time and frequency domain calculations, to provide an estimation of the level of consciousness.

Fourier Transformation and the Power Spectrum

Fourier analysis (also called spectral analysis) is based on the concept that complex waveforms can be approximated as a sum of sinusoids of various frequencies, amplitudes (power), and phase relationships, as shown in Figure 12–2. A discrete Fourier transformation (DFT) converts a sample of periodic brain waves from the "time domain" to the "frequency domain" and "phase domain." A fast Fourier transform (FFT) is an algorithm that very efficiently performs DFTs. Applied to an EEG, an FFT takes as an input the raw EEG waveform measured over time, and outputs the frequencies and phase of the component waves of the raw waveform. (A loose analogy for the FFT would be a prism separating out white light into individual colors of various wavelengths.)

The information about the frequency domain is often presented as a graph of power (the magnitude of the frequency contribution) versus frequency. The resulting "power spectrum" thus provides a measure of the extent to which various frequencies (corresponding to α-, β-, γ-waves, etc.) are present in the EEG.

Median Frequency and Spectral Edge Frequency

Early frequency-based analysis included simple parameters such as the peak frequency, the median frequency, or the spectral edge frequency.[18] The peak frequency is often the frequency with the greatest power in a given wave region. The median frequency is the frequency that divides the power in half, and the spectral edge frequency is calculated as the frequency below which the majority (often, 90% or 95%) of the power lies (Figure 12–3).

Nonlinearity and Phase Coupling

The cerebral cortex can be thought of as a system in which sinusoidal inputs (from neuronal triggers such as thalamic pacemakers) are entered into a "system" which outputs a certain EEG signal. Examination of the power spectrum alone provides information about the power and frequency, but not the phase relationships of the inputs. In a "linear" system, the output represents simple addition of each input, and the phase (time offset of the sinusoid) of the input does not matter.[3] The neuronal system is complex, however, and should be thought of as a non linear system. As consequence of non linearity, the phase of the output signal depends on the phases of the input signals. The phases are then considered to be "phase coupled."

As the degree of phase-coupling of various EEG frequency components is thought to reflect complex neurophysiological changes associated with various levels of consciousness, DoA monitors can use this phase coupling information to help predict the depth of anesthesia.

BIS Technology (Aspect Medical Systems)

Bispectral (BIS) technology is based upon an empirically determined proprietary algorithm developed by Aspect Medical Systems; it was approved by the U.S. Food and Drug Administration in 1996. It converts the recordings from a frontal EEG to a single number, the BIS index, which ranges from 0 (isoelectric) to 100 (awake) and represents the level of consciousness by the patient. The BIS system is the most widely used DoA monitor in the United States. According to information provided on the manufacturer's website as of

June, 2009, the BIS platform is installed in 75% of U.S. operating rooms, and 19% of procedures requiring general anesthesia or deep sedation use the BIS monitor. As such, most of the research pertaining to DoA monitors has been done on the BIS. In 2006, a PubMed search for the phrase "bispectral index" yielded 852 citations[8]; at the time of writing, the same search parameters revealed 1543 citations.

Following the earlier A-2000 and BIS VIEW monitoring platforms, the latest implementation of the BIS technology is the BIS VISTA system, which provides an option for bilateral monitoring. The BIS technology is available as a stand-alone system or can be incorporated into "BIS modules" for use with monitoring systems of external manufacturers (Figure 12–4).

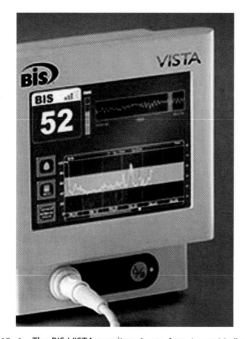

Figure 12–4   The BIS VISTA monitor. *(Image from Aspect Medical Systems. (website): http://www.aspectmedical.com/assets/Images/photos/right_column/bis-vista.jpg.) Accessed November 20, 2008.*

Underlying Principle: Bispectral Analysis

Bispectral analysis (also called two-dimensional spectral analysis) refers to the statistical process of quantifying quadratic nonlinearities of the system. The bispectrum, or bispectral value, represents the degree of phase coupling of two fundamental frequencies and a modulation frequency represented by the sum of the two frequencies (Figure 12–5). A related parameter is the bicoherence, which is obtained by normalizing the bispectrum to a 0% to 100% range, to reflect the effect of relative amplitudes of the component signals. Part of the BIS algorithm calculates the logarithm of the ratio of the sum of bispectrum peaks in the range from 0.5 to 47 Hz to the sum of the peaks from 40 to 47 Hz. This value, known as the "SyncFastSlow," is one of the many parameters used to calculate the BIS index. A full explanation of the calculation of the bispectral value is beyond the scope of this chapter, but can be found in the primer by Sigl and Chamoun.[15]

The overall premise behind bispectral analysis is that changes in the clinical state are represented by changes in phase coupling. The neurophysiological significance of a large bispectral value being generated by two particular frequencies is not clear, but may represent the degree of shared EEG pacemaker elements.[14]

What It Measures

Single Zipprep electrodes were initially developed for use with the BIS monitor, but the more recent versions have up to four single-use proprietary electrodes (BIS-XP Quatro) embedded in a single sensor. More recently, the BIS Vista bilateral monitoring system features four-channel EEG monitoring with two channels of information obtained from either side of the forehead to allow for hemispheric comparisons.

Of note, one study in 2002 found that BIS values obtained using generic ECG electrodes (costing 10 cents each) and proprietary BIS electrodes (costing $10 to $20) had acceptable limits of agreement.[20] A study in 2007 similarly found no statistical difference in the signal quality index obtained from ECG electrodes compared with an unspecified version of BIS electrodes.[21] Cost-effectiveness analysis regarding the newest iterations of the BIS electrodes is not currently available.

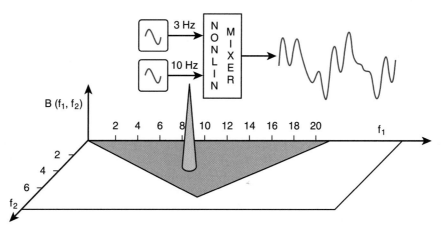

Figure 12–5   The linear combination of two frequencies (f_1 = 10 Hz, f_2 = 3 Hz) results in a new waveform that contains the sum of the original waves. Bispectral analysis of these waveform results in a peak bispectral value, B (f_1, f_2), which reflects the phase-locked constituent frequencies. *(Image from Rampil IJ. A primer for EEG signal processing in anesthesia. Anesthesiology 1998;89:980-1002.)[14]*

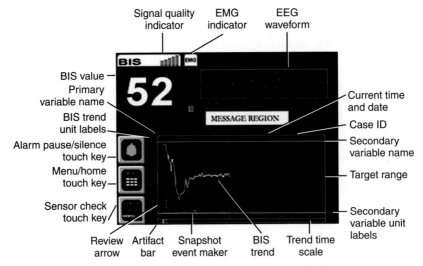

Figure 12–6 The BIS VISTA display shows the BIS index value and trend and the raw EEG waveform and EMG indicator. *(Image from Aspect Medical Systems. BIS VISTA Monitoring System Operating Manual, website: http://www.aspectmedical.com/ Files/file/Doc/BISVISTAmanual.pdf.) Accessed July 21, 2010.*

What It Outputs

To be useful for the clinician, the information resulting from the bispectral analysis is converted into an easily interpretable and clinically meaningful value.

For the BIS monitor, this value is the "BIS index," which is calculated using a proprietary algorithm. The formula was empirically developed by correlating clinically assessed depths of anesthesia with features of the EEG including information from the frequency domain (i.e., power spectrum, bispectrum, and bicoherence) and the time domain (burst-suppression analysis).

The BIS VISTA display shows the BIS index value and trend and the raw EEG waveform and EMG indicator (Figure 12–6).

The BIS bilateral system provides the option of a density spectral array (DSA) to be displayed (Figure 12–7). This displays the trend of the power spectrum from each hemisphere simultaneously.

Clinical Utility

Although one study suggested that bispectral analysis does not give any additional information beyond information provided by the power spectrum,[22] it is nonetheless worth examining the large body of literature regarding the clinical utility of the device. Of note, of the devices mentioned in this chapter, only the BIS monitor has been subjected to large-scale randomized clinical trials to assess whether usage of the monitor decreases the incidence of awareness. Despite the many studies to date, much remains controversial with respect to the clinical benefits of BIS monitors.

It is important to bear in mind that the BIS algorithm was empirically developed by the analysis of EEG effects of commonly used anesthetics such as propofol, midazolam, and isoflurane. The BIS index thus does not necessarily accurately represent the effects of all drugs. For example, the BIS Index has been shown to be unchanged upon administration of nitrous oxide,[23] while ketamine has been shown to increase the BIS value.[24] Although the traditional belief was that BIS indices do not accurately reflect xenon,[25] a recent study using

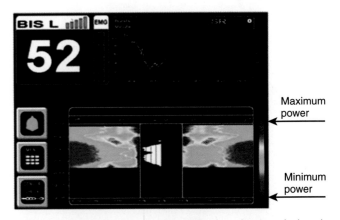

Figure 12–7 The density spectral array (DSA) can be viewed when the BIS bilateral system is used. The frequency scale with a range of 0-30 Hz is on the *horizontal axis*, with the *vertical axis* representing the time progression. The area to the midline with respect to the white spectral edge line contains 95% of the power. *(Image from Aspect Medical Systems. BIS VISTA Monitoring System Bilateral Monitoring Addendum, website: http://asrs. aspectms.com/Manuals/Vista/070-1024%20VISTA%20Op%20Man%20Bilat%20 Add.pdf.) Accessed July 21, 2011.*

single-agent xenon anesthesia demonstrated that while the BIS index showed a delay to detect loss of response during induction, the BIS monitor was able to distinguish between consciousness and unconsciousness during steady state anesthesia.[26]

Also, the BIS index may have lower values in patients with neurological conditions, such as cerebral ischemia,[27] dementia,[28] and severe hypoglycemia.[29] The probability of explicit recall decreases below a BIS index of 70 and becomes extremely small below 60.[8] Persistent BIS indices above 60 thus conservatively indicate that the patient may be at risk for intraoperative awareness, while levels below 40 may indicate unnecessarily excessive anesthetic administration. Although the generally accepted target range is 40 to 60, a recent study suggested that in opioid-heavy anesthetic cases, targeting a BIS value less than 60 may "result in an unnecessarily deep anesthetic state."[30]

Awareness-Related Outcomes

Given the low incidence of awareness, studies examining the impact of BIS monitoring on awareness reduction require large sample sizes. In 2004, Ekman et al[31] performed a prospective cohort study of 4945 surgical patients who were monitored with the BIS, using a protocol to keep the BIS index between 40 and 60. Using a historic control, the study found a statistically significant reduction in awareness (0.04% in the BIS group compared with 0.18% in the control group).

In the same year, Myles et al[32] conducted the "B-Aware" study, randomizing 2643 patients at high risk of awareness to either routine care or BIS-guided anesthesia. Two of the 1225 patients assigned to the BIS-guided anesthesia group and 11 patients of the routine care group reported awareness, resulting in a statistically significant reduction in the relative risk of awareness by 82% and a number needed to treat (NNT) of 138 patients. The study did not show any significant difference in death rate, satisfaction, or postoperative complications.

In early 2008 a highly publicized study (the "B-Unaware" study) was published by Avidan et al.[33] Two thousand patients were randomly assigned to BIS-guided anesthesia (targeting a BIS value of 40 to 60), or to a protocol based on end-tidal anesthetic gas (ETAG), for which the target ETAG range was 0.7 to 1.3 MAC. Two cases of definite awareness were found in each group (with 967 patients and 974 patients in the BIS and ETAG groups, respectively), for an absolute difference of 0% (95% CI −0.56% to 0.57%).

There has been considerable controversy over the conflicting conclusions given by the B-Aware and the B-Unaware study. In a letter to the editor, representatives of Aspect have criticized the B-Unaware for an inadequate sample size calculation.[34] However, appropriate interpretation of confidence intervals may be more meaningful than posthoc criticisms of power analysis. Regardless of the statistical power of the study, the results show that within the 95% confidence interval, the "best case" scenario in favor of the BIS is a −0.56% difference in the rate of awareness. Another criticism is that the choice of the ETAG-based alert system as a standard of comparison does not reflect a routine "standard of care" in most practices. The conclusion drawn from the study by the B-Unaware trial should be that the BIS monitor does not appear to provide an additional benefit over ETAG monitoring.

Summarizing the available evidence, a 2007 Cochrane review[35] examined 20 studies with 2056 participants, and concluded that BIS-guided anesthesia significantly reduced the incidence of intraoperative recall awareness in surgical patients with high risk of awareness (OR 0.20, 95% CI 0.05 to 0.79). In contrast, the 2006 ASA Practice advisory cautioned that despite the results of the B-Aware trial, "there is insufficient evidence to justify a standard, guideline, or absolute requirement that (depth of anesthesia) devices be used to reduce the occurrence of intraoperative awareness in high-risk patients undergoing general anesthesia."[2]

The aforementioned studies have focused on BIS usage in a population at high risk for awareness, and there is no current evidence regarding whether or not BIS monitoring helps reduce the incidence of awareness in routine cases.

Secondary Outcomes

Monk[36] provides a review of the evidence for improved patient outcomes with BIS usage and concludes that EEG monitoring appears to provide a "modest reduction in intraoperative primary anesthetic agent dosing of approximately 20% to 25%," which was linked to other benefits such as a reduction in early recovery time, postoperative nausea and vomiting, and possibly long-term outcomes following major surgery. Similarly, the 2007 Cochrane review[35] found that the use of BIS statistically significantly reduced propofol requirements by 1.30 mg/kg/hr and volatile anesthetic use by 0.17 MAC. BIS also reduced the recovery times, including time for eye opening, response to verbal command, time to extubation, and orientation by 2 to 3 minutes. The duration of postanesthesia care unit stay decreased by 6.8 minutes but time to home readiness remained the same. The review concluded that "anesthesia guided by BIS within the recommended range (40 to 60) could improve anesthetic delivery and postoperative recovery from relatively deep anesthesia." However, the ASA Task Force on Intraoperative Awareness suggested that "brain function monitoring is not routinely indicated for patients undergoing general anesthesia, either to reduce the frequency of intraoperative awareness or to monitor depth of anesthesia."[2]

In addition, a study by Monk et al[7] found that prolonged deep anesthesia (defined as the time during which the BIS value was less than 45) was a significant independent risk factor for 1-year postoperative mortality. However, a recent follow-up study by Lindholm et al[37] found that the relationship between either 1- or 2-year mortality and the time of deep anesthesia was not significant when preexisting malignancy was included as a covariate. Further work is required on the relationship of anesthetic depth, malignancy, and mortality.

S/5 Entropy Module (GE Healthcare)

The S/5 Entropy module (M-Entropy) was originally developed by Datex-Ohmeda; the technology is now owned by GE Healthcare. The module takes the raw EEG and frontal EMG signals and applies an algorithm that quantifies the irregularity of the signal to provide a measure of depth of consciousness. Bein[38] provides a good overview of the principles behind the Entropy module.

Underlying Principle: Entropy

Entropy, in general, is a measure of disorder. In 1948, Shannon[39] developed the concept of information entropy for use with signal processing and analysis. This concept is also called the "Shannon Entropy" or "Spectral Entropy," and reflects the irregularity, or predictability, of frequencies present in a signal. Given that the EEG is composed of a range of various frequencies as revealed by the power spectrum, information entropy of an EEG can be calculated to reflect the degree of frequency variability. The Entropy module calculates an "entropy number," which ranges from 0 (minimum entropy, such an isoelectric EEG) to 1 (maximum entropy, or white noise). A deeper level of anesthesia, which causes burst suppression and highly regular patterns, would result in a lower entropy number. The algorithm as implemented in the original Datex-Ohmeda S/5 Entropy module from 2004 is described by Viertiö-Oja et al.[40]

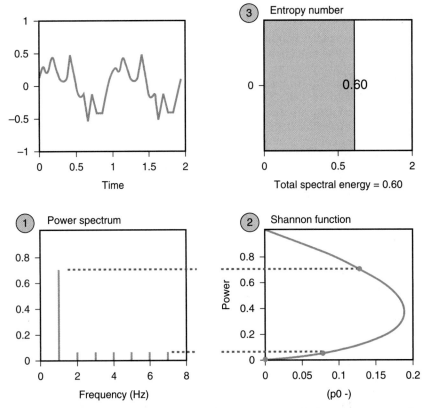

Figure 12–8 White noise is superimposed upon a sine wave (Top Left). After normalization, the frequency spectrum shows high power corresponding to the frequency of the original sine wave, with small amounts of power resulting from the noise (Bottom Left). The Shannon function yields values representing the power from the sine wave (.12) and the noise frequencies (6 × 0.08) (Bottom Right), which together provide the total entropy (0.12 + 6 × 0.08 = 0.60) (Top Right). *(Image from GE Healthcare. Entropy algorithm. (website): http://www.gehealthcare.com/usen/patient_mon_sys/mon_systems/products/s5_pat_mon/products/mentropyalgorithm.html.) Accessed October 19, 2008*

The Entropy number is calculated as follows:
1. The power spectrum P(F) is adjusted to produce a normalized power spectrum, Q(F), that is equal to 1.
2. The Shannon function f(x) = x log (1/x) is applied to the normalized power spectrum, Q(f), to yield a function, H(f), representing the transformed components.
3. The summed transformed components are normalized to yield an "entropy number" E that ranges from 0 (indicating complete regularity, like a sine wave) to 1 (indicating complete irregularity, like white noise.) Figure 12–8 demonstrates this process for a sample sinusoid with superimposed noise.

The Entropy monitor calculates two different entropy numbers: State Entropy (SE), calculated over the 0.8 Hz to 32 Hz band to reflect cortical processes, and Response Entropy (RE), calculated over the 0.8 Hz to 47 Hz range, which includes the high frontal EMG-dominated frequencies. The RE ranges from 0 to 100 (awake), while the SE ranges from 0 to 91 (awake). The target range for both values is 40 to 60. If the SE is above 60, the anesthetic dose should be increased. A rise in the RE of 5 to 10 points above the SE, despite an SE of less than 60, may be a sign of inadequate analgesia.[38] Of note, unlike the BIS monitor, the EMG is treated as a component signal, rather than as an artifact. Inouye et al[41] and Bruhn et al[42] provide good explanations of these entropy measures.

What It Measures

Like the BIS monitor, the M-entropy monitor uses proprietary, single-use, multielectrode sensors applied to one side of the forehead to collect EEG and frontal EMG signals.

What It Outputs

The S/5 Modular multiparameter anesthesia monitor screen can display the respective values and 5 or 30 minute trend of the RE, SE, and burst suppression ratio (Figure 12–9). The EEG waveform can be displayed, and trending is available up to 24 hours. During induction, there will be frontal EMG activity, resulting in a difference between the RE and SE; as RE and SE both decrease, the difference becomes minimal during maintenance. A quick rise in RE is caused by frontal EMG activity, which may be an early indication of possible arousal.

Clinical Utility

The central premise of the Entropy index is that EMG activity is not an EEG artifact, but instead a source of useful information for impending arousal that reflects a patient's attempt to respond to stimuli. To test this premise, one study[43] administered either remifentanil or esmolol in patients receiving propofol-nitrous oxide general anesthesia, holding the state

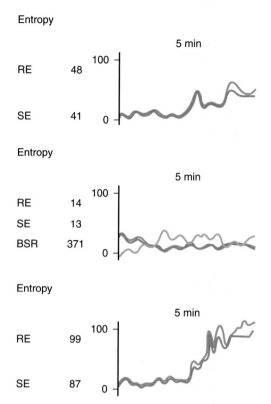

Figure 12–9   Display of entropy module, showing the value and trend for response entropy (RE), state entropy (SE), and burst suppression ratio (BSR). *(Image from GE Healthcare. M entropy module. (website): http://www.gehealthcare.com/usen/patient_mon_sys/mon_systems/products/s5_pat_mon/products/mentropymodule.html.) Accessed September 28, 2008.*

	Narcotrend stage	Narcotrend index
Awake	A	95–100
Sedated	B_0	90–94
	B_1	85–89
	B_2	80–84
Light anesthesia	C_0	75–79
	C_1	70–74
	C_2	65–69
General anesthesia	D_0	57–64
	D_1	47–56
	D_2	37–46
Deep General anesthesia	E_0	27–36
	E_1	20–26
	E_2	19–19
General anesthesia with increasing burst suppression	F_0	5–12
	F_1	1–4

Figure 12–10   Narcotrend stages with the respective index values. *(Table from Kreuer S, Bruhn J, Larsen R, et al. Comparability of Narcotrend index and bispectral index during propofol anaesthesia. Br J Anaesth 2004;93:235–240.)*[51]

with neurological disorders, trauma, and psychoactive medications. Like the BIS index, the state and response entropy values are increased by ketamine[47]; unlike the BIS index, however, the state and response entropy are decreased by nitrous oxide.[48] Similar to the BIS monitor, although the entropy monitor had difficulty detecting loss of response during single-agent xenon induction, it was able to distinguish between steady state anesthesia and return to responsiveness.[26]

Narcotrend (MonitorTechnik)

The Narcotrend system was originally developed at the University Medical School of Hannover, Germany, based on the principle of visual pattern recognition of EEG waveforms. A previous version of the system classified EEG traces from A (awake) to F (general anesthesia with increasing burst suppression) with 16 alphanumeric substages, with a level of D or E corresponding to a BIS of 40 to 65[49] (Figure 12–10). The newer version developed in 2004 produces a dimensionless Narcotrend index that ranges from 0 (isoelectric signal) to 100 (fully awake). Kreuer et al[50] provides a good review of the development and technologies behind the monitor. The device has been FDA approved and has recently become commercially available in the United States.

What It Measures

Right and left frontal electrodes are placed at least 8 cm apart, and a midline frontal lead acts as the reference electrode. The standard setup is a single-channel lead, but 2 channel recordings are possible. Of note, the Narcotrend system works with standard ECG electrodes, rather than proprietary sensors.

What It Outputs

Measures from both the time and frequency domain, such as spectral variables and entropy measures, are incorporated into an unspecified multivariate statistical function to produce the Narcotrend index.[9] Age-related changes of the EEG are also incorporated.[52]

entropy constant by adjusting the propofol infusion. If the RE reflected muscle activation, the analgesia provided by the remifentanil would theoretically reduce muscle responsiveness and movement, resulting in a decreased EMG (and lower RE) compared with the esmolol group. The study showed no difference in RE between the two groups, although all patients in the esmolol group and no patients in the remifentanil group moved. In addition, although Vakkuri et al[44] suggested that RE detects emergence 11 seconds earlier than SE and 12.4 seconds earlier than BIS, another study using physical stimuli instead of verbal commands indicated no advantage of the RE over SE in detecting emergence.[45] This calls into question the benefit of EMG monitoring specifically using RE, but the overall benefit of the Entropy monitor should be evaluated on the basis of clinical outcomes. There are no studies demonstrating the effect of entropy monitoring on the incidence of intraoperative awareness. A single-blinded randomized control trial showed that patients randomized to anesthetic care with the entropy values shown, with SE targeted to 45 and 65, resulted in less propofol consumption, especially during the last 15 minutes of the case, compared with patients randomized to anesthetic care for which entropy values were hidden; this translated to faster recovery times for the entropy group.[46] The Pk values for "anesthesia versus first reaction" to stimulus during propofol-remifentanil anesthesia were 0.82, 0.85, and 0.91 for SE, RE, and BIS, respectively, suggesting the BIS monitor was better able to detect lightening of anesthesia.[45]

As with other monitors, patient movement can cause artifacts, and entropy readings may be inaccurate in patients

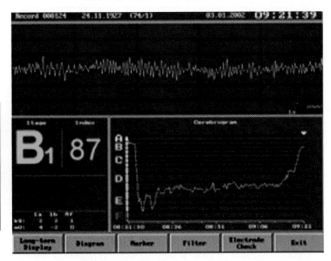

Figure 12–11 The Narcotrend display shows the value and trend of the Narcotrend index and stage and the raw EEG. *(Image from Narcotrend. (website): http://www.narcotrend.de/home_e.htm.) Accessed October 19, 2008.*

The Narcotrend monitor can display the raw EEG, the alphanumeric Narcotrend stage, and the Narcotrend index. It can also show the power spectrum for each hemisphere, and derived EEG parameters such as the median frequency and the 95% spectral edge frequency (Figure 12–11).

Clinical Utility

There is a modest amount of literature pertaining to the Narcotrend monitor, but there have been no studies examining its utility in reducing the incidence of awareness. The Pk for predicting the awake state versus steady state anesthesia was 1.0 for both the Narcotrend index and the BIS index, while the Pk for Narcotrend for steady state anesthesia versus first reaction (i.e., emergence) was 0.94 compared to 0.79 for BIS.[53] However, a later study found that that the Pk for differentiating between awareness and unconsciousness by Narcotrend was 0.501 (i.e., the device did not perform better than chance).[54] Furthermore, the study found that Narcotrend values were not independent of the anesthetic regimen.

A study using artificially generated EEG signals to compare the time delay of index calculation of the BIS index, Narcotrend index, and cerebral state index found time delays between 14 and 155 seconds for all indices; the delays depended on the particular starting and target index values, and no consistent pattern of delay was found suggesting that one index was generally slower than another.[55]

Cerebral State Monitor (Danmeter)

The cerebral state monitor, launched in 2004, is a battery powered portable device, capable of wireless communication with a patient monitor. Using fuzzy logic, the device calculates a cerebral state index (CSI) scaled from 0 to 100. The values of 40 to 60 indicate an optimal target for surgical anesthesia. According to the manufacturer's website,[4] over the past 10 years more than 150,000 devices have been sold.

Underlying Principle: Fuzzy Logic

Fuzzy logic is a type of "multivalued logic" that considers gradations in attributes, or "degrees of truth" rather than strictly binary values. This approach is often useful for the analysis of nonlinear, complex systems that have vague or contextual decision-making rules. As such, fuzzy logic has a broad range of applications, including digital image processing, subway control systems, and even rice cookers. In binary logic, temperature might be described by a "yes" or "no" value for a variable representing "hot." In fuzzy logic, a number is assigned to represent the degree to which the variable is true. A lukewarm temperature may be represented by a value of 0.7 for the variable "hot." (This number is called the "set membership value" in the context of fuzzy set theory.) Membership does not have to be exclusive: the lukewarm temperature may have a 0.3 value for the variable "cold." Various combinations of values for "cold" and "hot" can be defined to create categories such as "very hot" (e.g., 1.0 hot, 0 cold) or "somewhat cold" (e.g., 0.4 hot, 0.6 cold). Logical statements (e.g., "if-then" rules) could then be easily created based on these categorical definitions, effectively creating context-dependent algorithms.

Similarly, the cerebral state monitor processes the parameters characterizing the EEG into fuzzy logic classifications, using an empirically developed algorithm.[10] It calculates the α-ratio (log of the ratio of the power in the 30 to 42.5 Hz to the 6 to 12 Hz band), the β-ratio (log of the ratio of the power in the 30 to 42.5 Hz band to the 11 to 21 Hz band), the difference between the two ratios (β-ratio and α-ratio), and the amount of burst suppression (BS%) in the preceding 30 seconds. These parameters are processed using fuzzy logic analysis to yield the CSI.

What It Measures

The cerebral state monitor acquires a single-channel EEG signal using standard ECG electrodes with snap connectors placed on the forehead. Of note, one Swedish study found that the use of generic ECG electrodes, compared with proprietary Danmeter EEG electrodes, provided comparable signal acquisition for the cerebral state monitor with no difference in impedance, noise, or artifacts, at a tenth of the cost.[56]

What It Outputs

The display of the cerebral state monitor displays the CSI, scaled from 0 to 100, the degree of burst suppression, EMG activity in the 75 to 85 Hz range, and the quality of the signal (Figure 12–12). Other display options include 3 hour and 5.5 minute CSI trends, and display of last 3 seconds of EEG waveform.

Clinical Utility

There have been a limited number of studies of the CSI, with no studies examining the efficacy of the monitor in reducing the incidence of awareness. One study showed that both the CSI and BIS had high prediction probabilities (Pk values >0.9) for "awake versus loss of verbal contact," "awake versus loss of response (to physical stimuli)," and "loss of verbal contact versus loss of response" during propofol infusions.[57] A study

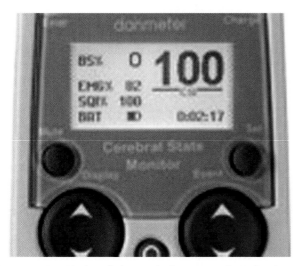

Figure 12–12 Display of the cerebral state monitor, showing the cerebral state index (CSI), burst suppression (BS%), electromyography (EMG%), and signal quality index (SQI%). *(Image from Danmeter. CSM monitor. (website): http://www.danmeter.dk/products/neuromonitoring/ csmmonitor/screendumps/index.html.) Accessed September 10, 2008.*

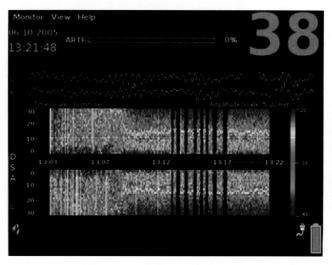

Figure 12–13 The SEDLine display, showing the raw EEG tracing, the patient state index (PSI) value, and the dual color density spectral array (DA) showing the dominant frequencies in the EEG. *(Image Courtesy Hospira.)*

comparing the performance of the cerebral state monitor to the BIS monitor found that they had similar performance during propofol induction, but suggested that the BIS may be better for the evaluation of intermediate anesthetic levels and the CSI may be better for evaluating deeper anesthetic levels.[58]

SEDLine/Patient State Analyzer (Masimo)

The patient state analyzer (PSA) technology was developed by Physiometrix, which was acquired by Hospira in 2005, and subsequently by Masimo in 2010. Initially presented as the PSA4000 EEG Monitor, the most recent implementation of the PSA technology is the SEDLine System. The PSA system uses a proprietary algorithm to calculate a dimensionless number called the Patient State Index (PSI) that ranges from 0 to 100 (awake) to reflect the depth of sedation.

The proprietary algorithm was empirically developed using electrophysiological databases and incorporated information regarding the EEG power, frequency, and coherence comparing bilateral brain regions and the anteriorization of power and uncoupling of anterior and posterior regions that occurs during loss of consciousness.[59] Drover[60] provides a good overview of the PSA technology.

What It Measures

The SEDLine system uses a disposable five-electrode sensor (the SEDtrace electrode set) placed on the forehead, which allows for a four-channel EEG system. The PSA 4000 system uses a similar electrode set called the PSArray.

What It Outputs

The SEDLine system displays the electrode status, EEG wave forms, PSI trend plots, and a dual color density spectral array (DSA), which provides a concise spectral time history from

both frontal hemispheres simultaneously (Figure 12–13). The newest system also can store up to 50 hours of raw and processed data.

Clinical Utility

The SedLine system and patient state index have not been as well studied as the BIS monitor, and there is no published literature demonstrating the ability of the PSI to decrease the incidence of awareness. One study of surgical patients showed that the Pk for "consciousness" versus "unconsciousness" for the PSI was 0.69 compared to 0.70 for the BIS.[61] This is consistent with a study that concluded that both PSI and BIS predicted depth of sevoflurane anesthesia equally well.[62]

The initial clinical validation of the PSI took the form of a prospective study of propofol, alfentanil, and nitrous oxide, wherein PSI-guided anesthesia resulted in patients receiving significantly less propofol and emerged from anesthesia more quickly.[63] Another study showed both PSI and BIS predicted sevoflurane effect site concentration equally well during sevoflurane anesthesia[62] and predicted failure to respond to stimuli equally well.[64] An early study using a variety of anesthetic drugs found weak concordance between BIS and the PSI.[65] A subsequent study suggested that BIS and PSI numbers generally track together, although the PSI appeared to respond slower and with greater variability when BIS values were low (<40).[66]

SNAP II (Stryker)

The SNAP II, introduced in 2002 by Nicolet Biomedical Monitors, was the first PDA-based DoA monitor, designed to emphasize portability and speed of processing (Figure 12–14). Currently sold by Stryker, it assesses high and low frequency EEGs and outputs a SNAP index that ranges from 0 to 99 (awake). A SNAP index range of 58 to 70 has been found to be equivalent to a BIS index range of 40 to 60.[67] Bischoff and Schmidt[68] provide a good overview of the SNAP II device.

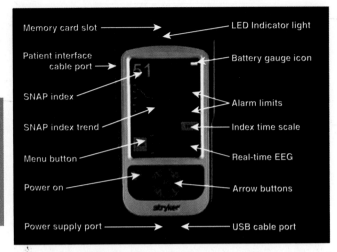

Figure 12–14 The portable SNAP II device, displaying the value and trend of the SNAP and the real-time EEG. *(Image from ORLive. (website): http://www.orlive.com/anesthesiaawareness/assets/pdfs/SNAP2_Monograph_STR026.pdf.) Accessed October 23, 2008.*

What It Measures

The SNAP II system measures frontal EEG using a single-lead disposable sensor that attaches to the center of the forehead, above the arch of the eyebrow, and near the temple.

What It Outputs

The SNAP II device calculates a SNAP index every second based on a 15-point moving average, using variables representing the energy in the high frequency (80 to 420 Hz) and low frequency (0.1 to 40 Hz) bands. Gamma frequency waves (40 to 80 Hz) are ignored. The algorithm behind the SNAP Index has been previously published.[69]

Clinical Utility

There has been very little research regarding the clinical utility of the SNAP device. The SNAP index has been shown to be significantly but weakly correlated to the BIS index with a positive bias of about 10 points.[70] Another study showed that the SNAP index (Pk of 0.91) and BIS (Pk of 1.0) reliably distinguished between awake and unconscious states, but the SNAP index did not reflect the analgesic potency of remifentanil during a propofol infusion.[71]

The manufacturer suggests that the device is a faster and more sensitive indicator of return to consciousness than the BIS monitor, based on a study finding that the SNAP II index returned to baseline 1 minute before awakening following general anesthesia with sevoflurane or sevoflurane/nitrous oxide, while the BIS XP index remained at baseline at awakening.[72] However, there is no further evidence that the SNAP is better than other devices at detecting states of consciousness.

It should be noted that Bischoff and Schmidt expressed concern that EMG power of high and lower frequencies changes to different degrees during induction and suggested that the effect of muscle paralysis and EMG must be better studied before widespread clinical adoption of the SNAP II device.[68]

AEP Monitor/2 (Danmeter)

Brain function monitoring using auditory evoked potentials (AEP) is based on the premise that hearing is the last retained sense during deepening anesthesia. Thus, measurement of the brain's reaction to acoustic stimuli provides useful information regarding the state of anesthesia. The A-LINE AEP Monitor, commercially introduced in 2000 by Danmeter, was the first commercially available device to use the principle of AEP to monitor awareness. In 2003, the A-Line AEP Monitor/2 was introduced, which combines AEP signal processing with EEG information to produce a composite A-Line autoregressive index (AAI), scaled from 0 to 100. An AAI greater than 50 corresponds to the awake state, and the suggested range for surgical anesthesia is 15 to 25. Although AEP is suppressed during deep anesthesia, AEP monitoring purportedly allows for fast detection of awakening during moderate levels of consciousness. Plourde[73] provides a good review of the physiology and utility of AEP monitoring.

Underlying Principle: Auditory Evoked Potentials

The AEP is produced by electrical activity that passes from the cochlea to the cortex in response to an acoustic stimulus and comprises a series of response waves that can be categorized by the time window.[74] The brainstem response waves, called the brainstem auditory evoked potential (BAEP), occur within 10 ms of the stimulus and are relatively insensitive to the effects of anesthetics. Middle latency waves (middle latency auditory evoked potential, or MLAEP) occur 20 to 80 ms following a stimulus and represent transmission from the thalamus to the auditory cortex. This is often referred to as the middle-latency auditory evoked response (mLAER). Because increased concentrations of general anesthetics result in increased latency and decreased amplitude of the mLAER, this signal can be extracted to provide information about the depth of anesthesia. Late latency evoked potentials (LLAEP) reflect the activity of the frontal cortex and association areas. LLAEP occur 80 ms following the stimulus and disappear during sedative concentrations of general anesthesia. Figure 12–15 shows the progression of electrical activity as a function of time elapsed following an auditory stimulus.

What It Measures

Three disposable forehead electrodes measure the EEG. Bilateral acoustic stimulation is administered 9 times a second using reusable earphones or clamshell-style headphones.

What It Outputs

The extraction of the mLAER signal from the EEG is performed by the AEP Monitor/2 using a proprietary process called "ARX modeling," which reduces the amount of time needed to obtain the AEP from 2 minutes (using the traditional moving time average method, which required 1000 stimuli repetitions), to a few seconds. The AAI represents a linear combination of parameters from the AEP and from the EEG, which includes measures of burst suppression and the shift of power from higher to lower frequencies.

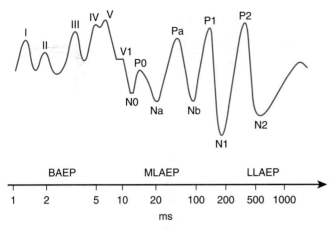

Figure 12–15 Schematic figure showing the various phases of the brainstem response *(y-axis)* as a function of time *(x-axis)* after an auditory stimulus. *(From Danmeter. The AEP monitor/2. (website): http://www.danmeter.dk/products/neuromonitoring/aepmonitor2/index.html.) Accessed September 10, 2008.*

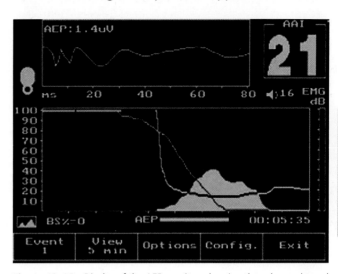

Figure 12–16 Display of the AEP monitor, showing the value and trend of the autoregressive index (AAI) and auditory evoked potential (AEP) and the burst suppression (BS%) and electromyographic potential (EMG). *(Image from Danmeter. The AEP monitor/2. (website): http://www.danmeter.dk/products/neuromonitoring/aepmonitor2/screendumps/index.html.) Accessed September 20, 2008.*

Decreased signal to noise ratios result in increased weighting of the EEG parameters. The AAI ranges from 0 to 99, but a 0 to 60 range can be selected, which results in fewer oscillations while a patient is awake, and increased graphical resolution of lower index values. According to the AEP manual provided by the manufacturer, the recommended AAI values for surgical anesthesia are 15 to 25. However, authors of a recent study suggested that targeting an AAI less than 30 may "result in an unnecessarily deep anesthetic state."[30]

Figure 12–16 shows the display of the AEP Monitior/2. The system is capable of displaying the EEG, AEP and AAI with trend views of 5 and 30 minutes, AAIS (smoothed AAI, which is the average of the previous 12 AAI values), EMG, and burst suppression expressed as the percentage of the previous 30 seconds that had an isoelectric EEG.

Clinical Utility

There are no studies examining the effect of AEP monitoring on the incidence of awareness. AEP monitoring has been shown to reduce time to extubation and orientation.[75] Monitoring with the AEP and BIS equally decreased maintenance anesthetic requirements, resulting in a shorter PACU length of stay and improved self-reported quality of recovery.[76]

The Pk values of the AEP vary depending on the study design and anesthetic regimen used. The Pk for the ability of the AEP index to predict responsiveness after discontinuation of remifentanil was 0.63,[77] while the Pk for predicting movement after skin incision during sevoflurane anesthesia was 0.91 compared with 0.537 for the BIS monitor.[78] While both the BIS index and AAI had identical Pk values (0.87) for predicting loss of consciousness during propofol anesthesia, neither was able to predict explicit or implicit postoperative recall.[79] The ability of both monitors to predict sedation but not memory formation illustrates the fundamental difficulty of using Pk values to assess the function of an "awareness" monitor.

It should be noted that although the AEP is insensitive to the effects of ketamine[24] and nitrous oxide, it is suppressed by xenon.[80]

Emerging Technologies and Research

There have been a number of very recent publications on the value of approximate entropy and permutation entropy calculations.[81-83] Approximate entropy (AE) is a statistic that quantifies the randomness of fluctuations by reflecting the predictability of future EEG amplitudes based on *previous* amplitude values. It is a slightly different concept from Shannon entropy (used in the Entropy module), which measures the predictability of future amplitudes by measuring the probability distribution of amplitudes observed in the *current* signal.[42] Permutation entropy (PE) is another measure of the irregularity of the signal, which measures the relative occurrence of various patterns of the EEG. Jordan et al[81] and Li et al[82] provide more details regarding these concepts, and demonstrate the potential for AE and PE to estimate anesthetic drug effects. More clinical research is needed if and when these mathematical techniques are incorporated into a commercially available product.

There is also a relatively new DoA monitor developed in 2008 by Morpheus Medical called the IoC-view. EEG information can be transmitted from the IoC view device to a PDA via Bluetooth wireless technology (Figure 12–17). The index of consciousness is a unitless scale that ranges from 0 to 99, calculated using symbolic dynamics, which is a process by which the EEG signal is described using abstract symbols corresponding to certain states (or time intervals) of the system. At the time of writing, the peer-reviewed literature demonstrating the validity of the device is very limited, but one study concluded that the IoC index and the BIS performed equally well at predicting levels of consciousness using the Observer's Assessment of Alertness and Sedation Scale.[84] Independent verification of the validity and reliability of this new technology will be needed.

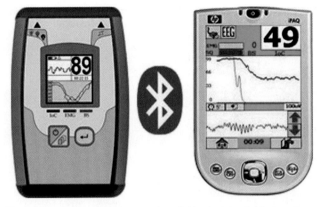

Figure 12–17 The IoC View monitor *(left)* calculates the index of consciousness and transmits information wirelessly to a PDA. *(Image from Morpheus Medical, website: http://www.morpheus-medical.com/index.php?id=4258.)* Accessed October 1, 2008.

Conclusion

In the context of competing industrial interests and public pressure to use brain monitoring devices, the anesthesia community must remain vigilant in producing and analyzing outcome-oriented evidence to enable informed policy decisions (e.g., protocols calling for the routine use of a particular monitor). Future research should focus on the demonstration of cost-effective benefits, and on determining the appropriate indications for DoA monitor use. Also, in the absence of clear and convincing evidence of the general superiority of one device over another, the practitioner's familiarity with the device being used is probably more important than the actual choice of the device.

Performance data about monitors are useful for generalized decision making regarding the use of a device, but it is worth reemphasizing that each index value, like any physiological value, must be considered in the clinical context. As mentioned earlier, DoA monitors should be used to help modify the individual pretest probability of awareness as determined by the clinician. In response to the release of the ASA Practice Advisory for Intraoperative Awareness, Dr. Orin Guidry, then ASA president, aptly cautioned "the most important monitor in the operating room is the anesthesiologist."[5] Anesthesiology providers can make the best individual practice decisions only by understanding the technological and physiological principles underlying the tools used in the operating room.

1 Adapted from Dr. Steven Barker, "Nuts and Bolts of Brain Function Monitoring," ASA 2008 Annual Meeting. October 18, 2008.

2 Mathematically stated, Pk = (Pc + 0.5*Pt)/(Pc + Pd + Pt), where Pc, Pd, and Pt are the respective probabilities that two data points selected are concordant, discordant, or tied.

3 Mathematically, a system is linear if an input x1(k) results in an output y1(k), and x2(k) results in an output y2(k), then a*x1(K) + b* x2(k) would output a*y1(k) + b*y2(k).

4 http://www.danmeter.dk/products/index.html.

5 http://www.asahq.org/news/news102505.htm. Accessed November 28, 2008.

Suggested Reading

Best Pract Res Clin Anaesthesiol 2006;20(1). *Edited by Peter Tonner and Jens Scholz, an issue focused on the theme "monitoring consciousness." Contains general articles pertaining to consciousness and EEG utilization and has individual articles each describing the technologies of a particular DoA monitor.*

Bowdle, T.A. 2006. Depth of anesthesia monitoring. Anesthesiol Clin 24, 793–822. *A broad overview of depth of anesthesia monitors, focusing on considerations relating to the clinical usage of the BIS monitor, such as the effects of individual drugs or artifacts on the BIS index.*

American Society of Anesthesiologists Task Force on Intraoperative Awareness 2006. Practice advisory for intraoperative awareness and brain function monitoring: a report by the American Society of Anesthesiologists task force on intraoperative awareness. Anesthesiology 104, 847–864. *A comprehensive overview that synthesizes the evidence regarding the brain function monitors discussed in this chapter. The practice advisory provides a task force consensus regarding the use of brain function monitors for preventing intraoperative awareness and also discusses recommendations based on surveys of ASA members and consultants.*

Jameson, L.C., Sloan, T.B. 2006. Using EEG to monitor anesthesia drug effects during surgery. J Clin Monit Comput 20, 445–472. *An overview of DoA monitoring technologies that provides additional background on the neurophysiology of general anesthesia, memory formation, and anesthetic effects on the EEG.*

Sigl, J.C., Chamoun, N.G. 1994. An introduction to bispectral analysis for the electroencephalogram. J Clin Monit 10, 392–404. *An excellent primer clearly explaining the basic mathematical foundations of bispectral analysis used in the BIS monitor.*

References

1. Joint Commission, Sentinel event alert No. 32: preventing, and managing the impact of, anesthesia awareness, (website). http://www.jointcommission.org/SentinelEvents/SentinelEventAlert/sea_32.htm2008 Accessed October 23.

2. American Society of Anesthesiologists Task Force on Intraoperative Awareness, 2006. Practice advisory for intraoperative awareness and brain function monitoring: a report by the American Society of Anesthesiologists task force on intraoperative awareness. Anesthesiology 104, 847–864.

3. Samuelsson, P., Brudin, L., Sandin, R.H., 2007. Late psychological symptoms after awareness among consecutively included surgical patients. Anesthesiology 106, 26–32.

4. Osterman, J.E., Hopper, J., Heran, W.J., et al., 2001. Awareness under anesthesia and the development of posttraumatic stress disorder. Gen Hosp Psychiatry 23, 198–204.

5. Pollard, R.J., Coyle, J.P., Gilbert, R.L., et al., 2007. Intraoperative awareness in a regional medical system: a review of 3 years' data. Anesthesiology 106, 269–274.

6. Errando, C.L., Sigl, J.C., Robles, M., et al., 2008. Awareness with recall during general anaesthesia: a prospective observational evaluation of 4001 patients. Br J Anaesth 101, 178–185.

7. Monk, T.G., Saini, V., Weldon, B.C., et al., 2005. Anesthetic management and one-year mortality after noncardiac surgery. Anesth Analg 100, 4–10.

8. Bowdle, T.A., 2006. Depth of anesthesia monitoring. Anesthesiol Clin 24, 793–822.

9. Bruhn, J., Myles, P.S., Sneyd, R., et al., 2006. Depth of anaesthesia monitoring: what's available, what's validated and what's next? Br J Anaesth 97, 85–94.

10. Jameson, L.C., Sloan, T.B., 2006. Using EEG to monitor anesthesia drug effects during surgery. J Clin Monit Comput 20, 445–472.

11. Smith, W.D., Dutton, R.C., Smith, N.T., 1996. Measuring the performance of anesthetic depth indicators. Anesthesiology 84, 38–51.

12. Weber Jensen, E., Rodriguez, B., Litvan, H., 2005. Pk value does depend on the fineness of the observer scale. Acta Anaesthesiol Scand 49, 427, author reply 8.

13. Gibbs, F.A.G.L, Lennox, W.G., 1937. Effect on the electro-encephalogram of certain drugs which influence nervous activity. Arch Intern Med 60(1), 154–166.

14. Rampil, I.J., 1998. A primer for EEG signal processing in anesthesia. Anesthesiology 89, 980–1002.

15. Sigl, J.C., Chamoun, N.G., 1994. An introduction to bispectral analysis for the electroencephalogram. J Clin Monit 10, 392–404.

16. Lee, U., Mashour, G.A., Kim, S., et al., 2008. Propofol induction reduces the capacity for neural information integration: implications for the mechanism of consciousness and general anesthesia. Conscious Cogn 18(1), 56–64.

17. Niedermeyer, E., Lopes da Silva, F.H. (Eds.), 2004. Electroencephalography: basic principles, clinical applications, and related fields, ed 5. Lippincott Williams & Wilkins, Philadelphia.

18. Tonner, P.H., Bein, B., 2006. Classic electroencephalographic parameters: median frequency, spectral edge frequency etc. Best Pract Res Clin Anaesthesiol 20, 147–159.

19. Dressler, O., Schneider, G., Stockmanns, G., et al., 2004. Awareness and the EEG power spectrum: analysis of frequencies. Br J Anaesth 93, 806–809.

20. Hemmerling, T.M., Harvey, P., 2002. Electrocardiographic electrodes provide the same results as expensive special sensors in the routine monitoring of anesthetic depth. Anesth Analg 94, 369–371.

21. Akavipat, P., Dumrongbul, K., Neamnak, P., 2006. Can electrocardiogram electrodes replace bispectral index electrodes for monitoring depth of anesthesia? J Med Assoc Thai 89, 51–55.

22. Miller, A., Sleigh, J.W., Barnard, J., et al., 2004. Does bispectral analysis of the electroencephalogram add anything but complexity? Br J Anaesth 92, 8–13.

23. Barr, G., Jakobsson, J.G., Owall, A., et al., 1999. Nitrous oxide does not alter bispectral index: study with nitrous oxide as sole agent and as an adjunct to i.v. anaesthesia. Br J Anaesth 82, 827–830.

24. Vereecke, H.E., Struys, M.M., Mortier, E.P., 2003. A comparison of bispectral index and ARX-derived auditory evoked potential index in measuring the clinical interaction between ketamine and propofol anaesthesia. Anaesthesia 58, 957–961.

25. Goto, T., Nakata, Y., Saito, H., et al., 2000. Bispectral analysis of the electroencephalogram does not predict responsiveness to verbal command in patients emerging from xenon anaesthesia. Br J Anaesth 85, 359–363.

26. Laitio, R.M., Kaskinoro, K., Sarkela, M.O., et al., 2008. Bispectral index, entropy, and quantitative electroencephalogram during single-agent xenon anesthesia. Anesthesiology 108, 63–70.

27. Merat, S., Levecque, J.P., Le Gulluche, Y., et al., 2001. BIS monitoring may allow the detection of severe cerebral ischemia. Can J Anaesth 48, 1066–1069.

28. Renna, M., Handy, J., Shah, A., 2003. Low baseline bispectral index of the electroencephalogram in patients with dementia. Anesth Analg 96, 1380–1385.

29. Wu, C.C., Lin, C.S., Mok, M.S., 2002. Bispectral index monitoring during hypoglycemic coma. J Clin Anesth 14, 305–306.

30. Manyam, S.C., Gupta, D.K., Johnson, K.B., et al., 2007. When is a bispectral index of 60 too low? Rational processed electroencephalographic targets are dependent on the sedative-opioid ratio. Anesthesiology 106, 472–483.

31. Ekman, A., Lindholm, M.L., Lennmarken, C., et al., 2004. Reduction in the incidence of awareness using BIS monitoring. Acta Anaesthesiol Scand 48, 20–26.

32. Myles, P.S., Leslie, K., McNeil, J., et al., 2004. Bispectral index monitoring to prevent awareness during anaesthesia: the B-Aware randomised controlled trial. Lancet 363, 1757–1763.

33. Avidan, M.S., Zhang, L., Burnside, B.A., et al., 2008. Anesthesia awareness and the bispectral index. N Engl J Med 358, 1097–1108.

34. Kelley, S.D., Manberg, P.J., Sigl, J.C., 2008. Anesthesia awareness and the bispectral index. N Engl J Med 359, 427–428, author reply 30-1.

35. Punjasawadwong, Y., Boonjeungmonkol, N., Phongchiewboon, A., 2007. Bispectral index for improving anaesthetic delivery and postoperative recovery. Cochrane Database Syst Rev, CD003843.

36. Monk, T.G., 2006. Processed EEG and patient outcome. Best Pract Res Clin Anaesthesiol 20, 221–228.

37. Lindholm, M.L., Traff, S., Granath, F., et al., 2009. Mortality within 2 years after surgery in relation to low intraoperative bispectral index values and preexisting malignant disease. Anesth Analg 108, 508–512.

38. Bein B., 2006. Entropy. Best Pract Res Clin Anaesthesiol 20, 101–109.

39. Shannon, C., 1948. A mathematical theory of communication. Bell Syst Tech J 27, 623–656.

40. Viertio-Oja, H., Maja, V., Sarkela, M., et al., 2004. Description of the entropy algorithm as applied in the Datex-Ohmeda S/5 Entropy Module. Acta Anaesthesiol Scand 48, 154–161.

41. Inouye, T., Shinosaki, K., Sakamoto, H., et al., 1991. Quantification of EEG irregularity by use of the entropy of the power spectrum. Electroencephalogr Clin Neurophysiol 79, 204–210.

42. Bruhn, J., Lehmann, L.E., Ropcke, H., et al., 2001. Shannon entropy applied to the measurement of the electroencephalographic effects of desflurane. Anesthesiology 95, 30–35.

43. Valjus, M., Ahonen, J., Jokela, R., et al., 2006. Response entropy is not more sensitive than state entropy in distinguishing the use of esmolol instead of remifentanil in patients undergoing gynaecological laparoscopy. Acta Anaesthesiol Scand 50, 32–39.

44. Vakkuri, A., Yli-Hankala, A., Talja, P., et al., 2004. Time-frequency balanced spectral entropy as a measure of anesthetic drug effect in central nervous system during sevoflurane, propofol, and thiopental anesthesia. Acta Anaesthesiol Scand 48, 145–153.

45. Schmidt, G.N., Bischoff, P., Standl, T., et al., 2004. Comparative evaluation of the Datex-Ohmeda S/5 Entropy Module and the bispectral index monitor during propofol-remifentanil anesthesia. Anesthesiology 101, 1283–1290.

46. Vakkuri, A., Yli-Hankala, A., Sandin, R., et al., 2005. Spectral entropy monitoring is associated with reduced propofol use and faster emergence in propofol-nitrous oxide-alfentanil anesthesia. Anesthesiology 103, 274–279.

47. Hans, P., Dewandre, P.Y., Brichant, J.F., et al., 2005. Comparative effects of ketamine on bispectral index and spectral entropy of the electroencephalogram under sevoflurane anaesthesia. Br J Anaesth 94, 336–340.

48. Hans, P., Dewandre, P.Y., Brichant, J.F., et al., 2005. Effects of nitrous oxide on spectral entropy of the EEG during surgery under balanced anaesthesia with sufentanil and sevoflurane. Acta Anaesthesiol Belg 56, 37–43.

49. Kreuer, S., Biedler, A., Larsen, R., et al., 2001. The Narcotrend—a new EEG monitor designed to measure the depth of anaesthesia. A comparison with bispectral index monitoring during propofol-remifentanil-anaesthesia. Anaesthesist 50, 921–925.

50. Kreuer, S., Wilhelm, W., 2006. The Narcotrend monitor. Best Pract Res Clin Anaesthesiol 20, 111–129.

51. Kreuer, S., Bruhn, J., Larsen, R., et al., 2004. Comparability of Narcotrend index and bispectral index during propofol anaesthesia. Br J Anaesth 93, 235–240.

52. Schultz, B., Kreuer, S., Wilhelm, W., et al., 2003. The Narcotrend monitor. Development and interpretation algorithms. Anaesthesist 52, 1143–1148.

53. Schmidt, G.N., Bischoff, P., Standl, T., et al., 2003. Narcotrend and bispectral index monitor are superior to classic electroencephalographic parameters for the assessment of anesthetic states during propofol-remifentanil anesthesia. Anesthesiology 99, 1072–1077.

54. Schneider, G., Kochs, E.F., Horn, B., et al., 2004. Narcotrend does not adequately detect the transition between awareness and unconsciousness in surgical patients. Anesthesiology 101, 1105–1111.

55. Pilge, S., Zanner, R., Schneider, G., et al., 2006. Time delay of index calculation: analysis of cerebral state, bispectral, and Narcotrend indices. Anesthesiology 104, 488–494.

56. Anderson, R.E., Sartipy, U., Jakobsson, J.G., 2007. Use of conventional ECG electrodes for depth of anaesthesia monitoring using the cerebral state index: a clinical study in day surgery. Br J Anaesth 98, 645–648.

57. Zhong, T., Guo, Q.L., Pang, Y.D., et al., 2005. Comparative evaluation of the cerebral state index and the bispectral index during target-controlled infusion of propofol. Br J Anaesth 95, 798–802.

58. Cortinez, L.I., Delfino, A.E., Fuentes, R., et al., 2007. Performance of the cerebral state index during increasing levels of propofol anesthesia: a comparison with the bispectral index. Anesth Analg 104, 605–610.

59. John, E.R., Prichep, L.S., Kox, W., et al., 2001. Invariant reversible QEEG effects of anesthetics. Conscious Cogn 10, 165–183.

60. Drover, D., Ortega, H.R., 2006. Patient state index. Best Pract Res Clin Anaesthesiol 20, 121–128.

61. Schneider, G., Gelb, A.W., Schmeller, B., et al., 2003. Detection of awareness in surgical patients with EEG-based indices—bispectral index and patient state index. Br J Anaesth 91, 329–335.

62. Soehle, M., Ellerkmann, R.K., Grube, M., et al., 2008. Comparison between bispectral index and patient state index as measures of the electroencephalographic effects of sevoflurane. Anesthesiology 109, 799–805.

63. Drover, D.R., Lemmens, H.J., Pierce, E.T., et al., 2002. Patient state index: titration of delivery and recovery from propofol, alfentanil, and nitrous oxide anesthesia. Anesthesiology 97, 82–89.

64. White, P.F., Tang, J., Ma, H., et al., 2004. Is the patient state analyzer with the PSArray2 a cost-effective alternative to the bispectral index monitor during the perioperative period? Anesth Analg 99, 1429–1435.

65. Schneider, G., Mappes, A., Neissendorfer, T., et al., 2004. EEG-based indices of anaesthesia: correlation between bispectral index and patient state index? Eur J Anaesthesiol 21, 6–12.

66. Anderson, R.E., Jakobsson, J.G., 2006. Cerebral state monitor, a new small handheld EEG monitor for determining depth of anaesthesia: a clinical comparison with the bispectral index during day-surgery. Eur J Anaesthesiol 23, 208–212.

67. Ruiz-Gimeno, P., Soro, M., Perez-Solaz, A., et al., 2005. Comparison of the EEG-based SNAP index and the bispectral (BIS) index during sevoflurane-nitrous oxide anaesthesia. J Clin Monit Comput 19, 383–389.

68. Bischoff, P., Schmidt, G., 2006. Monitoring methods: SNAP. Best Pract Res Clin Anaesthesiol 20, 141–146.

69. Wong, C.A., Fragen, R.J., Fitzgerald, P.C., et al., 2005. The association between propofol-induced loss of consciousness and the SNAP index. Anesth Analg 100, 141–148.

70. Casati, A., Putzu, M., Vinciguerra, F., 2005. A clinical comparison between bispectral index (BIS) and high frequency EEG signal detection (SNAP). Eur J Anaesthesiol 22, 75–77.

71. Schmidt, G.N., Standl, T., Lankenau, G., et al., 2004. SNAP-index and bispectral index during induction of anaesthesia with propofol and remifentanil. Anasthesiol Intensivmed Notfallmed Schmerzther 39, 286–291.

72. Wong, C.A., Fragen, R.J., Fitzgerald, P., et al., 2006. A comparison of the SNAP II and BIS XP indices during sevoflurane and nitrous oxide anaesthesia at 1 and 1.5 MAC and at awakening. Br J Anaesth 97, 181–186.

73. Plourde, G., 2006. Auditory evoked potentials. Best Pract Res Clin Anaesthesiol 20, 129–139.

74. De Cosmo, G., Aceto, P., Clemente, A., et al., 2004. Auditory evoked potentials. Minerva Anestesiol 70, 293–297.

75. Maattanen, H., Anderson, R., Uusijarvi, J., et al., 2002. Auditory evoked potential monitoring with the AAITM-index during spinal surgery: decreased desflurane consumption. Acta Anaesthesiol Scand 46, 882–886.

76. Recart, A., Gasanova, I., White, P.F., et al., 2003. The effect of cerebral monitoring on recovery after general anesthesia: a comparison of the auditory evoked potential and bispectral index devices with standard clinical practice. Anesth Analg 97, 1667–1674.

77. Muncaster, A.R., Sleigh, J.W., Williams, M., 2003. Changes in consciousness, conceptual memory, and quantitative electroencephalographical measures during recovery from sevoflurane- and remifentanil-based anesthesia. Anesth Analg 96, 720–725.

78. Kurita, T., Doi, M., Katoh, T., et al., 2001. Auditory evoked potential index predicts the depth of sedation and movement in response to skin incision during sevoflurane anesthesia. Anesthesiology 95, 364–370.

79. Hadzidiakos, D., Petersen, S., Baars, J., et al., 2006. Comparison of a new composite index based on midlatency auditory evoked potentials and electroencephalographic parameters with bispectral index (BIS) during moderate propofol sedation. Eur J Anaesthesiol 23, 931–936.

80. Hirota, K., 2006. Special cases: ketamine, nitrous oxide and xenon. Best Pract Res Clin Anaesthesiol 20, 69–79.

81. Jordan, D., Stockmanns, G., Kochs, E.F., et al., 2008. Electroencephalographic order pattern analysis for the separation of consciousness and unconsciousness: an analysis of approximate entropy, permutation entropy, recurrence rate, and phase coupling of order recurrence plots. Anesthesiology 109, 1014–1022.

82. Li, X., Cui, S., Voss, L.J., 2008. Using permutation entropy to measure the electroencephalographic effects of sevoflurane. Anesthesiology 109, 448–456.

83. Olofsen, E., Sleigh, J.W., Dahan, A., 2008. Permutation entropy of the electroencephalogram: a measure of anaesthetic drug effect. Br J Anaesth 101, 810–821.

84. Revuelta, M., Paniagua, P., Campos, J.M., et al., 2008. Validation of the index of consciousness during sevoflurane and remifentanil anaesthesia: a comparison with the bispectral index and the cerebral state index. Br J Anaesth 101, 653–658.

Chapter 13

Alarms in Clinical Anesthesia

F. Jacob Seagull and Richard P. Dutton

Principles of Alarm Systems

A well-implemented clinical alarm system can save a patient's life. During clinical care, the monitor's alarm system is always vigilant and, when an alarm is triggered, provides a clear signal that a notable event has occurred. The signal can draw attention to the event and facilitate timely treatment. Alarms can cue action that can save lives; however, they are far from perfect. They function as a combination of technology and a human operator, built to capitalize on a machine's ability to detect a change, and the human's ability to interpret its meaning.[1] While alarms alert the clinician to an event, they cannot distinguish between clinically relevant and trivial occurrences.[2] They have very limited ability to (1) understand the context of the situation, (2) reason out the cause of a problem, and (3) determine clinical relevance. Because of these limitations, alarm systems are often plagued by high rates of false alarms.[2,3] False alarms interrupt care during critical junctures[4] and cause stress and frustration to care providers.[5,6] By understanding the principles of alarm systems, a well-prepared clinician can manage them efficiently and thus maximize the value of the monitors, ease workload, and increase patient safety.

To understand alarm systems, we must understand the principles underlying the determination that an "event" has occurred. It is rarely possible to measure an event of interest directly. In normal circumstances, we measure some aspect of the environment that reflects the underlying state of the system. For example, during open heart surgery, one can see the heart beating directly, but we more often measure the electrical signals at a patient's skin via an electrocardiogram (ECG). When a situation is "normal" (i.e., when no event such as a change in the patient's state has occurred), measures taken from the environment tend to cluster around a particular "normal" value. Similarly, when a particular event has occurred, measures of the environment tend to cluster around a different value. In most systems, there is overlap between the values associated with a normal situation and an event situation (Figure 13-1). Many values could indicate either an event or a normal situation. The value or threshold at which an alarm is sounded is called the decision criteria in signal detection theory, or "β" ("beta").[7] Given any reading from the environment, a monitoring system will make a determination of whether the parameter (patient) is normal or abnormal, and the resulting action by the monitoring system can be classified into one of four categories: a hit (true alarm), which occurs when the system detects an event when an event has occurred; a correct rejection (true normal), in which the monitoring system does not detect an event when no event has occurred; a false alarm, where the monitoring system detects an abnormal situation when the situation is in fact normal; and a miss, in which an abnormal situation arises, but the monitoring system fails to detect it (Table 13-1).

From the four states, we can derive two important characteristics of a monitoring system: sensitivity and specificity. *Sensitivity* represents the likelihood that when an event (abnormal situation) occurs, it will be detected (i.e., the "hit rate") (equation 13-1). The *specificity* signifies the likelihood that when the situation is normal, no event will be indicated (i.e., the correct rejection rate) (equation 13-2).

$$\text{Sensitivity} = \frac{\text{hits}}{\text{hits} + \text{misses}} \qquad (13\text{-}1)$$

$$\text{Specificity} = \frac{\text{correct rejections}}{\text{correct rejections} + \text{false alarms}} \qquad (13\text{-}2)$$

The sensitivity and specificity of a system is determined by:
- *The characteristics of the signal:* Every signal has inherent variability, such as normal variations in heart rate or in blood pressure. Some signals have a very clear dividing line between normal and abnormal, such as the presence or absence of ventricular fibrillation (VFib). Others are more indistinct, such as end-tidal CO_2 levels or oxygen saturation levels. The extent to which the normal and abnormal states are distinct affects the overlap between the two curves in Figure 13-1.

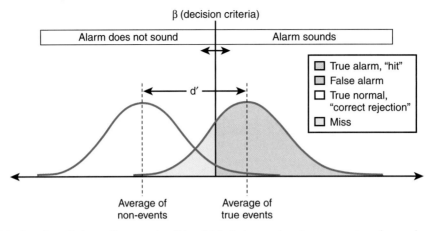

Figure 13–1 A signal-detection view of alarms. True events will be distributed around a given parameter value, and normal, nonevents (random noise) distributed around a different value. Most often these distributions overlap.

Table 13–1 Classification of Alarm-Related Situations

		The Monitoring System Response	
		Sound Alarm	**Do Not Sound Alarm**
True state of the world	Situation is normal	False alarm	Correct rejection (specificity)
	Situation is abnormal	"Hit" (sensitivity)	Miss

- *The mechanics of the sensor:* The mechanics of the sensor determine its ability to detect the underlying state of the system. Each type of sensor has inherent advantages and disadvantages. For example, invasive monitoring often is less susceptible to artifacts, and may provide a more direct measure of the underlying state than a noninvasive measure. However, invasive monitors are associated with higher risk of complications and cause insult to the patient.
- *Mechanics of the artifact rejection:* Monitoring devices are often hard-wired with the ability to sense degradation in the quality of the signal and can sometimes filter out noise that does not indicate a true change in patient state. The degree to which these filtering techniques are successful affects the specificity of the alarm system.
- *Programming by the user:* Adjustable alarm limits (decision criteria) can shift the proportion of hits to misses and, correct rejections to false alarms. These shifts occur without changing any of the inherent qualities of the alarm system's ability to detect state changes. Changes in decision criteria should reflect the relative value placed on detecting an event as compared with missing an event or sounding a false alarm.

The process of determining the relationship between the measure and the state of the world is as follows. Alarm systems typically monitor a single value or monitor for signs of a single event. When the measure/parameter reaches a certain decision criteria, β, the alarm is sounded. A system's

effectiveness (hit rate, false-alarm rate, etc.) is determined by two factors. One is the difference between the two populations (i.e., how much overlap there is in the curves in Figure 13-1), which is a type of signal-to-noise ratio known as the discriminability index, d' ("dee prime"). The second determining factor for effectiveness is the decision criterion (i.e., the point at which the alarm goes off, or β). Setting the decision criteria determines the effectiveness of the alarm system, as much as the inherent difference between the population of "true events" and "normal situations." As the decision criteria is made more stringent (higher threshold for an alarm), the number of false alarms decreases, but the number of misses increases as well. The discriminability index, d', indicates how easy it is to distinguish a true event from a nonevent and is a function of the characteristics of the parameter being measured and the technology used to measure it. The decision criterion β is set by the operator, and determines at what point an alarm will sound. For a given system, the value of β will determine proportion of true alarms to misses, and the proportion of false alarms to true normal reading. The value of d' will determine the proportion of true alarms to false alarms for a given β.

Concepts and Components of an Alarm System

A number of key definitions for basic concepts and terms that facilitate an understanding of alarm systems are listed next.

1. Alarm annunciators: The auditory signal (bell, buzzer, chime), visual indicator (flashing display, light, marquee), or tactile signal (vibration) that indicates that an alarm has been triggered. Annunciators can be separate from the clinical monitoring device itself, such as with a pager, mobile phone, or hand held device.
   a. Visual annunciator: The element of the visual display that indicates that an alarm is sounding. An annunciator can consist of text or graphical icons. Visual annunciators often are color coded in red or yellow, may also blink to indicate severity or attract attention, and may include highlighting on the monitor or even on a device separate from the monitor itself (Figure 13-2).

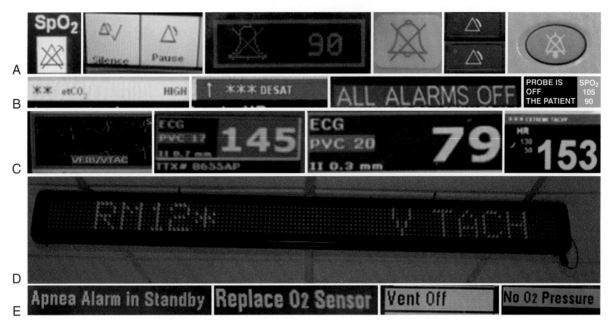

Figure 13–2 Row A. (from left to right) Icons indicating a disconnected sensor (first), and for silencing and pausing alarms on monitor screens (second and third). Physical buttons for alarm management (fourth through end) may include backlighting or other visual annunciators to indicate that their status. **Row B.** Two levels of visual annunciation (first, second) for parameter alarms (third), as well as system-status alarms, highlighted (fourth) or nonhighlighted (fifth). **Row C,** Different styles of visual annunciations including border highlighting, parameter highlighting, and text highlighting. **Row D,** Visual annunciators may be installed separate from the clinical monitor, such as in hallway marquees on critical care or telemetry units. Similarly, phone or paging systems may be used for auditory, visual, and tactile annunciation of alarms. **Row E,** System-status indicators from an Ohmeda monochrome ventilator display. System-status alarms may be presented as plain text or highlighted and may flash to indicate priority level.

b. Auditory annunciator: A sound produced by the monitoring system to indicate that an alarm is sounding. The sound may include a pattern of or repetition of tones to indicate severity, such as single tone for low priority alarms, and repeated tones for higher priority alarms.

c. Haptic/tactile annunciator: A touch-based signal produced to indicate that an alarm is sounding. Most commonly, pagers in "silent" mode annunciate by vibrating.

2. Alarm states: Terminology for alarm states can be confusing, with the original terms coming from early electronics systems in which an alarm would sound when a current in an alarm circuit ceased to flow, or "went off." The terminology has remained, as an alarm "going off" indicates that an alarm is sounding. In clinical monitoring, there are terms describing the state of the annunciator, and the state of the alarm system as a whole.

a. Enabled/disabled: Enabled/disabled describes an alarm system, not an individual alarm's activity. Enabling or disabling an alarm system indicates that the system as a whole will or will not detect events, respectively. When an alarm is enabled, it will detect events as they occur.

b. Sounding/not sounding: Sounding describes the activity of an individual annunciator. With an alarm system enabled and an event detected, an alarm will "sound." An enabled system will not sound when no event is detected.

c. Alarm suppression: Alarms that are sounding can be acknowledged, and the annunciator silenced or suspended. In the "silenced" state, alarm states are actively detected, but annunciators not actuated. Alarms can be silenced or suspended for a brief period (e.g., 30 seconds to 2 minutes). Alarm systems can silence the auditory annunciators permanently, while leaving the visual annunciators active. Some alarms must be "dismissed" from a monitor (see "latched" alarms in Alarm Types section).

3. Alarm Types

a. Latched: Once it is triggered, a latched alarm will continue to sound until silenced. For example, a burglar alarm sounds if a door is opened, and will sound until reset. In clinical monitoring, crisis-level alarms are often "latched." When a latched alarm sounds, it must be "dismissed" through interaction with the monitor.

b. Unlatched: Unlatched alarms will sound only as long as criteria for sounding are met. An example is the auditory alarm that indicates that you have left lights on in the car—the alarm stops when the lights are turned off. In clinical monitoring, the pulse oximeter will sound an alarm when saturations drop below the alarm threshold, but the alarm stops when saturations return to normal.

c. Tiered: An alarm system that assigns a relative priority to the various alarms that may sound. Typically there are three to four levels of alarm annunciation, ranging from informational alerts and messages at the low levels, to crisis alarms at the highest level (see later discussion).

4. Classification of alarm events: When an alarm sounds, it is typically classified into one of the first four categories below. The four terms are commonly used, but in practice the classification of alarms may not capture the subtlety of the clinical domain. The fifth category, "nuisance alarm," can be an informal classification of a true or false alarm.

   a. True alarm: An alarm caused by a change in the underlying state of the system being monitored. Note that because of the highly contextual nature of monitoring, a "true" alarm may have no clinical relevance (see "nuisance alarm").

   b. False alarm: An alarm that sounds when the underlying state being monitored is normal. False alarms can be caused by an increase in the "noise" contained within the monitored signal (artifacts) or can be a natural function of the decision criteria (alarm thresholds) set on the monitoring system.

   c. Miss: A true event occurs but an alarm does not sound.

   d. Correct normal: When the situation is normal (no event occurs) and an alarm does not sound. The term "correct rejection" is often used in signal detection theory to indicate the rejection of the hypothesis that a signal is present.

   e. Nuisance alarm: Alarms that sound often or predictably, but provide no useful information to the practitioner. Nuisance alarms can be true alarms or false alarms. They can indicate a true change in the state of the patient or equipment that either has no clinical significance, or that may already be known, such as an apnea alarm that sounds during the process of tracheal intubation. When alarm thresholds are set inappropriately, nuisance alarms may indicate a trivial change that does not represent a threat to the patient. False alarms caused by artifacts such as electrocautery or patient movement can also be nuisance alarms.

5. Characteristics of Alarm Systems

   a. Sensitivity: The probability that a true event will be detected. For alarms, it is the probability that an alarm sounds when an event has occurred

   b. Specificity: The probability that no event will be detected when no event is present. For alarms, it is the probability that an alarm will not sound when an event has not occurred.

   c. False-alarm rate: The probability that when an alarm sounds, it does not indicate a true event.

   d. Alarm limits, alarm thresholds: The value or level at which an alarm will sound. See also decision criteria, β.

   e. Default parameters: Alarm limits that have been preset to typical, acceptable, standard values. Default parameters are at default values upon initiating clinical monitor, and typically return to default values when the patient is discharged from the monitor.

6. Signal Detection Theory

   a. Signal-to-noise ratio: The clarity of a signal, as measured by the strength of the desired signal compared with the random disruptions present in the signal. In clinical monitoring, it can relate to the relationship between the underlying physiology being measured and the measured parameter representing it.

   b. d' ("dee prime"): The discriminability index or sensitivity index indicating how discernable a true event is from a nonevent. This is a specific type of signal-to-noise ratio determined by the characteristics of the monitored parameter and the technology used to monitor it. The value is calculated using the magnitude of the difference in the parameter's value between normal and abnormal states (separation), and the variability in each state (spread).

   c. β ("Beta"): The decision criteria. The threshold at which a monitored parameter is considered abnormal. It is determined by the operator of the system. In clinical monitoring, changes in the β are expressed as changes in alarm limits, which determine the proportion of false alarms to true alarms, and the proportion of misses to correctly identified nonevents.

   d. Base rate: The prevalence or frequency of a condition or event within a given population, often expressed as the probability of an event occurring. In clinical monitoring, it may be the *a priori* probability that a particular clinical condition will arise during a given case or epoch.

Clinical monitoring systems indicate more than the presence or absence of an alarm. They additionally classify its severity. In most systems, a *tiered* or graded classification of events is used, where alarms are classified into classes such as message, advisory, warning, or crisis. Each class of alarm may have a unique annunciation pattern (Table 13-2). Such tiered responses can help clinicians respond appropriately to the urgency of an event (Table 13-3). Alarms at a particular tier can trigger automatic actions in the monitoring system. All crisis alarm events, for example, may initiate permanent archiving of the alarm log in the central monitoring database, while warnings would be stored only until a patient is discharged. Arrhythmia alarms can trigger automatic printouts of ECG strips.

The potential consequence of a miss—death or serious injury of the patient—is much greater than the potential consequence of a false alarm: distraction or annoyance of the healthcare provider. For this reason most medical monitors are set up with a high sensitivity for events, leading to a relatively high rate of false alarms. In some clinical situations, the provider can adjust decision thresholds to reduce the incidence of false alarms (e.g., increasing the threshold for counting premature ventricular contractions [PVCs]). In other situations this is not possible, especially when the false alarm is due to an abrupt change in the clinical situation (e.g., cessation of spontaneous ventilation with induction of anesthesia). To reduce distractions, therefore, most clinical alarms offer the ability to pause the alarm before it sounds or silence (suspend or disable) the alarm when it does sound. In these situations the alarm has served its purpose—the provider has acknowledged it—and distraction can then be reduced. Message, advisory, and warning alarms can usually be permanently disabled by the user (e.g., the PVC alarm when the patient has a pacemaker). Latched critical alarms can usually only be paused or suspended (e.g., the low tidal volume alarm on a ventilator).

Table 13–2 A Prototypical Example of Visual and Auditory Coding Showing a Tiered Response to Events of Differing Severity

Alarm Level	Visual Coding	Auditory Coding
Message	Flashing text in yellow	No auditory component
Advisory	Flashing text or parameter in red	One beep, not repeated
Warning	Flashing text or parameter value in red highlighting	Two beeps, repeated for 3 min
Crisis	Flashing text or parameter value in red highlighting	Three beeps, repeated until silenced (latched)

Table 13–3 Examples of a Typical Classification of Events at Different Levels of Urgency/Severity

Crisis	Warning	Advisory	Message
Asystole Ventricular fibrillation (VFib) Ventricular tachycardia (VTach)	Heart rate high CO_2 no breath Spo_2 low	CO_2 high	Leads fail Bigeminy Premature ventricular contraction (PVC)

Though typical, the classifications are not standardized. Many of these specific events can be assigned by the user to a given type of alarm as appropriate on a per-unit basis.

Strategies for Interacting with Alarm Systems

In a given monitoring situation, there are only two fundamental techniques for improving the performance of an alarm system. The first is to improve the signal-to-noise ratio. The second is to adjust the decision criteria.

The signal-to-noise ratio is changed either by (1) reducing the amount of noise or (2) improving the sensing of the true event. In practical, clinical terms, the way to improve discrimination is to eliminate artifacts in the data; ensure that the contact between the patient and the sensors is good, and that other events within the clinical environment do not impinge upon the sensors. For electrocardiography (ECG), lowering the impedance of the electrode by using an abrasive skin prep can reduce artifacts and "noise," as will making sure the leads are placed correctly (see also Chapter 9). Adjusting the position or location of the pulse oximeter probe can improve the signal and reduce artifacts. Appropriate maintenance and periodic testing of equipment is useful as well (see Chapter 3).

An alternative method of improving the signal-to-noise ratio is to change the technology used to sense events. Changing from a noninvasive monitor such as a pulse oximeter to an invasive monitor such as an arterial line will fundamentally change the distribution of the signal and noise. These efforts may make the true event less like the nonevent, improving the signal-to-noise ratio and improving the d'.

The second general strategy for changing the ratio of false alarms to true alarms is to adjust the decision criteria, β, which signifies the threshold of what constitutes an "event." Unlike changing the d', which can improve a system's overall performance, adjusting the decision criteria involves a tradeoff between high sensitivity (not missing a true event) and high specificity (not having false alarms). Interaction with the alarm system should be managed to establish optimal alarm limits. When initiating monitoring on a patient, it is likely that the default alarm limits preset on the monitor should be adjusted to reflect the patient's baseline physiology and any relevant clinical indications (Figure 13-3). For example, healthy, athletic patients may have different resting heart rates than "average" patients; patients at risk of hemorrhagic stroke require more conservative limits for blood pressure.

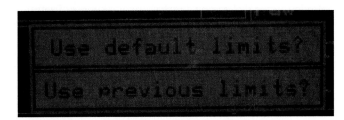

Figure 13–3 Alarm limits should be set upon initiation of monitoring and adjusted as needed. Many anesthesia machines provide the option of using default or previous alarm limit settings upon initiation of monitoring. *(From Ohmeda.)*

Many care providers find alarms to be a nuisance and will react by disabling them or setting detection thresholds inappropriately high or low. This removes any benefit that might derive from an alarm system. More experienced clinicians will make the small investment of effort to adjust monitors and alarms appropriately, on the basis that this will increase the predictive value of alarms, reduce nuisance alarms, and ultimately improve the margin of safety.

Common Alarms

In monitoring, it is useful to differentiate parameter alarms from alarms regarding the monitoring system itself. Parameter alarms indicate patient status and are designed to indicate clinically relevant change to the patient. System alarms may relate to the status or function of system components, such as a vaporizer, ventilator, gas supply, breathing circuit, or others. When these alarms sound, they do not indicate an immediate clinical problem with the patient, although they may indicate the potential for one. They can indicate an equipment malfunction, or the absence of data regarding the patient. Some monitoring systems differentiate system and parameter alarms by using different annunciator patterns for each.

In general, system alarms can be avoided through good maintenance and careful preanesthesia machine checkout [8-10] (see Chapter 3). System alarms may indicate a true failure of equipment, or may require recalibration or resetting of some component of the monitoring and anesthesia system.

Ideally, parameter alarms would indicate only true clinically relevant conditions that have arisen in the patient. Often, however, parameter alarms result from poor signal-to-noise ratio of the monitored parameter, and do not indicate a clinically relevant event. Appropriate responses to these alarms may be to adjust the transducer to improve the signal-to-noise ratio, or to adjust the alarm thresholds to optimize the decision criteria, β.

In responding to alarms, the initial goal should be to determine the validity of the alarm, discerning whether the alarm truly indicates a malfunction of equipment or a meaningful change in patient status. The number of possible alarms in anesthesia monitoring is large. However, a relatively small number of equipment and parameter alarms will comprise the majority of alarms encountered by practitioners. A compendium of typical alarms is provided (Table 13-4), listing for each alarm the potential causes for a true and false alarm and appropriate responses to such an alarm to determine the validity. While by no means exhaustive, it can serve as a foundation for developing a repertoire of responses useful in responding to alarms.

Responding to Critical Alarms

The anesthesia provider's job is to ensure the patient's safety and comfort throughout a surgical procedure. As such, the provider has a close and continuous interaction with monitoring and therapeutic technology. Responding to alerts and alarms is a significant part of this job.

First, of course, the experienced provider will set alarm limits before starting the case, or at the earliest appropriate point after monitoring is started. This task can be simplified for every case if the clinical engineers set defaults when the monitoring system is installed that will provide consistent sensitivity and specificity for the average patient having a common procedure. For some alarms (low F_iO_2, hypoxia, line isolation failure) these are relatively absolute across all cases. For others (high heart rate, respiratory rate, blood pressure) the kind of patients and cases being done will affect the ideal default settings. Pediatric patients, for example, will routinely and safely experience high heart rates that would be disastrous in an adult vascular surgery population. Some alarm limits should be set individually at the start of the case: ventilation parameters, for example, or blood pressure boundaries. Even with attentive advance efforts, however, surgery and anesthesia are physiologically dynamic and it is likely that there will be alerts and alarms throughout any case. The following is a simplified approach to a provider response.

First step: Determine reality. When an alarm occurs in the operating room (OR), the anesthesia provider should immediately determine which device is reacting and what change of state is being indicated. This will determine the priority of the provider's response, relative to other activities. Some alarms, such as a ventilator disconnection or loss of oxygen inflow, require an immediate response, whereas others, such as an elevated heart rate or a fluid warmer overheating, can be dealt with once other priorities have been managed. Changes in patient state, such as cessation of spontaneous breathing with the induction of anesthesia, produce predictable nuisance alarms that can be ignored until homeostasis is restored, the patient is intubated, and mechanical ventilation is started. Watching for these alarms to resolve spontaneously is one indicator that the case is going well.

Experienced providers will assess where on the spectrum of severity the alarm lies, ranging from pure artifacts through true alarms that are physiologically inconsequential to true alarms that indicate a real risk. This assessment is usually accomplished through rapid correlation of the information from the alarming monitor with all of the other information available.

Alarms disrupt the workflow and increase tension throughout the clinical environment,[6,11] and experienced providers often rapidly silence alarms as an early step in the diagnostic process of determining the alarm's cause. This is different from not paying attention to the alarm; rather, it is removing a distraction to allow one to think clearly about its causation.

Indications that an alarm is most likely due to an artifact include:

- Sudden changes in value from an established baseline, without an obvious inciting event
- Transient changes, with rapid return to normal
- A change indicated on only one monitor (e.g., oximeter heart rate but not ECG heart rate)
- Occurrence only during electrocautery use (suggests electrical interference) or NIBP cycling (transient vascular occlusion distally)

Indications that an alarm is due to a real change which is *not* clinically significant include:

- Values on a single monitor only slightly different than normal
- Variations within the normal measuring error of the device
- Transient variations associated with surgical maneuvers or change in bed position
- Variations associated with baseline patient characteristics (e.g., frequent unifocal PVCs)

Indications that an alarm is real and relevant include:

- Multiple alarms at the same time, from different devices
- Alarms associated with sudden changes on the field (e.g., rapid bleeding)
- Alarms occurring at predictable high-risk moments (e.g., ST segment changes after aortic cross-clamping)
- Alarms with a very high specificity (e.g., loss of wall oxygen pressure)

Second step: Assess and treat the patient. Once the reality of the alarm has been assessed, the provider should check the patient and the state of the surgical procedure, while responding to the alarm based on the most serious and most common possible causes. For some alarms, physical examination of skin color and temperature, chest rise and fall, carotid and radial pulse, and bilateral breath sounds can rapidly rule in or out the most serious changes in physiology. Physical examination should proceed to treatment as needed for changes that are determined to be real and significant. These may include suctioning secretions or changing ventilator settings, adjustment of anesthesia depth or agents, administration of fluids or blood products, or other indicated care up to and including the initiation of cardiopulmonary resuscitation (CPR) and advanced cardiac life support (ACLS) protocols.

Sometimes it is not possible to determine whether or not an alarm is real and significant. An example might be moderate hypoxia (SpO_2 of 92%) occurring in a high-risk patient. This might be due to real hypoxemia, or it might be a monitoring error due to poor peripheral circulation. An event like this requires further testing, usually by sending a blood sample for

Table 13–4 Alarms, with True and False Causes

Alarm	True Alarm	False Alarm	Response to Alarm
ECG	Tachycardia	Agitation of ungrounded cable; electrocautery interference	Confirm with oximeter and palpate pulse
	Bradycardia	Failure to sense	Check leads and cable; confirm with oximeter and palpate pulse
	PVCs, ventricular beats	Motion artifact, pacer, unusual native rhythm	Readjust sensitivities and alarm threshold
	ST segment elevation/depression	Bad lead placement or monitor settings	Confirm lead placement and monitor settings; assess clinical significance
OXIMETER	Tachycardia	Double counting of P or T waves; electrocautery interference	Confirm with ECG and palpate pulse
	Bradycardia	Failure to capture, cold	Confirm with ECG and palpate pulse, move sensor to a different site
	Hypoxemia	Cold patient, NIBP cycling or other transient vascular obstruction	Check ventilator function; send ABG; move sensor to different site
VENTILATOR	Low F_iO_2	Bad Clark electrode	Check oximeter and ventilator settings; recalibrate/replace electrode
	Low tidal volume	Bad flowmeter; circuit or machine leak	Clean or replace flowmeter; tighten circuit connections and CO_2 canister; replace circuit; check ETT for leak
	High pressure	Circuit obstruction; kinking or biting ETT	Suction patient; check circuit visually; redose muscle relaxant or add bite block
CAPNOMETER	Hypercapnia	Always real	Check ventilator settings; clinical correlation, including ruling out malignant hyperthermia; readjust alarm parameters
	Hypocapnia/no breath	Tubing disconnect or occlusion; sensor misposition or failure	Check ventilator; listen for breath sounds; replace monitoring pathway/cables
	Tachypnea	Partial occlusion of circuit or tubing	Suction patient, check ventilator settings and muscle relaxant level
IV PUMP	Occlusion	Temporary obstruction, bolus IV injection	Check line from bag to patient, check IV site, restart
	Air in line	Microbubbles, bad sensor contact	Visually inspect line; flush with fluid; clean and reseat sensor; restart
NONINVASIVE BP	Hypertension	Inappropriately small cuff; extreme vasoconstriction	Check cuff placement, repeat measure
	Hypotension	Inappropriately large or mispositioned cuff; temporary or chronic isolated vascular obstruction	Check cuff placement, check pulse distal to cuff, change arms
	Failure to measure	Mispositioned cuff, hose disconnection, leak in hose or cuff, or obstruction	Check pulse, check cuff position, check tubing, change arms, remove external pressure on cuff or tubing (e.g., move surgeon)
ARTERIAL LINE	Hypertension	"Whip," bad calibration, dropped transducer	Check transducer position and rezero; flush line; remove extra segments of tubing. If "whip," consider deliberate introduction of small air bubble to damp
	Hypotension	Bad calibration; elevated transducer; damping from air bubble; thrombosis in artery	Flush catheter; check transducer position and rezero; aspirate blood
FLUID WARMER	Overheating	Low water level, tipping or sloshing; no flow through heater	If water bath warmer, check water level, turn off and allow to cool before restarting
LINE ISOLATION MONITOR	Ground fault	"Gremlins"	Unplug last device plugged in and reset alarm; repeat as needed; send failed device for service
ICP MONITOR	High ICP	Loss of calibration; obstruction of measuring line; stopcock misdirected	Rezero; check fluid path from brain to sensor; consult neurosurgery to flush catheter

ABG, Arterial blood gas; *ECG,* electrocardiograph; *ETT,* endotracheal tube; *F_iO_2,* fraction of inspired oxygen; *ICP,* intracranial pressure; *IV,* intravenous; *NIBP,* noninvasive blood pressure; *PVC,* premature ventricular contraction.

analysis of arterial blood gases, hemoglobin concentration, or electrolyte levels. An alternative approach is provocative testing with a low-risk treatment, to see if the problem is resolved. In the example given, an increase in PEEP on the ventilator from 5 to 10 would resolve hypoxia if it was due to developing atelectasis. Use of a fluid bolus to address a fall in blood pressure is another example. This kind of real-time "experimentation" is common and important in anesthesia practice, but has two important pitfalls. First is the use of "temporizing" therapies that cover up the underlying pathology without identifying it. In the example given previously, hypoxia could be addressed by an increase in the F_iO_2. This would very likely silence the alarm, but would not address the most likely underlying physiological problem: developing atelectasis. A better "experiment" would be to perform a manual recruitment maneuver and increase the PEEP. This would also improve oxygen saturation and silence the alarm, but in a much more productive fashion. The second pitfall with "experimentation" is making too many changes at once, thus making it impossible to know which was the most beneficial. An example would be responding to a fall in blood pressure by simultaneously administering an inotropic agent, decreasing the anesthetic dose, and administering fluid. While likely to be successful in silencing the alarm, the provider will not know if the underlying problem was hypovolemia, anesthetic overdose, or impaired myocardial contractility.

Third step: Reset and readjust the alarms. Finally, once appropriate patient care has been provided, the provider should consider the alarm itself. In general, the more real and significant the alarm was, the less need there is to readjust it. Correcting the underlying physiology should cause the alarm to resolve. For artifacts or clinically irrelevant alarms, it may be useful to reset the alarm parameters to prevent repeated indicators from creating a distraction. Remember that there are primarily two ways to influence false-alarm rates in a case: adjusting your decision criteria (β) by adjusting alarm limits; and improving your discrimination (d') by making sure your transducers are getting good readings, thus improving the signal-to-noise ratio.

Challenges in Clinical Monitoring

The complexity of physiology, the nebulous definitions of "normal," and the difficulty posed by monitoring a safe process are three core challenges for clinicians. Compared with clinical monitoring, monitoring in manufacturing is simple because the parameters in manufacturing are generally stable for a given industrial process; in clinical monitoring, patient physiology varies from patient to patient, and is homeostatic—influencing vital signs independent of the clinician's actions.[12] Furthermore, the definition of normal and abnormal clinical values for vital signs is not uniform across patients. Even for a given patient, the targeted or "normal" values for vital signs can change drastically depending on context.[13] For example, heart rate may be kept depressed because of the depth of anesthesia before the initial incision, knowing that the surgical stimulation will raise the level of arousal; a care provider may want end-tidal CO_2 levels to be high during emergence to stimulate spontaneous breathing. Values that indicate a clinically significant event under certain circumstances may be expected and considered normal in other situations.

This lack of consistent criteria for normal and abnormal values creates a difficult problem for interacting with alarm systems: high false-alarm rates. False-alarm rates of 70% to 95% have been reported. While this statistic may seem unacceptable, it may be more a function of the inherent safety of anesthesia monitoring rather than an indication of the poor quality of the monitoring systems. In examining the relative rates of true alarms and false alarms, it is important to consider the underlying prevalence of true "event" that an alarm is intended to indicate, the base rate. Even with high sensitivity and specificity, in situations where a true "event" is rare, the proportion of true alarms to false alarms will often be unacceptably high.

Consider two examples with an alarm system that has 99% sensitivity (i.e., misses 1 of every 100 true alarm situations) and 99% specificity (only has 1 false alarm in 100 nonalarm situations).

When monitoring for an event with a base rate of 50% (i.e. a true event occurs in half of the cases that are monitored), for every 10,000 possible alarm situations, there will be 5000 true events, and 5000 nonevents. Of the 5000 events, 4950 will be correctly identified as events—the alarm will sound—and 50 of those events will be missed. Similarly, of the 5000 nonevents, 4950 will be recognized as nonevents, and 50 will be misdiagnosed as true events (false alarms). Thus the probability of an alarm indicating a true event would be (4950 true events causing alarms)/(4950 true positive + 50 false positive)], which is 99%.

With those same numbers but an event base rate of 1% instead of 50%, of the 10,000 possible alarm situations, there will be only 100 true events. Ninety nine of those will be identified as events correctly, and one will be missed. In comparison, 9900 will be nonevents, and 1% (99) will be misdiagnosed as true events (false alarms). In this scenario, even with the same 99% specificity and sensitivity, the probability of a true event when an alarm sounds is only 50% (99 true alarms/[99 true alarms + 99 false alarms]).

When the base rate is 1 in 1000 (0.1%), the probability of a given alarm indicating a true event drops to only 1%, which is a false-alarm rate of 99%.

Thus, even with well-implemented alarm systems, monitoring a generally safe process (i.e., low base rate of true events) will inevitably lead to a high proportion of false to true alarms.

The above fact reveals another paradox of clinical monitoring. Ironically, assigning more patients to monitored beds "just to be safe" will have the opposite effect. Having healthier patients on monitors will lower the base rate of true clinically relevant events, which will increase the probability of a false alarm.

There is also a "cry wolf" problem that arises from such situations.[14] Human behavior is such that if an alarm is perceived to be a false alarm 60% of the time, people will "probability match" their response to the perceived rate, discounting or ignoring the alarm 60% of time,[15] even though this strategy may lead to suboptimal results. With a higher false-alarm rate, there will be a larger "cry wolf" effect, and care providers are less likely to respond to a true alarm when it does occur.[16]

The legal system in which modern medicine is practiced also has an impact on alarm systems. Manufacturers are likely to be held accountable for clinical monitors that miss true events. Therefore, they will drive the sensitivity of their systems toward its maximum value. Manufacturers have much less incentive to maximize specificity.

Future Trends

The solution to the problem of false alarms, as previously discussed, is largely a structural problem: the safer the overall system, the lower the base rate of true events, and the higher the probability of a false alarm. However, there are promising technologies that may help to reduce false alarms. Simple techniques have shown some efficacy, such as simply delaying the onset of alarms sounding by a few seconds to reduce transient alarms.[17,18] More fundamentally, better transducers or new monitoring technologies may be developed, leading to better signal-to-noise ratios. Various forms of artificial intelligence are being developed using techniques such as neural network programming and fuzzy logic to filter false alarms more effectively.[19,20] In some proposed systems, alarm thresholds are defined partly as deviations from the current patient state as opposed to strict numerical limits.[21,22] Using artificial intelligence, monitoring systems can concentrate or collect information from various sources ("data fusion") and develop contextual models of patients, effectively troubleshooting potential alarm situations before an alarm is sounded, thus reducing nuisance alarms.[23,24] For example, using arterial blood pressure waveform as a reference to verify the veracity of critical ECG alarms reduced false alarms by nearly 60%.[5] While the literature is replete with proposed technological solutions dating back nearly two decades, adoption of intelligent alarm filtering into current patient monitors has been slow. No matter how effective the filtering becomes, any system that decreases sensitivity would likely be rejected for legal reasons: the cost of missing a true event is often unacceptable.

Improvements are also still needed to address the problem of alarm cascades that result from sudden and dramatic changes in patient state. At such times, multiple alarms can obscure the primary source from its antecedents. Intelligent alarm systems should prioritize alarms and present a diagnosis of the problem's source, as opposed to a list of observed problems. As alarm systems become more sophisticated, they may evolve to resemble decision support systems for diagnosis and treatment.

In principle, a future alarm would be part of an integrated patient monitoring solution (see also Chapter 30). In such a system, the information from the suite of instrumentation in the care environment (ventilators, anesthesia machines, IV pumps, patient monitors, electrocautery, etc.) would all be considered by a central alarm management system. That system could perform many of the initial status checks and verifications that the care providers currently perform. Such a system could sense not only the state of the patient and the equipment being used, but also create a model of the events external to the patient to intelligently adjust alarm limits appropriately. While the literature is full of demonstrations of individual components of this vision, the realization of such a vision seems quite distant. Care providers can expect incremental improvements in sensitivity and specificity, but should not anticipate a full technological solution in the near term.

In the interim, great benefits can be attained by sticking to the basics: ensure a good signal from transducers to improve the signal-to-noise ratio, and set alarm thresholds appropriately to optimize your decision criteria.

References

1. Sorkin, R.D., Woods, D.D., 1985. Systems with human monitors, a signal detection analysis. Hum Comput Interact 1, 49–75.
2. Kestin, I.G., Miller, B.R., Lockhart, D.O., 1988. Auditory alarms during anesthesia monitoring. Anesthesiology 69 (1), 106–109.
3. Meredith, C., Edworthy, J., 1995. Are there too many alarms in the intensive care unit? An overview of the problems. J Adv Nurs 21 (1), 15–20.
4. Block, F.E., Schaaf, C., 1996. Auditory alarms during anesthesia monitoring with an integrated monitoring system. Int J Clin Monit Comput 13 (2), 81–84.
5. Grumet, G.W., 1993. Pandemonium in the modern hospital. N Engl J Med 329 (3), 211–212.
6. Topf, M., Dillon, E., 1988. Noise-induced stress as a predictor of burnout in critical care nurses. Heart Lung 17, 567–573.
7. Green, D.M., Swets, J.A., 1966. Signal detection theory and psychophysics. Wiley, New York.
8. Subcommittee of ASA Committee on Equipment and Facilities 2008. Recommendations for pre-anesthesia checkout procedures (2008). ASA. Available at http://www.asahq.org/clinical/finalcheckoutdesignguidelines02.08-2008.pdf.
9. Cooper, J.B., Newbower, R.S., Kitz, R.J., 1984. An analysis of major errors and equipment failures in anesthesia management: considerations for prevention and detection. Anesthesiology 60, 34–42.
10. The Association of Anaesthetists of Great Britain and Ireland 2004. Checking anaesthetic equipment, 3. AAGBI, London. See www.aagbi.org/pdf/Check_Anae_Equip.pdf.
11. Donchin, Y., Seagull, F.J., 2002. The hostile environment of the intensive care unit. Curr Opin Crit Care 8 (4), 316–320 (review).
12. Botney, R., Gaba, D.M., 1995. Human factors issues in monitoring. In: Blitt, C.D., Hines, R.L. (Eds.), Monitoring in anesthesia and critical care medicine, ed 3. Churchill Livingstone, New York.
13. Seagull, F.J., Sanderson, P.M., 2001. Anesthesia alarms in context: an observational study. Hum Factors 43 (1), 66–78.
14. Bliss, J.P., Gilson, R.D., Deaton, J.E., 1995. Human probability matching behavior in response to alarms of varying reliability. Ergonomics 38 (11), 2300–2313.
15. Breznitz, S., 1984. Cry wolf: the psychology of false alarms. Lawrence Erlbaum Associates, Hillsdale, NJ.
16. Xiao, Y., Seagull, F.J., Nieves-Khouw, F., et al., 2004. Organizational-historical analysis of the failure to respond to alarm problem. IEEE Trans Syst Man Cybern A Syst Hum 34 (6), 772–778.
17. Görges, M., Markewitz, B.A., Westenskow, D.R., 2009. Improving alarm performance in the medical intensive care unit using delays and clinical context. Anesth Analg 108 (5), 1546–1552.
18. Rheineck-Leyssius, A.T., Kalkman, C.J., 1998. Influence of pulse oximeter settings on the frequency of alarms and detection of hypoxemia: theoretical effects of artifact rejection, alarm delay, averaging, median filtering or a lower setting of the alarm limit. J Clin Monit Comput 14, 151–156.
19. Lowe, A., Harrison, M., Jones, R., 1999. Diagnostic monitoring in anaesthesia using fuzzy trend templates for matching temporal patterns. Artif Intell Med 16 (2), 183–199.
20. Orr, J.A., Westenskow, D.R., 1994. A breathing circuit alarm system based on neural networks. J Clin Monit 10 (2), 101–109.
21. Charbonnier, S., Gentil, S., 2007. A trend-based alarm system to improve patient monitoring in intensive care units. Control Eng Pract 15 (9), 1039–1050.
22. Connor, C.W., Gohil, B., Harrison, M.J., 2009. Triggering of systolic arterial pressure alarms using statistics-based versus threshold alarms. Anaesthesia 64 (2), 131–135.
23. Clifford, G.D., Aboukhalil, A., Sun, J.X., et al., 2006. Using the blood pressure waveform to reduce critical false ECG alarms. Comput Cardiol 33, 829–832.
24. Blum, J.M., Kruger, G.H., Sanders, K.L., et al., 2009. Specificity improvement for network distributed physiologic alarms based on a simple deterministic reactive intelligent agent in the critical care environment. J Clin Monit Comput 23 (1), 21–30.
25. Aboukhalil, A., Nielsen, L., Saeed, M., et al., 2008. Reducing false alarm rates for critical arrhythmias using the arterial blood pressure waveform. J Biomed Inform 41 (3), 442–451.

Suggested Reading

Sorkin, R.D., Woods, D.D., 1985. Systems with human monitors, a signal detection analysis. Hum Comput Interact 1, 49–75. *This early paper provides a further introduction to signal detection theory and applies the theory to situations, such as clinical monitoring, where the operator relies on the alarms for alerting to potential problems. A "dual signal detection" model is presented, which introduces the idea that the alarm is but one source of information, taken with other sources of information available. It presents an interesting way of envisioning the monitoring system as a combination of technology and human judgment working together, as opposed to two independent sources of vigilance over the patient. The accuracy of the monitoring system, it notes, should be measured by the end actions of the operator, not the alerting actions of the monitor.*

Kestin, I.G., Miller, B.T., Lockhart, C.H., 1988. Auditory alarms during anesthesia monitoring. Anesthesiology 69, 106. *This often-cited study was among the seminal efforts to document the scope of the alarm problem. In this in situ study, observations within the operating room were classified alarms as artifact, nuisance, or true issues of patient risk. Results emphasized the low predictive value that alarms carry and the degree to which alarms typically fail to achieve their canonical function of alerting a clinician to a real problem.*

Takla G., Petre J.H., Doyle D.J., et al., 2006. The problem of artifacts in patient monitor data during surgery: a clinical and methodological review. Anesth Analg 103, 1196–1204. *Because artifacts are a major contributor to false alarms in monitoring, this work provides a broad view of artifacts for a number of parameters that are typically monitored. Largely technical, the review provides more in-depth coverage of the approaches to artifact reduction used in current monitor systems and discusses types of filtering strategies and artificial intelligence techniques.*

Chapter 14

Equipment for Regional Anesthesia and Acute Pain Management

Reuben Slater and Lisa Warren

Regional anesthetic techniques are used to render a portion of the body insensate for the purposes of operative anesthesia or postoperative analgesia. The basis of regional anesthesia is selective neural blockade with local anesthetics. A precise knowledge of anatomy is required to locate the neural structures, and an understanding of pharmacology is required to manipulate the density and duration of blockade. A range of equipment is available to aid in anatomic location and delivery of local anesthetic agents.

Anatomical Classification of Regional Anesthetic Techniques

Regional anesthetic techniques can be classified based on anatomical regions:
  Neuraxial: Spinal and epidural
  Truncal: Paravertebral, transversus abdominis plane
  Peripheral: brachial plexus, lumbo-sacral plexus, distal nerves, intravenous regional anesthesia
Location of specific neural structures has traditionally relied on a solid understanding of surface anatomy and eliciting paresthesia. Use of nerve stimulators and ultrasound may play a role in improving safety and efficiency of block performance.[1]

Delivery of local anesthetics during nerve blocks may be performed with a simple hypodermic needle; however, many modifications of needle design have been made to facilitate performance and potentially improve safety. This chapter will not discuss intravenous regional anesthesia, and we refer you to the following reference.[2]

General Considerations

Treating Early Complications

Early complications of regional anesthesia, though rare, may be life-threatening and require immediate medical intervention. They include intravascular injection of local anesthetic leading to systemic toxicity and complete spinal anesthesia (which is most commonly seen in neuraxial techniques but may also be a complication of interscalene, paravertebral, or ophthalmic blockade). Patients undergoing regional anesthesia may be exposed to anaphylactic triggers, and vasovagal reactions are not uncommon. To perform regional anesthesia safely, all patients should be monitored as defined in the American Society of Anesthesiologists standards,[3] and sufficient resuscitation equipment should be available to provide advanced cardiac life support.

Recent animal experiments and human case reports suggest that lipid emulsion (Intralipid 20%) may reverse the cardiac toxicity of local anesthetics.[4] Although this use of intralipid is "off-label," it is currently stocked as part of standard resuscitation supplies in many hospitals practicing regional techniques.

Preventing Infectious Complications

Strict aseptic technique should be followed when practicing regional anesthesia, to prevent infectious complications. Commercially available sterile solutions including alcohol, povidone-iodine, and chlorhexidine gluconate (with and without isopropyl alcohol) are available for skin disinfection, although none is specifically FDA approved for use in regional anesthesia (spinal, epidural, or peripheral nerve block) povidone-iodine has been used safely for many years, provided that it is allowed to dry on the skin before needle insertion. Recent research demonstrates that alcohol-based chlorhexidine solution has superior antimicrobial coverage and bactericidal activity compared to that of povidone-iodine solution. The use of chlorhexidine is now currently recommended for peripheral nerve and epidural blocks.[5] Due to concerns about possible neurotoxicity of chlorhexidine, and given the paucity of clinical studies, the FDA has not formally approved its use for skin antisepsis before lumbar puncture. There is no current data to support the use of sterile gowns to reduce the incidence of infection associated with regional anesthesia, and their use should be adopted based on individual or institutional guidelines. However it would seem prudent to use full aseptic technique when performing catheter-based techniques. Careful hand hygiene and sterile surgical gloves must be used to protect patients from contamination and healthcare workers from blood-borne pathogen exposure.

Providing Equipment

Specific carts for peripheral or neuraxial blockade allow practitioners to bring all the required equipment to the patient in an efficient manner. By having carts that can be locked one can protect valuable equipment and allow medications to be securely colocated.

Sterile kits containing the equipment to perform specific blocks may be purchased. Typically these kits contain skin preparation, drapes, and the needles and syringes required to deliver local anesthetic superficially and perform the block itself. Preprepared kits may be an efficient and economical way of providing equipment to an anesthesia practitioner (Figure 14–1).

Needles

A large variety of needles are available for regional anesthesia (Figure 14–2). The features used to describe a needle are its hub type, length, diameter, and tip shape. Special features unique to regional anesthesia are insulation (to facilitate nerve stimulation) and echogenicity (to improve visualization under ultrasound).

HUB

In 1925 B&D introduced the Luer slip and Luer lock system for attaching needles to syringes. This system is now the standard in the United States and is described by the International Standards Organization.[6] The system involves a tapered (6% taper) male attachment, and matching female component made of metal or plastic. The taper allows the components to be held together by friction in the Luer slip system, whereas the Luer lock system has a built-in screw mechanism (Figure 14–3).

LENGTH

The length of needle chosen is determined by the anatomic location in which it is to be used. Needle length is typically described in either centimeter or inch long measurements. Longer needles are more difficult to control as a small

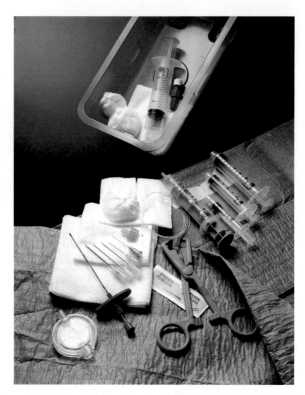

Figure 14–1 A prepackaged regional anesthesia kit. *(From Al-Shaikh B, Stacey S, editors. Essentials of anaesthetic equipment, ed 3, Philadelphia, Churchill Livingstone, 2007, Figure 12.8.)*

movement at the hub is amplified at the tip. They are also more likely to flex. This may contribute to uncertainty about the position of the tip and increased likelihood of needle fracture. Needles may also be designed with length markings (typically in cm along the shaft), which are especially useful in determining the distance a needle or catheter has been inserted.

DIAMETER

The outer diameter of medical needles is typically represented using the Stubbs Iron Wire Gauge system (which is also known as the Birmingham Wire Gauge System). In this system of measurement, gauge is inversely proportional to the outside diameter of the needle. The diameter of the needles lumen is determined by the manufacturing process. Inner needle diameter determines resistance to flow on injection (Table 14–1).

The French gauge system, denoted by Fr, FR, or F, is also used to measure the outer diameter of needles and catheters. In this system, dividing the French gauge measurement by 3 gives the outer diameter in millimeters. For example, a 12-Fr catheter would have a 4-mm outer diameter.

TIP SHAPE

The key feature of most needles is the shape of the tip, a wide variety of tip shapes are used during regional anesthetic techniques. A typical hypodermic needle is a metal tube cut obliquely at its distal end; this cut gives the needle its primary bevel, which determines the length of its end orifice (Figure 14–4). In turn the bevel is angled to make the needle sharp. Sharp-tipped, or "A" bevel (12- to 15-degree angle), needles pass through skin and underlying tissues with minimal disruption, decreasing pain associated with insertion and injection.

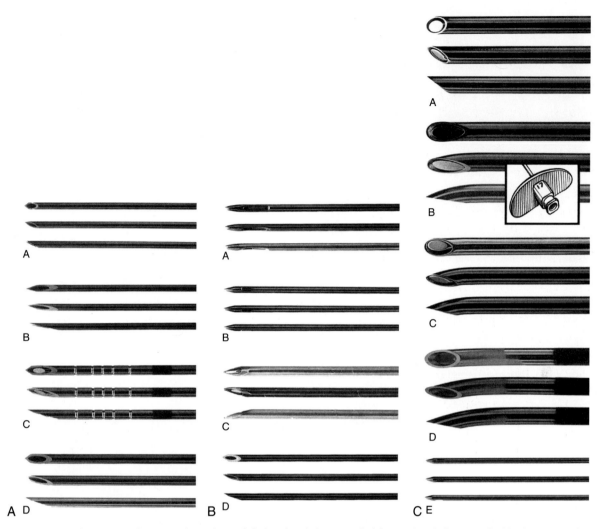

Figure 14–2 A range of needles used in regional anesthesia: **(A)** Blunt-beveled 25g needle (A), Long-beveled 25g needle (B), Ultrasonography Imaging needle (C), Short-beveled needle (D); **(B)** Sprotte needle (A), Whitacre needle (B), Greene needle (C), Quinke needle (D); **(C)** Crawford needle (A), Tuohy needle (B), Hustead needle (C), Curved 18g Epidural needle (D), Whitacre 27g Spinal needle (E). *(From Brown DL, Rosenquist W, Sites BD, Spence BC, Local Anesthetics and Regional Anesthesia Equipment. In Brown D. Atlas of regional anesthesia, ed 3, Saunders-Elsevier, 2006, Figures 1.6, 1.7, 1.8.)*

Short bevel needles (18- to 30-degree angle) disrupt tissue layers as they pass through, thus allowing the user to feel "clicks" and "pops" as the needle passes through fascial planes.

NEEDLE TIPS FOR SPINAL ANESTHESIA

Spinal needles come with a variety of tip shapes (Figure 14–5). The most simple tip is a cutting edge that resembles the "A" bevel hypodermic needle, this is also known as a "Quincke" tip. Pencil point spinal needles were introduced in an attempt to decrease the incidence of postdural puncture headache (PDPH).[7] These needles have a conical tip with a lateral distal aperture. Common examples are the "Sprotte" and "Whitaker" needles. These needle tips may also spread nerve fibers rather than cut them or may produce a traumatic hole in the dura, which acts as a focus for fibroblast activity.[8]

NEEDLE TIPS FOR EPIDURAL ANESTHESIA

The most popular styles of epidural needle have noncoring tips (Figure 14–6). Noncoring needles have an end that is curved so that the distal orifice is on the lateral aspect. The leading edge of the needle may be sharpened or rounded.

NEEDLE TIPS FOR PERIPHERAL NERVE BLOCKS

There is controversy about the appropriate needle tip for performing peripheral nerve blocks. Sharp needles have the benefit of causing less discomfort to the patient; however, some authors feel that sharp needles are more likely to pierce nerves, rather than laterally displace them. As mentioned previously, blunt needles provide better "feel" and may be more likely to deflect nerves rather than pierce them. However, if a blunt needle does penetrate a nerve, it may be more traumatic.[9]

ECHOGENICITY

The introduction of ultrasound-guided regional anesthesia has led to the development of a new group of needles that are more visible under ultrasound. These needles may have echogenic markers or etching at the tip (e.g., Echostim, Havel's Inc., Cincinnati) or may have a special coating, (e.g., Nanoline, Pajunk, Geisingen, Germany). The markers may be on the surface of the needle or may be on a removable stylet contained within the needle. The markers allow the user to confirm visualization of the needle tip under ultrasound.

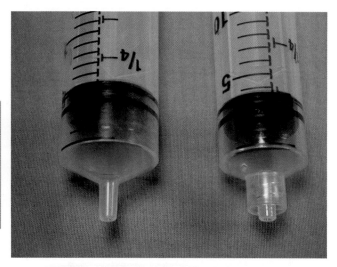

Figurer 14–3   Luer slip and luer lock systems.

Table 14–1   The Relationship Between Gauge and External Diameter for Common Needle Sizes

Gauge	Outside Diameter (mm)	Outside Diameter (in)
14	2.11	0.083
16	1.65	0.065
18	1.25	0.049
20	0.889	0.035
22	0.711	0.028
24	0.559	0.022

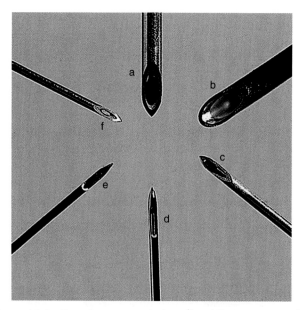

Figure 14–5   Tips of common spinal needles: **(A)** 18-gauge Quinke, **(B)** 16-gauge Tuohy, **(C)** 22-gauge Yale, **(D)** 24-gauge Sprotte, **(E)** 25-gauge Whitacre, (F) 25-gauge Yale. *(From Al-Shaikh B, Stacey S, editors. Essentials of anaesthetic equipment, ed 3, Philadelphia, Churchill Livingstone, 2007, Figure 12.11.)*

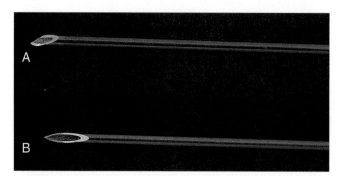

Figure 14–4   Figure demonstrating the **(A)** short beveled needle for nerve block; **(B)** a typical hypodermic (cutting) needle. *(From Checketts MR, Wildsmith JAW, Equipment for local anaesthesia. In Ward's Anaesthetic Equipment, 5th ed. Davet AJ, Diba A, Eds. 2005 Saunders LTD, London. Figure 15.1.)*

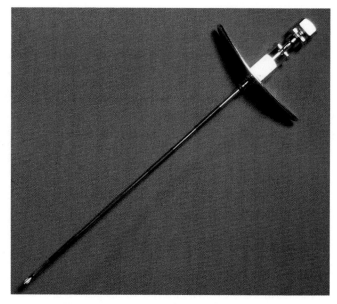

Figure 14–6   Tip of Weiss Tuohy epidural needle.

Catheters

Needles allow for single injection of local anesthetic drugs; however, in some instances neural blockade of longer duration may be required. Under these circumstances, catheters are placed in proximity to neural structures to allow infusion or episodic bolus dosing of local anesthetics and adjuncts.

Catheters for continuous epidural, spinal, or perineural infusions are made of small diameter, hollow polyvinyl, nylon, or silicon tubing that is placed using a through needle or over needle technique.

Typically these catheters are radiopaque and have either a single or multiorifice tip (Figure 14–7). Markings along the length denote distance from the tip. Catheters reinforced with coiled wire may be less prone to kinking. Still others may have a stylet inserted, either to stiffen the catheter to aid insertion, or to act as a conduit for current if nerve stimulation is to be used to aid placement.

At the proximal end of the catheter, a Luer lock attachment is either snapped or screwed into place to allow for easy connection to syringes or infusion pumps. Many commercial catheter kits contain a filter to limit injection of microscopic debris and also devices for securing catheters to the patient.

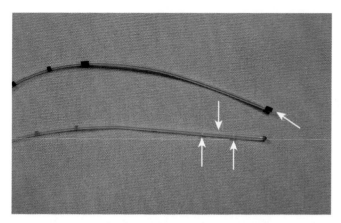

Figure 14–7 Typical catheters, demonstrating single versus multiorifice.

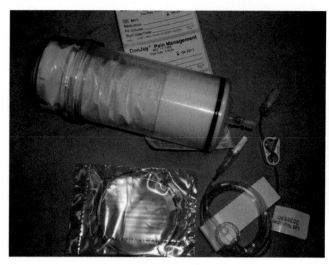

Figure 14–9 Elastomeric infusion device.

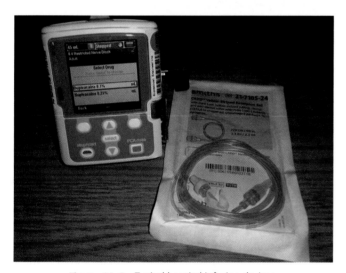

Figure 14–8 Typical hospital infusion devices.

Careful attention to placement technique is necessary to prevent shearing the catheter with the sharp needle end, resulting in a portion of the catheter being retained in the patient. In general, catheters should never be drawn back through a needle. The catheter and needle should always be withdrawn as a unit, even if this means recommencing the technique.

Pumps

Traditionally, catheter-based regional anesthetic techniques have relied on bolus dosing or use of standard hospital infusion devices (syringe drivers, peristaltic pumps). These pumps are often programmable allowing for constant infusion and intermittent boluses, which may be triggered by a medical practitioner or by the patient (Figure 14–8). An example would be patient-controlled epidural analgesia. Safety features of these infusion devices include locks that prevent alterations to the programming of the device, locked boxes to contain the infusate, and infusion tubing that does not contain injection ports.

The move toward same-day surgery has sparked a new wave of infusion devices for regional anesthesia. These devices are simple mechanical or elastomeric pumps that deliver constant infusions of drug through a catheter (Figure 14–9). Variations include the ability to adjust the infusion rate and give either physician or patient-controlled boluses.

Implantable pump devices are frequently used in the management of chronic pain to deliver local anesthetic, opioids, or antispasmodics, and are beyond the scope of this chapter.

Spinal Anesthesia

Spinal needles are available in 18- to 27-gauge diameters, and lengths of 5 to 15 cm; 10-cm needles are most commonly used for adults. Shorter needles are used for children and longer needles for obese patients and combined spinal epidural techniques. Tight-fitting internal stylets are necessary to prevent coring of tissue as the needle is advanced and to make needles less flexible. Once the dura is penetrated, the stylet is removed, and cerebrospinal fluid (CSF) flow confirmed before injection of local anesthetic.

Continuous Spinal Anesthesia

Continuous spinal anesthesia technique involves the placement of a catheter into the CSF and is useful for precise titration of local anesthetic to develop a spinal block of desired level and duration. Microcatheters in diameters of 28 to 30 gauge and variable lengths are available, and may be passed through spinal needles as small as 23 gauge. Epidural catheters may be used, but require larger gauge needles increasing the chance of post-dural puncture headache (PDPH).

Early use of continuous spinal techniques with microcatheters was associated with cauda equina syndrome.[9] However, it now appears that exposure of the nerve roots to high concentrations of local anesthetic (5% lidocaine) was the cause and not the microcatheters themselves. Multi-orifice rather than end-orifice catheters are probably better suited for continuous spinal infusion use.

Epidural Anesthesia

Epidural needles come in a variety of gauges, tip types, and lengths and may have "wings" (Weiss needle) at the hub to assist grip and stabilize the needle as it is inserted. The smallest

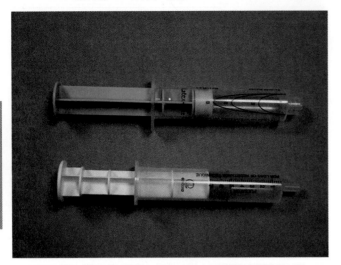

Figure 14–10 Examples of loss-of-resistance (LOR) syringes.

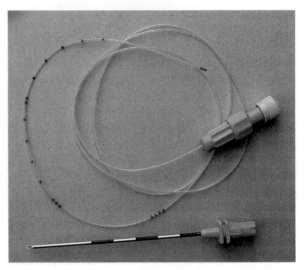

Figure 14–11 Image of epidural catheter markings. *(From Checketts MR, Wildsmith JAW. Equipment for local anaesthesia. In Ward's Anaesthetic Equipment, 5th ed. Davet AJ, Diba A, Eds. 2005 Saunders LTD, London. Figure 15.4.)*

gauge epidural needle of adequate tensile strength that will allow passage of appropriate catheters should be used. Typical needles for adult epidurals are available in 16- to 22-gauge diameters, with a smaller 25-gauge diameter available for pediatric patients. Needle lengths range from 0.9 to 15.5 cm, with the 10.5-cm length used most commonly for adults. In the 10.5-cm needle, the needle shaft is 8-cm long and the hub accounts for the other 2.5 cm.

The classic Tuohy needle has a sharp curved Huber tip, allowing the catheter to exit at a 20-degree angle to the shaft, and includes a stylet.[11] The curved tip facilitates passage of the catheter into the epidural space, and the stylet prevents clogging of the needle with tissue as it is advanced. Hustead improved on the Tuohy design by changing the bevel angle (12 to 15 degrees), dulling the tip to reduce the risk of dural puncture, and rounding the heel to reduce the chance of trapping the catheter should it have to be withdrawn. Although the most common epidural needle used is referred to as the "Tuohy," it more closely approximates the Hustead design.

Other tip designs include the Sprotte needle ("olive-shaped, rounded tip"), which has an internal ramp to deflect the catheter laterally and has been proposed to cause less tissue damage because it tends to spread rather than cut tissue fibers, and the short bevel (60 degree), straight-tip Crawford needle. The Crawford needle is often favored by practitioners of the "hanging-drop" technique, but unless positioned properly, the straight tip could direct the catheter toward the dura rather than the epidural space.

Entry of the needle tip into the epidural space is identified by "loss of resistance to injection," or the "hanging-drop technique" (Figure 14–10). These techniques are grounded in the premise of a negative pressure existing in the epidural space. In reality, the negative pressure in the epidural space results from impingement or "tenting" of the dura by the tip of the epidural needle.[11]

Both techniques require that the needle tip is firmly inserted into the interspinous ligaments. With "loss of resistance," the stylet is withdrawn and the needle advanced with a low resistance syringe (glass or plastic) filled with saline or air attached. Constant pressure is maintained on the syringe plunger as the needle tip is advanced through the dense ligamentum flavum into the loose connective tissue of the epidural space. As the

needle tip enters the space, the characteristic loss of resistance is perceived. The hanging-drop technique involves placing a drop of saline at the needle hub after the stylet is removed, and watching for movement of the drop into the hub of the needle after the epidural space is entered.

After the epidural space has been identified, either a bolus of drug can be given or a catheter can be placed. Typically around 5 cm of epidural catheter is left within the epidural space. The catheters are characteristically marked to demonstrate distance from the tip in centimeters (Figure 14–11). A common method of marking the catheters is to have marks at each centimeter with a thick mark at 5 cm, a double thick mark at 10 cm, a triple thick mark at 15 cm, etc.

As previously mentioned, catheters may have a hole at the tip or multiple side holes at a variable distance from the tip, although not usually further than 2.5 cm. Catheters should be threaded at least 3 cm into the epidural space to ensure that the side holes lie within the epidural space.

Combined Spinal/Epidural

The technique of combined spinal/epidural (CSE) has become popular, particularly within the realm of obstetric anesthesia. It allows for rapid onset via the spinal component and the flexibility of a catheter technique offered by the epidural component. The technique can be performed with the spinal and epidural components at the same or different interspaces; a long spinal needle can be passed through a standard epidural needle or a specialized kit can be used. One benefit of the specialized kits is that the spinal needle can be firmly locked in place once the dural space is identified. Specially designed CSE needles are available that have two holes: a small distal hole that only allows passage of a small diameter spinal needle, and the standard Huber tip for catheter passage.

If a standard Tuohy or Sprotte epidural needle is used, then the spinal needle follows the contour of the rounded Huber tip, and is then advanced further into the intrathecal space. The catheter should be displaced laterally, reducing the chance of being directed into the subarachnoid space (Figure 14–12).

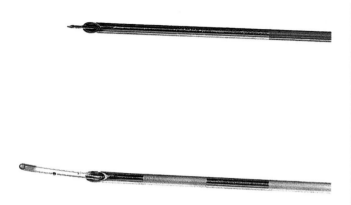

Figure 14–12   Detail of two-hole epidural needles. *(From Al-Shaikh B, Stacey S, editors. Essentials of anaesthetic equipment, ed 3, Philadelphia, Churchill Livingstone, 2007, Figure 12.6.)*

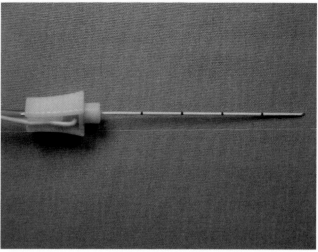

Figure 14–13   Image of stimulating needle. *(From Enneking FK, Equipment for Regional Anesthesia. In Sosis MB, editor. Anesthesia equipment manual, Philadelphia, Lippincott-Raven, 1997, Figure 3.)*

Peripheral Nerve Blocks

A large variety of peripheral nerve block needles are currently commercially available. The facet-tip, short-beveled needle has been traditionally used for increased safety, as discussed earlier in this chapter, while Tuohy and Sprotte tip needles have been used for the placement of peripheral nerve catheters. These side port needles may allow easier passage of catheters parallel to nerves; however, the distance of the side port from the Sprotte tip may actually cause the catheter to lie outside of a fascial plane, particularly if indirect methods of nerve localization are used.

Typical nerve block needles have a diameter of 22 to 24 gauge, and a length that varies from 25 to 150 mm. The length chosen depends on the depth of the target nerve from the skin, and the angle of needle insertion. Shorter needles are better for the more superficial nerves such as the interscalene brachial plexus; longer needles for the deeper structures such as the lumbar plexus or the sciatic nerve, and for larger, obese patients. With ultrasound guidance techniques, the needle is often inserted at a shallow angle, some distance from the transducer as a method to improve needle visualization (see Chapter 15). A longer needle is necessary so that target nerve(s) may be reached. Optimally, the smallest length needle possible should be chosen for the particular block and patient to minimize flex of the needle and the chance of penetrating organs and vessels.

Insulated Needles

Passage of an electrical current through a needle can be used to locate nerves. Electrical currents can depolarize nervous tissue causing an action potential, which leads to contraction of innervated muscle. Covering a stainless steel needle with an insulating material, such as Teflon, creates a small, dense field of current at the needle tip and increases the accuracy of nerve localization. Insulation may cover the needle shaft, leaving the bevel free, or may cover the bevel leaving only the tip exposed. Typically, needles with an exposed tip produce a higher current density,[12] but are less sharp (Figure 14–13).

Stimulating needles typically come with an integrated electrical connection that is compatible with available nerve stimulators. This connection must be long enough so that it sits outside of the sterile field. Frequently, a length of sterile tubing is attached to the nerve block needle, either directly or through a side arm port, thus allowing for injection of local anesthetic by an assistant at some distance from the needle. This may help to minimize movement of the needle and reduce the chance of block failure.

Nerve injury may result from mechanical trauma, ischemia, or neurotoxicity. High needle injection pressures (>20 psi) have been associated with a higher incidence of nerve injury and may indicate intraneural position of a needle.[13] A safety device, the BSmart (Concert Medical, Norwell, Mass.) syringe manometer was developed to help identify and limit elevated injection pressures. It is connected between the nerve block needle and syringe, allowing direct observation of injection pressure during administration of local anesthetic.

Catheters

Peripheral nerve catheters have become a popular method for increasing the duration of nerve blocks in both the inpatient and outpatient setting. Simple epidural catheters may be passed through insulated needles and placed adjacent to nerves, or stimulating peripheral nerve catheters may be used. The latter includes an electrode at the tip allowing for nerve stimulation during catheter passage, and ultimate confirmation of proper placement adjacent to the targeted nerve or plexus (Figure 14–14). The Arrow Stimucath and Pajunk Stimuplex catheters have a metallic spiral in their walls, and the Pandin catheter has an integrated braided conduction wire with a metal ball at the end (HDC Corp., Milpitas, Calif.) End-orifice catheters are probably better suited for the purpose since catheters with side orifices may fall outside of the nerve sheath or fascial plane, contributing to secondary block failure. In this case the initial block is successful since local anesthetic is injected through the needle, but the continuous infusion fails to maintain the block. Catheters typically have centimeter markings and connectors as described earlier for epidural catheters.

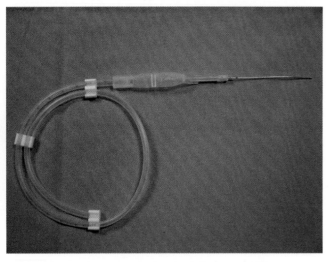

Figure 14–14 Image of a stimulating nerve catheter.

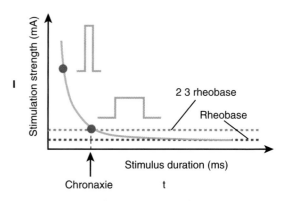

Figure 14–15 Diagram demonstrating rheobase an chronaxie. *(Lin C, Kieman M, Burke D, Bostock H, Assessment of Nerve Excitability Properties in Peripheral Nerve Disease. In Peripheral Nerve Diseases. Kimura J, ed. 2006. Elsevier Health Sciences, Philadelphia., Figure 17.3.)*

Locating Neural Structures

Regional anesthesia requires the placement of needles close to nerves to deliver local anesthetics accurately. Several techniques are used to guide needle placement and include the use of anatomic landmarks, paresthesia techniques, ultrasound guidance, and nerve stimulation.

Anatomic landmarks are used to estimate nerve positions, as in a field block where local anesthetic is infiltrated around a nerve distribution, or in the "fascia iliaca" block, where a blunt needle is used to pass through two layers of fascia to place local anesthetic in the plane of the lumbar plexus. In the axilla, the axillary artery can be used to guide needle placement in a transarterial technique, where the needle and local anesthetic is placed posterior and then anterior to the axillary artery to block the perivascular nerves of the brachial plexus. Paresthesia techniques assume that a needle is in close proximity to a nerve, when the patient describes a "pins and needles" sensation in the distribution of the targeted nerve or plexus. Local anesthetic is then injected after the needle is slightly repositioned.

Most contemporary nerve blocks are performed with technological aids to facilitate needle placement such as nerve stimulators and ultrasound, or a combination of the two techniques. In experienced hands, there is no evidence that any one technique exceeds the other in safety; however, ultrasound guidance improves efficacy and performance time[1] (see Chapter 15).

The remainder of this chapter will describe the principles of nerve stimulation; description of ultrasound can be found in a separate chapter.

Principles of Nerve Stimulation

In 1780 Luigi Galvani demonstrated that application of a current to the spinal cord of a frog caused a motor response in the frog's legs. This is the earliest demonstration of the same principles that underlie nerve stimulators used today.

Nerve membranes have a resting membrane potential of approximately 70 mV with the inside of the neuron negative relative to the extracellular fluid. If a current is applied to the nerve membrane it will depolarize to a threshold potential where an action potential is triggered. This action potential will be propagated along the nerve and in the case of a motor neuron cause a contractile response in associated muscle.

A nerve stimulator is a device that produces a constant, regulated current between a needle that forms a negative electrode, and a positive electrode that usually consists of an EKG pad placed on the skin. The nerve stimulator produces square waves of current typically lasting 0.1 ms that can be regulated between 0 and 2 mA. When a muscle response is noted in response to an appropriate current, the assumption is made that the tip of the needle is close enough to the nerve to allow effective delivery of local anesthetic for a nerve block to occur.

Sensitivity of Nerves to Current

The amount of energy delivered to a nerve is determined by the current measured in milliamperes, and the duration of the stimulus measured in microseconds.

$$\text{Energy Delivered (nC)} = \text{Current (mA)} \times \text{Time (μs)}$$

It is evident from this equation that both the current and the duration of the stimulus are important in determining whether a nerve membrane will depolarize to threshold. Two properties of nerves are used to describe sensitivity to depolarization:

Rheobase—The minimum current required to depolarize a nerve given an infinite duration of stimulation.

Chronaxie—The duration of current required to depolarize a nerve to threshold when the current is two times the rheobase.

Motor neurons tend to have a lower rheobase and shorter chronaxie than sensory or autonomic neurons, which may exist in the same nerve. This makes motor nerves more responsive to the current that is delivered (Figure 14–15).

In the phase immediately following the action potential, the neuronal membrane has an absolute and then a relative refractory period; during this time further administration of current will not induce an action potential. Typically nerve stimulators produce impulses at 1 or 2 Hz, ensuring that the nerve membrane has time to return to resting membrane potential between stimulations.

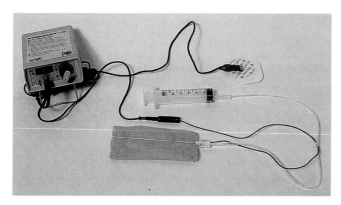

Figure 14-16 The Braun Stimuplex nerve stimulators connected to a nerve block needle and skin electrode. *(From Al-Shaikh B, Stacey S, editors. Essentials of anaesthetic equipment, ed 3, Philadelphia, Churchill Livingstone, 2007, Figure 12.15.)*

Energy Delivery to the Nerve

The distance between the positive and negative terminals of the nerve stimulator varies as the needle tip moves through the tissue, resulting in changes in resistance and therefore current flow. It is critical that the current at the end of the needle remain constant because it is being used to draw an inference about the distance of the needle tip from the nerve being studied. The nerve stimulator must alter its output voltage in response to changes in resistance to provide a constant current. This change is described by Ohm's law where

$$\text{Voltage (V)} = \text{Current (A)} \times \text{Resistance } (\Omega).$$

As a needle approaches a nerve, the delivery of energy is described by Coulomb's law:

$$E = K(Q/r^2).$$

Here E is the required stimulating current, k is a constant, Q is the minimum stimulating current, and r is the distance between the needle tip and the nerve. The key point is that the inverse square law applies; current is inversely proportional to the square of the distance between the needle tip and the neural target. At distances over about 8 mm, such high currents are required to produce a motor response that other systemic effects are likely to occur (at 2 cm a current of 50 mA is necessary to produce a response).

The polarity of the nerve stimulator circuit is critical. The skin electrode must be positive and the needle electrode negative. Switching the polarity leads to a threefold increase in the energy delivery required to stimulate the nerve, the consequence of this is that the needle could easily pass into or through the nerve before stimulation is obtained. The position of the skin surface electrode does not seem to make an impact on the ability to stimulate nerves.

The Ideal Characteristics of a Nerve Stimulator

An ideal nerve stimulator will provide current output in the form of a rectangular wave 0.1 ms in duration with a frequency of 1 to 2 Hz. The current output will be constant and not affected by changes in resistance between the needle and skin electrode. The current delivered should be controlled so that it can be decreased as the needle electrode approaches the

target nerve, and current output should be displayed. Safety alarms to warn of circuit discontinuity, low battery and internal faults should be integral, and the polarity of the output electrodes should be unambiguous (Figure 14-16).

Using a Nerve Stimulator

Preparation for performing regional blockade cannot be covered in detail here but should involve careful patient choice, consent from the patient, adequate cardiovascular monitoring, sedation as appropriate, and strict asepsis. Typically the initial current is set at 0.75 to 1.0 mA. This may need to be moderated if the stimulating needle has to pass through skeletal muscle as local stimulation of muscle can cause contraction that is uncomfortable for the patient. Once muscle contraction is noted in the distribution of the nerve being blocked, the current can be dropped. The goal is to stimulate the nerve at approximately 0.5 mA. At currents higher than this, there is a risk that the needle tip is too far from the nerve to allow effective local anesthetic spread. At currents of around 0.2 mA, there is a risk that the needle tip is actually inside the nerve itself and injection of local anesthetic could have adverse consequences.

Nerve stimulators may also be used for surface mapping of nerves, using a blunt tip electrode along anatomic landmarks rather than a percutaneous needle. Foot pedals and special hand controls have been developed for nerve stimulators, allowing the individual performing the block to adjust the stimulator current, rather than using an assistant to do so.

Ultrasound Guidance

Ultrasound-guided peripheral nerve blocks have gained increasing popularity over the last 10 years as a result of the development of affordable, portable, high-resolution systems. Multiple studies have shown a higher rate of success and a decreased time required to perform the block when ultrasound is employed. Although direct visualization of nerve block procedures would imply greater safety, no studies to date support its use over other techniques in experienced hands. For further information about ultrasound guidance, please refer to Chapter 15.

References

1. Sites, B.D., Brull, R., 2006. Ultrasound guidance in peripheral regional anesthesia: philosophy, evidence-based medicine, and techniques. Curr Opin Anaesthesiol 19, 630–639.
2. Van Zundert, A., Helmstadter, A., Goerig, M., et al., 2008. Centennial of intravenous regional anesthesia Bier's Block. (1908-2008). Reg Anesth Pain Med 33 (5), 483–489.
3. ASA, 2009. Standards for basic anesthetic monitoring." ASA.
4. Weinberg, G., 2006. Lipid rescue resuscitation from local anesthetic cardiac toxicity. Toxicol Rev 25 (3), 139–145.
5. Hebl, J., 2006. The importance and implications of aseptic techniques during regional anesthesia. Reg Anesth Pain Med 31 (4), 311–323.
6. International Organization for Standardization, "ISO 594." 2009. International Standards for Business, Government and Society.
7. Lambert, D.H., Hurley, R.J., Hertwig, L., et al., 1997. Role of needle gauge and tip configuration in the production of lumbar puncture headache. Reg Anesth Pain Med 22 (1), 66–72.
8. Turnbull, D.K., Shepherd, D.B., 2003. Post dural puncture headache, pathogenesis, prevention and treatment. Br J Anaesth 91 (5), 718–729.

9. Sosis, M .B., 1997. Equipment for regional anesthesia. Anesthesia equipment manual. Mitchel B. Sosis ed. Lippincott-Raven, Philadelphia.
10. Denny, N.M., Selander, D.E., 1998. Continuous spinal anesthesia. Br J Anaesth 81, 590–597.
11. Frolich, M.A., Caton, D., 2001. Pioneers in epidural needle design. Anesth Analg 98, 215–230.
12. Ford, D., Pither, C., Raj, P.P., 1984. Comparison of insulated and uninsulated needles for locating peripheral nerves with a nerve stimulator. Anesth Analg 63, 925.
13. Hadzic, A., Dilberovic, F., Shah, S., et al., 2004. Combination of intraneural injection and high injection pressure leads to fascicular injury and neurologic deficits in dogs. Reg Anesth Pain Med 29, 417–423.

Additional Reading

Hadzic, A., 2006. Textbook of regional anesthesia and acute pain management. McGraw-Hill, New York.

Tsui, B., 2007. Atlas of ultrasound and nerve stimulation-guided regional anesthesia. Springer.

Hadzic, A., Vloka, J., Hadzic, N., et al., 2003. Nerve stimulators used for peripheral nerve block vary in their electrical characteristics. Anesthesiology 98, 969–974.

Le-Wendling, L., Enneking, F.K., 2008. Continuous peripheral nerve blocks for postoperative analgesia. Curr Opin Anaesthesiol 21 (5), 602–609.

Chapter 15

Ultrasound for Regional Anesthesia and Vascular Access

Lisa Warren and Reuben Slater

Technological advances over the last decade, including improvements in image resolution, and the development of smaller, more manageable, laptop-sized systems have made ultrasound techniques more accessible for all medical practitioners.

Ultrasound allows immediate and dynamic visualization of anatomy, and it is an invaluable diagnostic used in prenatal screening, assessment of cardiac function, and assessment of intraabdominal and vascular pathology.

Ultrasound also has a role in facilitating performance of invasive procedures. In the field of anesthesiology, this predominantly means insertion of central venous lines and placement of neural blockade. Adopting ultrasound to guide procedures can improve safety and success rate and decrease performance time.[1-3]

Technology

An Overview of Ultrasound

Sound is transferred by mechanical waves of compression and rarefaction through a medium.[4] Audible sound has frequencies between 12 Hz and 20,000 Hz, sound with frequencies greater than 20,000 Hz is known as ultrasound. Ultrasound used in medical imaging applications typically has a frequency in the megahertz range.

Ultrasound is produced by piezoelectric crystals. Piezoelectricity is the ability of a material to generate an electric potential after application of a mechanical stress. The piezoelectric effect also occurs in reverse; application of an electric potential to a crystal will cause mechanical deformation. Both the direct and reverse piezoelectric effects are used in medical ultrasonography.

The basic premise of ultrasonography is that sound waves travel at different speeds in tissues of different density and that sound waves are reflected at tissue boundaries.[5] A short pulse of ultrasound created by a piezoelectric crystal can be conducted through tissues of interest (Figure 15-1). Ultrasound will reflect back from boundaries between tissues and cause deformation of the piezoelectric crystal, which via the direct piezoelectric effect will cause a potential difference to occur in the crystal. The potential difference in the crystal induces a current that is measured. The time gap between impulse generation and returning echoes is carefully measured. Making assumptions about the speed of ultrasound in tissue (on average 1540 m/sec) allows time gaps to be interpreted as distances. Complex postprocessing allows these data to be converted to images.

Ultrasound and Its Interaction with Tissue

To produce a single scan line an ultrasound machine passes a defined current through a piezoelectric crystal to produce a defined pulse of ultrasound. A pulse of ultrasound will typically be 1 to 2 cycles with a frequency of 2 to 15 MHz. The physical length of the pulse is determined by multiplying the number of cycles by the wavelength and is known as the spatial pulse length (SPL).

Once the pulse of ultrasound has been created and conducted into the tissue of interest, the transducer will wait a defined period of time to receive echoes. The amount of time the transducer waits is determined by the depth of field required to visualise the anatomical structure of interest and the average speed of sound in tissue. After the specified period of time, the next pulse of ultrasound is produced.

The time between pulses is known as the pulse repetition period (PRP), and its inverse is the pulse repetition frequency (PRf). This is distinct from the frequency of the ultrasound itself.

Ultrasound in Tissue

The speed at which ultrasound travels through tissue is determined by the compressibility and density of the tissue. It averages 1540 m/sec (Table 15-1).

Speed of sound in tissue (c) = 1 / compressibility × density

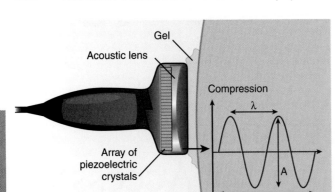

Figure 15–1 Representation of a linear ultrasound transducer and pulse of ultrasound. Note the linear array of piezoelectric crystals. The crystals are in sonic continuity with the tissue to be examined via the body of the transducer and a conductive gel. The wavelength and amplitude of a typical pulse of ultrasound are seen. *SPL,* Spatial pulse length.

Table 15–1 Property of Sound in Various Tissues and Air

Material	Speed of Transmission (m/s)	Acoustic Impedance (kg/m²/s × 10⁶)	Attenuation Coefficient (dB/cm at 1 MHz)
Water	1484	1.5	0.002
Blood	4080	1.62	0.18
Fat	1450	1.35	0.63
Lung	550	0.26	41
Muscle	1580	1.65-1.74	1.3-3.3
Bone	4080	7.8	20.0
Air	330	0.0004	3.3×10^6

The property of a tissue that determines the speed of ultrasound is known as acoustic impedance (z).

$$\text{Acoustic Impedance}\,(z) = \text{Density}\,(\rho) \times \text{Acoustic Velocity}\,(V)$$

Ultrasound is reflected back toward the transducer as it crosses tissue boundaries. The degree of reflection that occurs is dependent on the angle the pulse interacts with the boundary, the acoustic impedance of the tissues on either side of the boundary, and the size of the boundary.

There are three ways a sound wave can behave when it arrives at a tissue boundary: it can be transmitted, reflected, or refracted (Figure 15-2).

Transmission of a sound wave will occur if some or all of the wave passes directly across the tissue boundary. Refraction occurs when the direction of the ultrasound wave is altered as it is transmitted across a tissue barrier. The degree of deflection that occurs is determined by the acoustic impedance mismatch between the two tissues and the angle at which the wave strikes the tissue barrier. The degree of refraction is described by Snell's law:

$$\sin\theta1/\sin\theta2 = c1/c2$$

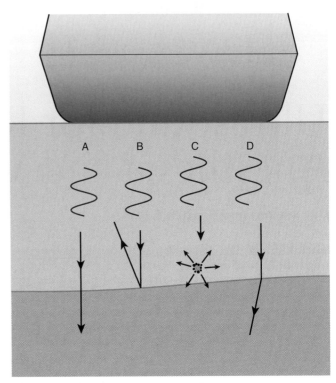

Figure 15–2 A, Transmission and attenuation of an ultrasound pulse. **B,** Reflection of an ultrasound pulse. **C,** Scattering of an ultrasound pulse. **D,** Refraction of an ultrasound pulse.

$\theta1$ is the angle of incidence of the sound approaching the interface, $\theta2$ is the angle of refraction and c1 and c2 are the propagation velocities of sound in either tissue (Figure 15-3).

No refraction will occur if sound waves are perpendicular to the tissue boundary.

The degree of reflection that occurs from a tissue interface is determined by the difference in acoustic impedance of the tissues that make up the interface. The fraction of energy reflected at an acoustic interface is known as the reflection coefficient (R).

$$R = (Z1 - Z2)^2/(Z1 + Z2)^2$$

Z1 and Z2 are the acoustic impedances of the tissues on either side of the interface.

The direction of reflected energy is determined by the angle of incidence, the angle formed between the propagating wave, and the normal, a line perpendicular to the reflecting surface. The angle of reflection will be a mirror of the angle of incidence.

Reflectors that follow these simple rules are known as specular reflectors and include structures such as the diaphragm and most vessel walls. Smaller structures do not obey these simple rules.

If a reflector has a diameter that is equal to one wavelength of the ultrasound pulse, the energy of the wave is scattered in all directions in a nonuniform fashion. Reflectors with a diameter less than one wavelength cause Rayleigh scattering, described as even scatter of the ultrasound energy in all directions.

Attenuation

Attenuation is the loss of ultrasound power as it passes through tissue. Attenuation is primarily due to the conversion of kinetic energy to heat energy as a result of friction.

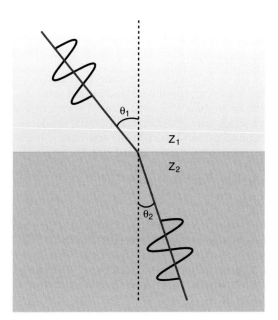

Figure 15–3 Refraction of a pulse of ultrasound: θ_1, angle of incidence; θ_2, angle of refraction; Z_1, a Acoustic impedance of superficial tissue; Z_2, a Acoustic impedance of deep tissue.

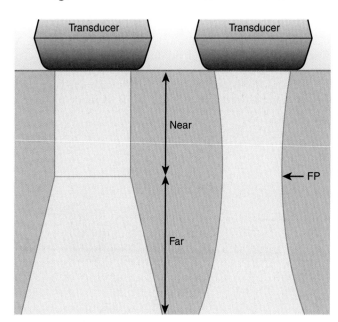

Figure 15–4 Demonstrating *(left)* a representation of unfocused ultrasound and *(right)* a representation of electronically focused ultrasound. *FP,* Focal point.

The result of attenuation is that the amplitude or power of the ultrasound wave is decreased.

Attenuation determines the degree of penetration of ultrasound waves into tissue; as a result it determines the depth to which imaging can occur. High frequency ultrasound attenuates more quickly than low frequency ultrasound. To examine deep structures—the sciatic nerve in the gluteal region, for example—a low frequency probe should be used.

The benefit of high frequency probes is that they provide improved resolution. This means that a balance between depth of field and resolution should be considered for any given scan.

Resolution

When applied to ultrasonography, resolution is the ability of a system to distinguish between two objects. Two small objects, beyond the limit of resolution, will appear as one on the screen.

Spatial Resolution

Axial resolution is the ability of the system to distinguish objects that are in line with the ultrasound pulse (Figure 15-4). Generally axial resolution is better than lateral resolution. The major determinant of axial resolution is the spatial pulse length; in fact axial resolution is equal to half the spatial pulse length (SPL) and does not vary with depth. Objects that are separated by a distance greater than one half the SPL will produce echoes completely distinct from each other and will be visualized as two separate structures. If two objects are separated by less than one half of the SPL, then the returning echoes will overlap and the objects will be visualized as a single structure. A high frequency ultrasound wave with a short pulse length results in better axial resolution than a low frequency wave.[6]

Lateral resolution is the ability of an ultrasound system to distinguish objects in a plane perpendicular to the ultrasound

pulse. It varies depending on the depth of imaging and frequency of the probe. Generally resolution is best at the focal point of the ultrasound beam.

Focal Points

An unfocused ultrasound beam has a near zone where waves travel directly and a far zone where waves begin to diverge (Figure 15-5). As the waves diverge, lateral resolution is lost. Modern machines electronically focus the ultrasound waves so that the user can alter the depth of the narrowest point, where the resolution is highest.

Temporal Resolution

Temporal resolution is the ability of an ultrasound system to detect movement. Temporal resolution is dependent on the frame rate of the system. A higher frequency of frames will increase the probability of seeing a quick movement. Frame rate is determined by the speed of sound in tissue, the depth of field, and the number of scan lines required per field.

Temporal resolution is improved by optimizing the depth of field and narrowing the frame to the object of interest.

Creating an Ultrasound Picture

A single pulse of ultrasound returns to the transducer as a series of reflected wave fronts with different amplitudes. The time between the creation of the pulse and reception of the wave is the time for the pulse to travel into the tissue and get reflected back to the transducer (Table 15-2). Given that the speed of sound in tissue is relatively constant, 1540 m/sec, careful timing of the wavefronts allows distance to tissue planes to be calculated. The amplitude of returned waves can also be measured.

Complex interpretation and filtering of the returning signals occur before the results are displayed on a monitor. A single pulse of ultrasound produces a single vertical scan line.

To create an M-mode picture, a single scan line is plotted against time; however, to produce a 2-D, B-mode picture, a series of consecutive scan lines need to be obtained. A series of scan lines together produce a frame, or a single image. The process is repeated to produce frame after frame; this will give the illusion of movement.

There are several styles of ultrasound transducer, common styles include linear, curvilinear, and phased array.

In a linear probe a series of crystals fire in turn, each producing a single scan line; here each crystal produces a pulse of ultrasound perpendicular to the transducer. If a series of crystals are placed along a convex front, the result is a curved array transducer. This produces a series of divergent pulses, which give a large field of view.

A phased array transducer uses complex electronic synchronization of ultrasound pulses from a group of piezoelectric crystals to produce a wave front. The resultant wave can be electronically "steered" and focused at different depths. Phased array transducers can have a relatively small footprint and a large field of view. They are ideal for imaging structures, such as the liver or heart or between the ribs.

In B-mode, ultrasound images are displayed as a 2-D matrix of grayscale pixels. An area on the screen that is bright represents an area of tissue from which there was strong reflection, a hyperechoic area.[7] Dark-colored areas represent tissue from which there was little or no reflection, anechoic or hypoechoic areas (Figure 15-6). A specular reflector is hyperechoic when perpendicular to the ultrasound wave. Fluid-filled areas are typically anechoic or hypoechoic and appear dark.

A particular feature of some neural structures is that the amount of ultrasound they reflect is determined by the angle

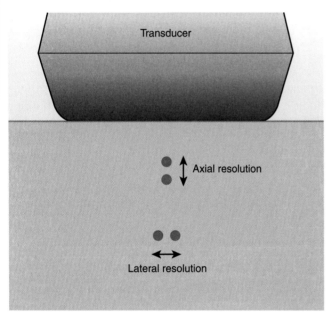

Figure 15–5 Demonstrating the concept of axial and lateral resolution.

Table 15–2 Different Ultrasound Image Formats

Ultrasound Mode	Summary	Variables	Use
A-Mode	A-mode is the simplest form of interpretation. An ultrasound wave is sent along a single scan line, and the depths and intensities at which echoes occur are represented on the screen as a line graph.	1. Distance to tissue boundary 2. Amplitude of reflected waves (gray-scale)	The A scan in ophthalmology is used to assess the axial length of the eye.
M-Mode	The M is short for motion. M-mode ultrasonography is used to demonstrate changes along a single scan line with time.	1. Distance to tissue boundary 2. Amplitude of reflected waves (gray-scale) 3. Time on the x-axis 4. Inference of motion (from 1 and 3)	M-mode is typically used as part of an echocardiographic examination to assess function of rapidly moving parts of the heart.
B-Mode	The B is short for brightness. B-mode ultrasonography is used to give 2-D representations of "slices" of tissue by summation of the returns from multiple scan lines.	1. 2-D representation of "slice" of tissue 2. Amplitude of reflected waves (gray-scale) 3. Time 4. Motion	B-mode is used for anatomic diagnosis and ultrasound-guided invasive procedures.
Doppler	Doppler shift occurs when the frequency of sound waves is altered if either the reflector or receiver is moving relative to the other. In medical ultrasonography, this phenomenon is used to assess the velocity of tissue movement or blood flow. During placement of central venous lines for example, blood flow can be assessed with Doppler to differentiate between arterial and venous flow.	1. Velocity of flow 2. Direction of flow	In medical ultrasonography, this phenomenon is used to assess the velocity of tissue movement or blood flow. During placement of central venous lines, for example, blood flow can be assessed with Doppler to differentiate between arterial and venous flow.

of incidence of the ultrasound pulse. As the transducer is angled a nerve may change its appearance from hypoechoic to hyperechoic. This property is known as anisotropy.

Doppler

Doppler technology allows the characterization of blood flow and identification of blood vessels. The Doppler shift occurs as a result of frequency change when there is relative movement between the source of a sound and a receiver. Anyone standing on the street as a fire engine with siren blaring passes by is familiar with this phenomenon.

During Doppler examination of blood vessels, red blood cells act as the moving source of sound and the transducer as the stationary receiver. When a pulse of ultrasound is reflected from moving red blood cells, there is a change in the frequency of the returning echoes due to the relative motion between the sound source and the receiver. If the source of sound (RBC) is moving towards the transducer, the perceived frequency is higher; if the source is moving away from the receiver, the perceived frequency is lower. The change in frequency can be displayed using a color scale, with red to indicate flow toward the transducer and blue indicating flow away from the receiver (Figure 15-7).

Color Doppler detection is best when the transducer is parallel to blood flow and becomes less accurate at angles greater than 30 degrees to the structure under study.[5]

If the direction of blood flow is not important, color power Doppler can be used. This technique is a more sensitive way of discovering flow at the expense of information about direction of flow. Color power Doppler is useful during placement of neural blockade.

Advances in ultrasound technology include compound imaging, differential tissue harmonics, and 3-D and 4-D imaging. Spatial compound imaging techniques improve contrast resolution and reduce artifacts by obtaining multiple images from different viewing angles and then combining them into a single image.[4] Overlapping scans are acquired by electronically steering the beam of a transducer array. Harmonics imaging allows simultaneous transmission of two frequencies of ultrasound within the same pulse, thus permitting increased penetration without sacrificing resolution. Three-dimensional imaging takes multiple ultrasound images in rapid succession and displays a reconstructed image in near real time. Four-dimensional imaging is a 3-D motion video. These technological advancements have improved the diagnostic capabilities of ultrasound by rendering faster and more accurate images.

LIMITATIONS

Image Artifact

Several types of imaging artifacts, or display errors, may adversely affect image acquisition and interpretation.[8,9]

Acoustic shadow—occurs when the ultrasound beam penetration is severely impeded by a structure with a high attenuation coefficient, such as bone (Figure 15-8).

Reverberation—of the ultrasound beam can occur when it encounters a strong specular reflector, resulting in a "comet tail" acoustic signal deep to the specular reflector (Figure 15-9).

Air artifact—results in a "dropout" artifact, when the ultrasound beam encounters an air-filled space, or there is insufficient conduction gel between the transducer and the skin.

Acoustic enhancement—occurs as a hyperechoic region resulting when beam penetration passes through an area of low attenuation coefficient to an area of higher

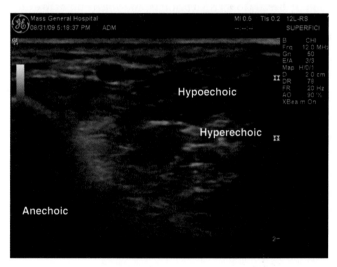

Figure 15–6 An example of an ultrasound displaying anechoic, hypoechoic, and hyperechoic regions.

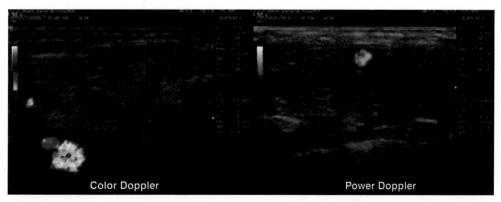

Figure 15–7. Color Doppler (left), power Doppler (right). Note that the image on the left is colored red and blue representing flow towards and away from the transducer. In the power Doppler image, no information about direction of flow is obtained.

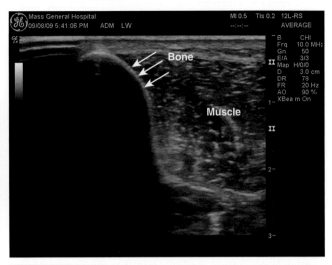

Figure 15–8 Example of acoustic shadowing or image dropout behind bony structure.

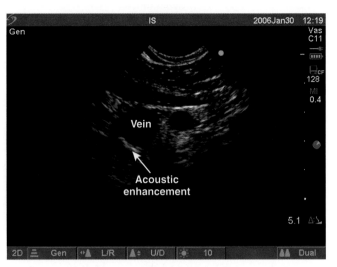

Figure 15–10 Acoustic enhancement artifact.

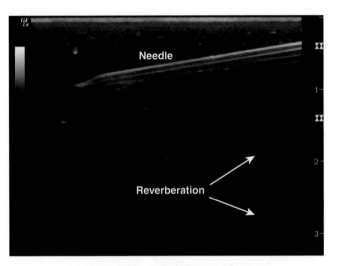

Figure 15–9 Reverberation artifact.

attenuation coefficient. This is commonly encountered when visualizing blood vessels (Figure 15-10).

Ghost (mirror image) artifact—occurs when sound waves bounce off a strong reflector, start to return, and then bounce off a lesser reflector, return to the strong reflector, and then reflect back to the transducer. The ultrasound computer calculates that the echo has taken longer to return, and therefore plots another echo image deeper than the real structure.

ULTRASOUND FOR REGIONAL ANESTHESIA AND VASCULAR ACCESS

The basic components of an ultrasound scanner include a pulser or transmitter, a transducer, a receiver, a display, and memory (Figure 15-11). The transmitter provides brief pulses of energy to the transducer. The transducer converts the pulses of energy into acoustic waves (ultrasound beams) and also serves as the receiver, converting the reflected sound waves back into electrical energy (Figure 15-12). The electrical signal is processed, amplified, and displayed in B-mode as a grayscale 2-D image where the degree of brightness is a function of the amplitude of the signal. Typically ultrasound

systems have internal memory that allows for archiving of static and dynamic (clips) images. The ability to save images to external memory devices varies by machine manufacturer. Typical systems have the capacity to save images via USB ports, Ethernet and wireless in DICOM format to PACS, to output directly to thermal printers, and video output to external recording devices.

General Preparation and Machine Care

Preparation for ultrasound scanning includes choosing the correct transducer for the anatomic structure to be studied, selecting the proper frequency depending on the depth of the structure, adjusting the gain to provide the best contrast, and adjusting the depth on the display and the focal zone to optimize resolution.

Many systems offer the ability to create "presets," or saved settings for structures that are frequently scanned (Figure 15-13). The visualization of structures is determined not only by the machine settings, the chosen transducer, and the structure under study, but also by the way in which the ultrasonographer handles the transducer. By altering the pressure placed on the transducer-tissue interface, and the alignment, rotation and tilt of the probe in real time, the operator can obtain the optimal image for the application.[10]

Additionally, most systems allow for the input of data concerning the patient and ultrasonographer along with the image. Images may also be saved with text labels, measurements, and markings for later analysis (Figure 15-14).

Accessories for ultrasound transducers include impermeable sheaths for sterile applications, biopsy guides to aid in the precise placement of needles for injection or aspiration of medications or fluids, and mechanical arms for hands-free positioning of the transducer (Figure 15-15).

Great care should be taken not to drop transducers, as piezoelectric crystals are easily broken, and image quality is severely affected as a result. Transducers should be cleaned between applications with nonalcohol-containing disinfectant solutions effective against bacteria and viruses.

Regional Anesthesia

In many practices, ultrasound guidance for regional anesthesia has quickly supplanted the older "blind techniques" of nerve stimulation and paresthesia. Direct visualization of

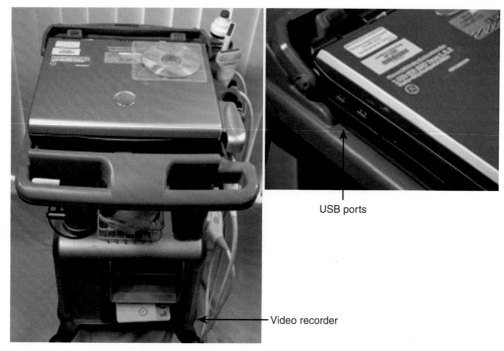

USB ports

Video recorder

Figure 15–11   Basic system with ports/recorders. *GE Logiq E, Fairfield CT.*

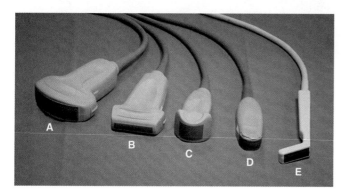

Figure 15–12   Transducers. *Sonosite, Bothell, WA.*

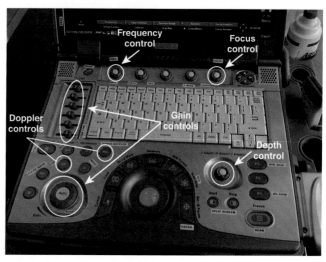

Figure 15–13   Knobology. *GE Logiq E, Fairfield CT.*

neural structures, and the spread of local anesthetics around the nerves, improves performance time and efficacy, and may reduce the failure rate and complications.[7] Ultrasound guidance can be combined with use of a nerve stimulator to confirm the identity of the nerve targeted. Whether this actually improves the success rate and safety of ultrasound-guided nerve blocks remains to be determined.

When structures are visualized under ultrasound, they may be seen in either cross-section, also called short-axis or transverse view, or along the long axis or longitudinal view (Figure 15-16). Likewise, an inserted needle may be seen in transverse view or out-of-plane with the transducer or in a longitudinal view or in plane with the transducer.[7]

The type of block, either single shot or continuous catheter technique, and the experience of the operator may determine the approach taken. Regardless of approach, the aim is to place the needle or catheter within the connective tissue sheath surrounding the nerve or plexus of interest and to deposit local anesthetic around this neural structure. The entire length of the block needle and circumferential spread of local anesthetic around nerves can be best appreciated with

the needle in plane with the transducer and the nerve in short axis view (Figure 15-17). Oblique "cuts" may also be useful to assist in visualization of the entire needle trajectory when placing continuous catheters for particular nerve blocks (sciatic and femoral). Before needle insertion, the targeted and surrounding structures should be studied for the presence of artifacts, anomalies, and pathology, and color Doppler should be used to assess for the presence of blood vessels nearby and in the likely path of the needle.

Vascular Access

Nearly 5 million central venous catheters are placed annually in the United States for the purposes of administering medications, such as chemotherapy and long-term antibiotics, delivering hyperalimentation or blood products, monitoring hemodynamic parameters, managing perioperative

Figure 15–14 P-A-R-T. Maneuvers to optimize visualization under ultrasound. **A,** Pressure. **B,** Alignment. **C,** Rotation. **D,** Tilt.

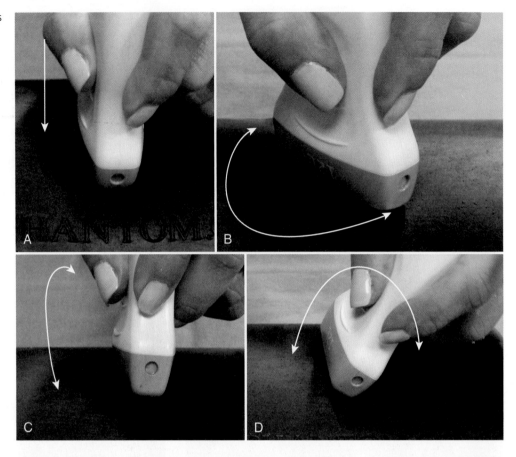

Figure 15–15 Transducer holder, sheath, biopsy guide. **A,** Biopsy guide, CIVCO Medical Solutions, Kalona, Iowa. **B,** Sterile transducer sheath. **C,** Transducer holder, ultra-Stand, Wellan Medical, Lebanon, N.H.

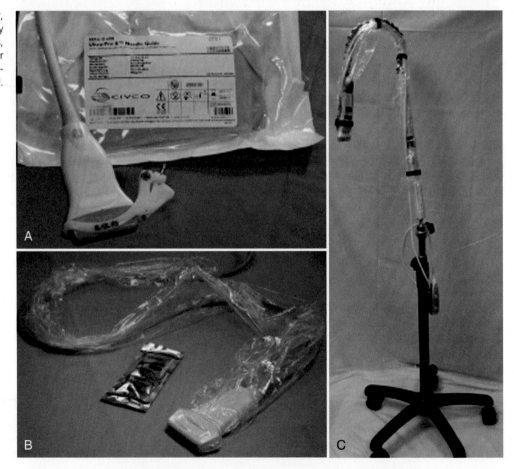

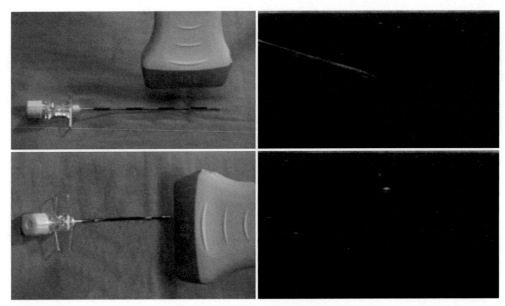

Figure 15–16 Transverse versus longitudinal, in-plane versus out-of-plane. Upper frames: *(left)* needle in-plane with transducer; *(right)* needle visualized in longitudinal axis. Lower frames: *(left)* needle out-of-plane; *(right)* needle visualized in transverse or short axis.

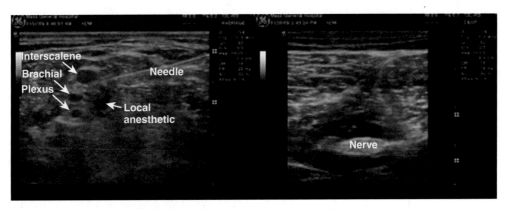

Figure 15–17 Image of nerves after injection of local anesthetic. Two examples of hypoechoic local anesthetic surrounding nerves.

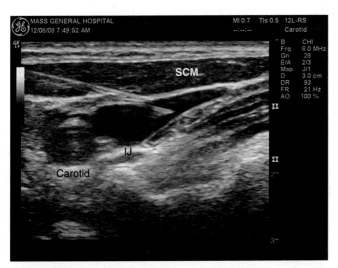

Figure 15–18 Image of vascular access. Oblique visualization of the internal jugular vein and access needle.

fluids, and for hemodialysis.[11] Typical sites for central venous access include the internal jugular, femoral, and subclavian veins. Traditionally landmark techniques have been used to achieve vein puncture by passing the needle along the anticipated trajectory of the vein. The rate of failure of attempted central venous cannulation depends upon patient characteristics and is higher in obese, pediatric, or repeatedly accessed patients.[12] Serious complications from central vein placement are not infrequent, vary by site, and include arterial puncture, hematoma, pneumothorax, hemothorax, injuries to the thoracic duct, and thrombus formation.[13]

In 2001, ultrasound guidance for central venous access was endorsed by the Agency for Healthcare Research and Quality because of compelling evidence that the frequency of complications is reduced when used over landmark techniques.[14] Direct visualization of the vascular structure of interest reduces the failure rate and allows identification of anomalies and pathology. Ultrasound guidance is best used

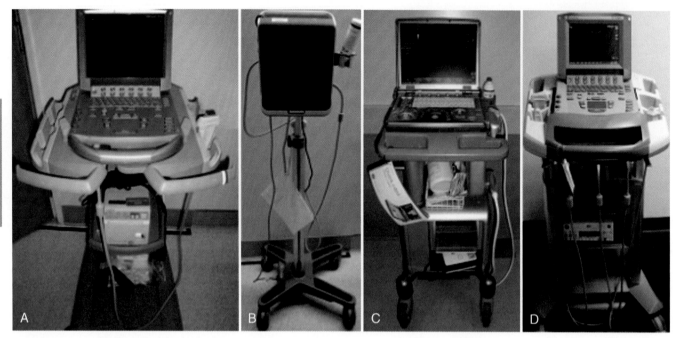

Figure 15–19 Examples of portable ultrasound machines. **A,** SonoSite Micromax, SonoSite, Bothell, Wash. **B,** SonoSite S Nerve. **C,** GE Logiq E, GE, Waukesha, Wis. **D,** SonoSite Titan.

in a dynamic fashion, locating the vascular target and guiding cannulation.

Most commonly a transverse approach to real-time guidance is used where the needle and vein are visualized in cross-section. The vessel is centered under the transducer, and the needle is inserted at the midpoint of the transducer. Care must be taken not to lose visualization of the needle tip and thus penetrate deeper into unintended structures.[15] In some patients the carotid artery may lie directly behind the internal jugular vein, and may be inadvertently punctured and accessed mistakenly (Figure 15-18). Once the vessel is punctured and blood return verified, additional confirmatory tests, such as color comparison, manometry, or blood gas analysis, are recommended.

Oblique scanning techniques can provide a longitudinal view of needles and vessels, thus providing visualization of the entire shaft and tip of the needle as it is inserted into the targeted vein, potentially reducing the chance of unintended puncture of nearby structures.[16] Furthermore, once the guidewire is passed via Seldinger technique, it too can be visualized, and proper placement confirmed.

Performance of ultrasound-guided central venous access must include strict adherence to sterile technique. Standardized patient skin preparation and draping, and the use of prepackaged "Line Access" kits may help to reduce the incidence of line-associated infection, a source of significant patient morbidity. As mentioned above, sterile transducer sheaths and conduction gel are commercially available.

Choosing a System

When choosing a system, several factors must be considered, such as simplicity, image quality, ergonomic design, data management, portability, cost, durability, training, and customer service (Figure 15-19). Systems that perform multiple applications (echocardiography, obstetric imaging, vascular access, and regional anesthesia guidance) may

be more desirable than single-purpose designs. Ultimately, objective evaluation reflecting one's own clinical practice is necessary.[17]

Conclusion

Ultrasound technology is a versatile modality for diagnostic and interventional purposes. It has become an ever increasingly popular tool for anesthesiologists performing regional anesthesia and central venous access. With the development of smaller and simpler systems, ultrasound machines are becoming more affordable and available to most practitioners, providing faster performance and improved success, and the safety of techniques traditionally performed in a blind fashion.

References

1. Hadzic, A., Sala-Blanch, X., Xu, D., 2008. Ultrasound guidance may reduce but not eliminate complications of peripheral nerve blocks. Anesthesiology 108 (4), 557–558.
2. Orebaugh, S.L., Williams, B.A., Kentor, M.L., 2007. Ultrasound guidance with nerve stimulation reduces the time necessary for resident peripheral nerve blockade. Reg Anesth Pain Med 32 (5), 448–454.
3. Koscielniak-Nielsen, Z.J., 2008. Ultrasound-guided peripheral nerve blocks: what are the benefits? Acta Anaesthesiol Scand 52 (6), 727–737.
4. Hangiandreou, N.J., 2003. AAPM/RSNA physics tutorial for residents. Topics in US. Radiographics 23 (4), 1019–1033.
5. Sites, B.D., Brull, R., Chan, V.W., et al., 2007. Artifacts and pitfall errors associated with ultrasound-guided regional anesthesia. Part I: understanding the basic principles of ultrasound physics and machine operations. Reg Anesth Pain Med 32 (5), 412–418.
6. Bushberg, J.T., Seibert, J.A., Leidholdt, E.M.,Boone, J.M. 2002. Ultrasound. The essential physics of medical imaging, 2nd ed. Lippincott Williams & Wilkins, Philadelphia.
7. Sites, B.D., Brull, R. 2006. Ultrasound guidance in peripheral regional anesthesia: philosophy, evidence-based medicine, and techniques. Curr Opin Anaesthesiol 19, 630–639.
8. Huang, J., Triedman, J.K., Vasilyev, N.V., et al., 2007. Imaging artifacts of medical instruments in ultrasound-guided interventions. J Ultrasound Med 26, 1303–1322.

9. Sites, B.D., Brull, R., Chan, V.W., et al., 2007. Artifacts and pitfall errors associated with ultrasound-guided regional anesthesia. Part II: a pictorial approach to understanding and avoidance. Reg Anesth Pain Med 32 (5), 419–433.

10. Sites, B.D., Chan, V.W., Neal, J.M., et al., 2009. The American Society of Regional Anesthesia and Pain Medicine and the European Society of Regional Anaesthesia and Pain Therapy joint committee recommendations for education and training in ultrasound-guided regional anesthesia. Reg Anesth Pain Med 34 (1), 40–46.

11. Hind, D., Calvert, N., McWilliams, R., et al., 2003. Ultrasonic locating devices for central venous cannulation: meta-analysis. BMJ 327, 7411–7417.

12. Kilbourne, M.J., Bochicchio, G.V., Scalea, T., et al., 2009. Avoiding common technical errors in subclavian central venous catheter placement. J Am Coll Surg 208, 104–109.

13. Mansfield, P.F., Hohn, D.C., Fornage, B.D., et al., 1994. Complications and failures of subclavian-vein catheterization. N Engl J Med 331, 1735–1738.

14. US Dept of Health and Human Services 2001. Evidence report/technology assessment number 43: making health care safer: a critical analysis of patient safety practices. Agency for Healthcare Research and Quality, Rockville, Md., US Dept of Health and Human Services AHRQ publication 01–E058.

15. Blaivas, M., Adhikari, S., 2009. An unseen danger: frequency of posterior vessel wall penetration by needles during attempts to place internal jugular vein central catheters using ultrasound guidance. Crit Care Med 37 (8), 2345–2349.

16. Blaivas, M., Brannam, L., Fernandez, E. 2003. Short-axis versus long-axis approaches for teaching ultrasound-guided vascular access on a new inanimate model. Acad Emerg Med 10 (12), 1307–1311.

17. Wynd, K., Smith, H.M., Jacob, A.K., et al., 2009. Ultrasound machine comparison. An evaluation of ergonomic design, data management, ease of use, and image quality. Reg Anesth Pain Med 34, 349–356.

Additional Reading

Abrahams, M.S., Aziz, M.F., Fu, R.F., et al., 2009. Ultrasound guidance compared with electrical neurostimulation for peripheral nerve block: a systematic review and meta-analysis of randomized controlled trials. Br J Anaesth 102, 408–417.

Chan, V.W.S., 2008. Ultrasound imaging for regional anesthesia: a practical guide. Toronto Printing, Toronto, Canada.

Ban, C.H.T., 2007. Atlas of ultrasound and nerve stimulation-guided regional anesthesia. Springer, New York.

Reeves, A.R., Seshadri, R., Trerotola, S.O., 2001. Recent trends in central venous catheter placement: a comparison of interventional radiology with other specialties. J Vasc Interv Radiol 12, 1211–1214.

Chapter 16

Intravenous Therapy, Fluid Delivery Systems for Resuscitation, and Cell Salvage Devices

Vanessa G. Henke and Warren S. Sandberg

Fluid Delivery Systems for Resuscitation

Infusion Devices

Background

Determinants of Fluid Flow Rate

Numerous factors determine the flow rate of IV fluids, including characteristics of the fluid itself, characteristics of the IV circuit that are extrinsic to the patient, and patient-driven determinants of the driving pressure for fluid flow (Figure 16–1).

Characteristics of the infusate that affect flow rate include its viscosity and temperature, its potential to form air locks or overwhelm closed air filters (with air derived either from the fluid source or from spontaneous bubble formation as a cold solution spontaneously warms within the IV circuit), or its potential to occlude the administration set with particulate matter (such as clot, emulsifiers, or precipitates resulting from incompatible infusates) (Table 16–1).

Features of the IV circuit that affect fluid flow include the inner diameter of the IV catheter, tubing, injection ports

and Luer- locks, the length of each circuit component (particularly the narrowest components), the distensibility of the tubing[1] and its propensity to kink, whether the fluid delivery system is pressurized, and the vertical distance between the fluid source and the target vein. When multiple fluid sources funnel into the same IV catheter, the carrier flow rate, the relative pressurization of each fluid source, and the competency of any one-way valves at the convergence of two fluid streams can also profoundly affect the forward flow rate for each infusate.[2,3] Lastly, fluid flow rate also reflects patient-specific factors such as the back-pressure in the cannulated vein (intrinsic or extrinsic [i.e., from a noninvasive blood pressure cuff]) and the pressure gradient between the vein containing the IV cannula and the right atrium.[4]

Determinants of Drug Delivery

Drug delivery through an IV administration set is a function of the concentration of the stock solution of drug given as an infusion through a piggyback into a carrier infusion, and the flow rates of both infusions (Figure 16–2). Another important factor is the size of the dead space volume (V) that lies between the convergence of the carrier and drug infusions

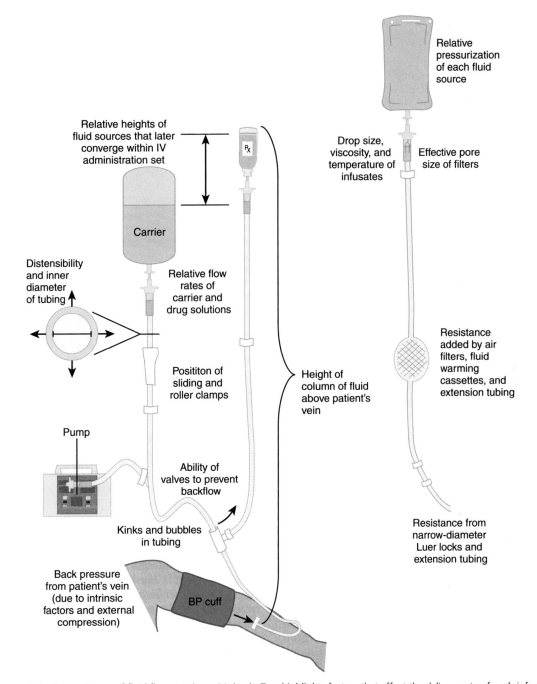

Relative heights of
fluid sources that later
converge within IV
administration set

Carrier

Distensibility
and inner
diameter
of tubing

Relative flow
rates of
carrier and
drug solutions

Posititon of
sliding and
roller clamps

Pump

Ability of
valves to prevent
backflow

Kinks and bubbles
in tubing

Back pressure
from patient's vein
(due to intrinsic
factors and external
compression)

BP cuff

Relative
pressurization
of each fluid
source

Drop size,
viscosity, and
temperature of
infusates

Effective pore
size of filters

Height of
column of fluid
above patient's
vein

Resistance
added by air
filters, fluid
warming
cassettes, and
extension tubing

Resistance from
narrow-diameter
Luer locks and
extension tubing

Figure 16–1   Determinants of fluid flow rate in an IV circuit. Text highlights factors that affect the delivery rate of each infusate.

and the tip of the IV cannula. To avoid fluctuations in drug delivery, the carrier flow rate within IV tubing should be kept constant and the dead space of the infusion system should be minimized. Avoid using concentrated solutions of potent drugs to minimize the risk of complications if carrier flow changes abruptly.[3]

Experimental and mathematical models[3] demonstrate that it takes 1 to 3 time constants for the drug concentration volume (V) throughout the dead space to reach a new steady state after a change in carrier or drug flow rate. The time required for a new drug infusion to reach the patient at the desired concentration also varies significantly, depending on the dead space volume of the side port that must be primed.[3]

CHARACTERIZING FLUID FLOW WITHIN THE IV CIRCUIT

The impact of length and inner diameter on fluid flow rates (through both catheters and IV cannulas) has long been appreciated.[5] Historically, fluid flow through IV catheters and tubing was considered laminar (and therefore has been described by the Poiseuille formula) (Figure 16–3, *A*). However, the Poiseuille formula does not fully describe pressure loss for fluid flow through IV cannulas and IV tubing. Laminar flow through an IV catheter is prevented by the short length and abrupt decrements in tubing diameter (i.e., where the IV administration set meets the catheter), which create eddies.

Table 16–1 Combinations Known to Occlude IV Administration Sets

Mechanism of Occlusion	Examples
Clot formation	Calcium-containing solutions (lactated Ringer's, Hetastarch) with blood products
Precipitate formation	Thiopental with vecuronium/pancuronium; heparin, amiodarone, and numerous antibiotics with a variety of anesthesia drugs
	Bicarbonate with calcium/many local anesthetics
Clogged filter	Any of the above; air; emulsifiers such as those in propofol, intralipid

To reduce the risk of precipitate formation within the IV tubing, flush the IV tubing thoroughly after bolus doses and verify drug compatibility, particularly when using amiodarone, protamine, or unfamiliar drugs, particularly antibiotics.

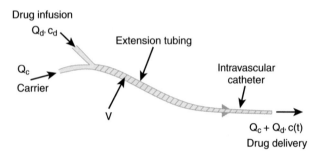

Figure 16–2 Determinants of drug delivery in a system with a carrier infusion. The mass of drug within the dead space volume (V) of IV tubing that lies beyond the convergence of the carrier and the drug infusion (see *shaded area*) equals $t \times c_d \times Q_d$, where the time constant $(t) = V/(Q_d + Q_c)$, Q_d is the infusion rate of the stock solution of the drug, and Q_c is the carrier flow rate. The concentration of drug exiting the IV catheter, $c(t)$, varies with time after any of the variables change. If the flow rate suddenly increases (as often happens when a previously unrecognized empty bag of carrier is replaced), this mass of drug is given as a rapid bolus to the patient, which can be clinically significant. *(Image from Lovich MA, Kinnealley ME, Sims NM, et al. The delivery of drugs to patients by continuous intravenous infusion: modeling predicts potential dose fluctuations depending on flow rates and infusion system dead volume. Anesth Analg 2006;102:1147-1153.)*

In reality, flow through IV tubing and catheters has both laminar and turbulent characteristics.[6–8] Accordingly, the prevailing model for flow through IV catheters and infusion systems incorporates both types of flow by using a quadratic equation (Figure 16–3, *B*) to describe the relationship between radius and flow, rather than Poiseuille's quadratic relationship. For IV catheters, the laminar component of pressure loss (which has a linear pressure-flow relationship) is consistent with what the Poiseuille formula would predict, while the turbulent component reflects pressure loss due to flow disturbances at the inlet, and where the catheter changes shape. For IV tubing, there is an additional component of turbulent-flow pressure loss that is proportional to tubing length. Recent research indicates that while radius is the most powerful determinant of flow rate through an IV catheter, the effect of changing radius on flow rates through 14- to 20-gauge IV catheters is less than commonly believed.[9]

Regulations from the International Organization for Standardization require the disclosure of maximal IV flow rates through all catheters. These quoted rates describe the flow through a perfectly straight cannula into an open receptacle, from an IV fluid source located 100 cm above the receptacle.[10] While these idealized conditions approximate neither conditions in the operating room nor the maximum flow rates obtained clinically, the quoted rates are helpful for making comparisons among various IV catheters.

IV Catheters
Overview

IV cannulation devices consist of a tapered catheter threaded over a hollow-bore needle. Most are latex-free, radio-opaque, and nonpyrogenic. While no venipuncture system can eliminate the risk of unintended needlesticks, self-retracting safety systems eliminate the risk of needlesticks after a needle is withdrawn from its catheter.

Because of its comparatively shorter length (and lower resistance), a large-bore, well-functioning peripheral IV is considered superior to a central venous catheter for large volume fluid resuscitation. For example, as highlighted in Table 16–2, manufacturer-quoted maximum flow rates are significantly lower for central venous catheters, as compared with peripheral IV catheters with the same inner diameter. This difference is fivefold when comparing the flow through a 16-gauge peripheral IV (approximately 330 mL/min) to that through the 16-gauge proximal port of a triple lumen central line (63 mL/min) (Table 16–2).

OTHER FEATURES OF IV CANNULATION SYSTEMS

Other important design features include the conformation of the orifice on the needle tip and the distance between this orifice and the catheter tip (see Figure 16–5). A flash of blood appears (whose location may vary, see Figure 16–4) when the tip of the needle orifice enters the vessel lumen; the needle must then be advanced further to project the catheter tip into the vessel lumen before the catheter can be threaded. Because unfamiliarity with these product-specific spatial relationships can predispose one to transect or tear a vein during attempted cannulation, it is useful to become facile with a variety of IV cannulation systems.

Other product-specific features also affect the cannulation process (Figure 16–5). These include the needle penetration force required (which can range from 50 to 150 g) during cannulation (which is largely determined by the needle bevel), the type of hub used to advance the catheter, and the degree to which the catheter tapers (which affects catheter penetration force, a force that typically exceeds needle penetration force by onefold to twofold).[11] Material memory can cause severe kinks to persist, even after extrinsic forces are removed.

Rapid Infusion Catheters
Rationale

The rapid infusion catheter is designed to replace an in situ 20-gauge (or larger) peripheral IV catheter, to facilitate large volume rapid infusions (Figure 16–6). RIC lines allow for more rapid infusion rates as compared to central and conventional peripheral catheters, owing to their larger

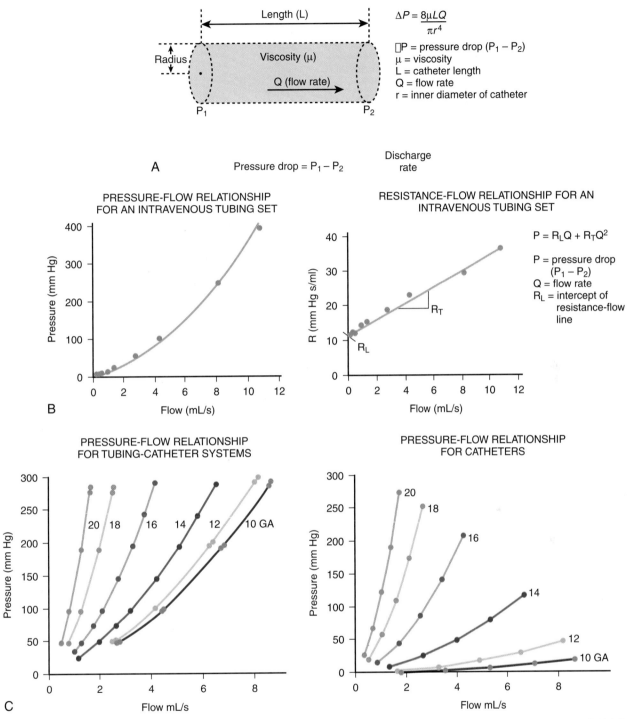

Figure 16–3   Formulae describing fluid flow through tubing. **A,** The Poiseuille formula describes the laminar flow rate of a Newtonian fluid (whose viscosity depends only on temperature and pressure) through a straight cylinder with a circular cross-section. When the Reynolds number of the fluid is less than 2000-2300, laminar flow is predicted. **B,** Experimentally derived data show that flow through IV catheters has both laminar and turbulent characteristics, and the pressure-flow relationship in plastic tubing and cannulas is nonlinear (see graph on *left*). The coefficient of flow (R_L) and coefficient of the square of flow (R_T) are (respectively) the intercept and slope of the resistance flow plot (see graph on *right*). The relationship between length and each of the parameters of flow is linear. Therefore the quadratic equation $P = R_LQ + R_TQ^2$ describes the pressure-flow relationship for plastic intravenous tubing and cannulas. **C,** Experimentally derived data show that the pressure-flow relationships for both tubing-catheter systems and isolated catheters are nonlinear; both systems are described by the equation shown in **B**. *(Figures in* **B** *taken from Philip BK, Philip JH. Characterization of flow in intravenous infusion systems. IEEE Trans Biomed Eng 1983;30:702-707. Figures in* **C** *taken from Philip BK, Philip JH. Characterization of flow in intravenous catheters. IEEE Trans Biomed Eng 1986;33:529-331.)*

Table 16–2 Characteristics of Commonly Used IV Catheters

Gauge	Inner Diameter (mm)	Length	Manufacturer-Quoted Flow (mL/min)
14 Jelco	2.25 mm	50 mm	315
Introcan	2.2 mm		345
16 Jelco	1.85 mm	50 mm	210
Introcan	1.7 mm		
18 Jelco	1.35 mm	45 mm	100
Introcan	1.3 mm		
20 Jelco	1.15 mm	32 mm	63
Introcan	1.1 mm		60
22 Jelco	0.9 mm	25 mm	33
Introcan			35
24 Jelco	0.7 mm	16 mm	24
Introcan		19 mm	22
7F Triple-lumen arrow central catheter for use only with 8.5 or 9F percutaneous sheath introducer (PSI)			
16 (proximal)		140 mm	76
18 (medial)			35
18 (distal)			36
7F Triple-lumen arrow central catheter for use only with MAC two-lumen central venous access device			
16 (proximal)			63
18 (medial)			26
18 (distal)			25

Overview of key parameters for commonly used peripheral IV catheters (Jelco Smiths Medical, St Paul, Minn; Introcan B. Braun Medical, Bethlehem, Pa), including inner diameter, catheter length, and manufacturer-quoted flow rates (derived using ISO standards). For comparison, the maximal flow rates through representative central venous catheters (Arrow International Corp, Reading, Pa.) are also shown.

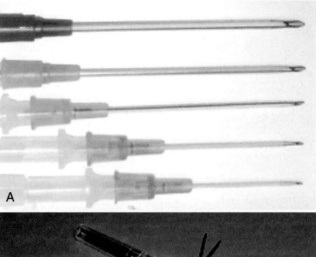

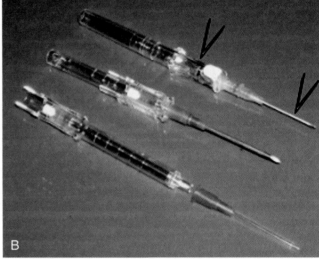

Figure 16–4 Examples of self-retracting and "unprotected" IV cannulation devices. **A,** Unprotected cannulation sets (*top to bottom*): 14-, 16-, 18-, 20-, 22-gauge sets (Jelco, Smiths Medical, St. Paul, Minn.). **B,** Safety cannulation systems: *Top:* 22-gauge catheter set ready for use (needle retracts when white button is pressed), *carets* point to sites where the flash of blood is visible during cannulation; *middle:* 14-gauge catheter set ready for use; *bottom:* 14-gauge catheter fully deployed with needle manually retracted. *(Insyte Autoguard 22-gauge, Becton Dickinson Infusion Therapy Systems, Sandy, Utah; PROTECTIV Jelco 14-gauge, Smiths Medical, St. Paul, Minn.)*

diameter and shorter length. Relative to central lines, RIC lines can be easier or faster to place (and even have a role in pediatrics), although central access can be easier to obtain and more reliable when peripheral veins are small or friable. Because of the dire consequences of intra-arterial infusion of air, pharmacologic agents or fluids (especially under pressure), it is critical to confirm that the RIC is intravenous before using it.

Technique

To place a RIC, the guidewire is advanced through an in situ IV catheter (with limited force, to avoid damaging the vein), and the preexisting IV catheter is removed. Next, the skin opening is enlarged, by advancing the scalpel away from the guidewire, carefully to avoid cutting the guidewire or creating a skin bridge. The dilator is then threaded over the guidewire, grasped close to the skin incision, and advanced through the skin and subcutaneous tissues into the vein with a slight twisting motion. Finally, the dilator is removed, and the infusion catheter is inserted, connected to IV tubing, and sutured into place.

To achieve maximal flow rates with the RIC, standard-gauge stopcocks and any small-diameter or unnecessary lengths of IV tubing should be removed from the IV

administration set. The maximal flow rate through a RIC doubles when IV tubing with a large inner diameter is used.[12]

Intraosseous Needles
Rationale

Sometimes intravenous access is impossible. However all patients have long bones, and the bone marrow space is connected to the circulation. In fact, the bone marrow space, or intraosseous compartment, is considered to be connected to the central circulation and is suitable for administration of fluids for resuscitation and potent vasopressors.

Intraosseous cannulation has been described using various needles, typically as a technique of last resort. Pain on insertion, pain on injection, and concerns about osteomyelitis have limited use of the technique in the past. Recently available commercial kits and changes in technique have effectively addressed most of these concerns these obstacles.

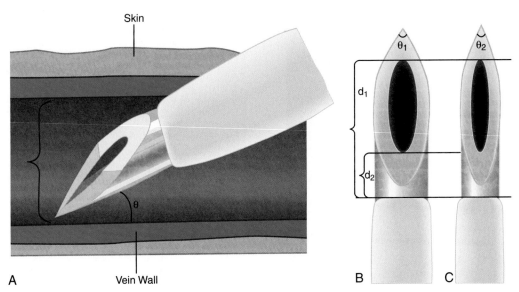

Figure 16–5   Product features affecting the cannulation process. Several factors determine how far a needle must be advanced after obtaining flashback before attempting to advance the catheter. These include **(A)** the inner diameter of the vessel *(bracket),* the angle of the needle relative to the vessel (θ), and **(B)** the distance between the proximal tip of the needle opening and the distal tip of the catheter *(as indicated by the distance d1, as well as the distance between the proximal opening of the needle and the distal tip of the catheter, as indicated by the distance d₂).* Because the bevel of the needle (θ₁>θ₂) is sharper and the needle diameter is narrower, less force would be required to use the cannulation set in **(C)** as compared to the set in **B**.

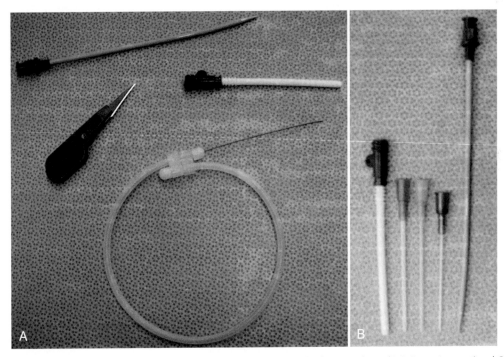

Figure 16–6   RIC equipment. **A,** This 8.5F × 2.5″ (6.4 cm) radiopaque, latex-free rapid infusion catheter (RIC, Arrow International Corp, Reading, Pa.) is characteristic of those available in North America. A 7F × 2″ (5.08 cm) is also available. The kit also includes a dilator, a 13.125″ (33 cm) spring-wire guide and a #11 scalpel. **B,** Relative sizes of *(from left to right)* an 8.5F RIC, various peripheral IV catheters (14g, 16g, 18g) and the dilator supplied for use with the 8.5F RIC catheter.

Technique

A commercially available intraosseous access kit is illustrated in Figure 16–7. The kit contains all of the items needed to make the technique safe and relatively painless. The skin over the selected bony prominence should be disinfected with a germicidal, persistent solution, such as chlorhexidine in alcohol (shown as part of the kit in Figure 16–7). Local anesthesia is provided at the skin puncture site. The appropriate length of needle is chosen; typically only one diameter is available. The needle is inserted with a powered driver, shown in Figure 16–8. Use of a powered driver to spin the needle shortens the duration of painful stimulus, reduces the insertion force required, and adds an element of control in placement. Pain from injection is alleviated by first giving a dose of local anesthetic such as lidocaine. After lidocaine administration, the

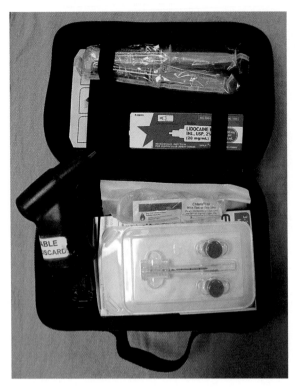

Figure 16–7 Intraosseous needle insertion kit. This commercially available kit has been customized so that it contains all items needed to obtain intraosseous access, including the needle and driver, a disinfectant applicator, lidocaine to blunt the pain of injection, and syringes of flush solution. Hidden behind the drugs is a graphic instruction card showing sites and insertion technique.

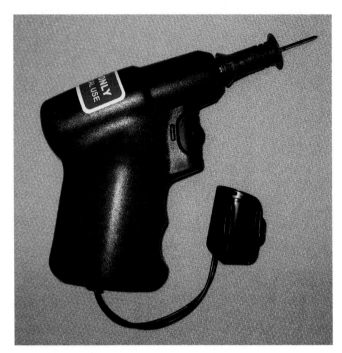

Figure 16–8 Intraosseous needle mounted on powered driver, ready for insertion.

needle should be flushed under pressure, with one or more 10-mL syringes of sterile normal saline to establish flow.

Confirmation of successful insertion hinges on a constellation of "soft" findings, including a firmly seated needle, potential (but not certain) ability to aspirate blood from the needle, easy flow of fluids under pressure, and expected responses to pharmacological agents. Because the intramedullary pressure is higher than venous pressure (typically 35 to 50 mm Hg), fluids must be given under pressure to achieve high flow rates.

Intraosseous administration provides quick access to the circulation and should be considered when access is difficult. This is particularly true when difficulty obtaining intravenous access is delaying administration of resuscitation drugs. Even in elective settings, the intraosseous route may be preferable to repeated attempts at starting a peripheral IV. Common insertion sites include the distal and proximal tibia and the proximal humerus. All of these have the key feature of being palpable even in obesity, and well removed from any major nerves or blood vessels.

Contraindications include: infection at the potential insertion site, fracture of the target bone, and recent procedures involving the target bone.

IV Tubing Sets
Overview

Simple fluid administration sets typically consist of a dripper, a drip chamber, a rolling side-clamp to adjust flow, sliding clamps to occlude flow, and, typically, some kind of injection

port (Figure 16–9, *A*). Manufacturer-quoted drop size (often 15 gtt/mL for adult sets, 60 gtt/mL for pediatric sets) describes the flow rate of a standard crystalloid infusate at room temperature. The internal diameter of tubing typically ranges from approximately 0.1 to 0.3 mm. Many sets also contain an air filter (typically capable of sequestering less than 5 mL of air).

While injection ports are sometimes left out of administration sets designed to be piggy-backed onto other infusion tubing, most sets contain stopcocks and/or swabbable injection ports (Figure 16–9, *B*). The advantage of swabbable injection ports is that they can be effectively cleaned with an alcohol wipe before each use, which reduces the risk of introducing bacteria into the fluid stream and causing infection. In contrast, stopcock injection ports leave the fluid path open to air when the cap is removed, and, if contaminated, the caps and edges of the port cannot be effectively cleaned without compromising the sterility of the fluid stream. However, an advantage of these ports is that the stopcock can be easily closed to prevent backflow, which is a distinct advantage when relative pressurization of part of the fluid stream (i.e., by manual boluses or use of a pressure infuser) is anticipated.

In practice, drop size and fluid flow rates also reflect intrinsic fluid properties, such as viscosity and temperature. Dilution alone allows a fivefold increase in the gravity flow rate of refrigerated packed red blood cells through standard IV tubing,[13,14] and is achieved by simply adding a 250-mL bag of warmed normal saline to each unit of blood (see Figure 16–10 for technique). This technique reduces viscosity (hematocrit drops by approximately 50%) and increases temperature (from 18° to 26° C).[15]

To allow further increases in flow rate, fluid administration sets (designed to accommodate red blood cell products) may have a larger inner diameter and contain a pressure reservoir

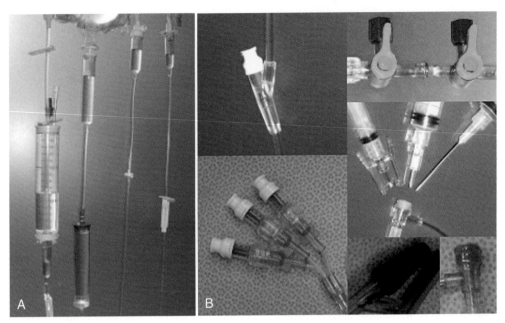

Figure 16–9   Various types of IV tubing and injection ports. **A,** Various drip sets. *Left-to-right:* pediatric burette (60 gtt/mL dripper; burette has access point for aspiration of air or injection of exogenous fluids); administration set with pressure reservoir, helpful for administration of viscous infusates (15 gtt/mL dripper); standard administration set (15 gtt/mL dripper); piggyback tubing (60 gtt/mL dripper). **B,** Various types of injection ports. *Clockwise from top right:* (1) Two-gang stopcock capped injection ports; (2) injection port compatible for use with lever-locking blunt connectors, blunt connectors and sharps (arranged from *left to right* above the port); (3) close-up of aforementioned injection port; (4) injection port with female Luer lock, also compatible for use with sharps; (5) set of three parallel injection ports (commonly used in TIVA) with female Luer locks, which funnels distally through narrow-bore tubing to terminate with a male Luer lock; (6) swabbable injection port built into a standard IV administration set.

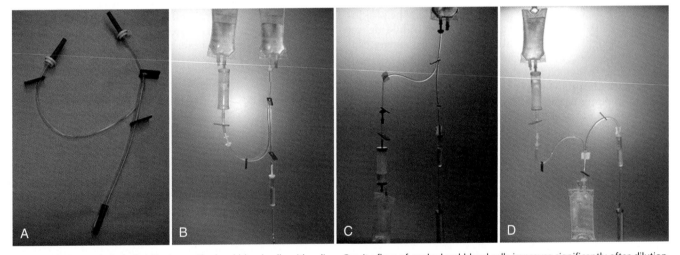

Figure 16–10   Technique for diluting packed red blood cells with saline. Gravity flow of packed red blood cells improves significantly after dilution with normal saline (preferably warmed). **A,** Y-set extension tubing: tubing set consists of two proximal spikes and one distal female connector; each limb has a clamp (Arrow International Inc, Reading, Pa.). **B,** Step 1: attach packed RBC *(left side)* and deaired bag of normal saline *(right side)* to proximal limbs of extension tubing, with the distal limb clamped shut. **C,** Step 2: drop the RBC bag *(left)* below the axis of the saline bag *(right)*, allowing normal saline to enter the RBC bag. **D,** Step 3: to infuse diluted blood, hang RBC bag *(left)*; the empty saline bag may be left hanging (as shown in *middle*) or simply clamped shut; open clamp on distal limb *(right)* to allow infusion to begin.

that often holds 50 to 60 mL. A one-way ball valve at the proximal end of this reservoir allows for manual boluses of the infusate. To convert the one-way valve into a two-way valve (for instance, to evacuate air from the reservoir during priming or air derived from an IV bag), the ball is manually displaced before the reservoir is squeezed. Specialized tubing designed for platelet administration is optimized to minimize priming volume.

Specialized IV Tubing

When running low-volume infusion pumps, rigid tubing is useful. Its limited distensibility and low priming volumes (generally <1 to 2 mL) facilitate accurate titration of important infusates, such as narcotics and vasoactive drugs, and minimize the volume needed to flush through bolus doses of medication in pediatric cases (Figure 16–11, *A, B*). For

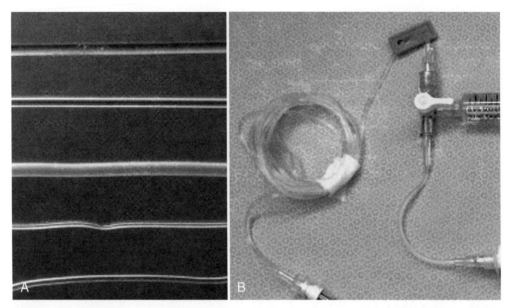

Figure 16–11   Specialized IV tubing. **A,** Diameters of various types of IV tubing. *Top to bottom*: Conventional IV tubing (Arrow, Reading, Pa.), pressure tubing (Edwards Lifesciences, Irvine, Calif.), level 1 high flow extension line tubing (Smiths, Rockland, Mass.), high pressure microbore tubing (Churchill Medical Systems Inc, Horsham, Pa.), and microbore extension tubing (which adds significant resistance when used as a link between the IV cannula and the administration set; (Hospira, Lake Forest, Ill.). **B,** Rigid tubing: microbore extension tubing with stopcock, often used in pediatrics to minimize the dead space volume of IV tubing that must be flushed after each bolus is delivered: 78" set; ~0.8 mL priming volume; the syringes connected to the stopcock *(top)* and terminus of the tubing *(bottom)* represent an intended bolus dose of a drug and the flush solution, respectively. *(Churchill Medical Systems, Horsham, Pa.).*

intermediate-volume infusions, specialized gravity sets are useful, including burette sets, which are especially helpful in pediatrics. For infusions through a resuscitation fluid-delivery device, high-flow tubing with a larger inner diameter can be used to connect the resuscitation device tubing directly to the IV catheter to maximize the flow rate.

Warm fluids soften most IV tubing, making it more susceptible to kinking. In cases where positioning will limit access to IV tubing and warmed fluids might be used, it is helpful to place tape over curves in IV tubing (i.e., near the catheter insertion site), to prevent kinks from forming later.

Pressurized Infusions

To increase fluid flow through a gravity IV set, simple pressure infusion devices and specialized pressure-generating machines are available (Figure 16–12). Pressurization of saline-diluted packed red blood cells to 150 to 300 mm Hg yields at least a threefold increase in the flow rate when compared with gravity administration.[16,17] Simple pressure bags can be inflated manually using the built-in hand-operated pressure bulb. Although it is faster to connect a length of oxygen tubing to the stopcock on the pump apparatus and fill the bag with air or oxygen from a pressurized source, such as the oxygen supply on the anesthesia machine. Some pressurization machines come with an air compressor, while others rely on an exogenous pressurization source, such as the wall air supply. A gauge shows the pressure within the bag.

Pressurizing an infusion increases the risk of both air embolism (which is discussed further below) and compartment syndrome (a rare complication). Compartment syndrome (requiring fasciotomy) has been reported after infusion of just

1 L of crystalloid pressurized to 150 mm Hg during trauma surgery.[18] To recognize an infiltrated IV early (and avoid precipitating compartment syndrome), vigilant surveillance of the IV site is necessary whenever pressurized infusions are delivered, especially since the IV site is often obscured by drapes.

Air Embolism

The incidence of air embolism (both venous and arterial) increases during the perioperative period, especially when large volumes are rapidly infused during periods of intense clinical activity. As little as 200 mL of intravenous air has been proven to trigger cardiac arrest and death.[19,20] Significantly less air is needed to cause a clinically significant outcome from arterial air embolism. Any venous air embolism has the potential to cause arterial air embolism, even when there are no pathological right-to-left shunts. The risk of secondary arterial air embolism correlates with the size of the venous air embolus. Intracerebral arterial air emboli often consist of bubbles with a diameter of just 30 to 60 microns, and cause ischemic stroke with cerebral ischemia and vasogenic edema.[21]

Entrained air may derive from the IV solution bag itself, or from room air if the integrity of the IV circuit is disrupted. Another important source of air in IV tubing results from the phenomenon of "outgassing," in which air bubbles develop and expand as fluids warm. As they warm, fluids accommodate less dissolved gas. Specifically, Henry's law ($p = k_{\mathrm{H}}c$) describes how the amount of a gas dissolved in a liquid is a function of the partial pressure of that gas in contact with the liquid and the solubility coefficient (which is defined for each gas-liquid pair, and drops at higher temperatures), and Charles' law ($V_1 / T_1 = V_2 / T_2$) describes the proportionality

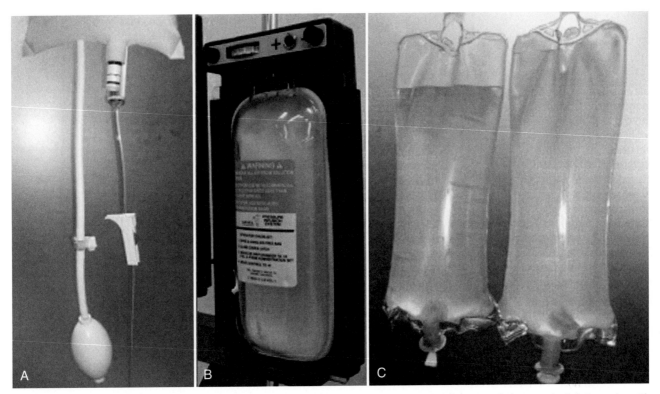

Figure 16–12 Pressure infusers. **A,** Manually operated pressure infusion setups contain a three-way stopcock that permits inflation using either the bulb or via tubing connected to a pressurized air source and a gauge that displays the pressure within the bag. **B,** Automated pressure infusion device. **C,** Before using a pressure infuser, IV bags must be de-aired *(right)* to remove the significant amount of air included by the manufacturer in each bag *(left)*.

between temperature and the volume occupied by a given quantity of gas (causing bubbles to expand as temperature rises).[22]

Outgassing becomes clinically significant as cool solutions (such as premixed refrigerated solutions) passively warm to room temperature within the IV tubing set, when room temperature fluids are infused inside a heated room, or when fluids are passed through a warmer. To minimize the degree of outgassing that occurs within the IV tubing, one can allow cool solutions to equilibrate to room temperature, before de-airing and attaching them to the IV administration set. When large volumes of fluid are delivered through fluid warmers, outgassing results in large amounts of air. Consequently, fluid warming systems incorporate a variety of air detection and air evacuation systems, which are described further in the section on fluid warmers.

Preventing Venous Air Embolism from the IV Administration Set

Most IV solution bags contain 40 to 100 mL of air as packaged, and priming volumes for standard IV tubing sets are in the range of 5 to 20 mL (plus the volume contained by any reservoirs, burettes, or extension tubing). Nearly all air can be removed with careful technique. After spiking the IV bag, air is removed by withdrawing the spike, compressing the IV bag to evacuate all the air, and respiking the air-depleted bag. The drip chamber should be filled to approximately to the two-thirds level, and all ports should be primed and tightly recapped. To prevent entrainment of room air into the system (and backup of intravenous blood), all capped ports and Luer connections should be tightly closed.

Preventing Arterial Air Embolism in High-Risk Patients

Even minuscule bubbles can cause clinically significant air embolism when they reach the arterial circulation. Therefore, air filters are used to reduce the risk of venous air embolism in patients at risk of arterial embolism via a right-to-left shunt. The patients at highest risk are those with baseline right-to-left intracardiac or intrapulmonary shunts, and those with the potential to develop such shunts during the stress of the perioperative period (approximately 25% of the population is estimated to have a patent foramen ovale;[23,24] right-to-left shunt flow is more likely to occur in the setting of pulmonary hypertension and other conditions frequently encountered or exacerbated in the perioperative setting).

An in-line air filter reduces the risk of venous and secondary arterial air emboli, though this risk reduction is limited by the capacity of the filter. Most air filters hold less than 3 mL of air, and flow slows and ultimately halts as air accumulates within the filter. Autoventing filters, which use a microporous membrane that can continuously vent air, are more costly, and the surface area of the microporous membrane limits the rate at which air can be vented. Filters can fail, and when placed backwards some air filters allow air to pass indiscriminately.

To reduce the risk of air embolism, an air filter should be attached close to the patient to prevent inadvertent administration of air when medications are given through a distal port (Figure 16–13). A three-way Luer lock or injection port placed downstream of the filter can be used to give air-free substances that exceed the 0.2-micrometer diameter of conventional air filters (i.e., propofol, any poorly soluble substances, or any blood products). Maximum flow rates are significantly lower

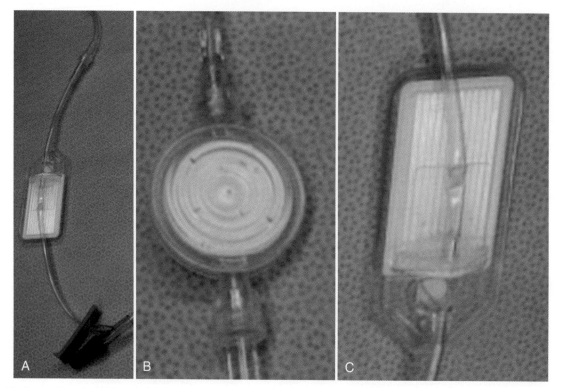

Figure 16–13 Preventing arterial air embolism in high-risk patients. **A,** Air filter in line, with distal injection port, which can be reserved exclusively for boluses of medications (such as propofol) and cellular blood products that would clog the filter. **B,** Air filter 7″ set: 0.2-μm filter. **C,** Macrobore extension set: 0.2-μm filter; distal injection port. *(B, Medex, Dublin, Ohio; C, Hospira, Lake Forest, Ill.)*

through air filters because of added resistance from the filter membrane and extension tubing.

Filtration of Blood Products

Overview of Blood Product Filters

To prevent administration of clots or other particulate debris, a particulate filter must be used for administration of blood products (including RBCs, platelets, granulocytes, FFP, and cryoprecipitate) (Figure 16–14). Typical particulate filters for this purpose have a pore diameter of 170 to 260 microns. The efficacy of filters designed for blood products depends upon pore size of the filter, the load of aggregates already deposited in the filter (which reflects the age, handling, and amount of the blood products given), and the speed and pressure at which products have been driven through the filter.

Standard screen filters for blood products consist of a screen with a pore diameter of 170 microns, designed to remove particulate debris. In contrast, microaggregate filters (which are not generally used in the perioperative setting) trap smaller particles in a synthetic unwoven mesh with a smaller effective pore size.

Administering Blood Products hrough the Filter Set

General Guidelines for Perioperative Administration of Blood Products

To prepare for a transfusion, the IV tubing should be primed with the blood component itself, or with sodium chloride (0.9%) or other isotonic, calcium-free blood-compatible solutions, such as albumin (5%) or plasma protein fraction.

The IV tubing must be flushed to eliminate calcium, since clot forms within the IV line if the calcium content overwhelms the buffering capacity of the citrate anticoagulant.[25] Examples of calcium-containing solutions capable of inducing clot formation include lactated Ringer's (which contains 3 mEq/L of ionized calcium) and hetastarch 6%, which is diluted in lactated Ringer's. Since they would cause hemolysis, hypotonic solutions must also be avoided when transfusing cellular blood products.

A stopcock should be positioned close to the IV cannula to permit infusion of normal saline in the event of a transfusion reaction. Most potentially life-threatening transfusion reactions occur within the first 15 minutes of a transfusion.[26]

Specialized leukocyte-reduction filters are not indicated for routine administration of blood products in the perioperative setting. For appropriate patients, third-generation leukocyte reduction filters are often used in the blood bank to decrease the incidence of febrile transfusion reactions, HLA alloimmunization, and CMV transmission. The use of such filters at the bedside is limited by an increased risk of dramatic hypotension, particularly among patients on angiotension-converting enzyme (ACE) inhibitors.[27]

Erythrocytes

Normal erythrocytes are less than 7 microns in diameter. Erythrocyte transfusions should be given through a 170- to 260-micron particulate filter. The technique for packed red cell dilution is described previously in Figure 16–10.

Because the filter traps coagulated proteins, cell aggregates, and cellular debris, the milieu at the filter surface promotes bacterial growth and slows flow through the filter. For this reason, the American Association of Blood Banks recommends that a reasonable time limit for the use of a particulate

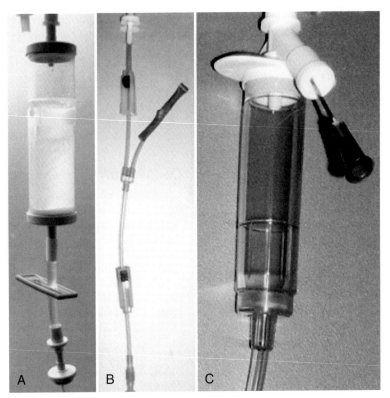

Figure 16–14　Blood product filters. **A,** Filter for erythrocytes and plasma products, with pore size 170-260 μm; approximately 15 gtt/mL when used for blood **B,** Filter/tubing for platelets, with small priming volume and Y-site to permit storage of aliquots (common for pediatric patients); 80-μm filter is located at the bottom of the photo. **C,** Filter/tubing for albumin, with 15-μm filter and membrane (punctured with supplied 19-gauge needle) to vent air: 20 gtt/mL for 5% albumin; 25 gtt/mL for 25% albumin. *(A, Baxter, Deerfield, Ill.; B, Baxter Healthcare Corp, Deerfield, Ill.; C, Accellent Inc, El Paso, Tex.)*

filter is 4 hours (standard filters are designed to filter 2 to 4 units of blood). For optimal performance and flow rates, filters should be fully wetted, and the filter drip chamber should be less than half full.[28]

When microaggregate filters are employed (i.e., in pediatric cases where their small priming volume can be advantageous), caution must be exercised to prevent generating negative pressure, since negative pressure filtration of stored red blood cells through a microaggregate filter can cause hemoylsis.[27]

Positive-pressure erythrocyte infusions can also cause varying degrees of hemolysis, particularly when given through a small-bore IV, and when the viscosity and hematocrit of the infusion are high. Dilution of packed red cells with saline improves delivery rate via syringe pump. At pressures of greater than 300 mm Hg, the seams of a blood bag may leak or rupture.

Platelets

Normal platelets measure 2 to 4 microns in diameter. Platelet infusion sets (and sets for granulocytes and other low volume blood products) have a small priming volume and tubing inner diameter to minimize waste. Platelet filters typically consist of a 170- or 260-micron particulate filter (though filters with smaller pores, such as 80 microns, are also acceptable).

Platelet products must be handled with care to prevent triggering aggregation or introducing contamination (platelets, the only blood product stored at room temperature, are the most likely blood products to become contaminated, typically by gram-positive skin flora). To prevent aggregation, platelets should be administered through unpressurized tubing

primed with normal saline or albumin, with no traces of calcium, which has not been used for red blood cells (which leave behind fibrin and cellular debris).

Fluid Warmers

Background: Intraoperative Hypothermia

Intraoperative hypothermia stems from patient-mediated processes (that alter thermoregulation and redistribute heat from core to periphery, and alter metabolic rate), and processes extrinsic to the patient (such as conductive and convective losses, and infusion of hypothermic fluids). Induction of anesthesia leads to hypothermia due to redistribution, with peripheral vasodilation and transfer of core body heat to the cooler periphery. Mean body temperature decreases on the order of 0.25° C for each unit of refrigerated blood (stored at 4° C to 6° C) or each liter of room temperature crystalloid infused intraoperatively.[28]

Intraoperative hypothermia is a significant cause of morbidity. Prospective, randomized trials show that a 2° C drop in core body temperature triples the relative risk of perioperative myocardial complications[29] (largely via sympathetic nervous system activation) and surgical wound infection.[30] Intraoperative hypothermia also affects pharmacokinetics and pharmacodynamics,[31,32] contributes to negative nitrogen balance and shivering,[33] and increases duration of recovery, patient discomfort, and need for hospitalization.[34,35] Recent murine biochemical data even implicates hypothermia as a necessary precondition for the τ-hyperphosphorylation associated with postoperative cognitive dysfunction, a phenomenon that occurred independent of the type of anesthesia used.[36]

Finally, hypothermia also worsens hemostasis, since it impairs both platelet function (primarily by impairing the release of thromboxane A_2 and the subsequent formation of platelet plugs) and coagulation cascade function (even when coagulation parameters derived from blood samples warmed to room temperature suggest normal clotting function). PTT increases significantly below the 34° C threshold, and both coagulation factor activity and platelet function decline significantly below 33° C.[37,38] A drop in core temperature of just 0.8° C, according to a recent meta-analysis, is associated with statistically significant increases in blood loss (16%, range 4% to 26%) and relative risk for transfusion (22%, range 3% to 37%).[39]

Significant heat is lost from warmed IV fluids as they pass through IV tubing to the patient; especially at lower flow rates. Passively prewarming IV fluid bags before infusion (without concomitant use of a fluid warmer) offers limited benefits if the infusion rate is slow: at flow rates less than 1.2 L/hr (20 mL/min), warmed fluids traveling through noninsulated IV tubing cool by as much as 8° C before they reach the patient.

Overview of Fluid Warming Systems

The primary purpose of IV fluid warmers is to warm infused fluids to near body temperature or slightly above to prevent hypothermia due to infusion of cold fluids. Risks associated with the use of fluid warmers include air embolism, heat-induced hemolysis and vessel injury, current leakage into the fluid path, infection, and pressurized infiltration.[42]

A fluid warmer is also absolutely indicated for the rapid infusion of cold blood products, due to the risks of cardiac arrest and arrhythmia (especially when the sinoatrial node is cooled to less than 30° C). Cardiac arrest has been demonstrated when adults receive blood or plasma at rates greater than 100 mL/min for 30 minutes.[40] The threshold for inducing cardiac arrest is far lower if the transfusion is delivered centrally and in the pediatric population.

Fluid warmers can be broadly categorized into devices designed to warm fluids for routine cases and more complex devices designed for large volume resuscitation. While all fluid warmers contain a heater, a thermostatic control, and, in most cases, a temperature readout, resuscitation fluid warmers are optimized for higher flows, and stop flow to the patient when significant air is detected in the tubing. Simple fluid warmers deliver warmed fluids at rates up to 150 mL/min (and sometimes at higher rates, with specialized disposable sets and pressurized infusions), in contrast to resuscitation fluid warmers that effectively warm fluids at flow rates up to 750 to 1000 mL/min (one resuscitation fluid warmer even eliminates the need for pressurization).

Heating of IV fluids can be accomplished by dry heat exchange, countercurrent heat exchangers, fluid immersion, or (less effectively) by placing part of the fluid circuit in the proximity of a separate heater (such as a forced-air device or heated water mattress).

Dry Heat Warmers

Many fluid warmers use dry heat, which can be delivered by metal plates or blocks, a magnetic induction heater, or an infrared lamp. Designs strive to maximize the interface for energy transfer while minimizing the amount of energy stored in the heat exchanger to prevent overheating of the infusate in the event of an abrupt decrease in flow. Most dry heat warmers introduce a disposable cassette and additional tubing into the IV circuit to maximize the surface area of the fluid-heater interface, while minimizing the additional resistance caused by a longer fluid path. Many new simple fluid warmers place a small heating unit as close as possible to the patient to minimize heat loss through the IV tubing.

Countercurrent Heat Exchangers

Countercurrent heat exchangers use specialized coaxial tubing that surrounds the IV tubing. The coaxial tubing pumps heated fluids around the IV tubing that carries the infusate. By actively heating the infusate almost to the point where it enters the IV cannula, these designs significantly mitigate heat loss distal to the main heating unit. The bulky, stiff coaxial tubing creates ergonomic challenges; since it is designed to be attached close to the IV cannula, a falling loop of coaxial tubing can even pull the IV cannula out of the patient's vein.

Water Immersion Heaters

Immersion bath fluid warmers have largely been supplanted by other technologies for the delivery of normothermic fluids. Their capacity to warm fluids at high rates is limited, lag time is long due to the time needed to preheat or change the temperature of the bath solution, maintenance is more labor-intensive, and bath solutions are associated with increased risks of infection and equipment colonization.

Other Methods

IV tubing can be diverted through a convective heating device (such as a forced air heater or heated mattress) to deliver warmed fluid at low flow rates.

Simple Fluid Warmers
Overview of Simple Fluid Warmers

With most pole-mounted fluid warmers (for which the heating unit is usually separated from the patient by at least 2 feet of IV tubing), heat loss is significant at flow rates less than 2 L/hr (33 mL/min). In such cases, forced air warming is a more effective means of targeting normothermia. Increasingly, however, simple fluid warmer designs (Table 16–3) mitigate the magnitude of heat loss within the IV tubing distal to the heating unit, even at low flow rates, by placing the heating unit very close to the IV catheter site. Because some models can even function on batteries, warmed fluids can now be delivered even during transport (at flow rates up to 150 mL/min). On the other hand, is a cost-effective means of reducing the degree of hypothermia at infusion rates greater than 2 L/hr, if a simple fluid warmer is not available.

Comparison[41] of several simple fluid warmers (which are described in Table 16–3 and Figure 16–15) highlights the impact of pressurization and flow rate on the temperature of fluid measured at the end of the IV administration set. Room temperature (22° C) bags of crystalloid were pressurized to 300 mm Hg and run through a 1-m fluid head. The temperature and flow

Table 16–3 Comparison of Several Fluid/Blood Warmers

	Features	Air Embolism Risk
FMS 2000 Dry heat (electromagnetic induction) Up to 750 mL/min	Achieves flow rates up to 750 mL/min without need for pressurization, via roller peristaltic pump. Line pressure regulator. Optional 3-L fluid reservoir. Touch screen displays input and output fluid temperature, volume given, line pressure and flow rate.	Two air detectors. If reservoir drains, the patient line automatically shuts off, and machine prompts with instructions (repriming takes <13 sec). Automatic air purging after every 500 mL.
Level 1 H1200 Dry heat (plates) and countercurrent water jacket Up to 1000 mL/min	Delivers warm fluids at rates from 75-1000 mL/min (pressurization required for highest rates).	An improved air detector/clamp unit (previously sold separately, older units without this component were recalled by the FDA in 2006) is integrated into all currently manufactured units. Air must be removed manually.
Ranger Dry heat (plates) Up to 500 mL/min	Cassettes for standard, neonatal, pediatric, and large-volume cases. Optional 150-μm filter. Dual-chamber pressure infusor available.	Automatic venting: air trap removes up to 3000 mL/min of air from the system. Vent whistles as air is vented.
Medi-Temp III FW600 Dry heat (plates) Up to 500 mL/min	Lower recommended maximum flow rates for refrigerated fluids (300 mL/min) or if using standard set (150 mL/min).	Bubble trap with port for manual air removal.
Buddy Dry heat (plates) Up to 100 mL/min	Small (7 oz) heating unit resides close to patient. Disposable has a 7-mL priming volume, a pressure-regulating valve, and a check valve.	Anti-air entrainment valve. Relatively large microporous membrane within disposable automatically vents air from crystalloids.

rate of the exiting fluid through a 14-gauge IV catheter were reported. In contrast to their performance under gravity flow, under pressurization to 300 mmHg, no device warmed the fluid to 37° C. The Ranger (with gravity flow and a standard disposable) and the Fluido (with both gravity and pressurized flow) achieved the highest output temperature: 35° C. The Bair Hugger 241 and Hotline (with both gravity and pressurized flow) and the Ranger (with pressurized flow), achieved only 24° C to 31° C. The authors went on to extrapolate that at the maximum recommended flow rates specified by the manufacturers, all four devices should achieve close to 37° C (17, 83, 150, and 800 mL/min for the Bair Hugger 241, Hotline, Standard Ranger, and Fluido, respectively). Earlier comparisons[42,43] have indicated that the Hotline, Buddy, and Ranger appear to have equal warming capacity at flow rates less than 50 mL/min, and for gravity administration of crystalloid, colloid, and packed RBC. At flow rates greater than 100 mL/min, the Ranger and Buddy are more effective, and at flows greater 180 mL/min, the Ranger is most The Medi-Temp was not included in these studies.

Mechanisms to Reduce Risk of Air Embolism

Simple fluid warmers lack the capacity to automatically vent large quantities of air. They also have no means of increasing the infusion rate beyond that achievable by gravity. While pressurization of the infusate increases flow through simple fluid warmers, it can also compromise their safety. Due to the heightened risk of clinically significant air embolism when large volume rapid infusions of warmed fluid are anticipated, it is best to use a purpose-built resuscitation fluid warmer for such cases.

Resuscitation Fluid Warmers

Resuscitation fluid warmers again contain an electric heater and thermostat, but the control circuits and the heaters are more sophisticated to allow precise heating of large volumes

of fluid delivered at high rates.[43-45] They also have an air detector and a control system that automatically interrupts the flow when air is detected.

Resuscitation fluid warmers are clearly indicated when the anticipated fluid requirement is approximately 1 blood volume (in adults) or greater. The device acquisition costs and disposable costs are substantially greater than for simple fluid warmers. High flow rates are achieved by either pressurization or a roller pump. The roller pump allows for quantitative flow control and infused volume measurements.

Once the anticipated blood loss (and fluid administration requirement) approaches one blood volume, resuscitation warmers with a reservoir offer another advantage, namely that 1 to 3 L of fluid can be kept ready for high flow infusion at all times. When using a reservoir, it is advantageous to keep the fill level between one fourth to one half of the total reservoir volume, so that the composition of the infusate can be readily adjusted to best meet the patient's needs with changing situations. Some disposable sets contain "prefilters" (with pore size of approximately 300 microns) designed to decrease the burden on conventional downstream blood filters. Flow rates improve when packed red cells are diluted before entering the fluid warmer tubing.

Cell Salvage Systems
Overview

Cell salvage (CS) consists of scavenging of blood from operative fields or wound sites for reinfusion into the patient, typically after noncellular matter is reduced by saline dilution followed by centrifugation, a process termed "washing." CS is best suited for cases in which large volume, rapid blood loss into a clean surgical field is anticipated (since these factors maximize the quality of the salvaged blood, and minimize the risks of hemolysis and contamination). In a rapidly bleeding patient, CS can deliver the red cell mass equivalent to

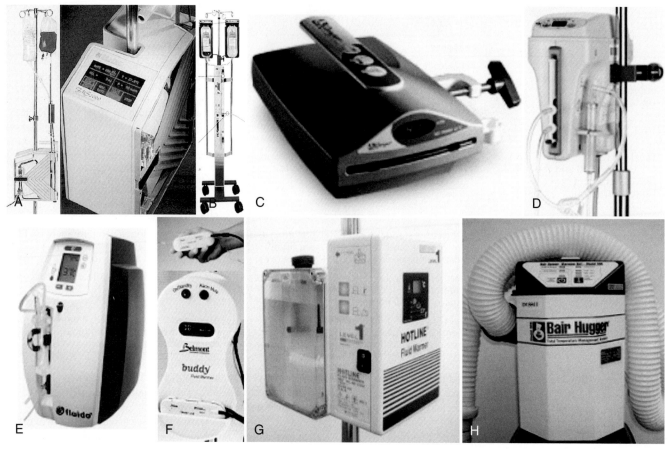

Figure 16-15   Fluid warmers. Purpose-built resuscitation fluid warmers:
A, FMS-2000: this purpose-built resuscitation fluid/blood warmer reliably delivers fluids at physiological temperature at rates up to 750 mL/min. The roller peristaltic pump delivers these flow rates without the need for pressurization, and the robust air detection system automatically shuts off the patient line and triggers an alarm. **B,** Level 1 H1200: this purpose-built resuscitation fluid/blood warmer heats via dry heat (plates) and countercurrent water jacket tubing to deliver fluids at physiological temperature at 75-1000 mL/min. Pressurization is required to deliver the highest flow rates. An improved air detector/clamp unit (which was previously sold separately and had been recalled by the FDA in 2006) is integrated into all currently manufactured units. Air must still be removed manually, in contrast to the FMS-2000 and Ranger.
(**A,** Belmont Instruments, Billerica, Mass.; **B,** Smiths Medical, Rockland, Mass.).
Simple fluid warmers:
C, Ranger: when equipped with a large-volume disposable set, the Ranger effectively warms at infusion rates from KVO-500 mL/min at temperatures of 33° C-41° C (several disposable sets are available, including neonatal). At low flow rates, heat loss within the tubing distal to the pole-mounted heating unit is significant. It withstands pressurization up to 300 mm Hg. **D,** Medi-Temp III FW600: when used with a high-flow disposable set, the manufacturer reports effective heating of room temperature fluids at flow rates up to 500 mL/min. At low flow rates, heat loss within the tubing distal to the pole-mounted heating unit is significant. It withstands pressurization up to 300 mm Hg. **E,** Fluido. Warms fluid by infrared dry heat, with manufacturer-reported effective warming at flow rates from KVO-800 mL/min. The amount of heat delivered is modulated automatically, depending on the temperature of the incoming fluid.
(**C,** Arizant Healthcare, Eden Prairie, Minn.; **B,** Gaymar Industries, Orchard Park, N.Y. C, TSCI, Amersfoort, The Netherlands).
Simple fluid warmers optimized for lower flows:
F, Buddy: at flow rates from KVO-100 mL/min, the manufacturer reports the capacity to warm cold fluids to 38° C. The small heater unit (weighing just 7 oz) heats fluids as they pass through a disposable that connects near the IV catheter, while the power module attaches to an IV pole. (The Buddy Plus model gives the option of running on a rechargeable battery.) **G,** Hotline. Countercurrent heat exchange from coaxial water jacket tubing minimizes heat loss distal to the primary countercurrent heating unit, which mounts to an IV pole. According to manufacturer data, this device provides very effective warming at low fluid flow rates (up to 75 mL/min). **H,** Bair Hugger 241: the disposable warming coil fits inside the hose of a Bair Hugger forced air warmer to provide adjunctive fluid warming when flow ranges from KVO to 50 mL/min.
(**F,** Belmont Instruments, Billerica, Mass.; **G,** Smiths Medical, Rockland, Mass.; H, Arizant Healthcare, Eden Prairie, Minn.). (Photos A-F are from manufacturer's websites.)

12 units of banked blood per hour.[46] The risks of CS include air embolism, nephrotoxicity, coagulation disorders, leukocyte activation with resulting lung damage, and dissemination of microaggregates, infectious matter, cytokines, and malignant cells.[47] Due to the risk-benefit ratio and the considerable up-front costs of preparing for cell salvage, intraoperative cell salvage is generally only considered when blood loss is expected to exceed 20% of the patient's blood volume, or when greater than 10% of comparable patients require transfusion of more than 1 unit of packed RBCs.[48]

A Cochrane review from 2006 concluded that in 51 randomized controlled trials of adult patients undergoing cardiac, orthopedic, and vascular surgery, intraoperative and postoperative washed cell salvage reduced the overall need for transfusions of donated blood (with a 39% relative risk reduction, and a 23% absolute risk reduction), did not appear to cause any adverse clinical outcomes, and that evidence is sufficient to support the use of washed CS in cardiac and orthopedic cases (where risk reductions were even higher). For each patient, washed CS yielded an average savings of 0.67 units of allogeneic RBC. Study quality, however, was compromised by the unblinded nature and small size of most randomized clinical trials included in the review.[49] Because unwashed CS confers significantly greater risks, the same reviewers have likened it to "a very laborious means of obtaining an autologous volume expander,"[49] and intraoperative unwashed CS is generally discouraged.

Contraindications to Cell Salvage

Cell salvage is relatively contraindicated in situations involving heightened risk of contamination, whether the contaminant is exogenous or endogenous. Hemolysis can be exacerbated by CS,[50] and must be minimized since free hemoglobin is nephrotoxic. Consequently, blood products with a free hemoglobin concentration greater than 1% should not be transfused.

CS is generally avoided whenever there is likely contamination with bacteria or malignant cells, or when there is reason to suspect significant hemolysis (i.e., due to use of hypotonic solutions or detergents, significant hemolysis before collection, or excessive turbulence and suction pressures[56] during collection) or crenation (from hypertonic solutions). Additional risk stems from contamination with fat (which in sufficient quantities causes postoperative cognitive dysfunction and even fat embolism syndrome), proteolytic enzymes (i.e., from gastric or pancreatic secretions), methylmethacrylate (which can trigger circulatory collapse, and once hardened also tends to clog the salvage circuit) or clot.[52]

Triggers for clot formation include calcium-containing irrigants, clotting agents (such as thrombin, Thrombostat, and thrombogen) and activators of the clotting system (such as Gelfoam, Surgicel, hemofoam, and Nu-Knit). Contamination with agents that also increase the risks of platelet aggregation (microfibrillar agents such as Avitene, Gelfoam, Instat, Helitene, and Oxycel) are stronger contraindications to CS. Other reasons to avoid CS include carbon monoxide contamination (i.e., from electrocautery smoke), thalassemia or sickle cell disease (which increase the risk of hemolysis), or excess levels of catecholamines (i.e., in blood collected during pheochromocytoma resection, or contaminated with epinephrine from the surgical field). The use of blood that is potentially mixed with amniotic fluid or malignant cells is controversial, and a third-generation leukocyte reduction filter is often used for cell salvage under these circumstances.

Equipment for Cell Salvage

Intraoperative cell salvage requires a dedicated perfusionist, a dedicated suction apparatus, and a cell salvage system, including disposable components. The system is continually anticoagulated (typically with heparinized saline), to prevent clotting during collection or processing. To minimize

hemolysis, blood should be aspirated from the surgical field, ideally with carefully modulated suction force and a large-diameter suction catheter tip submerged in a pool of blood. These measures reduce the formation of air bubbles that increase the surface area of the air-water interface, where hemolysis tends to occur. Specialized suction apparatuses are marketed for this purpose.

Blood passes through a microaggregate filter (with a 20-to 40-micron effective pore size) to remove debris such as foreign matter, fibrin, and cell clumps. Centrifugation separates the noneryerythrocyte components (Figure 16–16), which are channeled into a waste container. In most cell salvage systems, the filtered aspirate collects in a single-use "bowl," and centrifugation commences after 70 to 250 mL accumulates. In contrast, in continuous autotransfusion systems, centrifugation commences with as little as 30 mL of solution and continues until blood collection is complete.

While autotransfusion devices that use intermittent centrifugation are incapable of removing all the fat from salvaged blood, specialized 40-micron leukoreduction filters can eliminate 80% to 97% of fat globules and leukocytes, and eliminate the need for a separate microaggregate filter after washing is complete.[53] In contrast, continuous centrifugation systems permit near-complete removal of lipids without a leukoreduction filter.

After the initial centrifugation step, an isotonic wash solution is introduced to carry away remaining activated coagulation factors, free hemoglobin, heparin, and proteolytic enzymes during further centrifugation. Once washing is complete, the red cells are pumped into an infusion bag for use, and air is evacuated from the bag. A typical yield ranges from 50% to 95.8% of all RBC retrieved,[54-56] with

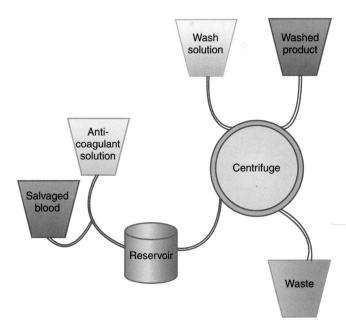

Figure 16–16   Cell salvage overview. Schematic of a cell salvage system. Salvaged blood, mixed with anticoagulant, can be held in a reservoir until it is needed; the washing process takes place in a centrifuge, and the washed product can be held for later use or transfused immediately. Commonly used intraoperative cell salvage systems include the Cell Saver 5+ [Haemonetics, Braintree, Mass.], the BRAT2 and Electa Essential Concept [Sorin Medical, Arvada, Colo.], and the Continuous Autotransfusion System [Terumo Cardiovascular Systems Corp, Ann Arbor, Mich.]

a final hematocrit typically in the 50% to 60% range, or higher for systems that use continuous centrifugation. In comparison to banked red blood cells, washed salvaged red blood cells have close to normal 2,3-diphosphoglycerate levels, and longer intravascular survival. The quality of the salvaged product reflects the collection methods and the quality of the cells collected. While most cell salvage systems have default programs to control processing, they also enable the perfusionist to intervene throughout, manually or via operator-designed programs, to maximize the quality of the product.

References

1. Weiss, M., Neff, T., Gerber, A., et al., 2000. Impact of infusion line compliance on syringe pump performance. Paediatr Anaesth 10, 595–599.
2. Lovich, M.A., Kinnealley, M.E., Sims, N.M., et al., 2006. The delivery of drugs to patients by continuous intravenous infusion: modeling predicts potential dose fluctuations depending on flow rates and infusion system dead volume. Anesth Analg 102, 1147–1153.
3. Lovich, M.A., Doles, J., Peterfreund, R.A., 2005. The impact of carrier flow rate and infusion set dead-volume on the dynamics of intravenous drug delivery. Anesth Analg 100, 1048–1055.
4. Flack, F.C., White, T.D., 1974. Behaviour of standard gravity-fed administration sets used for intravenous infusion. BMJ 3, 439–443.
5. Kestin, I.G., 1987. Flow through intravenous cannulae. Anaesthesia 42, 67–70.
6. Philip, B.K., Philip, J.H., 1983. Characterization of flow in intravenous infusion systems. IEEE Trans Biomed Eng 30, 702–707.
7. Philip, B.K., Philip, J.H., 1986. Characterization of flow in intravenous catheters. IEEE Trans Biomed Eng 33, 529–331.
8. Philip, B.K., Philip, J.H., 1987. Pressure-flow relationships in intravenous infusion systems. Anaesthesia 48, 776.
9. McPherson, D., Adekanye, O., Wilkes, A.R., et al., 2009. Fluid flow through intravenous cannulae in a clinical model. Anesth Analg 108, 1198–1202.
10. British Standards Institute, 1997. Sterile, single-use intravascular catheters, over-needle peripheral catheters. British Standards Institute, London.
11. Smiths Medical. (website): http://www.smiths-medical.com/upload/products/PDF/va406.pdf. Accessed May 1, 2009.
12. Dutky, P.A., Stevens, S.L., Maull, K.I., 1989. Factors affecting rapid fluid resuscitation with large-bore introducer catheters. J Trauma 29, 856–860.
13. Zorko, M.F., Polsky, S.S., 1986. Rapid warming and infusion of packed red blood cells. Ann Emerg Med 15, 907–910.
14. De la Roche, M.R., Gauthier, L., 1993. Rapid transfusion of packed red blood cells: effects of dilution, pressure, and catheter size. Ann Emerg Med 22, 1551–1555.
15. Zorko, M.F., Polsky, S.S., 1986. Rapid warming and infusion of packed red blood cells. Ann Emerg Med 15, 907–910.
16. De la Roche, M.R., Gauthier, L., 1993. Rapid transfusion of packed red blood cells: effects of dilution, pressure, and catheter size. Ann Emerg Med 22, 1551–1555.
17. Floccare, D.J., Kelen, G.D., Altman, R.S., 1990. Rapid infusion of additive red blood cells: alternative techniques for massive hemorrhage. Ann Emerg Med 19, 129–133.
18. Willsey, D., Peterfreund, R., 1997. Compartment syndrome of the upper arm after pressurized infiltration of intravenous fluid. J Clin Anesth 9, 428–430.
19. Yeakel, A.E., 1968. Lethal air embolism from plastic blood-storage container. JAMA 204, 267–269.
20. Toung, T.J.K., Rossberg, M.I., Hutchins, G.M., 2001. Volume of air in a lethal venous air embolism. Anesthesiology 94, 360–361.
21. Muth, C.M., Shank, E.S., 2000. Gas embolism. N Engl J Med 342, 476–482.
22. Tovar, E.A., Del Campo, C., Borsari, A., et al., 1995. Postoperative management of cerebral air embolism: gas physiology for surgeons. Ann Thorac Surg 60, 1138–1142.
23. Hagen, P.T., Scholz, D.G., Edwards, W.D., 1984. Incidence and size of patent foramen ovale during the first 10 decades of life: an autopsy study of 965 normal hearts. Mayo Clin Proc 59, 17–20.
24. Meissner, I., Whisnant, J.P., Khandheria, B.K., et al., 1999. Prevalence of potential risk factors for stroke assessed by transesophageal echocardiography and carotid ultrasonography: the SPARC study. Stroke prevention: assessment of risk in a community. Mayo Clin Proc 74, 862–869.
25. Dickson, D.N., Gregory, M.A., 1980. Compatibility of blood with solutions containing calcium. S Afr Med J 57, 787–797.
26. Sink, B.L. 2008. Administration of blood components. In: Roback, J.D., Combs, M.R., Grossman, B.J. (Eds.), Technical manual, ed 16. American Association of Blood Banks, Bethesda, Md.
27. Longhurst, D.M., Gooch, W., Castillo, R.A., 1983. In vitro evaluation of a pediatric microaggregate blood filter. Transfusion 23, 170–172.
28. Sessler, D.I., 1994. Consequences and treatment of perioperative hypothermia. Anesthiol Clin North America 12, 425–456.
29. Frank, S.M., Fleisher, L.A., Breslow, M.J., et al., 1997. Perioperative maintenance of normothermia reduces the incidence of morbid cardiac events. A randomised clinical trial. JAMA 277, 1127–1134.
30. Kurz, A., Sessler, D.I., Lenhardt, R.A., 1996. Perioperative normothermia to reduce the incidence of surgical wound infection and shorten hospitalisation. N Engl J Med 334, 1209–1215.
31. Heier, T., Caldwell, J.E., 2006. Impact of hypothermia on the response to neuromuscular blocking drugs. Anesthesiology 104, 1070–1080.
32. Leslie, K., Sessler, D.I., Bjorksten, A.R., et al., 1995. Mild hypothermia alters propofol pharmacokinetics and increases the duration of action of atracurium. Anesth Analg 80, 1007–1014.
33. Camus, Y., Delva, E., Cohen, S., et al., 1996. The effect of warming intravenous fluids on intraoperative hypothermia and postoperative shivering during prolonged abdominal surgery. Acta Anaesthiol Scand 40, 779–782.
34. Sessler, D.I., 2001. Complications and treatment of mild hypothermia. Anesthesiology 95, 531–543.
35. Lenhardt, R., Marker, E., Goll, V., 1997. Mild intraoperative hypothermia prolongs postanesthetic recovery. Anesthesiology 87, 1318–1323.
36. Planel, E., Richter, K.E., Nolan, C.E., et al., 2007. Anesthesia leads to tau hyperphosphorylation through inhibition of phosphatase activity by hypothermia. J Neurosci 27, 3090–3097.
37. Rohrer, M.J., Natale, A.M., 1992. Effect of hypothermia on the coagulation cascade. Crit Care Med, 20 1402–1405.
38. Wolberg, A.S., Meng, Z.H., Monroe D.M., III, et al., 2004. A systematic evaluation of the effect of temperature on coagulation enzyme activity and platelet function. J Trauma 56, 1221–1228.
39. Rajagopalan, S., Mascha, E., Na, J., et al., 2008. The effects of mild perioperative hypothermia on blood loss and transfusion requirement. Anesthesiology 108, 71–77.
40. Boyan, C.P., Howland, W.S., 1963. Cardiac arrest and temperature of bank blood. JAMA 183, 58–60.
41. Turner, M., Hodzovic, I., Mapleson, W. W., 2006. Simulated clinical evaluation of four fluid warming devices. Anaesthesia 61, 571–575.
42. Yamakage, M., Satoh, J.I., Saijoh, H., et al., 2005. Performance of four systems for warming intravenous fluids at different flow rates. Anesthesiology 103, A854.
43. Maani, C.V., Mongan, P.D., 2005. Relative efficiency of Hotline, Buddy, and Ranger blood/fluid warming devices. Anesthesiology 103, A856.
44. Zhang, R.V., Posey, R.J., Schmeck, A., et al., 2005. Evaluation and comparison of the Hotline fluid warmer and the Belmont Instrument Buddy fluid warmer. Anesthesiology 103, A855.
45. Comunale, M.E., 2003. A laboratory evaluation of the Level 1 Rapid Infuser (H1025) and the Belmont Instrument Fluid Management system (FMS 2000) for rapid transfusion. Anesth Analg 97, 1064–1069.
46. Williamson, K.R., Taswell, H.F., 1991. Intraoperative blood salvage: a review. Transfusion 31, 662–675.
47. Huet, C., Salmi, L.R., Fergusson, D., et al., 1999. A meta-analysis of the effectiveness of cell salvage to minimize perioperative allogeneic blood transfusion in cardiac and orthopedic surgery. International study of perioperative transfusion (ispot) investigators. Anesth Analg 89, 861–869.
48. Uhl L , 2009,. Alternative to transfusion: perioperative blood management. In Simon, T.L., Snyder, C.L., Stowell, C.P., et al, editors. Rossi's principles of transfusion medicine, ed 4, Blackwell Publishing.
49. Carless, P.A., Henry, D.A., Moxey, A.J., et al., 2006. Cell salvage for minimizing perioperative blood transfusion. Cochrane Database Syst Rev (4), CD001888 (review).
50. Waters, J.H., Williams, B., Yazer, M.H., et al., 2007. Modification of suction-induced hemolysis during cell salvage. Anesth Analg 104, 684–687.
51. Gregoretti, S., 1996. Suction-induced hemolysis at various vacuum pressures: implications for intraoperative blood salvage. Transfusion 36, 57–60.

52. Water, J.H., 2004. Indications and contraindications of cell salvage. Transfusion 44 (suppl. 1), 40S–44S.

53. Booke, M., Van Aken, H., Storm, M., et al., 2001. Fat elimination from autologous blood. Anesth Analg 92, 341–343.

54. Waters, J.H., 2005. Red blood cell recovery and reinfusion. Anesthesiol Clin North America 23, 283–294.

55. Gombotz, H., Kulier, A., 1999. Intraoperative autotransfusion of RBC and PRP. Transfus Altern Transfus Med 3, 5–13.

56. Haemonetics. Cell Saver 5+, (website): http://www.haemonetics.com/site/pdf/cs5plus-product-brochure.pdf. Accessed May 5, 2009.

Chapter 17

Drug Infusion Pumps in Anesthesia, Critical Care, and Pain Management

Nathaniel Sims, M. Ellen Kinnealey, Rick Hampton, Gayle Fishman, and Harold DeMonaco

The purpose of this chapter is to provide a framework for *anesthesiology clinicians to understand drug infusion technology devices and their safe use.* Intravenous infusion of fluids and drugs during the practice of anesthesia has commonly been viewed as mundane and straightforward. In reality, a well-constructed integrated system is required to provide a seamless transition from the clinician's intent, to the safe and effective administration of drugs and fluids into the patient, as the patient moves through the process of care in multiple care settings. The history of how this systems approach to drug infusion technology has evolved since the simple "analog" infusion devices of the 1970s is briefly detailed.

In this chapter we will describe an approach and the thoughts behind an integrated system for intravenous fluid and drug delivery and the implications of such a system to a practicing anesthesiologist. Infusion pumps are best viewed not just as isolated devices, but within an overall context: a provider organization's comprehensive, *end-to-end system of safe IV medication delivery* in *multiple care settings* (operating room, critical care, pediatrics, pain management, labor, and delivery). Infusion pumps are probably the most ubiquitous medical devices in the patient care setting, and have become a critical part of anesthesia practice. With the emergence of the new generation of modern "smart" infusion pumps, many safety features have been added to decrease adverse events and improve patient safety. Infusion pumps are used for administering bolus, continuous or long-term medication and fluids, ranging from anesthesia to pain management and enteral feeding.

Despite the increasing sophistication of infusion devices, users must recognize their own *responsibilities* as part of a

safety assurance system. All devices have distinctive *risks* and *failure modes* that can be triggered in specific situations. Comprehensive training of users must include enumeration of risks, and how to recognize and respond to failure modes. Some risks and failure modes can be mitigated by application of *technology*; the remaining risks require mitigation by *user education.*[1-6]

Systems Approach to Infusion Technology

Infusion technology must be seen as a component of an integrated system, not as a collection of "stand-alone" devices. Drug infusion pumps are but one element of a safety assurance system for IV drug delivery in a particular healthcare provider organization. In many healthcare provider organizations, a key objective of a safe IV medication system is a *seamless digital pathway from clinician order or intent, to the patient vein.* Infusion system functional requirements and capabilities must be viewed in light of two key considerations: (1) *patient safety* and (2) *efficacy* in a particular *environment of use* (patients, therapies, caregivers, support systems) over the *life cycle* of a device within the organization.

A safe IV medication delivery system is a combination of "*standardization*," *hardware, software,* "*connectivity*," *user education,* and "*peopleware*" integrated into a single system under a singular institutional philosophy. Each element, while important in its own right, is merely a part of a larger systems approach.

Standardization

In some quarters, standardization is a four letter word. Many clinicians view the imposition of institutional standards as just that, an imposition. In reality, most professional organizations have recognized the value of standards and the inherent reduction in risk accompanying their adoption. An ideal institutional system is one that is transportable across all care settings. Drug names, drug ordering, drug preparation and labeling, drug libraries, clinical practice, and education must be as standardized as possible. In those instances where multiple approaches are legitimate or recognized by competing professional organizations, every attempt should be made to reduce variability whenever possible. The reality is that modern institutions have many functional domains that intersect the drug supply chain and each must be integrated into a standardized framework. For example, suboptimum outcomes would be likely if clinicians were guided to order vasopressin for diabetes insipidus in units per hour in a computerized provider order entry, while infusion pump drug libraries for vasopressin for diabetes insipidus protocol offered only units per kilogram per hour as the mandatory dose rate unit, and the pharmacy provided the drug, labeled only in milligrams per milliliter.

Standardization should be viewed as an enabling process that allows institutions to apply additional technologies that would otherwise be beyond the reach of clinicians. For example, a simple bar code that supplies the drug generic name, concentration, and volume could be used to automate record keeping related to drug administration. Bar coding of drug containers would also allow for immediate recognition of the container contents by sophisticated infusion device and automatic provision of the drug library file. The value of such an approach has previously been demonstrated and is discussed below.[7]

Another advantage of standardization is exemplified in the ability to transfer and transport patients easily and efficiently across domains within an institution. Standardized platforms such as pictured below allow critically ill patients to be transported with minimal perturbation of their ongoing treatments (Figure 17-1).

Hardware

Infusion pumps, while an important component of an intravenous drug and fluid deliver system, are not stand alone devices. Infusion devices are currently available to deliver solutions and drugs from multiple containers, including syringes and IV bags. Each company producing devices provides a host of functionalities designed to meet as many institutional needs as possible. Each manufacturer provides a distinct user interface and recently unique drug library functionality. A systems approach to hardware acquisition requires a complete understanding of the tradeoffs inherent in multifunctionality devices. The complexity of the user interface, and the risk of user error, may increase as the device sophistication increases. Studies of computer-based medical devices used in critical care and operating room settings have found a variety of human-device interaction problems, such as poor or nonexistent feedback to users; complicated sequences of operation; multiple poorly distinguishable operating modes; and confusing alarms. Human factor deficiencies are important because

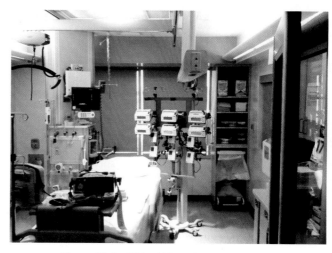

Figure 17–1   ICU cubicle and transport system.

they have been shown to increase the likelihood of errors. One approach used by institutions is to deploy an overall strategy for infusion devices that provides clinicians with the correct device for the correct functionality and reduces reliance on multifunctional devices. Additional comments on this approach are provided later in this chapter.[8-11]

Software

Infusion device software consists of two basic elements. Infusion pump software converts the user's instructions, regardless of the format, into a simple algorithm of fluid delivery, regardless of the type of infusion pump (syringe, large volume, peristaltic, etc.) In more recent years, these simple algorithms have been augmented with sophisticated drug libraries that provide the clinician with additional information at the time of drug or fluid administration. Based on institutional and local practices, these drug libraries have been shown to improve efficiency and reduce some types of errors. The drug libraries for a particular institution must initially be developed in close collaboration with end users. At the same time, there must be a standardized and transparent process for iterative changes in the libraries and their implementation. It should be obvious that the management of embedded sophisticated drug libraries requires an institutional commitment to a standard compendium of drugs, including standard container format, drug concentration, drug container labeling, and the like. The value of drug libraries is reduced without attention and ongoing reevaluation to a standardized drug compendium.

Connectivity

Drug infusion pumps now have the capability to be electronically networked together for the two-way dissemination of information, such as updated drug libraries. In a few leading institutions, wireless networks are being optimized to communicate *patient-specific IV medication orders*, in near real time, to drug infusion pumps (a form of *autoprogramming*). In the near future (in the United States), software in drug infusion pumps will likely include algorithms to permit the administration of intravenous anesthetics using TIVA (total intravenous anesthesia) or TCI (target-controlled infusion). These goals are, however, difficult to achieve without a standardized communication platform that encompasses all relevant devices.

Peopleware

No discussion of a systems approach would be complete without comments on the need for a coordinated approach to stakeholder needs. A systematic approach requires an understanding of the roles and responsibilities of pharmacists, drug library managers, biomedical engineers, nurses, physicians, educators, and information technology specialists, and also the development of an operational team dedicated to establishing and maintaining the system approach. The team establishes, guides, monitors, and adapts the end-to-end IV medication delivery system in relation to clinical practice changes and advances in treatment paradigms.

Infusion Pump History: From "Stand-Alone Pumps" to "Intelligent Infusion Devices"

Recently, infusion pump technology has focused on improving medication safety, creating user-friendly designs, developing closed-loop drug administration systems, and facilitating complete integration of smart pumps with other medical information systems used by clinical facilities. Wireless pumps are being used by healthcare facilities transitioning to high tech healthcare information systems. These programmable "smart" pumps have dose-calculation/ error reduction software (DERS) and drug libraries. Another emerging technology is bar-coded medication administration (BCMA), which allows for point-of-care verification to make sure the right patient receives the prescribed medication.

We will now provide a very brief history of improvements to drug infusion pumps.

"Analog" Infusion Pumps

Until relatively recently (1970s through early 1990s), drug infusion pumps were stand-alone devices whose only settings were related to the *flow rate and volume of a medical fluid* leaving a container and proceeding to a patient through a tubing conduit. If a *drug* was contained within the medical fluid, this was of no concern to the manufacturer of the device, as the user interface of the device did not provide any guidance or information to assist the caregiver in making the *complex calculations* that relate drug concentration, units of drug delivery, (such as micrograms per kilogram per minute) with fluid flow rate.

Early "Microcomputer" Infusion Pumps

During the period from the early 1980s through the mid-1990s, infusion pumps evolved from "analog and discrete logic digital" devices using simple thumbwheel or "up/down" controls and light-emitting diode (LED) one-line displays to adjust the rate of a pumped medical fluid to "computerized" devices. These contained microprocessors, memory that could store a software application and data, larger liquid crystal display (LCD) informational displays (numbers, text, or graphical objects) that formed the basis for a user interface, and a keypad (typically with up to 20 buttons or lights in a flush-mounted configuration to permit thorough cleaning).

Some of the earliest dose-computing infusion pumps, exemplified by the Baxter AS20G and the IVAC 770, allowed a user to numerically enter the concentration (mg/mL) of drug in a fluid, the weight of a patient (in kg), and adjust not the flow rate, but rather the dose rate of the pump in clinically-relevant units (μg/kg/min or μg/min). Many of these devices were quite power-efficient, with batteries that could operate the device for 12 to 20 hours, an AC power supply mounted in a cord, and DC stepper or DC servo motors powering the lead screw of a syringe pump or the mechanism of a large volume pump.

These early microcomputerized pumps provided advanced capabilities. The Baxter AS20G and the IVAC 770 syringe pumps offered dose computation, and the Minimed Medsystem III could be customized from a PC-based editor allowing multiple "personalities" tuned to the needs and ranges of diverse care settings. Both of these features would eventually merge together with "drug libraries" to form the essential features of "smart pumps." This era also marked the appearance and disappearance of the only true closed loop blood pressure system[12] —the IVAC 10K "Titrator" —which married a digital servo control box, an invasive arterial pressure sensor, and a microcomputer controlled pump providing clinicians with the ability to set a target mean arterial pressure and let the control loop maintain the patient at this level automatically, by regulation of a continuous infusion of sodium nitroprusside.[12]

Early Dose Error Reduction Systems (1992-2002)

In 1992, working under a sponsored research contract and in collaboration with *Baxter Healthcare*, a team at Massachusetts General Hospital (MGH) developed a prototype of a drug infusion pump with a microprocessor and 128K of system memory, capable of housing a user-customized *drug library* of commonly used drugs, drug concentrations, units-of-delivery, and default starting dose rates of each of 40 drugs commonly used in anesthesia and critical care. Two U.S. patents, one for an infusion pump with an electronically loadable drug library, and one for a personal computer-based toolkit for creating an electronically loadable drug library, were issued to MGH and Baxter, and nonexclusive licenses to these patents were granted to drug infusion pump manufacturers worldwide. The Baxter-MGH prototype syringe pump was called the AS40, and was marketed briefly during 1993. As sold, the pump contained a factory-supplied drug library, but no separate PC-based software toolkit ("drug library editor") was ever created by Baxter for use with the AS40 (Figure 17-2).

The first commercially available drug infusion pump with drug library editor software and a pump capable of being electronically loaded with several hundred drugs in a user-customized drug library, was a dual-channel syringe infusion pump ("Harvard 2") sold beginning in 1997 by *Harvard Clinical Technology* (HCT) of Natick, Massachusetts. This pump's drug library software was capable of storing a range of safe dose rates defined by upper and lower "limits" of safe operation of the drug. Exceeding these limits would trigger an alert to the user. The user's response to the alert could be to override the limit, reprogram the pump to a "permitted" dose rate value, or abandon the programming of the infusion. About 1000 of these devices were implemented widely at MGH and

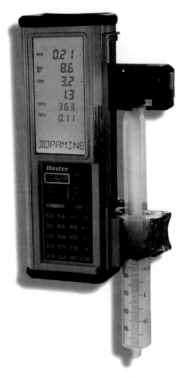

Figure 17–2   Baxter AS40.

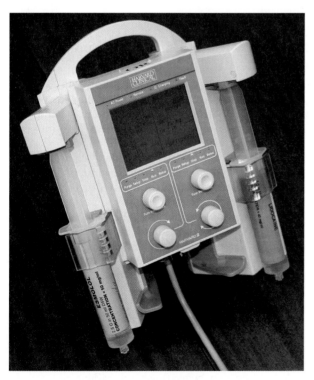

Figure 17–3   HCT Dual Channel Syringe Pump.

other hospitals globally. HCT was later acquired by Alaris Medical Systems (Figure 17-3).

In 2001, *Alaris Medical Systems* introduced a configurable, four-channel, drug infusion pump initially called the "Medley" (later renamed "Alaris System"). Over time, the Alaris System became available with five types of modules that could be mechanically engaged with a central

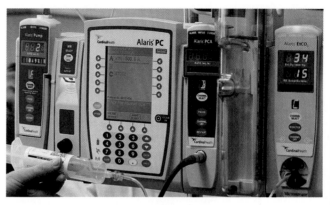

Figure 17–4   Carefusion Alaris System.

programming/control unit, the "Patient Controller" (PC). The five modules were a large volume pump (LVP), a syringe module (SP), a patient-controlled-analgesia syringe module (PCA), a bar-code-reader module, and two physiological monitoring modules. The physiological monitoring modules had the capability of pulse oximetry and capnography. Software resident in the PC was technically capable of "pausing" an opioid infusion in response to a measured physiological value crossing a limit such as a low respiration rate or low oxygen saturation. The Carefusion Alaris System, like the HCT pump, featured a user-customizable drug library editor program, but the "dose-error-reduction-system" (DERS) capability was strongly highlighted under the name "Guardrails." "Guardrails" consisted of not just dose limit alerts, but also the pump's capability to store within its memory all instances of dose limit overrides and their resolution for later analysis. This component of the technology, called "CQI" (continuous quality improvement) permitted basic information and data-mining tools to be applied to the problem of IV dosing errors. For example, the CQI analytic tools could be used to provide an understanding, in a particular hospital, of the medications most frequently involved in programming errors, and in what settings they occurred, so that error-mitigation responses could be developed (usually involving changes to the drug library values, or by education of users) (Figure 17-4). The features of the current generation of "smart" and "intelligent" drug infusion pumps evolved over time as a result of multiple parallel developments from various manufacturers and academic efforts. For example, in 1995, *Alaris Medical Systems* launched the Signature Edition single and dual channel large volume pumps. These contained a factory-installed drug library of several dozen possible drugs, a subset of which could be configured for use through the pump's user interface. This pump did not support "limits" on a per-drug basis. In 2004, a firmware upgrade together with PC editor software became available as an option for the Signature Gold® family of products, which already possessed EPROM memory and serial communication. With this option, the pump possessed multiple user-defined "profiles" or care areas and a large user-defined library of drugs together with attributes such as units, weight or BSA dose, and limits. Years prior, about 1997, a similar software upgrade option had become available for the (now CareFusion) Alaris MSIII pump.

In October, 2002, ECRI Institute, a nonprofit organization that tests and reports on biomedical equipment, identified

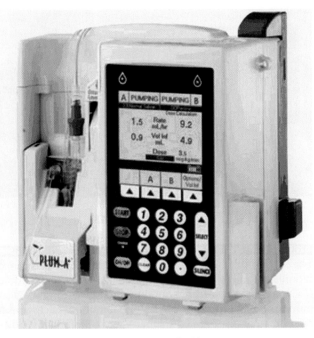

Figure 17–5   Hospira PlumA.

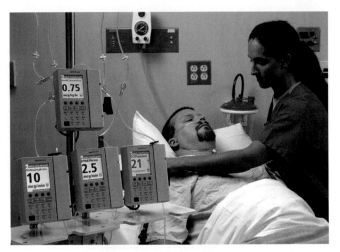

Figure 17–7   Sigma Spectrum.

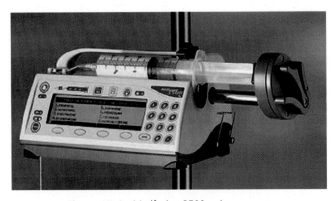

Figure 17–6   Medfusion 3500 syringe pump.

dose error reduction systems as a "leapfrog advance" and cautioned provider organizations to address IV medication safety by this means, and to retire older generation drug infusion pump technology.

In 2004-2005, additional manufacturers introduced drug infusion pumps with DERS, including the Hospira PlumA+ large volume pump (Figure 17-5), the Medfusion/Smiths Medical Medfusion 3500 syringe pump (Figure 17-6), and the SIGMA Spectrum large volume infusion pump (Figure 17-7).

Drug Infusion Pumps And The U.S. Food And Drug Administration

In 2010, the U.S. Food and Drug Administration identified drug infusion pumps as a *critical technology*. The FDA reported an unacceptable number of recalls, incidents, and patient deaths during the 5-year period (2005-2010). An "Infusion Pump Improvement Initiative" commenced in April 2010. At the same time, the FDA put in place new guidance documents that marked the introduction of significant

changes in how drug infusion pumps should be designed, tested, and assessed by the FDA before being approved for commercial sale. Changes were also being implemented with respect to sourcing and management of information about problems and adverse incidents reported by users, hospitals, and companies. The goal of increased attention to "postmarket" issues is to rapidly mitigate issues arising in the field.

Technology Matched to Functional Clinical Requirements

Many considerations pertain to the selection, use, and management of drug infusion devices. These may include cost, size, weight, ease-of-use, disposables, alarms, connectivity, precision, and range of flow rates, suitability for various medical fluids, methodology for drug recognition, method of identifying a device to a particular patient, and connectivity to a clinical information system. Provider organizations may have varying "strategic" approaches to standardized care protocols for specialty patients, such as those requiring *fluid restriction*, including populations of pediatric patients, and patients with various organ system failures, including (renal, hepatic, pulmonary, and neurological/neurosurgical). Choices made by provider organizations about fluid restricted patients will impact, for example, the balance of syringe pumps, large volume pumps, and other technologies across the spectrum of care settings.

There is an inherent tension between the clinician's need to individualize intravenous treatments and an institutional desire to standardize. This tension is best addressed institutionally and in a transparent fashion. Every attempt should be made to recognize legitimate individual needs and to integrate nonstandardized devices into the mainstream. At any given point in time, the details of provider organization needs, and the functional capabilities of devices that are available commercially, will be a moving target, as technology evolves. There are several different models of device acquisition under which a provider organization may operate, with respect to *choice of IV drug infusion technology*. For example, in an extreme ("ad-hoc technology") example, *each care setting* (such as the operating room, or a neonatal

ICU) of a provider organization might be permitted to select its "own" drug infusion technology and clinical practices. Patients transitioning from one care area to another, such as from an operating room to a critical care unit, may require an infusion pump equipment exchange after arriving in the new care setting. In another example, a provider organization may standardize with a *single vendor strategy* for drug infusion technology. Under a single vendor strategy, clinical practices will necessarily adapt to the vendor's offering in each given application, such as patient controlled analgesia, as the vendor's product offerings evolve over time, in response to marketplace demands, the vendor's business model, and/ or changes in the regulatory (FDA) agenda. In a third example, a provider organization may adopt a *set of core principles* that serve to inform both the evolution of clinical practice, and also the provider organization's search for "best-of-breed" technology. These core principles may be adopted by a group or steering committee and ultimately ratified by a pharmacy and therapeutics committee. Arising out of a consensus process, they comprise a formal codification of the practice of medicine at that institution, and the basis of the assumption of liability for provision of optimum quality care. Institutions that make decisions based on core principles are likely to adopt a "best-of-breed" approach to acquisition of technology in any given domain, such as pain management, neonatal care, cancer infusion, ambulatory infusion, or total intravenous anesthesia.

Examples of core principles or issues that may form the basis for an institution's search for best of breed technology might include conservation of administered fluid volume, cost (both capital and operating), device portability for patients on multiple infusions, standardization of packaging and labeling, standardization of concentrations, sufficient number of pumps to meet clinical need, nonproprietary tubing set disposables, ease of patient transport, cost, ease-of-use, risks, and failure modes. Once established, the institution's consensus priorities should be used as a guide for technology acquisition and related implementation activities.

Later in the chapter we have enumerated a list of questions that a new clinician might ask at a particular institution to understand "the systems" that underlie the technology and clinical protocols in use. It should not be necessary to ask these questions if the rationale for the institution's system technology choices is transparent and understood by all; unfortunately this is not always the case.

While not obvious to the casual observer, there is a distinct advantage to having a variety of infusion devices resident in a single institution. The rationale is that sophisticated devices require a sophisticated user interface as noted previously. In some instances, the sophisticated device is mandatory due to the complexity of the clinical circumstance and drugs administered (e.g., anesthetic drugs, cardiovascular drugs, and the like). However, not all drugs need to be administered with equally high precision or in vendor-supplied containers. Anesthetics, life-support drugs, and neonatal/ infant infusions require a high level of accuracy and consistency ($\pm$ 3% to 5%). Total parenteral nutrition and basic fluid administration can be given safely at a medium level of accuracy ($\pm$ 10%). Intermittently administered drugs, such as the majority of antiinfectives, can be given at even lower accuracy level ($\pm$ 20%). The resultant assessment of technology needs based on accuracy requirements can be used to

Table 17–1　MGH Classification of IV Drug Precision

Description/Attributes	Red	Yellow	Green
Accuracy of drug delivery time/%	High/ $\pm$3%–5%	Medium/ $\pm$ 10%	Low/ $\pm$20%
Degree of technology	High	Medium	Low
Estimate of cost of use	High	Medium	Low
Examples	Vasoactive drugs	Total parenteral nutrition	Antibiotics

develop realistic projections of how many devices of each type or level of accuracy will be needed in any given care setting (Table 17-1).

Technology Moves to Site of Care

Ideally, medical device technology, including infusion technology, should be available at the care location optimal for the management of a given patient's clinical condition. For example, in the United States, typically syringe pumps have been restricted for use only in pediatric intensive care units and operating rooms/interventional locations. But in reality, the precision of syringe pump infusion and the capability of reducing administered fluid to patients with organ system failure may be required in other locations, such as intermediate or step-down care, or even in general care floors. Out of necessity, a transparent and standardized systems approach is required. This allows for the migration of a standardized technology that has been proven and validated in a primary location in an institution to be flexibly applied in additional care settings as patient needs change over time.

Needless to say, dynamic flexibility in on-demand *user education* is a necessary correlate of the principal of flexibility of technology availability in all care areas where such flexibility is required.

Learning Environment and Institutional Self-Assessment

Regardless of the level of detail and the rigor with which a system is designed and implemented, errors will be made. These errors are an important feedback loop for the system and should be viewed as important pieces of information that should be evaluated in a formal fashion by stakeholders. Errors should be viewed as opportunities for improvement. To understand *efficacy in a particular environment of use*, representative clinical scenarios should be developed and periodically tested in a monitored, realistic environment, such as a simulation center, and an education program developed where users can be certified by the provider organization that employs them.

The authors are unaware of any comprehensive resources for the education of clinicians in the safe use of drug infusion technology in various environments of use, beyond that provided by manufacturers during initial installation. As the technology becomes more sophisticated, and particularly as more advanced TIVA/TCI devices are introduced from Europe into the United States, this will need to be remedied. At Massachusetts General Hospital, the rudiments of a comprehensive education system are emerging, with the establishment of a biomedical engineering web page containing policies and procedures, drug infusion pump manuals, interactive simulators, and up-to-date spreadsheet representations of the drug libraries resident in the hospital's drug infusion pumps. Specific educational modules, incorporated into the Anesthesiology Residency Training Program, are being developed for key issues that clinicians must understand to mitigate risks of unintended overinfusion or underinfusion of drugs in critically ill patients, particularly where rapid-acting vasoactive drugs are involved. One such issue is highlighted here, concerning the matter of "the infusion system fluid pathway and the 'dead volume'"

The Infusion System Fluid Pathway And The Dead Volume

A set of tubing connects the reservoir (syringe or bag) of fluid for infusion to the intravascular catheter. In a typical infusion set up, there is a carrier or mainline fluid infusion of a solution such as normal saline (NS) or lactated Ringer solution (LR). A syringe pump or large volume pump propels this fluid through the tubing at a user-defined rate into the patient's circulation. Drug infusions join the mainline fluid flow at a junction point, such as a sideport or a manifold. The *dead volume* of the system (also known as the *dead space*) is defined as the total volume of the intravascular catheter, any IV tubing, and connectors or manifolds from the point where a drug infusion joins the carrier flow, up to the patient's blood stream. Figure 17-8 illustrates the dead volume of a typical peripheral intravenous tubing set.

There are several operational and safety implications of the dead volume:

1. The dead volume serves as a reservoir of drug that is available for inadvertent bolus. The clinical impact of that bolus depends on the drug and the amount of that drug residing in the dead volume.

2. The dead volume interacts with total system fluid flow rates to influence the time course of delivery of drug to the patient's circulation when starting a new infusion or when increasing the dose of an ongoing infusion. Achieving steady state delivery of a dose of drug at the intended infusion rate can take much longer than expected.

3. The dead volume is also a reservoir of drug that enters the patient even when attempting to reduce the dose of an infusion or discontinue the infusion. Eliminating, or reducing, delivery of a drug can also take much longer than expected depending on the interaction of the dead volume and system fluid flow rates.

4. For drug infusions requiring precise control of drug delivery (e.g., an infusion of norepinephrine), the drug infusion should join the main fluid pathway as close to the circulation as possible (farthest downstream junction point).

These considerations are particularly important when "microinfusion" techniques are used to conserve total fluid volume delivery and also when delivering drugs by infusion to infants and small children.

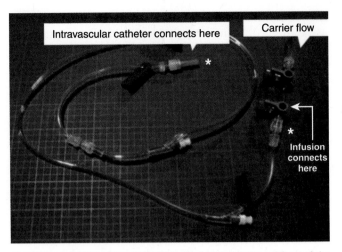

Fig 17-8 Infusion tubing "dead volume." The direction of flow of the mainline infusion/carrier is indicated. An infusion might enter the fluid pathway at the manifold port (stopcock) as indicated. The dead volume with this system architecture is approximately 5 mL.

Clinicians can influence the kinetics of drug delivery to the circulation by their choice of fluid flow rate for the carrier/mainline infusion. While higher flow rates can reduce the time to achieve new steady states of drug delivery, this comes at the expense of volume delivery to a patient. Over time, the accumulation of volume in the form of carrier fluid can be significant—liters per day. A dilute stock solution of drug must be infused at a higher flow rate than a concentrated stock solution of drug to achieve the same delivered dose. This again comes at the expense of volume delivery to the circulation.

Clinicians can also influence the kinetics of drug delivery by their design of the infusion system architecture, in particular the choice of manifold. Figure 17-9 illustrates a traditional manifold with a high dead volume (particularly for upstream access points) and a manifold designed to reduce the contribution of the manifold to the dead volume.

Implications for Anesthesia and Anesthesiology

Anesthesiology practice, for the purpose of this chapter, is intended to encompass the operating room, critical care, labor and delivery, procedural medicine, ambulatory, and general care settings. Thus anesthesiologists, while their practice is often centered on interventional environments and operating rooms, also practice or respond to emergent situations in *numerous clinical settings (pain clinic and pain service consults, pediatric and adult ICUs, and general care)*, each with highly *customized care protocols*.

In these settings, syringe pumps, large volume pumps, and PCA (patient-controlled-analgesia) pumps will be the principal devices used.

Devices commonly used for TIVA are briefly mentioned, but target-controlled infusion is not addressed because the technology is not sold in the United States, and it is well-described in other monographs and chapters in textbooks of anesthesiology.

With respect to anesthesia drugs, it has been the practice in the United States to implement TIVA with available syringe pumps, such as the Bard/Baxter InfusOR, the Medfusion 3500, or the syringe modules of the Alaris/Carefusion Medley

MICROINFUSION MANIFOLD   CONVENTIONAL STOPCOCK MANIFOLD

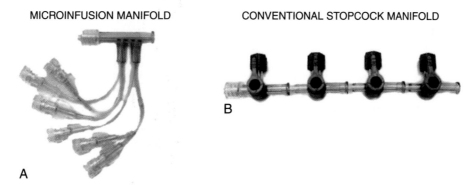

Figure 17–9 Manifolds for joining drug infusions to a fluid pathway. *Left,* Microinfusion manifold with minimal dead volume (Multi Line Extension Set; Summit Medical Products Inc., Worcester, Mass, Product No. MC8001). *Right,* Conventional stopcock manifold (Hi-Flo Manifold (Arrow International, Reading Pa, Product No. W21122).

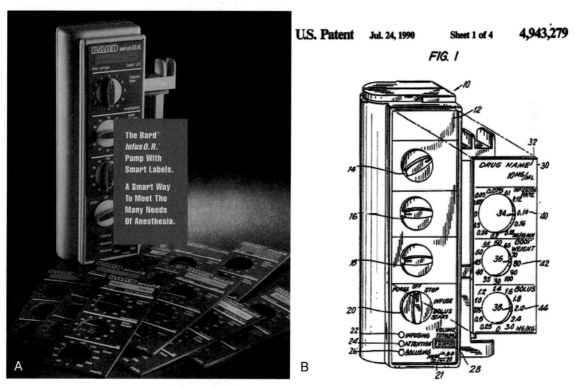

Figure 17–10 Baxter InfusOR.

System, using drug library entries that are custom-configured by each hospital for these anesthesia applications. Disadvantages of these devices for the TIVA application include maximum flow (bolus/loading dose) rates that are slower than manual bolus injection, and the absence of any commercially available devices to implement TCI. TCI is a widely used strategy (outside the United States) for administration of intravenous anesthesia, but TCI has not been approved by the U.S. Food and Drug Administration for sale in the United States.

Drug infusion pump technology is in a state of *rapid technological evolution.* There is a great *diversity of devices.* The regulatory environment (U.S. Food and Drug Administration; www.fda.gov) is also changing rapidly; see FDA (http://www.fda.gov/MedicalDevices/ProductsandMedicalProcedures/GeneralHospitalDevicesandsupplies/InfusionPumps/default.htm; accessed 8/5/10). "Infusion Pump Improvement

Initiative." For this reason, any detailed enumeration of the features and user interface of today's (May 2010) infusion devices available from vendors, is likely to be outdated almost immediately. Therefore, we are limiting the discussion of specific devices to a set of general questions for which every clinician should obtain updated answers.

With these considerations in mind, therefore, this chapter provides a *"toolkit of questions"* that a trainee (or an educator in a residency training program) may use to create a customized *self-education* program for use during the clinician's tenure at the particular institution. We emphasize the *responsibility for ongoing self-education* because of the practical likelihood that no standardized curriculum (as typically taught to incoming employees) will ever be complete, comprehensive, or up-to-date. Hence the concept, in this chapter, of providing a "toolkit of questions."

Table 17–2 Baxter AS40 Infusion Pump Standard Drug Library (1993)

Drug	Pump Drug Name	Conc. mg/mL	Infusion Rate Units	Low Dose Infusion Rate	Def Dose Infusion Rate	High-Dose Infusion Rate	Max Bolus Infusion Rate	Bolus Dose Units	Low Bolus Dose	Default Bolus Dose	High Bolus Dose
Alfentanil Pedi	ALFENTAN	0.25	µg/kg/min	0.5	1.5	3	50	µg/kg	25	75	175
Alfentanil	ALFENTAN	0.5	µg/kg/min	0.5	1.5	3	50	µg/kg	25	75	175
Amrinone	AMRINONE	5	µg/kg/min	5	7.5	10	250	µg/kg	100	500	2000
Atracurium Pedi	ATRACURIE	2	µg/kg/min	2	7	15	400	µg/kg	150	300	550
Atracurium	ATRACURIE	10	µg/kg/min	2	7	15	400	µg/kg	150	30	550
Dobutamine Pedi	DOBUTAMI	1	µg/kg/min	2	3	15					
Dobutamine	DOBUTAMI	5	µg/kg/min	2	3	15					
Dobutamine	DOBUTAMI	5	µg/min	50	200	1000					
Dopamine Pedi	DOPAMINE	0.8	µg/kg/min	1	3	20					
Dopamine	DOPAMINE	4	µg/kg/min	1	3	20					
Dopamine	DOPAMINE	4	µg/min	50	200	1000					
Dopamine	DOPAMINE	8	µg/min	50	200	1000					
Epinephrine Pedi	EPINEPHR	0.01	µg/kg/min	0.005	0.1	0.2					
Epinephrine	EPINEPHR	0.02	µg/kg/min	0.005	0.1	0.2					
Epinephrine	EPINEPHR	0.02	µg/min	0.1	1	8					
Esmolol	ESMOLOL	50	µg/kg/min	50	100	200	500	µg/kg	125	250	1000
Fentanyl Pedi	FENTANYL	0.025	µg/kg/min	0.02	0.05	0.2	2.5	µg/kg	1	5	50
Fentanyl	FENTANYL	0.05	µg/kg/min	0.02	0.05	0.2	2.5	µg/kg	1	5	50
Fentanyl	FENTANYL	0.05	µg/min	0.2	0.5	2					
General	GENERAL										
Heparin	HEPARIN	200	Units/hr	300	1000	1600					
Insulin	INSULIN	1	Units/hr	1	4	20					
Isoproterenol Pedi	ISOPROTE	0.01	µg/kg/min	0.01	0.025	0.1					
Isoproterenol	ISOPROTE	0.02	µg/kg/min	0.01	0.025	0.1					
Isoproterenol	ISOPROTE	0.02	µg/min	0.1	1	5					
Lidocaine	LIDOCAIN	40	µg/min	500	1000	4000	50000	mg	30	70	110
Mivacurium Pedi	MIVACURI	0.5	µg/kg/min	4	8	15	100	µg/kg	100	150	350
Mivacurium	MIVACURI	2	µg/kg/min	4	8	15	400	µg/kg	100	150	350
Nitroglycer-ine	NITROGLY	1	µg/kg/min	0.5	1	5					
Nitroglycer-ine	NITROGLY	1	µg/min	10	30	1000					
Nitroprusside	NITROPRU	0.2	µg/kg/min	0.01	0.1	3					
Norepineph-rine	NOREPINE	0.02	µg/min	0.25	1	10					
Prostaglandin Pedi	PGE1	0.005	µg/kg/min	0.025	0.05	0.2					
Phenyleph-rine	PHENYLEP	0.2	µg/min	3	10	30					

Table 17–2 Baxter AS40 Infusion Pump Standard Drug Library (for devices with serial numbers ending in "D1"—cont'd

Drug	Pump Drug Name	Conc. mg/mL	Infusion Rate Units	Low Dose Infusion Rate	Def Dose Infusion Rate	High-Dose Infusion Rate	Max Bolus Infusion Rate	Bolus Dose Units	Low Bolus Dose	Default Bolus Dose	High Bolus Dose
Procainamide	PROCAINA	40	µg/min	500	1000	4000	50000	mg	100	250	800
Propofol	PROPOFOL	10	µg/kg/min	25	100	200	1000	µg/kg	200	1000	2500
Sufentanil Pedi	SUFENTAN	0.005	µg/kg/min	0.01	0.025	0.1	1.5	µg/kg	0.1	1	5
Sufentanil	SUFENTAN	0.05	µg/kg/min	0.01	0.025	0.1	1.5	µg/kg	0.1	1	5
Vecuronium Pedi	VECURONI	0.2	µg/kg/min	0.7	1	1.3	50	µg/kg	40	75	150
Vecuronium	VECURONI	1	µg/kg/min	0.7	1	1.3	50	µg/kg	40	75	150

A "Toolkit" Of Questions To Assess A Provider Organization's IV Medication Safety System

Each hospital or provider organization creates a customized drug delivery infrastructure sanctioned by a "pharmacy and therapeutics committee." For these reasons, all infusion systems are "local," and ultimately the educational resource for a particular anesthesiology clinician will therefore need to be "local." Ultimately, the only way that a newly arrived clinician may deduce or infer the underlying assumptions that form the basis for a system of care is to ask questions that will elicit the underlying assumptions:

Pumps: Single-vendor or "best-of-breed"? What pumps are used for what applications?

Microinfusion: How are fluid-restricted patients cared-for here (pediatrics, organ-system failure)?

Training: Is there a website where I may teach myself how to use the devices we use here?

Drug libraries: Are our drug libraries posted somewhere online? Who manages them? Who would I call to add a new drug?

Piggyback (secondary) infusions: How are workhorse intermittent drugs given here?

Incident reporting: Whom do I call if I am involved in a "near miss," or incident involving a drug infusion pump? How do I "sequester" an incident pump? Who will analyze the pump logs?

Physiological monitoring: Are there any requirements for vital signs monitoring of patients receiving infusions of particular drugs, such as opioids, prostaglandins, and vasoactive drugs? Does the infusion technology integrate with physiological (vitals signs) monitoring devices? If so, how?

Patient transport: What systems are in place to facilitate transport of a patient with multiple drug infusion pumps, who must emergently return to the operating room (e.g., a "reexploration")?

Multidrug infusions/manifolds: What systems are in place to reduce *tubing dead volumes* and *inadvertent drug boluses/lapses*, where a patient is receiving multiple vasoactive drugs? Are there standard protocols for "carrier" solutions?

Containers: What standard containers are used? When the drug containers are IV bags, what is their overfill volume? Does the pharmacy compensate for this, if so, how? If the containers are bottles or semirigid containers, how are these containers vented? If the containers are syringes, what syringe manufacturers are used? What are the effects of using larger syringes on drug flow startup and shut off times, on time to detect occlusions, and on "bolus release volume" after occlusion detection? Are antisiphon mechanisms devices employed to prevent inadvertent flow when a syringe pump is elevated at a significant head height above the patient?

Secondary infusions: Is a "secondary" (or "piggyback") mode ever employed? For what medications? What is the practice? Is it aligned with the infusion device manufacturer's guidance?

TIVA: Are there any standardized *IV anesthesia* protocols here?

Analytics/Informatics/"Continuous Quality Improvement": How are incidents and problem reports examined to find opportunities for improvement in our "clinical practice"? For example: is there a designated "point person" to coordinate user feedback?

References

1. Institute Of Medicine. *Preventing medication errors:* quality chasm series, (website): http://www.iom.edu/Reports/2006/Preventing-Medication-Errors-Quality-Chasm-Series.aspx. Accessed August 5, 2010.
2. Joint Commission. *National patient safety goals,* (website): http://www.jointcommission.org/NR/rdonlyres/F71BC4E9-FEB6-495C-99D8-DB9F0850E75B/0/09_NPSG_General_Presentation.ppt. Accessed August 24, 2009.
3. Taxis, K., Barber, N., 2003. Ethnographic study of the incidence and severity of intravenous drug errors. BMJ 326 (7391), 684–687.
4. Husch, M., Sullivan, C., Rooney, D., et al., 2005. Insights from the sharp end of intravenous medication errors: Implications for infusion pump technology. Qual Saf Health Care 14 (4), 80–86.
5. Rothchild, J.M., Keohane, C.A., Cook, E.F., et al., 2005. A controlled trial of smart infusion pumps to improve medication safety in critically ill patients. Crit Care Med 33 (3), 533–539.
6. Bane, A.D., Luppi, C.J., Mylott, L., et al., Using Technology to Help Nurses Improve medication Safety. In Cina L, Clarke S, editors. The nurses role in medication safety: using technology to help nurses improve medication safety, Joint Commision Resources, Oakbrook Terrace, IL 2007.

7. Poon, E.G., Cina, J.L., Churchill, W., et al., 2006. Medication dispensing errors and potential adverse drug events before and after implementing bar code technology in the pharmacy. Ann Intern Med 145 (6), 426–434.

8. Leape, L.L., 2005. "Smart" pumps: a cautionary tale of human factors engineering. Crit Care Med 33 (3), 679–680.

9. Cook, R.I., Potter, S.S., Woods, D.D., et al., 1991. Evaluating the human engineering of microprocessor-controlled operating room devices. J Clin Monit 7 (3), 217–226.

10. Nunnally, M.E., Brunetti, V.L., O'Connor, M.F., et al., 2002. Lost in menuspace: variability among users programming infusion devices under controlled conditions. Anesthesiology 97 (3A).

11. Nemeth, C.P., Conran, A., Nunnally, M.E., et al., 2004. Laying traps: how infusion device interface design contributes to adverse events. Anesthesiology 101, A1296.

12. Chitwood Jr., W.R., Cosgrove, D.M., 1992. Multicenter trial of automated nitroprusside infusion for postoperative hypertension. Ann Thorac Surg 54 (3), 517–522.

Disclosure Statement

Dr. Sims, Mss. Fishman and Kinnealey, and Mr. DeMonaco are recipients of personal shares of institutionally distributed royalty revenues for patents owned and nonexclusively licensed by the Massachusetts General Hospital relative to various patient safety technologies.

Chapter 18

Devices for Cardiac Support

Michael G. Fitzsimons, Stephanie Ennis, and Thomas MacGillivray

The era of cardiovascular support began in the midtwentieth century. In 1952, Dr. Paul Zoll invented the first external cardiac pacemaker.[1] Dr. John Gibbon culminated 19 years of research on cardiopulmonary bypass when he performed a closure of an atrial septal defect in an 18-year-old girl at Thomas Jefferson Hospital in Philadelphia in 1953. In 1954, the American Society for Artificial Internal Organs (ASAIO) was founded.[2] Over the next 50 years surgeons such as Michael DeBakey, Denton Cooley, Domingo Liotta, and O.H. Frazier, along with brave patients such as Dr. Barney Clark reached many of the milestones in the development of devices to support the failing heart (Table 18-1).

Today, nearly 5 million Americans suffer from heart failure and 500,000 develop congestive heart failure every year.[3] Drugs alone cannot control the health and financial consequences. Those who develop end-stage heart failure, generally defined as persistent NYHA class IV symptoms, despite maximal medical therapy must hope for the "gold standard" treatment—heart transplantation.[4] Unfortunately only a small percentage of patients will receive a heart.[5] Mechanical support provides certain individuals awaiting heart transplantation, such as critically ill patients with temporary severe cardiac dysfunction along with others who do not qualify for transplantation, with hope.

Anesthesiologists performing procedures on patients coming for cardiac surgery will encounter a myriad of devices for cardiac support on a regular basis. These include cardiopulmonary bypass, temporary percutaneous support devices, temporary ventricular support, and long-term ventricular assist devices. The anesthesiologist must be familiar with the indications for such devices, their anesthetic implications, and common problems encountered in patients with cardiac support devices.

Anesthesiologists may also find themselves responsible for the placement and management of other devices used for temporary support, such as intraaortic balloon pumps, temporary pacing devices, and defibrillators.

Devices for Hemodynamic Support

Direct hemodynamic support for the heart can be either temporary (cardiopulmonary bypass, intraaortic balloon counterpulsation, temporary ventricular assist devices, extracorporeal membranous oxygenation) or permanent (left, right, or biventricular assist devices).

Cardiopulmonary Bypass

Cardiopulmonary bypass is primarily used during procedures of the heart to allow the surgeon to operate on the external blood vessels (coronary artery bypass grafting), aorta (ascending or arch replacement), pulmonary arteries, or within the chambers of the heart (valve repair or replacement) while avoiding excessive blood in the operative field or risk of myocardial injury due to ischemia. The bypass circuit must accomplish four basic functions: (1) oxygenation of the blood and removal of carbon dioxide, (2) circulation of blood, (3) cooling and warming of the blood, and (4) maintenance of a "bloodless" field. The bypass circuit consists of several key components: venous or atrial cannulae, venous reservoir, pump system, oxygenator, heater/cooler, anesthetic vaporizer, gas analyzer, cardioplegia delivery system, aortic cannula, and other types of venting and suction.[6]

Components

Venous Cannulae and Reservoir

The wire reinforced, flexible **venous cannula** is placed within the right atrium or vena cava and drains blood returning to the heart into a venous reservoir. For many operations only one cannula is needed. This cannula is positioned with its distal tip in the inferior vena cava and a proximal port in the right atrium (**two stage cannula**). In circumstances where the right heart chambers must be opened or the heart must be retracted and manipulated extensively, separate canulae are placed into both the superior vena cava and inferior vena cava (**single stage cannula**). Surgical tape and tourniquets around such cannulas serve to ensure that no blood returns to the right atrium. Drainage of the heart into the reservoir is commonly by gravity. Mechanisms do exist to provide "vacuum assist" or suction drainage, commonly referred to

Table 18–1 Milestones in Cardiovascular Support

Year	Milestone
1810	Le Gallois proposes extracorporeal support
1920s	Charles Lindbergh expresses interest in cardiovascular support
1937	Demikhov implants the first "artificial heart" in a dog
1952	First external pacemaker
1953	First use of cardiopulmonary bypass
1954	American Society for Artificial Internal Organs (ASAIO) conceived
1954	Cross circulation first used by Dr. Walt Lillehi
1959	First successful use of an internal cardiac pacemaker
1962	Dr. Clarence Dennis describes technique for removal of blood from the left atrium and return to the femoral artery via pump
1963	First successful implantation of a pneumatic ventricular assist device (VAD) by Dr. Michael DeBakey
1964	National Heart, Lung, and Blood Institute begins to sponsor development of mechanical support devices
1966	First successful use of an LVAD as a successful bridge to recovery
1967	First heart transplantation by Dr. Christian Barnard
1968	First use of the intraaortic balloon pump (IABP) by Dr. Adrian Kantrowitz
1969	First implantation of an "artificial heart" by Dr. Denton Cooley
1970	Invention of first internal defibrillator
1971	Dr. Michael DeBakey published landmark article outlining challenges to development of heart support devices
1976	FDA begins regulating medical devices—Medical Device Amendment to the Food, Drug, and Cosmetic Act
1979	First percutaneous implantation of an IABP
1980s	Introduction of cyclosporine leads to resurgence of heart transplantation
1982	Dr. Barney Clark became first patient to receive a permanent implant of an artificial heart as a destination device (Jarvik-7)
1984	Thoratec ventricular support device developed as a bridge to transplantation
1984	Novacor VAD first implanted
1988	Dr. O.H. Frazier implants the first HeartMate device as a bridge to transplantation
1992	FDA approves the Abiomed BVS 5000 for short-term use
1994	FDA calls for heightening efforts at ventricular assist
2001	REMATCH trial demonstrates the benefit of mechanical support over medical treatment for patients with end-stage heart failure
2004	ASAIO celebrates 50th anniversary
2004	FDA approves the CardioWest Total Artificial Heart as a bridge to transplant

as **augmented venous return**.[6] Venous suction allows smaller cannulae to be used, primarily in minimally invasive cardiac procedures.

The **venous reservoir** may be either open (hard-shell) or closed ("collapsible bag").[6] The **open reservoir** is a large canister connected to the bypass machine that collects from the venous system (Figure 18-1). The capacity varies depending on the manufacturer but is generally 3000 to 4000 mL. The venous reservoir may also receive blood removed from the left ventricle (vent) and from drains placed into the operative field (cardiotomy suction). Open systems have the capability to allow suction application and may overall be safer. Closed systems also do not require that entrained air be removed from the reservoir.

The "collapsible bag" of a closed system is less likely to allow the introduction of gaseous micro emboli (GME) into the circulation and potentially there is less activation of inflammatory factors.[6]

Pump Systems

Two types of pump systems exist: roller pumps and centrifugal pumps. These are the "heart" of the bypass circuit. **Roller pumps** have a length of tubing located inside a curved "raceway."[6] The rollers intermittently compress the tubing, propelling the contents (blood) forward (Figure 18-2). Each rotation of the pump head propels a fixed volume forward. Advantages include the ability to reuse the pump, ease of sterilization, and easy flow calculation. The disadvantage is blood trauma, hemolysis or microfragmentation of the inner surface of the tubing, and the ability to generate excessive pressure because the roller pump does not have an intrinsic ability to respond to distal pressure or resistance.

Centrifugal pumps consist of an impella or series of cones within a polycarbonate structure. These cones are rotated magnetically by a motor, propelling the blood forward. Blood trauma is less, there is minimal risk of overpressurization, and the systems are disposable. There may be benefit to centrifugal pumps as far as decreased emboli, potentially improved neurological outcome, less damage to blood elements, and

improved safety, but the data supporting these contentions are not entirely clear.[7]

Considerable debate exists about the benefit of pulsatile versus nonpulsatile perfusion while on bypass, and no recommendation can be made supporting one over the other.[7]

ADDITIONAL PUMPS

Every bypass circuit will have additional pumps with which to perform other tasks. The **cardiotomy suction** allows the surgeon to remove any blood accumulating in the field and return it directly to the venous reservoir. Debate still exists about the benefits of cardiotomy suction because this blood contains fat, bone, lipids, and other debris that accumulates in the field.[7] Debris from cardiotomy suction may ultimately activate systemic inflammation when in contact with blood elements and serve as a major source of cerebral emboli while on bypass. The longer the duration or cardiopulmonary bypass, the greater the embolic load. The **cardioplegia pump** facilitates delivery of solution with which to directly induce electromechanical cardiac standstilll and to provide substrate to the myocardium. A separate pump allows suction to be directed preferentially into a specific area or chamber, commonly the left ventricle (**vent or drain**).

Tubing

The contact of blood with all the artificial components of the bypass circuit results in the activation of both humoral and cellular components including the coagulation cascade, kallikrein-kinin, fibrinolytic, complement, platelets, and leukocytes.[8] Heparinizing the surface of CPB tubing has the potential benefit of a reduction in platelet activation, decrease in inflammation, decrease transfusion, and neurological outcome, along with a reduction in cost, although studies are small.[7]

Oxygenator/Cooler/Heater System

The **oxygenator** and **heater/cooler systems** are generally one single unit (Figure 18-3). This is essentially the "lung" of the bypass circuit. Blood is directed through the

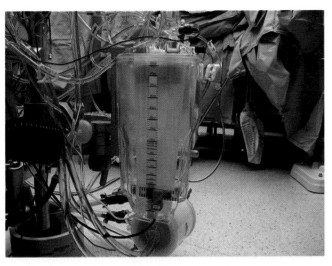

Figure 18-1   Venous reservoir.

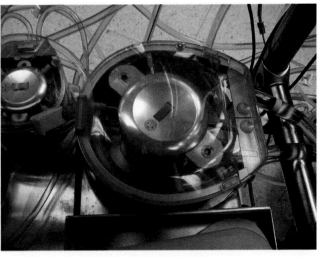

Figure 18-2   Roller pump.

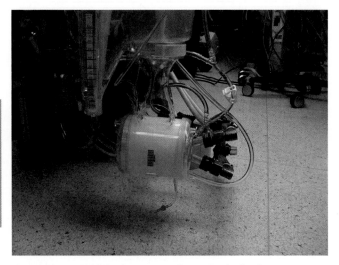

Figure 18–3   Combined oxygenator/heater/cooler fixed to venous reservoir.

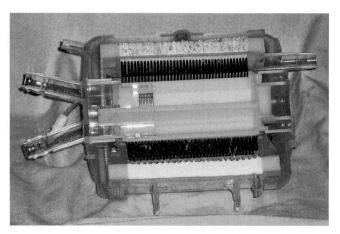

Figure 18–4   Oxygenator in cross-section.

oxygenator by the pump system. Venous blood enters into a mixing chamber where fresh gas is passed through in a **bubble oxygenator**. Small bubbles form allowing oxygen to enter the blood. This system is rarely used today because of the high occurrence of gaseous microemboli, platelet depletion, and hemolysis, all probably attributable to direct air-blood interactions.[8] The **membrane oxygenator** consists of series of hollow fibers with micropores through which the gas flows and is most commonly used today (Figure 18-4). Blood passes by in either a cross-current or counter current mechanism and diffusion occurs across the membrane. The gaseous microemboli are less than with a bubble oxygenator but such emboli are not entirely eliminated. The fraction of inspired oxygen and gas flow rate (equivalent to the minute ventilation) are controlled by the perfusionist with a device commonly referred to as a "**blender**." Heating and cooling are controlled by a circulating water system and occur via a countercurrent mechanism.

Anesthetic Vaporizer

All bypass circuits have an **anesthetic vaporizer** attached in the circuit. This allows maintenance of anesthesia while a patient is on cardiopulmonary bypass.

Arterial Filter

The **arterial filter** serves to remove both air and particulate matter from the bypass circuit before returning blood to the systemic circulation (Figure 18-5). Studies have shown that smaller filters (20 μm) are superior to larger (40 μm) and that larger embolic loads are associated with worsened neurological outcomes.[7,9]

In-Line Laboratory Analysis

Modern bypass machines have the capability of performing both arterial and venous real-time blood gas analysis or acid-base status and hemoglobin or hematocrit.

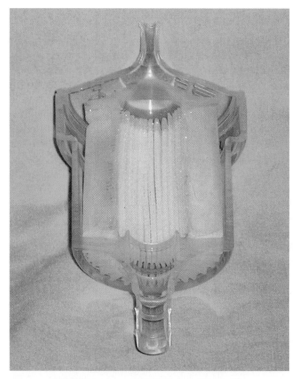

Figure 18–5   Arterial filter in cross-section.

Anesthetic Management on CPB

Close interaction between the anesthesiologist and perfusionist is critical immediately before initiation, during maintenance, and while transitioning from bypass back to native circulation. The anesthesiologist must continually monitor arterial pressure, the EKG, blood gas analysis, cardioplegia delivery, and temperature.

Arterial Pressure

Considerable debate exists regarding the appropriate blood pressure to maintain while on bypass. The optimal mean arterial pressure has not been established. A balance between myocardial protection and organ perfusion must be met. Proponents of higher pressure argue that a higher pressure is needed to perfuse certain areas of the heart that are not well protected by cardioplegia. Advocates of lower pressure argue that less trauma occurs to blood cells during CPB at lower pressure, and that noncoronary collateral blood flow to the heart is limited. Most centers maintain a mean arterial pressure of 50 to 70 mm Hg while on bypass. Often the dilemma focuses upon adequate perfusion pressure to the brain and kidneys, both of which are subject to autoregulation. It is believed that the normal brain maintains autoregulation at a mean pressure between 50 and 150 mm Hg, thus a lower limit of 50 mm Hg is felt to be reasonable.[7] Others argue that the lower limit of autoregulation is higher, especially in patients with hypertension, diabetes, or known cerebrovascular disease. Higher pressure may be necessary for such conditions.

The decision as to the ideal individual MAP while on bypass should be determined by the risks and benefits of higher and lower pressure, and the patient specific factors.

Systemic Flow Rates

Multiple factors determine the minimal safe flow rate during cardiopulmonary bypass, including body surface area, temperature, depth of anesthesia, and oxygen content of the blood.[7] Most centers will start with a flow rate of 2.2 to 2.5 L/min/m², which approximates the cardiac output of a normothermic, anesthetized individual. Lower flow rates may cause less trauma to blood cells and deliver less particulate emboli at the risk of potentially inadequate organ perfusion. There is no minimum, well-defined systemic flow rate.

ECG

The anesthesiologist must closely monitor the ECG while on bypass for three reasons: (1) assurance of electrical silence associated with adequate cardioplegia, (2) detection of ischemia during procedures performed "off-pump," and (3) to detect the return of an adequate cardiac rhythm before separation from bypass.[10,11] Adequate administration of cardioplegia is associated with complete electromechanical silence. The appearance of electrical activity after administration of cardioplegia should result in an immediate search for the cause. Electrical interference on the ECG is generally from the bypass circuit, although other sources have been reported. Interference often occurs at a very consistent rate equal to that of the roller pump. The ECG appears like ventricular tachycardia. This interference is often due to impedance mismatch caused by different impedances between skin ECG leads. The problem can often be rectified by replacement of skin leads and proper preparation of the skin site to ensure adequate contact.

Blood-Gas Management

The classic argument during cardiopulmonary bypass is whether to manage the acid-base status with an "**Alpha-stat**" technique or "**pH stat**."

Alpha-stat relies on the concept that intracellular pH must be normal at all temperatures. As the blood temperature decreases, CO_2 will dissolve in the blood. For instance at a temperature of 37° C the $Paco_2$ may be 40 mm Hg while at 20° C the $Paco_2$ may be 16 mm Hg. Alpha-stat management argues that this physiological "respiratory alkalosis" is appropriate. Proponents of pH-stat argue that neutrality is needed at all temperatures. To maintain neutrality, the perfusionist would add CO_2 to return the $Paco_2$ to 40 mm Hg with pH stat management.

Cardioplegia Delivery

Anterograde cardioplegia is administered into a small cannula placed in the ascending aorta or directly into the coronary ostia. **Retrograde cardioplegia** is delivered through a catheter placed through the right atrium into the coronary sinus. Cardioplegia is then delivered into the venous system of the heart.[12] The coronary sinus is a thin-walled structure located in the posterior atrioventricular groove of the heart. Damage to the sinus is difficult to repair and associated with significant morbidity.[13] The anesthesiologist must monitor the pressure with which the cardioplegia is delivered. Pressures exceeding 40 mm Hg may result in injury to the coronary sinus and an increase in myocardial edema.

Left Ventricular Pressure/Distention

The three components of myocardial protection are: (1) hypothermia and decrease in cellular metabolism, (2) induction of electromechanical silence, and (3) reduction of wall tension within the left ventricle. The left ventricle may be drained through a vent placed in the apex (rarely used), a vent placed in the right upper pulmonary vein and positioned in the ventricle across the mitral valve, via a cannula placed in the aortic root through which suction is applied, or through a cannula placed in the pulmonary artery. The anesthesiologist may monitor the pressure in the left ventricle directly through the cannula. Alternatively, pulmonary artery catheter pressure will reflect the pressure within the ventricle because electrical silence results in mitral valve incompetence and continual fluid column between the ventricle and pulmonary artery.

Temperature

Many believe that adequate myocardial and organ protection requires the induction of some degree of hypothermia, but this is debatable. Hypothermia may be mild (32 °C) or profound (<20 °C). The benefit of hypothermia is a reduction in cellular metabolism and oxygen consumption. Generally oxygen consumption is decreased 5% to 7% for every 1 °C reduction in body temperature. Decreased body temperature may allow lower systemic flow rates, less blood trauma, less emboli, and improved myocardial protection but at the risk of coagulopathy, especially platelet dysfunction.

Problem Solving on CPB

A concerted team effort among the surgeon, anesthesiologist, perfusionist, and other members of the cardiac care team is necessary when problems are encountered (Table 18-2).

Table 18–2 Problem Solving During Cardiopulmonary Bypass

Problem	Potential Cause	Correction
Hypotension (MAP <50 mm Hg)	Inadequate flow rate	Increase flows
	Inadequate roller head occlusion	Increase occlusion
	Excess anesthesia	Decrease anesthesia
	Vasodilation	Increase vascular tone
	Aortic catheter malposition	Reposition/rule out dissection
Hypertension (MAP >80 mm Hg)	Excess flow rate	Decrease flow
	Inadequate anesthesia	Increase anesthesia depth
	Excessive vascular tone	Add vasodilator
Low systemic flow rate (Flows <30 cc/kg/min)	Inadequate set flow rate	Increase flow
	Excessive vascular tone	Increase anesthesia add vasodilator
High systemic flow rate (Flow >70 cc/kg/min)	Vasoplegia	Increase vascular tone
	Excessive anesthesia depth	Decrease depth of anesthesia
Persistent electrical activity	Impaired cardioplegia delivery	Increase cardioplegia
		Increase potassium in cardioplegia
		Decrease temp of cardioplegia
		Check position of cannula
		Add retrograde
	Monitoring interference	Replace ECG leads
		Check interference from circuit
High retrograde pressure (>40 mm Hg)	Excessive flows	Decrease flows
	Catheter malposition	Reposition
Low retrograde pressure	Catheter malposition	Reposition
Excessive LV pressure (>5 mm Hg)	Inadequate vent rate	Increase vent
	Surgical retraction	Reposition or wait
	Excessive aortic regurgitation	Reposition cross clamp
Failure to decrease temperature	Cooling mechanism failure	Correct
Failure to warm	Heating failure	Correct

Intraaortic Balloon Counterpulsation (IABP)

Dr. Dwight Harkin first described the concept of counterpulsation as a means to improve coronary pressure and perfusion during diastole and decrease afterload during systole. The intraaortic balloon pump was first used clinically by Adrian Kantrowitz in 1968 as a means to provide temporary support to the failing heart after a myocardial infarction.[14] The underlying principle of the IABP is to provide a synchronized method to augment diastolic blood pressure while reducing afterload on the failing heart during systole.

Device

The IABP system consists of a balloon with a volume of 30 to 50 cc mounted on a flexible catheter, connected to a console with pressure wave and ECG displays, and a gas reservoir. The balloon may be inflated with either helium (low density) or CO_2 (high blood solubility and low risk of embolization). Carbon dioxide is rarely used anymore. The appropriate size of the IABP must be selected (Table 18-3) before insertion. The console allows the operator to select two different modes of control—autopilot or operator mode (Figure 18-6).[15] The autopilot mode allows the console to select the available trigger mode based upon the patient's condition and signal availability; all timing setting and adjustments are under control of the console.[15] Operator mode is the most common mode in clinical use. The clinician selects the trigger signal and then adjusts the appropriate timing.

Insertion Techniques

The most common site for IABP introduction is a percutaneous Seldinger technique through the femoral artery. The percutaneous technique was first demonstrated in 1979 and allowed more rapid placement by both surgeons and cardiologists.[16] The device may be placed with or without a sheath. The common femoral artery is localized in the standard

Table 18–3 Appropriate IABP Size Selection

IABP Volume	BSA	Height
30 cc	<1.8 m²	<162 cm (4'10"-5'4")
40 cc	>1.8 cm²	<182 cm (5'4"-6'0")
50 cc	>1.8 cm²	>182 cm (>6'0")

Adapted from Arrow International Educational Materials. *Counterpulsation applied: an introduction to intra-aortic balloon pumping,* Arrow International, Everett, MA, 2005.

Table 18–4 IABP Counterpulsation Indications

INCREASE DIASTOLIC CORONARY PERFUSION

Refractory angina refractory to medical management

Infarction or ischemia associated with PCI

Cardiogenic shock after MI

AFTERLOAD REDUCTION

Cardiogenic shock refractory to medical management

Acute ventricular septal rupture

Acute mitral regurgitation (chordae tendineae or papillary muscle rupture)

Bridge to transplant

Postbypass low cardiac output syndrome

PROPHYLACTIC INDICATIONS

Significant left main coronary artery disease before surgery

High risk PCI

High risk electrophysical intervention (i.e., ablation of ventricular fibrillation)

High risk patient undergoing noncardiac surgery

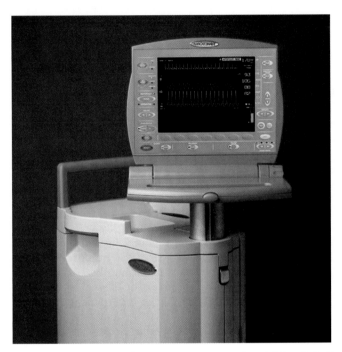

Figure 18–6 IABP console. *Used with permission from Teleflex Medical/Arrow International.*

Seldinger technique, generally at an angle not to exceed 45 degrees. The standard sheath is 6 cm. Markings every 1 cm on the IABP catheter indicate that the balloon itself is a certain distance from the tip of the sheath. The balloon is generally inserted with a goal of the tip being located 1 to 2 cm distal to the left subclavian artery and positioned above the renal arteries and celiac axis. Position may be confirmed during actual placement by transesophageal echocardiography, fluoroscopy, or after positioning by chest x-ray. The percutaneous route may be associated with more complications but has allowed use in more patients.[17] Alternative routes include the iliac, axillary, and subclavian arteries and the ascending aorta after bypass surgery.

Clinical Indications and Physiology

There are two major indications for IABP: augmentation of diastolic blood pressure and afterload reduction for the failing heart (Table 18-4).

Diastolic blood pressure augmentation occurs with inflation of the balloon in the descending thoracic aorta just distal to the left subclavian artery. Inflation may be triggered by one

of four means: The ECG, the arterial pressure waveform, off a pacing device, or in an asynchronous mode. Inflation is targeted to occur just after closure of the aortic valve (dicrotic notch) at the beginning of diastole. Inflation serves to displace blood proximal to the balloon and increase perfusion pressure within the coronary arteries.[14] Blood is also displaced distal to the balloon, improving perfusion to organs (mesentery, renal, etc.). Whether coronary blood flow actually increases with balloon inflation is subject to considerable debate. In the presence of critical coronary stenosis, the IABP does not appear to increase diastolic coronary pressure distal to the stenosis.[18] Deflation of the balloon is timed to occur just before opening of the aortic valve during the period of isovolumic contraction. Deflation creates a relative negative space in the aorta and reduction in afterload. This also decreases the time spent in isovolumic contraction, the most energy expensive part of the cardiac cycle. These overall effects depend upon the volume of the balloon, position in the aorta, aortic compliance, heart rate, and rhythm. The appropriate timing and characteristics of the IABP tracing are essential to ensure optimal clinical results (Table 18-5).

Afterload reduction during systole, primarily isovolumic contraction, may provide more benefits to the heart than diastolic pressure augmentation does. This occurs by decreasing myocardial work and the pressure against which the heart must pump. The overall effects increase the efficiency of the heart (Table 18-6).

Contraindications and Complications

Contraindications to the use of IABP include more than mild aortic insufficiency, severe aorta-iliac atheromatous disease, aortic dissection, or aortic aneurysm. Most complications related to the use of the IABP are either vascular, positional, or balloon related. Risk factors for vascular complications include diabetes mellitus, peripheral vascular disease,

Table 18–5 Appropriate IABP Timing Characteristics

INFLATION

Inflation at the dicrotic notch

Crisp "V" shape in inflation

PDP > PSP

DEFLATION

Crisp "V" shape in deflation

BAEDP < PAEDP (by 5-15 mm Hg)

APSP < PSP

PSP, Peak systolic pressure; *PDP,* peak diastolic pressure; *BAEDP,* balloon aortic end diastolic pressure; *APSP,* assisted peak systolic pressure; *PAEDP,* patient aortic end diastolic pressure.
Adapted from *Principles of counterpulsation intermediate IABP workshop,* St. Jude Medical Cardiac Assist Division, St. Paul, MN 1992.

Table 18–6 Physiological Effects of IABP Counterpulsation

Augmentation of diastolic blood pressure

Reduction of systolic blood pressure

Decrease heart rate

Decrease of pulmonary capillary wedge pressure

Increase in cardiac output

Increase in skin temperature

Decrease myocardial oxygen consumption and wall stress

Decrease pulmonary blood volume

Increase in ejection fraction

Decrease in systemic vascular resistance

Table 18–7 Clinical Criteria for IABP Removal

Signs of hypoperfusion absent

Urine output above 30 cc/hr

Minimal need for positive inotropic support

Heart rate less than 100 beats/min

Fewer than 6 ventricular ectopic beats/min

Cardiac index greater than 2 L/min/m^2 and does not drop more than 20%

LVEDP does not increase by more than 20%

Absence of angina

Adapted from Arrow International Educational Materials. *Counterpulsation applied: an introduction to intra-aortic balloon pumping,* Arrow International, 2005.

percutaneous insertion technique, smaller body surface area/height, and female sex.[17] Vascular complications include damage to the wall of the vessel, dissection, aneurysm development, or pseudoaneurysm.[17] Peripheral pulses must be monitored distal to the insertion site. Malpositioning of the IABP proximal into the aortic arch may compromise cerebral blood flow; distal malpositioning may result in mesenteric ischemia or renal insufficiency. Balloon related complications include balloon rupture, gas embolization, kinking, or platelet reduction from trauma. Platelet reduction is predictable and generally stabilizes after 4 days.[19] Recovery is prompt upon removal.

Weaning and Removal

Weaning generally occurs when myocardial performance is improving and dictated by the patient's hemodynamic status.[15] Weaning may be accomplished by decreasing the frequency of counterpulsation, volume within the balloon, or by a combination of the two. During full support, augmentation usually occurs in a 1:1 ratio with native rhythm. Weaning occurs by reducing the augmentation to 1:2, then 1:4 while monitoring the cardiac output, blood pressure, distal perfusion, and mental status and need for hemodynamic support. If hemodynamics are acceptable and cardiac performance at either 1:4 or 1:8 is stable, the IABP may be removed. Weaning may also occur through a gradual

decrease in the inflation volume. It is recommended that the volume delivered to the IABP not be less than two thirds of the total capacity of the balloon.[15] Addition of inotropic agents may be needed during the weaning process. Certain removal criteria are recommended (Table 18-7).[15] Most IABP may be removed by a closed technique where the balloon is simply pulled out and pressure applied to the site for 20 to 30 minutes.

Problem Solving with IABP

Problems are generally related to difficulty with the timing of inflation or deflation or positioning. Problems manifest as failure to augment or worsening of cardiac output or ischemia (Table 18-8). The individuals managing the IABP may be technicians, perfusionists, nurses, or physicians. Regardless, every individual responsible for these patients should be familiar with management of basic problems and possess the judgment to summon assistance when needed.

Extracorporeal Membranous Oxygenation (ECMO)

Extracorporeal membranous oxygenation is a means to provide temporary hemodynamic and/or respiratory support to critically ill patients who cannot be supported by less aggressive means, such as inotropes, vasopressors, an IABP, or advanced respiratory care interventions, such as high frequency jet ventilation. Success with ECMO has been demonstrated in the hemodynamic support of patients suffering from postcardiotomy shock who would otherwise have nearly a 100% mortality rate.[20]

Clinical Indications for ECMO

The indications for ECMO have expanded significantly since Hill reported the first use for hypoxic respiratory failure in 1972. Two primary indications for ECMO exist—respiratory failure and cardiac failure (Table 18-9). The highest success with ECMO has been among neonates and pediatric patients with respiratory failure. Lower rates of success have been seen among children and adults with primary or secondary cardiac failure. There are no set criteria for placement of a patient on ECMO but most adult centers have both "fast entry" and a "slow entry" criteria (Table 18-10).

Table 18-8 IABP Counterpulsation Problem Shooting

Failure of Augmentation	Solution
Balloon too small	Change IABP
Inflation volume too low	Increase volume
Early deflation	Adjust to deflate later in diastole
Misplacement	
False passage	Remove balloon (surgery consult)
Too distal	Advance balloon
Early inflation (before aortic closure)	Trigger after "R" wave/change trigger mode (i.e., arterial line)
Inability to appropriately trigger	
Atrial fibrillation/flutter	Pace ventricle
Tachycardiac	Treat tachycardia
Bradycardia	Pace (atrium or ventricle)

Table 18-9 Indications for ECMO

NEONATES AND CHILDREN	
Respiratory	**Cardiac**
Primary pulmonary hypertension	Cardiac failure after cardiac surgery
Congenital diaphragmatic hernia	Cardiomyopathy
Meconium aspiration	
Persistent fetal circulation	
Pneumonia	
ARDS	
Pulmonary hemorrhage	
ADULT PATIENTS	
Respiratory	Cardiac
ARDS	Cardiac failure posttransplant
Pneumonia	Right heart failure
Near drowning	Failure to wean from bypass
Amniotical embolization	Temporary support for high-risk PCI
Post–lung transplantation	Emergency resuscitation

Technique and Physiology

ECMO is similar to cardiopulmonary bypass consisting of cannula, a pump mechanism, and a gas exchange unit. Two major differences are the site of cannulation and the lack of a venous reservoir.

Venous Cannulas

All ECMO circuits must have venous cannulas. These cannulas are wire reinforced to reduce the risk of kinking and heparin coated to prevent clot formation. The most common sites are the femoral or jugular system. Support after cardiac surgery

Table 18-10 ECMO Treatment Criteria

FAST ENTRY
PaO_2 <50 mm Hg for >2 hr at FiO_2 1.0; PEEP ≥5 cm H_2O
SLOW ENTRY CRITERIA
PaO_2 <50 mm Hg for >12 hr at FiO_2 0.6
PEEP ≥5 cm H_2O
Maximum medical therapy >48 hr

may allow cannulation directly into the right atrium. Adult cannulas must be of sufficient size to allow flows up to 6 L/min.

Pump System

Most centers use a roller pump system similar to that on a bypass circuit while others use a centrifugal propulsion mechanism. Blood enters the pump mechanism by gravity and then is passed through the gas exchange unit.

Gas Exchange Unit

The gas exchange unit, which is matched to the patient's size, may consist of a means to remove carbon dioxide and water vapor while adding oxygen to the blood. Hollow fiber oxygenators are preferred.

Return Cannulas

ECMO differs from cardiopulmonary bypass in that return of blood may be either to the arterial circulation through the femoral or carotid (neonate) artery if oxygenation is needed or into the venous system if extracorporeal CO_2 removal is the primary goal.

Venovenous ECMO

ECMO support for respiratory failure is commonly venovenous. The right internal jugular vein is accessed for drainage while the femoral vein is used for the return blood. Flows are generally 80 to 100 mL/kg/min. Once flows are established, a ventilatory strategy aimed at resting the lungs is initiated. Gatinnoni recommends "rest settings" with a low respiratory rate (3 to 5 breaths/min) while all carbon dioxide is removed by the circuit.[21]

Venoarterial ECMO

Venoarterial ECMO is designed to primarily support a patient with cardiopulmonary failure. Venous sites include the femoral vein, jugular vein, or even the atrium. Other arterial sites include the right common carotid artery (neonates) or femoral artery in the adult patient. A graft attached to the axillary artery may also allow access.

Contraindications and Complications to ECMO

Most complications are either mechanical (due to the apparatus itself) or patient related. Mechanical complications include failure of the gas exchange unit, tubing disruption or disconnection, or inadequate flow. Patient-related complications include bleeding, emboli, organ failure, and metabolic disarray.

Weaning and Removal

The means to wean a patient from ECMO depends upon the indication. Weaning from ECMO when initiated for respiratory failure depends upon adequate recovery of normal lung function. The injured lung has often surrendered most of its vital functions to the ECMO circuit. Gradual increases in the respiratory rate allow the lung to resume CO_2 exchange and oxygenation. Reductions in the required FIO_2 follow.

Weaning from circulatory failure requires a reduction in the amount or support provided by the ECMO circuit while the heart resumes its circulatory function. Flows through the ECMO circuit are reduced allowing more blood to return to the right side of the heart. When support is no longer required and adequate organ perfusion is demonstrated, cannula may be removed. Predictors of reinsertion after removal include lower ejection fraction, cardiac index, or ventricular fractional shortening.[22]

Ventricular Assist Devices

Dr. Michael DeBakey pioneered research in the area of artificial hearts and mechanical-cardiac assist in the 1960s at Baylor College of Medicine.[2] He observed the benefits of occasionally prolonging bypass to allow the heart to recover function. He implanted the first pneumatically powered ventricular support device in a woman suffering postcardiotomy shock in 1963 and supported her for 4 days.[23] His efforts led the National Institutes of Health to establish the Artificial Heart Program in 1964. In 1966 he placed a more sophisticated device and supported a patient for 10 days before recovery explantation. The patient survived several years afterward.[23] Many devices have been developed for both temporary and long-term support of the failing heart and for surgical and percutaneous placement. Research and development will continue because the supply of hearts for transplantation may only reach 5% of the waiting population.

Destination, Indications and Inclusion Criteria

The ultimate goal of any ventricular support device is to provide support to the failing heart. Destination refers to endpoint of support.

A "**bridge-to-recovery**" refers to placement of a temporary support device with the goal of explantation after the native heart has had time to recover its function. Reversible heart failure caused by myocarditis, peripartum cardiomyopathy, or other cardiomyopathy often requires days to weeks to restore adequate function. These patients are often treated with β-blocking agents, thiazides, ACE inhibitors, and β$_2$-agonists in an attempt to improve the function of the heart and allow explantation.[24]

A "**bridge-to-transplant**" refers to a situation where a patient has developed irreversible heart failure, which ultimately is best served with transplantation. Nearly 30% of

Table 18–11 REMATCH Inclusion Criteria
INITIAL INCLUSION CRITERIA
Chronic end-stage heart failure
Ejection fraction <25%
NYHA IV for 90 days
Peak exercise oxygen consumption <12 mL/kg/min
BROADENED CRITERIA
NYHA class IV for 60 days
Peak exercise oxygen consumption <12 mL/kg/min
NYHA class III or IV for 28 days with intraaortic balloon pump or inotrope dependence (not weanable)

patients who receive a heart transplant will be on some form of mechanical support before the transplant. The placement of a ventricular assist device does not adversely affect 1-year transplantation survival and is effective as a bridge although cost-effectiveness is still debatable.[25,26]

True "**destination therapy**" means that long-term support by the device itself is the goal. The patient does not qualify for a transplant and does not have a reversible cardiac condition.[27]

A right ventricular assist device (RVAD) is most commonly placed as a "bridge to recovery" postcardiotomy, after transplantation, or for other indications when the right ventricle (RV) does not respond to more traditional management aimed at reducing RV afterload, such as optimizing preload and maintaining contractility of both the RV and LV.[28] Historically, more than 20% of patients who received an LVAD subsequently received and RV AD due to right ventricular failure. This incidence is lower today.[29]

The REMATCH (Randomized Evaluation of Mechanical Assist in the Treatment of Congestive Heart Failure) trial was the largest prospective, randomized trial comparing VAD to optimal medical management assessing the benefits of mechanical assist and included strict inclusion criteria (Table 18-11).[30] Broader criteria included those patients receiving inotropic support.

General Function

Surgically implanted left ventricular assist devices (LVAD) drain the ventricle through the apex or the left atrium and return blood to the systemic circulation through a conduit to the ascending aorta. Right ventricular assist devices drain blood from the right atrium and return blood to the pulmonary artery. Placement of two separate devices to support both ventricles simultaneously is referred to as **biventricular support** (BiVAD). Common features of all devices include unidirectional valves (either tissue or mechanical).

Physiological Benefits to Ventricular Assist

Recovery of mechanical function is often due to mechanical unloading of the heart.[31] These benefits may be mechanical and cellular (Table 18-12). The placement of an LVAD may acutely worsen the function of the right ventricle. The benefits of increased cardiac output associated with an LVAD

Table 18–12 Benefits of Chronic Mechanical Unloading of the Heart

CONTRACTILE PROPERTIES
Increased magnitude of contraction
Shorter time to peak contraction
Larger contraction
Greater response to ß-adrenergic stimulation
Regression of cellular hypertrophy
NEUROENDOCRINE EFFECTS
Decreased plasma renin
Decreased angiotensin II
Decreased epinephrine and norepinephrine
Decreased atrial natriuretic peptide
CELLULAR FUNCTION
Potentiation of endogenous nitric-oxide mediated regulation of mitochondrial function
APOPTOSIS
Reduction in indicators of cellular stress

Adapted from Nicolosi AC, Pagel PS. Perioperative considerations in the patient with a left ventricular assist device. Anesthesiology 2003;98:565-570.

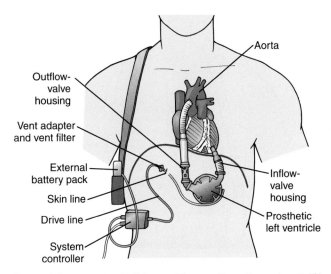

Figure 18–7 HeartMate XVE System (Thoratec Corp., Pleasanton, Calif.).

may include increased venous return to the RV, subsequently increasing RV preload. This may result in a shift of the interventricular septum to the left. The shifting of the septum causes RV distention, worsening of RV contractility, and increased tricuspid regurgitation.

Specific Devices
HeartMate XVE (Vented Electric)

The HeartMate XVE (Thoratec Corp.; Pleasanton, Calif.) is a pulsatile flow ventricular assist device.[32] This system uses a pusher displacement plate technology with a polyurethane diaphragm to propel the blood forward.[33] The XVE system contains an electric motor directly in the blood pump itself and is driven by an external electrical power source increasing portability (Figure 18-7). The pump is constructed of titanium and weighs 1150 grams. The internal surface of the pump is textured to allow the adherence of blood elements and creation of a pseudoneointima.[34] Porcine valves direct the flow.[33] This pump may be implanted below the left hemidiaphragm, either in the peritoneal cavity or abdominal wall.

Filling of the pump is passive. Upon complete filling, the device will eject its contents into the ascending aorta (83 mL). The pump rate can vary from 60 to 120 beats/min and flows from 1.6 to 11.6 L/min. The rate may either be fixed or automatic. The major advantage of this system is the low rate of thromboembolism.[35]

The HeartMate system has a **system controller**, which controls the speed and power while responding to performance and recording events. The **power base unit** (PBU) supplies the main power to the VAD along with the capability of charging and testing back-up batteries. The **system monitor** displays information about the performance and alarms

and allows the operational mode to be set. The HeartMate system has several alarms to indicate potential failures. A yellow battery on the controller indicates 15 minutes of power remaining while a red battery indicates 5 minutes. The primary means of treatment is restoring power to the device, although a manual hand pump may be used temporarily until power is restored. A red heart icon indicates that the pump is not filling to capacity, a low flow state or mechanical pump failure. Immediate assessment of causes of hypovolemia or arrhythmias is imperative as a hand pump will not support the system. Pneumatic support is available for the VXE VAD but only in the hospital.

Cardiac arrest presents a unique challenge to the team caring for a VAD patient. Chest compressions are contraindicated due to the risk of device displacement. One individual must use the hand pump while another searches for the problem or localizes electrical backup. Circulation is often maintained despite ventricular fibrillation or tachycardia and defibrillation is only indicated when a patient is symptomatic.

HeartMate II Left Ventricular Assist System (LVAS)

The HeartMate II Left Ventricular Assist System (Thoratec Corp.) is a valveless, axial-flow rotary device that consists of a blood pump, percutaneous lead, external power source, and a system driver.[36] The only moving part of the device is a blood pump impeller, which spins on blood-lubricated ceramic bearings. Fewer moving parts result in better durability.[33] The pump speed can vary from 6000 to 15,000 rpm and provide flows up to 10 L/min. The blood inflow to the device comes from a titanium cannula implanted thru the apex of the left ventricle while the outflow is directed into a Dacron graft sewn to the ascending aorta (Figure 18-8). The system is approved as a bridge to transplant and for destination therapy. The HeartMate II is small (375 grams) and measures 4 cm in diameter and 6 cm long.[37] It is easily implanted between the muscles of the abdominal wall or directly into the peritoneum (Figure 18.8 HeartMate II LVAD in situ).

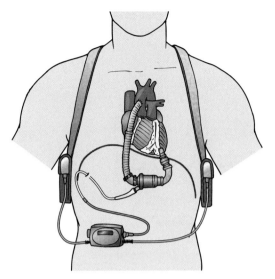

Figure 18–8 HeartMate II LVAD system. *(Used with permission from Bartley BP, Kormos RL, Borovetz HS, et al. HeartMate II left ventricular assist system: from concept to first clinical use. Ann Thorac Surg 2001;71:S116-S120.)*

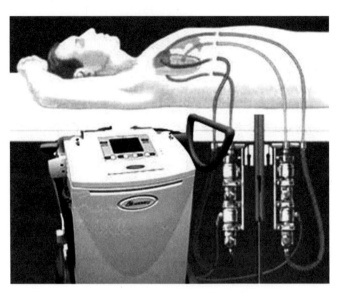

Figure 18–9 Abiomed BVS 5000.

The HeartMate II is a continuous flow system. Certain characteristics of the device include afterload sensitivity and pump output that varies over the cardiac cycle. Flow is determined primarily by the speed of the rotor and the pressure differential across the pump. The pump differential pressure equals the aortic pressure minus the left ventricular pressure, plus the combined pressure across the inlet and outlet cannula. A sufficient baseline flow must always be present or reverse flow could occur. One disadvantage of a continuous flow system such as the HeartMate II is that negative pressure can be generated if the inflow cannula becomes blocked (interventricular septum) or if flow into the left ventricle is compromised.

The HeartMate II can be very sensitive to fluid and physiological changes in the perioperative period. A manual speed control can be adjusted only by a clinician. During periods of significant physiological changes, lower pump speeds are safest. It is recommended that 8000 to 9000 revolutions per minute, a pressure differential of 80 to100 mm Hg, and a flow of 3 to 4 L/min be maintained.

The HeartMate II system has the ability to monitor cardiac function via the **pulsatility index** (PI). The PI reflects a pressure differential between the left ventricle (inflow cannula) and the ascending aorta (outflow cannula). The calculated differential reflects the contribution of the ventricle. The higher the PI, the more contribution of the patient's heart.

Abiomed BVS 5000

The Abiomed BVS 5000 (Abiomed, Inc.; Danvers, Mass.) was initially marketed by the ABIOMED Corporation in the United States in 1992 with the approach that a rheumatically driven device could be managed at the bedside by nursing and housestaff.[38] It is designed to provide temporary support to patients with potentially reversible cardiac conditions, including precardiotomy states (viral myocarditis, myocardial infarction) and postcardiotomy heart failure including acute rejection and cardiogenic shock after heart transplantation.[39] The heart is supported in an extracorporeal, pulsatile pneumatic manner (Figure 18-9). Each pump has two polyurethane chambers within plastic casing separated by a polyurethane valve.

Blood flows into the first chamber (atrial chamber) by gravity and then passively into the second chamber (ventricle), where it is then pneumatically expelled into the aorta or pulmonary artery depending on the heart ventricle being supported. The stroke volume is constant at 82 mL. Flow is limited to 4 to 6 L/min. The device is disposable after use and thus of low cost. Complications may include stroke, pulmonary insufficiency, renal insufficiency, sepsis, and bleeding.[39]

Abiomed AB 5000 Ventricular Support Device

The Abiomed AB 5000 ventricular support device (Abiomed, Inc.; Danvers, Mass.) is designed for short- and intermediate-term mechanical support and to provide improved patient mobility, blood pump durability, and overall versatility when compared with the BVS 5000.[38] The device consists of a fully automatic, vacuum-assisted console and a paracorporeal, pneumatically driven blood pump. The blood pump is contained in clear housing to allow the clinician to view blood elements (Figure 18-10). Flows up to 6 L/min can be delivered.

Centrimag/Levitronix

The Centrimag Ventricular Assist System (Levitronix; Waltham, Mass.) is a continuous flow, extracorporeal support system consisting of a bearingless pump, motor, and console. The pump itself consists of a magnetically suspended, bearingless pump head with a 31-cc priming volume driven by a small motor. The pump can reach a maximum speed of 5500 rpm and a maximum flow of 9.9 L/min and may support a patient for 2 weeks or longer. The primary console allows the operator to adjust the rotations per minute while observing the flow rate. A back-up console provides temporary support in case of failure of the primary system. The inflow to the system is from a cannula in the atrium or ventricle while the outflow is either into the pulmonary artery (RVAD) or aorta (LVAD). The pump causes very little damage to blood elements.[37]

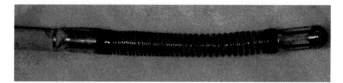

Figure 18–11   Impella Recover pVAD.

patients may be involved in the implantation, transportation, or management of such patients.

Impella Ventricular Assist Device

The Impella ventricular assist device (Abiomed, Inc. Danvers, Mass.) is a miniaturized axial pump within a flexible cannula for temporary mechanical cardiovascular support (Figure 18-11). The device is placed either in the ascending aorta through a small Dacron tube graft or via a percutaneous technique through a 13 Fr sheath placed into the femoral artery. The device is then positioned with its distal tip across the aortic valve. A proximal opening allows blood drawn from the distal tip to be ejected onto the aorta. Nonpulsatile flow rates of 4.5 to 5.0 L/min may be reached at a speed of 33,000 rpm. Generally these are used with a balloon pump. The device creates minimal hemolysis, may be placed with an "off-pump" technique, and requirement for minimal anticoagulation. The major disadvantage is limited blood flow and short-term use. The Impella may provide increased cardiac output when compared with an IABP.

TandemHeart Percutaneous Ventricular Assist Device (pVAD)

The TandemHeart Percutaneous Ventricular Assist Device (CardiacAssist, Inc.; Pittsburgh, Pa.) provides temporary mechanical support to the failing heart and is based upon the concept developed by Clarence Dennis. The device has three components, a transseptal cannula, arterial cannula, and a centrifugal pump. The transseptal cannula is placed into the femoral vein, up through the right atrium and across the intraatrial septum via a transseptal puncture.[40] The femoral artery catheter is placed into the femoral artery. Oxygenated blood is drawn from the left atrium, circulated by the centrifugal pump, and returned through the femoral artery to provide flow rates of up to 5 L/min[40] (www.texasheart.org). The pump relies upon adequate right ventricular function to perfuse the pulmonary vasculature. The major benefit is ease of implantation. The disadvantages are limited flow rates and provision of only temporary support. The device is designed only as a bridge to recovery or as a "bridge to bridge," meaning the device is placed until longer-term support is established, generally a few hours up to 14 days.[37] Complications include femoral artery injury, clot formation, dislodgement, and the creation of a large ASD with placement. A recent study demonstrated that the TandemHeart more effectively reversed the hemodynamic and metabolic parameters associated with cardiogenic shock than an IABP but complications such as severe bleeding and limb ischemia were more common.[41]

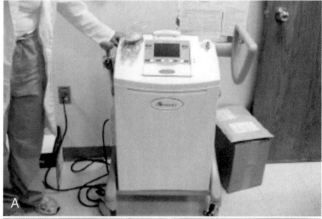
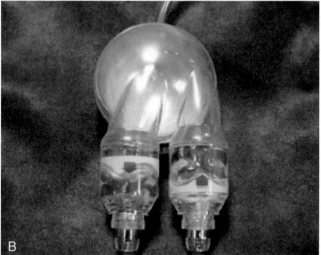
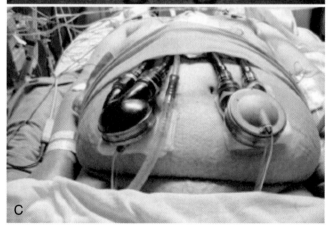

Figure 18–10   AB5000 system: **(A)** console, **(B)** blood pump, and **(C)** placement. (Used with permission from Samuels LE, Holmes EC, Garwood P, et al. Initial experience with the Abiomed AB5000 ventricular assist system. Ann Thorac Surg 2005;80:309-312.)

Percutaneous Ventricular Support Devices

Several temporary ventricular support devices are available for insertion either by a cardiologist in the catheterization laboratory under fluoroscopy or by surgeons in the operating room. Only rarely will the general anesthesiologist encounter these devices but anesthesiologists involved in the care of cardiac

Temporary Pacing Devices

The anesthesiologist is frequently called upon to provide temporary cardiac pacing either electively for patients with conditions that are associated with the development of complete heart block or significant bradycardia or for patients undergoing procedures that promote bradycardia. The common principle though is the provision of rate support from an external pulse generator via an electrode or electrodes, which can be removed easily after a short period of pacing or easily replaced by permanent pacing if necessary.[42]

Emergency Temporary Pacing

Temporary emergency pacing is indicated for any patient with an acute hemodynamic deterioration due to bradycardia, complete heart block, or asystole. In general medical treatment is attempted before the initiation of temporary pacing. Should atropine, glycopyrrolate, epinephrine, dopamine, or isoproterenol fail then temporary pacing must be initiated.

Elective Temporary Pacing

Elective temporary pacing is often initiated when patients are undergoing surgical procedures associated with significant bradycardia or in patients with a history of significant bradycardia or asystole with previous anesthetics. Often these patients have a history of second- or third-degree heart block or first-degree block associated with bifascicular block.

Modes of Temporary Pacing

Temporary pacing can be provided by either transcutaneous, transesophageal, transvenous, or via an epicardial route.

Transcutaneous Pacing

Transcutaneous pacing was originally developed by Paul Zoll in 1952. This mode may provide ventricular pacing for several hours while a condition promoting bradycardia resolves or while a more reliable mode is established. Transcutaneous pacing is easy to establish and reliable, but often requires that the patient receive sedation. Multifunction defibrillation electrode pads may be placed in either an anterior-anterior (right upper chest—left lower chest) position or in an anterior-posterior position. Such pads may be used for defibrillation, pacing, monitoring, or synchronized cardioversion. Pads are then connected to the monitor after placement. The pacing device must then be placed into the "pacing mode." A heart rate is set with an output sufficient to capture the ventricular myocardium. Complications include failure to capture and discomfort.

Transesophageal Pacing

Transesophageal pacing relies upon the anatomic position of the esophagus directly posterior to the left atrium. A small flexible electrode is placed either through the nose or mouth and positioned where atrial amplitude is maximal.

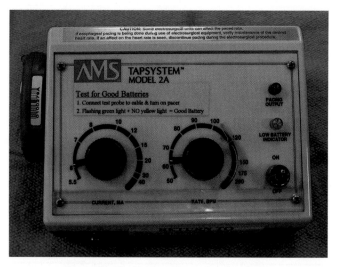

Figure 18–12   Transesophageal pacing device.

Output from 5.5 to 40 mAmp may be delivered with a heart rate between 50 to 200 beats/min. Success rate is up to 90%. Complications include failure to capture, patient discomfort, and esophageal injury. Transesophageal pacing is limited to asynchronous modes only (Figure 18-12).

Transvenous Pacing

Transvenous pacing may be applied either to the atrium, ventricle, or A-V sequential in a synchronous or asynchronous mode. Transvenous pacing is commonly initiated via a specially designed 8 Fr thermodilution pulmonary artery catheter placed through an 8.5 Fr minimum-sized introducer sheath. The catheter is designed with a port terminating approximately 19 cm from the distal tip of the sheath (ventricular pacing port) and a second port terminating approximately 27 cm from the distal tip (atrial pacing port). Such catheters have the advantage of bedside placement without the need for fluoroscopy. The appropriate position of the catheter is confirmed by hemodynamic pressure tracings. A specially designed balloon-tipped single lumen catheter is also available for placement of a right ventricle pacing lead.

After appropriate placement of the catheter, a flexible-tipped pacing probe designed either for the atrial port or ventricular port is necessary. The probe is placed in a sterile fashion and advanced through the appropriate lumen. After connection to a pacing-device, the pacing probe is advanced through until a pacing indicating "spike" is noted on the ECG and followed by either a "P" wave or "V" depending upon the chamber to be paced.

Transvenous pacing may also be initiated without the need for a pulmonary artery catheter. Such a setup requires a smaller introducer placed in either the internal or external jugular veins. A wire is floated through the catheter and generally guided into either the right atrium or ventricle via fluoroscopy.

The highest risk of transvenous pacing is related to obtaining appropriate vascular access and includes hematoma formation, arterial puncture, pneumothorax, or local trauma. Complications of transvenous pacing itself include malposition of the catheter, perforation of a chamber of the heart, diaphragmatic pacing, or in the case of a smaller patient, the inability to correctly position the correct lumen into the right ventricle. Later complications include infection, which may ultimately delay more permanent pacing when needed.[43]

Epicardial Pacing

Anesthesiologists do not place leads for epicardial pacing but are frequently called upon to control pacing after leads are placed by surgeons. Leads are directly placed on the epicardium of the right atrium or right ventricle into the myocardium by the surgeon. The wires are then directed through the skin. Capture is nearly 100% successful. Wires can be removed by gentle external traction. Complications include accidental dislodgement when the sternotomy or thoracotomy is closed leading to failure to capture. Removal may result in tamponade if bleeding occurs.

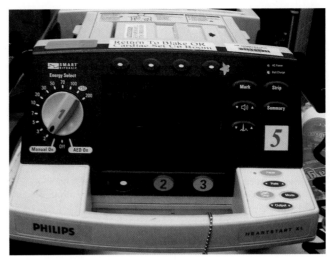

Figure 18–13   Phillips HeartStart LX biphasic defibrillator.

External Defibrillators

All anesthesiologists must be intimately familiar with the particular external defibrillators that are used within their individual hospital. Most of these devices have the ability to provide synchronous and asynchronous cardioversion or defibrillation through external or internal paddles or through multifunction defibrillator electrode pads. Many have an automatic external defibrillation mode and the ability to provide pacing either in a demand or fixed mode.

Modern defibrillators deliver energy in a biphasic fashion, meaning that the electrical current passes through the heart in one direction, reverses direction, and then passes through again. This ultimately results in a need for less energy than a monophasic waveform. It has been shown that biphasic defibrillation is as effective as conventional higher energy monophasic defibrillation and results in better myocardial function afterwards.[44,45]

The *manual output energy* determines the level of energy (Joules) that will be delivered and can be between 2 and 200 J. Energy is generally limited to 50 J for internal or epicardial defibrillation. A *synchronizer* button allows the operator to select whether defibrillation will occur immediately or only when synchronized with the cardiac cycle to prevent potential harm ("R-on-T" phenomenon). Additional features of the device include Liquid Crystal Display (LCD) of the single ECG lead. Leads I, II, or III may be selected when the external ECG cable is in place. The display also includes heart rate, synchronization mode, and energy to be delivered (Joules) (Figure 18–13).

The decision to select synchronized versus asynchronous cardioversion depends upon the clinical situation. Synchronous cardioversion is chosen for ventricular tachycardiac associated with a pulse, reentry supraventricular tachycardia, atrial fibrillation, or atrial flutter. A lower energy level is needed. Asynchronous defibrillation is selected when a patient does not have a pulse or in the setting of clinical deterioration.

Modern defibrillators are often simple to use but problems often develop and the operator must be able to trouble shoot (Table 18-13).

Table 18–13 Trouble shooting External Defibrillators

Problem	Potential Problems	Solution
Device will not display	Device on?	Select on
	Battery failed?	Plug in/obtain new device
Device will not synchronize	Synch on?	Push "synch" button
	ECG gain too low	Increase gain
	R-peak not prominent	Increase gain or select alternative lead
Device will not deliver shock	Inability to "synch"	Increase ECG gain
	Rhythm too erratic	Consider asynchronous
Device will not pace	Device in demand mode	Change to fixed mode
Fibrillation persists despite shock	Failure to cardiovert	Increase energy

Suggested Reading

Baskett, R.J., Ghali, W.A., Maitland, A., et al., 2002. The intraaortic balloon pump in cardiac surgery. Ann Thorac Surg 74, 1276–1287. *A very nice review of the utility of the IABP in cardiac surgery. Evidence from a MEDLINE search from 1966–2000 is reviewed and graded according to the ACC and AHA guidelines.*

Gammage, M.D., 2000. Electrophysiology: temporary cardiac pacing. Heart 83, 715–720. *A strong review of the various modes of temporary pacing including transvenous, transesophageal, and epicardial techniques.*

Lewandowski, K., 2000. Extracorporeal membrane oxygenation for severe acute respiratory failure. Crit Care 4, 156–168. *A comprehensive review article on the use of extracorporeal membranous oxygenation.*

Kern, M.J., 1991. Intra-aortic balloon counterpulsation. Coron Artery Dis 2, 649–660. *An older, simple to read review article on the use of the balloon pump.*

References

1. Brunwald, E., 2003. Cardiology: the past, the present, and the future. J Am Coll Cardiol 42, 2031–2041.
2. Joyce, L.D., Noon, G.P., Joyce, D.L., et al., 2004. Mechanical circulatory support—a historical review. ASAIO J 50. x-xii.
3. Friedrich, E.B., Bohm, M., 2007. Management of end stage heart failure. Heart 93, 626–631.
4. Task Force for Diagnosis and Treatment of Acute and Chronic Heart Failure 200b of European Society of Cardiology. ESC guidelines for the diagnosis and treatment of acute and chronic heart failure 2008 of the European Society of Cardiology. Developed in collaboration with the Heart Failure Association of the ESC (HFA) and endorsed by the European Society of Intensive Care Medicine (ESICM). Eur Heart J 29, 2388–2442.
5. Taylor, D.O., Edwards, L.B., Aurora, P., et al., 2008. Registry of the International Society for Heart and Lung Transplantation: twenty-fifth official adult heart transplant report - 2008. J Heart Lung Transplant 27, 943–956.
6. Davis, R.F., Gravlee, G.P., Kurusz, M. et al., (Eds.), 2000. Cardiopulmonary bypass principles and practice, ed 2. Lippincott Williams & Wilkins, Philadelphia.
7. Murphy, G.S., Hessel, E.A., Groom, R.C., 2009. Optimal perfusion during cardiopulmonary bypass: an evidence based approach. Anesth Analg 108, 1394–1417.
8. Hsu, L.C., 1997. Biocompatibility in cardiopulmonary bypass. J Cardiothorac Vasc Anesth 11, 376–382.
9. Paddyachee, T.S., 1988. The effect of arterial line filtration on GME in the middle cerebral arteries. Ann Thorac Surg 45, 647–649.
10. Saied, N.N., Helwani, M.A., Comunale, M.E., et al., 2007. A simple solution for electrocardiographic artifacts during cardiopulmonary bypass and in the intensive care unit. J Cardiothorac Vasc Anesth 21, 572–573.
11. Patel, S.I., Souter, M.J., 2008. Equipment-related electrocardiographic artifacts. Anesthesiology 108, 138–148.
12. Ruengsakulrach, P., Buxton, B.F., 2001. Anatomic and hemodynamic considerations influencing the efficiency of retrograde cardioplegia. Ann Thorac Surg 71, 1389–1395.
13. Economopoulos, G.C., Michalis, A., Palatianos, G.M., et al., 2003. Management of catheter-related injuries to the coronary sinus. Ann Thorac Surg 76, 112–116.
14. Kern, M.J., 1991. Intra-aortic balloon counterpulsation. Coron Artery Dis 2, 649–660.
15. Arrow International Educational Materials, 2005. Counterpulsation applied: an introduction to intra-aortic balloon pumping. Arrow International, Everett, MA.
16. Kale, P.K., Fang, J.C., 2008. Devices in acute heart failure. Crit Care Med 36, S121–S128.
17. Baskett, R.J., Ghali, W.A., Maitland, A., et al., 2002. The intraaortic balloon pump in cardiac surgery. Ann Thorac Surg 74, 1276–1287.
18. Yoshitani, H., Akasaka, T., Kaji, S., et al., 2007. Effects of intra-aortic balloon counterpulsation on coronary pressure in patients with stenotic coronary arteries. Am Heart J 154, 725–731.
19. Vonderheide, R.H., Thadhani, R., Kutter, D.J., 1998. Association of thrombocytopenia with the use of intra-aortic balloon pumps. Am J Med 105, 27–32.
20. Bakhtiary, F., Keller, H., Dogan, S., et al., 2008. Venoarterial extracorporeal membrane oxygenation for treatment of cardiogenic shock: clinical experiences in 45 adult patients. J Thorac Cardiovasc Surg 135, 382–388.
21. Gattinoni, L., Pesenti, A., Mascheroni, et al., 1986. Low-frequency positive pressure ventilation with extracorporeal CO_2 removal in severe acute respiratory failure. JAMA 256, 881–886.
22. Gunay, C., Cingoz, F., Kilic, S., et al., 2007. Reinsertion predictors of intraaortic balloon pumps. Heart Surg Forum 10, E463–E467.
23. DeBakey, M.E., 2005. Development of mechanical heart devices. Ann Thorac Surg 79, S2228–S2231.
24. Shams, O.F., Ventura, H.O., 2008. Device therapy for heart failure when and for whom? Am J Cardiovasc Drugs 8, 147–153.
25. Cleveland, J.C., Grover, F.L., Fullerton, D.A., et al., 2008. Left ventricular assist device as bridge to transplantation does not adversely affect one-year heart transplant survival. J Thorac Cardiovasc Surg 136, 774–777.
26. Clegg, A.J., Scott, D.A., Loveman, E., et al., 2005. Clinical and cost-effectiveness of left ventricular assist devices as a bridge to heart transplantation for people with end-stage heart failure: a systematic review and economic evaluation. Eur Heart J 27, 2929–2938.
27. Mehra, M.R., Uber, P.A., Uber, W.E., et al., 2004. Destination therapy in late-stage heart failure. Coron Artery Dis 15, 87–89.
28. Moazami, N., Pasque, M.K., Moon, M.R., et al., 2004. Mechanical support for isolated right ventricular failure in patients after cardiotomy. J Heart Lung Transplantation 23, 1371–1375.
29. Pavie, A., Leger, P., 1996. Physiology of univentricular versus biventricular support. Ann Thorac Surg 61, 347–349.
30. Aaronson, K.D., Patel, H., Pagani, F.D., 2003. Patient selection for left ventricular assist device therapy. Ann Thorac Surg 75, S29–S35.
31. Nicolosi, A.C., Pagel, P.S., 2003. Perioperative considerations in the patient with a left ventricular assist device. Anesthesiology 98, 565–570.
32. Frazier, O.H., Myers, T.J., Radovancevic, B., 1998. The HeartMate left ventricular assist system. Overview and 12-year experience. Tex Heart Inst J 25, 265–271.
33. Williams, M., Oz, M., Mancini, D., 2001. Cardiac assist devices for end-stage heart failure. Heart Dis 3, 109–115.
34. Rafii, S., Oz, M.C., Seldomridge, A.J., et al., 1995. Characterization of hematopoietic cells arising on the textured surface of left ventricular assist devices. Ann Thorac Surg 60, 1321–1327.
35. Slater, J., Rose, E., Levin, H., et al., 1996. Low thromboembolic risk without anticoagulation using advanced-design left ventricular assist devices. Ann Thorac Surg 62, 1321–1327.
36. Griffith, B.P., Kormos, R.L., Borovetz, H.S., et al., 2001. HeartMate II left ventricular assist system: from concept to first clinical use. Ann Thorac Surg 71, S116–S120.
37. Texas Heart Institute. (website): www.texasheart.org. Accessed July 24, 2009.
38. Samuels, L.E., Holmes, E.C., Garwood, P., et al., 2005. Initial experience with the Abiomed AB 5000 ventricular assist device system. Ann Thorac Surg 80, 309–312.
39. Petrofski, J.A., Patel, V.S., Russell, S.D., et al., 2003. BVS5000 support after cardiac transplantation. J Thorac Cardiovasc Surg 126, 442–447.
40. Kar, B., Adkins, L.E., Civitello, A.B., et al., 2006. Clinical experience with the TandemHeart percutaneous ventricular assist device. Tex Heart Inst J 33, 111–115.
41. Thiele Holger, Smalling, R.W., Schuler, G.C., 2007. Percutaneous left ventricular assist devices in acute myocardial infarction complicated by cardiogenic shock. Eur Heart J 28, 2057–2063.
42. Gammage, M.D., 2000. Electrophysiology temporary cardiac pacing. Heart 83, 715–720.
43. Rajappan, K., Fox, K.F., 2003. Temporary cardiac pacing in district general hospitals—sustainable resource of training liability? Q J Med 96, 783–785.
44. Tang, W., Weil, M.H., Sun, S., et al., 2001. A comparison of biphasic and monophasic waveform defibrillation after prolonged ventricular fibrillation. Chest 120, 948–954.
45. Reddy, R.K., Gleva, M.J., Gliner, B.E., et al., 1997. Biphasic transthoracic defibrillation causes fewer ECG ST-segment changes after shock. Ann Emerg Med 30, 127–134.

Chapter 19

Patient Warming Devices

Jennifer A. Chatburn and Warren S. Sandberg

Unintended perioperative hypothermia has been associated with multiple adverse effects. Numerous studies have found hypothermia to be associated with increased blood loss and transfusion requirements,[1] longer surgical wound healing times and increased wound infections, prolonged action of neuromuscular blocking agents and other medications, prolonged recovery in the postanesthesia care unit (PACU), postoperative shivering, and cardiac morbidity.[2,3] Hypothermia has been found to increase risk of a number of morbid cardiac events postoperatively, including ischemia, unstable angina, cardiac arrest, and myocardial infarction. Patients who experience hypothermia during the perioperative period may have longer hospital stays than patients who were normothermic during the perioperative period.[4,5]

The ACC/AHA 2007 Guidelines on Perioperative Cardiovascular Evaluation and Care for Noncardiac Surgery introduced a level I recommendation that body temperature should be maintained in a normothermic range for most procedures other than during periods in which mild hypothermia is intended to provide organ protection.[6] The maintenance of normothermia during the perioperative period has become a performance measure and is rapidly emerging as a standard of care.[7]

Causes of Hypothermia

The surgical patient is at risk for hypothermia for several reasons. Patient factors that increase the risk of hypothermia include preexisting hypothermia, extremes of age (e.g., neonates, infants, and older adults), trauma, extensive burns, low body weight, hypothyroidism, dysautonomia (e.g., diabetic neuropathy), and chronic antipsychotic or antidepressant use. Perioperative factors that increase the risk of hypothermia include a cold operating room environment, large open cavity surgery, intravenous infusion of larger volumes of unwarmed fluid or blood products, use of unwarmed irrigant solutions in body cavities, and use of pneumatic tourniquets.

Both general and neuraxial anesthesia reduce the body's heat production and impair thermoregulation. During general anesthesia, perioperative hypothermia develops in three stages. The most rapid decrease in core temperature occurs during induction and the first 30 to 60 minutes of anesthesia. This is due predominantly to redistribution of heat from the core to the peripheral body. Subsequently, a more gradual, linear decrease of core temperature occurs over several hours as heat loss from the body exceeds heat production by metabolic processes. Finally, core temperature plateaus and does not change for the remaining duration of anesthesia.[8]

Heat energy is transferred from the patient to the ambient operating room environment by radiation, conduction, convection, and evaporation. Surgical exposure and evaporation of water from the patient also contribute to heat loss; for every gram of water evaporated, 0.58 kcal of heat is removed from the patient.[9]

Preventing Hypothermia

Common methods to retard heat loss and warm patients in the perioperative setting include passive strategies and active strategies. Passive strategies include warming the ambient temperature of the operating room and covering the patient. Passive strategies slow heat loss but do not actively transfer heat to the patient or increase core temperature. In addition to slowing heat loss, active warming strategies may transfer heat to the patient and increase core temperature. Technologies that actively warm patients include convective warming devices and conductive warming devices. Convective warming devices transfer heat to the patient by circulating warmed air rapidly across the body surface. Conductive warming devices transfer heat to the patient through areas of direct contact. Radiant warming devices transfer heat to the patient by emitting infrared waves. Additional strategies for preventing perioperative hypothermia include administering warm intravenous fluids and using warm humidified inspired gases.

Passive Strategies

Passive strategies for keeping the patient warm perioperatively include reducing the temperature gradient between the patient and surroundings by raising the operating room temperature and insulating the patient with a single layer or multiple layers of coverings. These measures will not raise core temperature by transferring heat energy to the patient, but may help to decrease the risk of hypothermia by slowing heat loss.

Ambient Temperature

Patients are often exposed to cold operating room environments during the perioperative period. Lower ambient temperatures have been thought to create a more hostile environment for bacterial growth, and thus to reduce the risk of bacterial contamination or infection. This may be offset, however, by the increased risk of surgical wound infection associated with patient hypothermia. In addition, ambient temperature is often kept low for operating room personnel, who may be uncomfortable working in warmer temperatures, particularly when wearing sterile gowns or lead aprons for x-ray, CT, or fluoroscopy.

Certain situations may warrant increasing the ambient temperature to keep the patient warm or prevent hypothermia. One study found that increasing the operating room temperature to 26° C reduced the incidence of core hypothermia in at-risk younger and older patient populations. A warmer room temperature may improve patient satisfaction if the patient is awake in the operating room for any extended period of time, such as during surgery under local or regional anesthesia or during long periods of preparation before induction of general anesthesia. Patient populations at risk for hypothermia include pediatric patients, elderly patients, and patients with large total body surface area (TBSA) burns. Neonatal and pediatric patients have a large body surface area to volume ratio and lose heat faster than adult patients. Large TBSA burn patients lose both heat and water quickly because of epithelial barrier loss and are at significant risk for hypothermia and its sequelae.

Thermal Insulation

The most basic method of preventing heat loss is to avoid exposure and keep the patient covered. Sheets of various materials may be applied to the patient to cover the body. The head may be wrapped or covered with cloth or plastic sheets or with fitted reflective caps.[10] Passive coverings are inexpensive compared with electrically powered active warming systems. In most hospitals thermal insulators are often used in combination with active warming devices. While some studies have demonstrated coverings of certain materials to be more effective than others at preventing heat loss, one study found that a single layer of passive insulation reduced heat loss by about 30% regardless of the material. There are two types of thermal insulators, mass insulators and radiant insulators.

Mass Insulators

Mass insulators entrap air within a fiber matrix. Cotton blankets, cloth and paper surgical drapes, and plastic surgical drapes are all examples of mass insulators. Most of the insulation provided by mass insulators comes not from the fiber matrix itself, but from the still air entrapped between the insulator and the patient's skin surface. Still air is a very effective insulator, and the type of material used to trap the air is of less importance than the amount of air enclosed beneath the material.

Radiant Insulators

Radiant insulators reflect radiant heat back to the patient and emit little radiant heat to the exterior. Metallized "space blankets" and sheets are radiant insulators.[11] Radiant insulators have been found in experiments to be more efficient insulators than cloth surgical drapes and cotton blankets. The difference, however, is slight; one study found a "space blanket" to be only 13% more efficient than a cloth surgical drape. The minimal difference in effectiveness between a radiant insulator and ordinary mass insulators appears to have little clinical significance. Still air beneath the reflective blanket is still a large contributor to insulation, as it is with mass insulators. The effectiveness of radiant insulators appears to be reduced by the placement of other materials between the metallic surface and the patient's skin; the addition of a radiant insulator between layers of mass insulators does not reduce heat loss more than the addition of another mass insulator.

Other Considerations

Multiple layers are slightly more effective than a single layer of passive insulation in helping to prevent heat loss. One study found that a single cotton blanket reduced heat loss by about 33%, and that additional blankets to a total of three layers conferred an additional 18% reduction in heat loss. This was regardless of whether the blankets were warmed or kept at room temperature.

Cotton blankets are frequently stored in an oven in the operating room area to keep them warm. Prewarmed blankets often provide immediate comfort to the awake patient and may increase patient satisfaction. Prewarmed blankets do not, however, raise core temperature or transfer heat to the patient. Prewarmed cotton blankets also do not prevent heat loss more effectively than unwarmed cotton blankets stored at room temperature. One study found that although warmed blankets did reduce heat loss to some degree, this benefit dissipated after approximately 10 minutes, after which there was no significant difference between warmed and unwarmed blankets.[12]

Active Warming Devices

Active warming devices transfer heat to the patient and may raise core temperature. Heat may be transferred to the patient by convection, conduction, or radiation. Convective warming devices transfer heat by circulating warmed currents of air over the patient. Conductive warming devices transfer heat by direct contact with a warm surface. Radiant heating transfers heat by application of energy in the form of rays or waves.

Forced Air Warming Devices

Forced air warmers transfer heat to the patient by convection. They are effective at preventing hypothermia when used before induction of anesthesia, during anesthesia and surgery, and after emergence in the postanesthesia care unit. Forced air warmers are the most frequently used and studied active warming devices in the perioperative setting. Studies have shown that preinduction warming with forced air warmers also significantly reduces postoperative hypothermia and results in higher postoperative core temperatures.[13]

The forced air warmer consists of an electrically powered control unit, hose, and inflatable "blanket" (Figure 19–1). The control unit has an air filter and heater, which warms air entrained from the environment. The hose connects to a blanket. Small holes located throughout the blanket allow currents of warmed air to pass through and blow across the patient. Disposable forced air warming blankets have been manufactured in various shapes for placement under the patient as a mattress, over the upper body and arms, over the lower body and legs, or surrounding the head. Placement of a passive covering such as a cotton blanket, surgical drape, or sheet over the forced air blanket may help to warm the patient more rapidly than the forced air blanket alone.

Complications

Concern has been raised that forced air may seed the surgical site with bacteria from the environment, control unit, or hose. This has not been proven in any large studies, however, and some small studies have demonstrated no increase in wound or prosthesis infections associated with intraoperative use of forced air warming.[14,15] One small study found bacterial colonization in the hoses of forced air convection warmers and detected bacteria in the airstream flowing directly from unattached hoses, but no positive cultures from air which passed through the perforated forced air warming blankets when the hose was connected according to the manufacturer's intended design.[16] Forced air warmers have in-built filters to reduce microbial risk. Nonetheless, it remains a common practice to avoid turning on the forced air warmer until after surgical prepping and draping to avoid blowing air over the surgical site.

Burns from forced air warmers have been reported in certain settings. Forced air warming should not be applied to poorly perfused or ischemic areas, such as over the lower extremities during aortic or iliac cross-clamping in vascular surgery procedures. Second- and third-degree burns have been reported in neonatal and pediatric patients at risk for cyanosis or global ischemia, such as during cardiopulmonary bypass for surgical correction of cyanotic congenital heart disease.[17]

Burns may also occur when air flow is turned on at the control unit without attaching the hose to the appropriate forced air warming blanket (Figure 19–2). In 2002, the FDA cited several complaints in which burn injuries occurred from concentrated hot air blowing directly at the patient's skin from the unattached hose. These included first-, second-, and third-degree burns, with one case of severe muscle necrosis that resulted ultimately in above-the-knee amputation.[18] The American Society for Testing and Materials specifies that forced air warming devices should not exceed an average contact surface temperature of 46° C, and maximum contact surface temperature should not exceed 48° C under normal operating conditions. When the hose is not attached to the intended forced air warming blanket, concentrated air at the hose nozzle may exceed 48° C. In addition, the hose surface may be hot and may cause burns if it comes into direct contact with the patient's skin. It is recommended that a forced air warmer should always be used with the device's appropriately fitting blanket.[19,20]

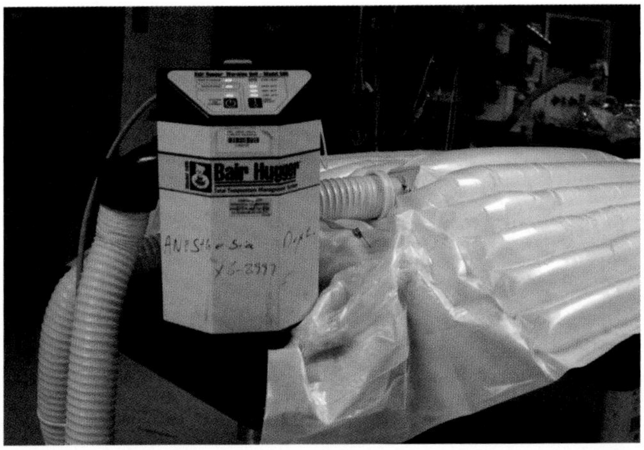

Figure 19–1   Forced air warmer. A typical forced air warmer consisting of a control unit, hose, and disposable blanket. Blankets are available in many sizes and configurations. Depending on patient and surgical needs, blankets may go above or beneath the patient, may cover the arms and torso or the lower body, or may surround the patient's sides.

Table 19–1   Summary of Patient Warming Devices

Passive devices to prevent heat loss

- Raise the room temperature
- Thermal insulation (cover the patient with cloth, paper, plastic or reflective sheets, blankets, or caps)

Active warming devices

- Forced air (convection) warming
- Circulating water garments, blankets, and mattresses
- Radiant heaters
- Resistive heating pads, blankets, and garments

Adjunct strategies

- Prewarm the patient before induction of anesthesia
- Warm intravenous fluids and blood products
- Heat and moisture exchangers (HMEs)
- Heated humidifiers
- Warm fluid for irrigation/lavage
- Warm gases for peritoneal insufflation

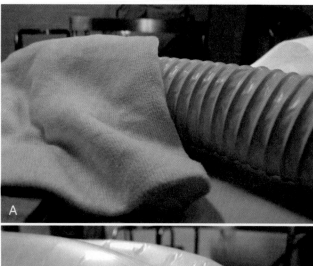

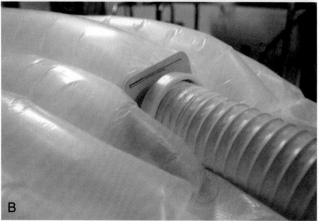

Figure 19–2 Incorrect **(A)** and correct **(B)** use of the forced air warming hose. To avoid burn injuries, the hose should always be attached to the proper forced air warming blanket. The forced air warming hose should never be used unattached to blow directly at the patient.

Liquid Circulating Devices

Liquid circulating devices transfer heat to the patient by conduction through points of contact between the patient and a mattress or blanket. The devices consist of a control unit that adjusts water temperature, and a device that contacts the patient (i.e., garments, a mattress, or a blanket), which is connected to the heater/control unit by tubing. Water warmed by the heating unit passes through the tubing and then circulates through the mattress or blanket. Figure 19–3 shows a simple underpatient warmer that uses circulating warmed water. The water is warmed by a resistive heater contained in a simple control unit that also includes a thermostat to regulate the temperature of the warmed water. Figure 19–4 shows a more sophisticated underpatient circulating water device. This system can be used both for active heating and cooling. The control unit contains both a heater and a refrigerator. The temperature may be sensed and controlled at the blanket or in the water reservoir.

Circulating water garments fitted over the patient have been found to be at least comparable in efficacy to forced air warming blankets placed over the patient, and several studies have found them to be actually superior in efficacy to forced air warming.[21,22] Figure 19–5 illustrates a water garment device, in this instance using self-adhesive disposable pads, applied to the patient's skin.

Table 19–2 **Thermal Injuries Caused by Patient Warming Devices**
Warmed IV fluid bags or bottles
• May cause burns when placed in contact with skin. • Should not be used for patient positioning or warming.
Forced air warmers
• May cause burns when placed over ischemic or poorly perfused areas (e.g., the lower extremities during aortic or iliac cross-clamping). • Severe burns may result from use of hose without warming blanket.
Circulating water mattresses
• Burns may occur at pressure points.
Radiant heaters
• May cause burns if heat lamp is placed closer to skin than specified by manufacturer's instructions. • High temperature heaters may cause burns when placed over ischemic or poorly perfused areas.

Numerous older studies comparing circulating water mattresses to forced air warming blankets such as Bair Hugger had found that forced air warming was more effective.[23,24] These studies, however, compared traditional circulating water mattresses placed underneath with forced air warming blankets placed over the patient. The effectiveness of circulating water mattresses placed beneath the patient may be limited by compression of the capillary beds in contact with the mattress by the weight of the body.

Complications

Potential hazards of liquid circulating devices include risk of burns at pressure points and areas of direct contact. Of 28 burns caused by devices intended to warm patients in an ASA Closed Claims analysis in 1994, 5 cases (18%) involved circulating water blankets. Circulating water blankets were second to oven-warmed intravenous fluid bags or bottles for burn claims from warming devices included in the analysis. The American Society for Testing and Materials' standard specification for liquid circulating devices mandates that the average contact surface temperature should not exceed 42° C, and the maximum contact surface temperature should not exceed 43° C under normal operating conditions.

Radiant Heaters and Heat Lamps

Radiant heaters are lamps that transfer heat to the patient by infrared radiation. The radiant heater consists of a heating unit, which emits infrared radiation, and a skin temperature sensor. The heat lamp is placed at a distance determined by the manufacturer from the chosen heating site. The skin temperature sensor is placed on the heating site and a target skin temperature is selected (37° C for infants and awake patients, 41° C for generally anesthetized adults). Radiant heaters emit primarily infrared B with minimal infrared A range radiation. Radiant heaters do not emit ultraviolet range radiation.

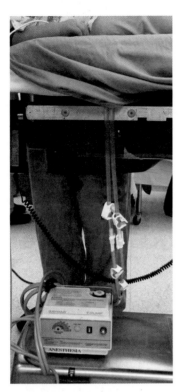

Figure 19–3 Under patient circulating hot water warming pad. The heater/control unit is conveniently placed under the OR table. However, in this arrangement, any air introduced into the water circulator raises to the top of the system—in this instance the warming pad itself—where it may cause an air lock that limits or eliminates the device's effectiveness as a warmer.

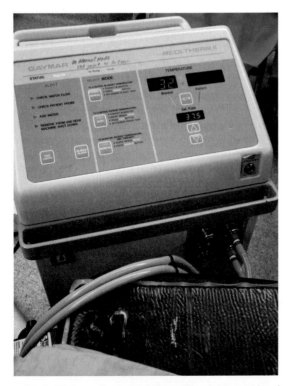

Figure 19–4 Under patient circulating water heater-cooler device. Note multiple temperature sensing points that can be used to control the device's performance.

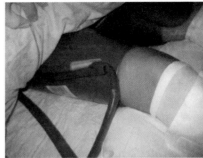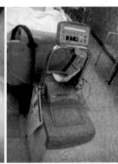

Figure 19–5 Circulating water garment device. *Left,* Illustrates pads applied to the patient's skin; *right,* illustrates controller. The device will apply or remove heat to achieve a set patient temperature—in this case 37.1° C.

Radiant heaters have been manufactured to emit infrared over the entire body, or over a smaller field covering a part of the body. For radiant heaters intended to warm just part of the body, the face, hands, and feet are the most effective areas to warm. These are well-perfused areas with a high concentration of arteriovenous anastomoses, which dilate rapidly when heated. The warmed blood is then carried to other parts of the body. When the distance from the heat lamp to the patient increases, the heat energy transferred to the patient decreases rapidly.

Simpler heat lamps lack the skin temperature sensor. They may also emit both infrared and visible light. An example of a simple heat lamp is shown in Figure 19–6.

Complications

Burns may occur during use of radiant heating devices if any body part is placed closer to the heat lamp than detailed by the manufacturer's instructions. Skin temperatures may also get excessively high if high temperature heating is applied to poorly perfused areas, such as the chest or back. Some radiant warmers may interfere with pulse oximeter function if the oximeter probe is placed near the heating unit.

Resistive Heaters

Resistive heaters transfer heat to the patient by conduction. A resistive heater is composed of a control unit, reusable blanket, and electric cable connection from the blanket to the control unit. Resistive heating devices generate heat by passing a low-voltage (12 to 15 V) current through a semiconductive fabric. Resistance in the fabric causes conversion of electrical energy to heat energy. Resistive heating blankets currently available are composed of carbon fiber material and come in multiple small segments instead of a single large sheet. The segments may be arranged on the patient in multiple configurations as permitted by surgical exposure and patient position. Several discontinuous parts of the body may be heated at once with different blanket segments. Because they transfer heat to the patient by conduction, direct skin contact is needed for maximal effectiveness.

Several studies have found currently available resistive heating devices to be as effective as, but not more effective than, forced air warming at maintaining normothermia. Resistive

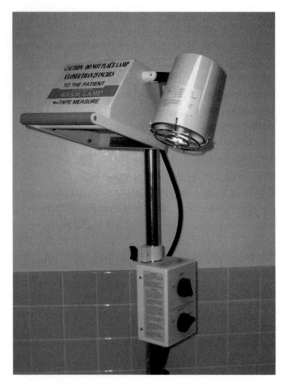

Figure 19–6 Simple heat lamp. Heat is applied as infrared radiation. Heat supplied varies as the square of the distance between the lamp and the object to be heated. This strong relationship means that the surgeon's hands can become uncomfortably hot while the device supplies inadequate heat to the patient. Conversely, placing the lamp too close to the patient by only a small amount can cause injury. Note user-generated safety signage on the device warning of this potential problem.

heating devices may offer several advantages when compared to forced air warmers. The flexibility of blanket positioning offered by current resistive heating devices may allow a greater surface area to be covered than can be achieved with a single forced air warming blanket. The blankets are reusable, so there is no continuing maintenance expenditure of purchasing new blankets. This may be somewhat offset, however, by the maintenance cost of cleaning the blankets regularly. Resistive heating devices may be particularly useful in prehospital settings where the high electrical requirements of forced air warmers limit their use.

Other Heat Loss Prevention Strategies

Prewarming

A warmer initial skin surface temperature may decrease the core-to-periphery temperature gradient and therefore decrease the temperature reduction that occurs from redistribution of heat from core to periphery during the first 30 to 60 minutes of anesthesia. Several studies have found that 15 to 30 minutes of prewarming with a forced air warming blanket immediately before induction of anesthesia results in higher intraoperative and postoperative core body temperatures.[25] It is often convenient for operating room staff to apply forced air warming blankets or circulating water garments to the patient's body after the induction of anesthesia. Active

warming devices may be applied earlier in the preoperative area and before induction of anesthesia to maximize their effectiveness at preventing hypothermia.

Intravenous Fluids

Rapid administration of intravenous fluids stored at room temperature or of cold blood products can contribute significantly to hypothermia when the amount infused is large. Blood products, colloids, and crystalloids may be warmed before intravenous administration. Heating of intravenous fluids usually does not actively warm the patient, but does help to prevent fluid-induced hypothermia in patients receiving large volumes of intravenous fluids. Many fluid warmers raise the infusate temperature to as much as 41° C. In the event of prolonged rapid infusion, such as during massive hemorrhage, active warming may occur, but this is an uncommon set of circumstances, and fluid warmers should not be considered active patient warming devices. Fluid warmers are addressed in Chapter 16.

Heat Loss from the Airway

Heat loss from the airway contributes only minimally to all heat loss and hypothermia, which occur during the perioperative period. Strategies for prevention of airway heat loss include use of low fresh gas flows, passive insulation of the airway with heat and moisture exchangers (HMEs), and active warming and humidification of inspired gases.

HMEs are disposable devices attached between the endotracheal tube and the breathing circuit (Figure 19–7). They consist of a hydrophobic or hygroscopic filter housed within a plastic case, with adaptors on either end allowing attachment to the endotracheal tube and the circuit. They may also contain an attachment port for an end-tidal expired gas sampling line. HMEs do not actively heat inspired gases, but retard heat and water vapor loss from the airway by insulation. They also provide some filtration of particles.

Water bath humidifiers actively warm inspired gases to a temperature as high as 37° C by passing them across a heating element. The warmed gases are humidified when passed through tubing containing water traps. To prevent cooling and condensation in the inspiratory limb of the breathing circuit, the warmed humidified gases must be delivered to the patient through a heated hose. Although water bath humidifiers are active warmers and thus more effective than HMEs, they are not enough to prevent hypothermia when used alone. Their use in operating rooms is limited by the cost of purchase and maintenance and by their significantly increased complexity compared with HMEs. They may increase the risk of infection and of accidental disconnection of the breathing circuit and interruption of oxygen and fresh gas delivery to the patient. There is a small theoretical risk of thermal injury to the airway in event of device malfunction.

Because the amount of heat loss prevented by HMEs and active inspired gas heater-humidifiers is minimal, the primary benefit of these devices is humidification rather than hypothermia prevention. Humidification of inspired gases helps prevent the sequelae of airway water loss. Airway temperature and water loss causes impaired ciliary function, thickened

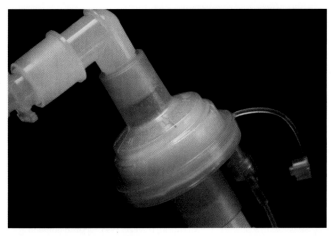

Figure 19–7 Heat and moisture exchanger (HME). HMEs do not actively heat inspired gases, but retard heat and water vapor loss from the airway by insulation.

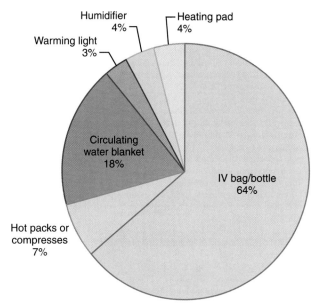

Figure 19–8 Burns from warming devices reported in an ASA closed claims analysis. The majority of burns caused by warming devices were from placement of oven-warmed intravenous fluid bags and irrigant fluid bottles in direct contact with the patient's skin. (Burns from forced air warming devices are not reported in this analysis.) *(Adapted from Cheney FW, et al. Burns from warming devices in anesthesia: a closed claims analysis. Anesthesiology 1994;80:806-810.)*

secretions, bronchoconstriction, coughing, and mucosal damage. The prevention of damage to the respiratory tract from airway drying merits the use of these devices despite their minimal impact on core body temperature.

Additional Methods

Warmed fluids may be used for body cavity lavage or for irrigation in the surgical field. Although the use of warmed fluid for irrigation will not raise core temperature, it may prevent the degree of heat loss that would occur with use of cold fluids. Warming of gases for peritoneal insufflation may help to prevent heat loss associated with laparoscopy.

Complications

Burn injuries may occur during the perioperative period from multiple electrical, chemical, or thermal sources. Patient warming devices are responsible for a portion of all thermal burns that occur during surgery and anesthesia. An ASA Closed Claims analysis found 54 burns among 3000 total claims collected from 1985 to 1993, of which 28 (52%) were caused by devices intended for patient warming.[26]

The majority of burns associated with patient warming devices reported in the Closed Claims analysis were caused by warm intravenous or irrigant fluid bags or bottles placed in direct contact with the anesthetized patient's skin (Figure 19–8). Oven-warmed fluid bags or bottles have been used to warm the awake patient's hands for comfort, or to warm the arm before intravenous catheter placement. Warm fluid containers such as bags or bottles should not be used to maintain patient position or to warm the anesthetized patient, as the patient is unable to complain about excessive heat or move him- or herself to safety.

Circulating water mattresses, a radiant heating lamp, a humidifier, hot packs or compresses, and a heating pad were responsible for the remaining injuries reported in the Closed Claims analysis. It should be noted that much of the data included in the Closed Claims analysis preceded the wide availability of forced air warming blankets.

Further Reading

Sessler, D.I., et al., 1991. Perioperative thermal insulation. Anesthesiology 74, 875–879. *A comparison of the effectiveness of various materials used to cover patients in the operating room at slowing heat loss.*

Sessler, D.I., Schroeder, M., 1993. Heat loss in humans covered with cotton hospital blankets. Anesth Analg 77, 73–77. *Discusses the effects of blanket temperature and multiple layers on the effectiveness of insulation with cotton blankets.*

Sessler, D.I., et al., 1995. Optimal duration and temperature of prewarming. Anesthesiology 82, 674–681. *Discusses how prewarming patients with forced air warming blankets before induction of anesthesia affects postoperative temperatures.*

Cheney, F.W., et al., 1994. Burns from warming devices in anesthesia: a closed claims analysis. Anesthesiology 80, 806–810. *Summarizes burn injuries analyzed in the ASA closed claims database before 1994. This article does not include burn injuries caused by forced air warmers.*

References

1. Rajagopalan, S., Mascha, E., Na Jie, et al., 2008. The effects of mild perioperative hypothermia on blood loss and transfusion requirement. Anesthesiology 108, 71–77.
2. Sessler, D.J., 1997. Mild perioperative hypothermia. N Engl J Med 336, 1730–1737.
3. Frank S.M., Fleisher L.A., Breslow M.J., et al., Perioperative maintenance of normothermia reduces the incidence of morbid cardiac events: a randomized clinical trial. JAMA
4. Schmied, H., Kurz, A., Sessler, D.I., et al., 1996. Mild intraoperative hypothermia increases blood loss and allogeneic transfusion requirements during total hip arthroplasty. Lancet 347, 289–292.
5. Kurz, A., Sessler, D.J., Lenhardt, R., 1996. Perioperative normothermia to reduce the incidence of surgical wound infection and shorten hospitalization. N Engl J Med 334, 1209.
6. Fleisher, L.A., et al., 2007. ACC/AHA 2007 guidelines on perioperative cardiovascular evaluation and care for noncardiac surgery. J Am Coll Cardiol 50, 1707–1732.
7. Hannenberg, A.A., Sessler, D.I., 2008. Improving perioperative temperature management. Anesth Analg 107 (5), 1454–1457.

8. Insler, S.R., Sessler, D.I., 2006. Perioperative thermoregulation and temperature monitoring. Anesthesiol Clin 24, 823–837.

9. Murphy, G.S., Vender, J.S., 2006. Monitoring the anesthetized patient. In: Barash, P.G., Cullen, B.F., Stoelting, R.K. (Eds.), Clinical anesthesia, ed 5. Lippincott Williams & Wilkins. Philadelphia, PA

10. Sessler, D.I., McGuire, J., Sessler, A.M., 1991. Perioperative thermal insulation. Anesthesiology 74, 875–879.

11. Brauer, A., Perl, T., Uyanik, T., et al., 2004. Perioperative thermal insulation: minimal clinically important differences? Br J Anaesth 92, 836–840.

12. Sessler, D.I., Schroeder, M., 1993. Heat loss in humans covered with cotton hospital blankets. Anesth Analg 77, 73–77.

13. Andrzejowski, J., Hoyle, J., Eapen, G., et al., 2008. Effect of prewarming on post-induction core temperature and the incidence of inadvertent perioperative hypothermia in patients undergoing general anaesthesia. Br J Anaesth 101, 627–631.

14. Dirkes W.E., Jr., Minton W.A., Sr., 1994. Convection warming in the operating room: evaluation of bacterial spread with three filtration systems. Anesthesiology 81, A562.

15. Huang, J.K.C., Shah, E.F., Vinodkumar, N., et al., 2003. The Bair Hugger patient warming system in prolonged vascular surgery: an infection risk? Crit Care 7, R13–R16.

16. Avidan, M.S., Jones, N., Ing, R., et al., 1997. Convection warmers—not just hot air. Anaesthesia 52, 1073–1076.

17. Siddik-Sayyid, S.M., Abdallah, F.W., Dahrouj, G.B., 2008. Thermal burns in three neonates associated with intraoperative use of Bair Hugger warming devices. Pediatr Anesth 18 (4), 337–339.

18. FDA encourages the reporting of medical device adverse events: free-hosing hazards. Anesth Patient Saf Found Newsl Fall 2002.

19. Arizant. Fact sheet: the dangers of "hosing," (website): http://www.arizant healthcare.com/arizanthealthcare/pdf/FactSheetHosing.pdf. Accessed on 2 August 2010

20. Burns from misuse of forced-air warming devices. FDA Patient Saf News October 2002.

21. Wadhwa, A., Komatsu, R., Orhan-Sungur, M., et al., 2007. New circulating-water devices warm more quickly than forced-air in volunteers. Anesth Analg 105, 1681–1687.

22. Taguchi, A., Ratnaraj, J., Kabon, B., et al., 2004. Effects of a circulating-water garment and forced-air warming on body heat content and core temperature. Anesthesiology 100 (5), 1058–1064.

23. Kurz, A., Kurz, M., Poeschl, G., et al., 1993. Forced-air warming maintains intraoperative normothermia better than circulating-water mattresses. Anesth Analg 77, 89–95.

24. Sessler, D.I., Moayeri, A., 1990. Skin-surface warming: heat flux and central temperature. Anesthesiology 73, 218–224.

25. Sessler, D.I., Schroeder, M., Merrifield, B., et al., 1995. Optimal duration and temperature of prewarming. Anesthesiology 82, 674–681.

26. Cheney, F.W., et al., 1994. Burns from warming devices in anesthesia: a closed claims analysis. Anesthesiology 80, 806–810.

Chapter 20

Point-of-Care Testing in the Operating Room

Marianna P. Crowley

Point of care testing (POCT), also known as near patient or bedside testing, is one of the most rapidly growing areas in the diagnostics industry. The key objective of POCT is the generation of a result quickly, so that treatment decisions can be made to improve medical or economic outcomes. The operating room presents unique opportunities to achieve both of these goals, particularly in rapidly changing medical situations, and when a rapid result may reduce the use of the expensive operating room time and resources. In addition, there are blood tests required during surgical procedures that must necessarily be performed at the point of care, such as activated clotting time. For some analytes, POCT is more accurate than core laboratory testing because of the delay in transport of the specimen or because of the transport process itself. Red blood cell metabolism can significantly change blood gases and glucose in a sample over time,[1] and even small air bubbles in a sample sent through a pneumatic tube can alter blood gas results.[2]

Utility and cost of point of care testing, compared with central laboratory testing, have been the subject of many studies over the past 20 years. In general, it has been shown that the per test cost of POCT is higher than the same test performed in a central lab, but the savings in terms of the entire hospital experience has been difficult to quantify. Point of care coagulation testing has been shown to reduce blood product use in cardiac surgery,[3] and intraoperative parathyroid hormone testing has been shown to reduce operative time,[4] but benefits of other forms of POCT are largely intuitive. For example, in a case of rapid hemorrhage, we would expect that a hemoglobin test that produces a result in 60 seconds would make management easier and safer than a result that takes 20 minutes from a central lab, and might prevent unnecessary, prophylactic transfusion.

There are several ways in which laboratory testing can be brought to or close to the point of care. A satellite laboratory may be placed in the operating suite, a testing device may be placed on a cart that is then taken into the operating room, or

hand-held or small desk top device may be brought literally to the patient's bedside. This chapter will focus on the latter two categories, those devices which are brought into the operating room and used by direct care givers, rather than by laboratory technicians.

What Can We Test?

Blood Gases, Electrolytes, and Metabolites

For the purpose of this discussion, these analytes are grouped together because most of the POCT devices measure them as part of a menu determined by the cartridge or device chosen. Most portable and hand-held instruments test whole blood samples, using electrodes or sensors and reagents, which are built into disposable cartridges or cuvettes. The number of tests available is determined by the reagents, chemicals, and enzymes on the cartridge and in the device. Cartridges may be single or multiple sample use, in some cases up to several hundred samples. Expiration dates are often several weeks after the cartridge is opened, so choosing the appropriate device and cartridge for expected testing volume is important for cost control. Figure 20–1 shows some of the many currently available POCT instruments for testing blood gases, electrolytes, metabolites, and other analytes.

Portable instruments range in size from larger desktop instruments to those to approaching the size of hand-held devices, which are somewhat larger than hand-held glucose meters. The larger devices may be brought to the patient's bedside on a cart. If a cart based system is used, it is important to make sure the device will run on batteries without interruption or require repeat calibration or quality control (QC) if unplugged from AC power.

Some POCT systems require that the operator manually place the sample in the cartridge using a syringe or capillary tube, while others aspirate the sample automatically from a syringe or tube. Manual entry may be a source of testing

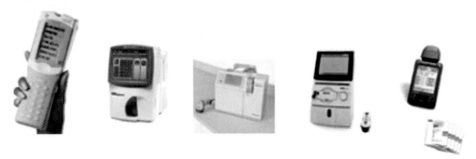

Figure 20–1   Some available devices for measuring blood gases and electrolytes.

error, from either over or under filling or introduction of air bubbles, though the devices will in many cases give an error message and require repeat testing.

Common analytic principles used in POCT instruments include potentiometry, amperometry, and optical methods.[5] In addition, conductometry is used to measure hematocrit, and will be discussed later.

Potentiometry is the measurement or electrical potential difference between two electrodes in an electrochemical cell. The potential difference is logarithmically proportional to the electrolyte concentration. One electrode is a reference, the other is specific for the ion being measured, an ion specific electrode (ISE). The ISE has a membrane that attracts the ion, creating a potential difference which can then be measured through the circuit of the reference and ISE. Potentiometry is used to measure pH, PCO_2, Na, Ca, Cl, K, and Mg.

Amperometry is measurement of the electric current flowing through an electrochemical sensor circuit when a constant potential is applied to the electrodes. The electrochemical sensor consists of an anode and a cathode, surrounded by a selectively permeable membrane, which prevents entry of proteins and other oxidants. When a sample is applied, the substrates and analyte diffuse through the membrane, an oxidation-reduction reaction occurs, electrons form a current under the electric potential applied. The amplitude of the current is proportional to the substrate level in the cell, and is measured by the device. Amperometry is used to measure PO_2, BUN, glucose, lactate, creatinine, and ketones.

Optical technologies used in POCT devices include optical reflectance, absorbance, fluorescence, and multilength spectrophotometry, which is used for co-oximetry testing. Optical reflectance and absorbance measure the change in color between incident light and absorbed or reflected light. As an analyte is oxidized by an oxidation-reduction reaction, electrons are generated, which oxidize a dye to create a color, the intensity of which is proportional to the concentration of the analyte. The device measures the reflectance or absorbance of a known incident wavelength of light. Optical reflectance has been used to measure glucose, PO_2, PCO_2, and pH. Optical fluorescence and luminescence technologies measure the photons emitted from molecules when exposed to light of a particular wavelength. For example, Na and K can be measured with fiber-optic optodes encased in a membrane that contains selective recognition elements, ionophores, linked to fluorescent dye. As the ions pass through the membrane, they bind the ionophores, and once exposed to light, fluoresce with an intensity that is proportional to the concentration of the ions.

The i-STAT (Abbott) device deserves particular mention because it uses microfabricated chip-based technology in its cartridges. i-STAT cartridges are approximately 1-inch square, 0.25-inch thick plastic. Channels are etched in the surface to draw the sample from a well to the sensors and electrodes. There are a number of cartridge types that allow a menu of testing, including blood gases, electrolytes, metabolites, cardiac markers, and hematologic parameters, using a variety of the technologies described above.

Most POCT devices measure some of the reported parameters and calculate others. For example, the instrument may measure PCO_2, pH, and electrolytes, and then calculate and display bicarbonate, total CO_2 base excess and anion gap.

Portable and handheld POCT instruments use a variety of methods for calibration and QC. Calibration for single use cartridges is usually automatically performed by the device just before use, while calibration on multiuse cartridges is performed periodically at intervals between sample measurements using reagent packages with the cartridge. Unlike larger laboratory instruments that use gas tanks to calibrate blood gas measurements, cartridges for POCT devices are packaged with pretonometered calibration solutions, or perform gas calibration using room air.

Liquid QC is performed on representatives from each cartridge lot as it is first used; typically known samples in a range over which testing will be performed are tested. In addition, many POCT systems are tested periodically using electronic QC, using a surrogate cartridge to assess the response of the sensors and to detect internal system failures.

Table 20–1 shows characteristics and specifications of a number of currently available and widely used POCT devices with capability of testing blood gases, electrolytes, and metabolites.

Blood Glucose

A large segment of the worldwide POCT market involves blood glucose testing, including the home, self-test devices, and the in-hospital devices. As ever increasing numbers of the patients who present for surgery are diabetic, and with relatively recent interest in intensive insulin therapy for some patient populations, the need for blood glucose monitoring is increasing. Many hospitals now have widespread POCT programs for blood glucose. Testing can be done with hand-held devices that use disposable strip technology, which will be discussed here, or on multianalyte machines that use cartridges, such as the i-STAT and Gem (Instrumentation Laboratories) systems, which will be discussed later.

Table 20–1 Specifications of Some Devices Available for Testing Blood Gases and Electrolytes

Device	Abbott i-STAT	IL Gem Premier 4000	Siemens Rapidpoint 405	Radiometer ABL80 Flex	Epocal Epoc
Test menu*	Po_2, Pco_2, pH, Na, K, Cl, iCa, Cl Glu, lactate, BUN, Hct, Crea, ACT, PT/INR, cardiac markers	Po_2, Pco_2, pH, Na, K, Ca, Cl Glu, lactate, Hct, tHb, O_2Hb, COHb, MetHb, HHb (co-ox)	Po_2, Pco_2, pH, Na, K, iCa, Cr, Glucose, Hct, Hb (co-ox))	Po_2, Pco_2, pH, Na, K, iCa, Cl, Glu, Hct, tHb, O_2Hb, COHb, MetHb, HHb (co-ox)	Po_2, Pco_2, pH, Na, K, iCa, Hct
Sample size	17-95 µL	150 µL	100-200 µL	105 µL	100 µL
Report time	130-200 sec except for ACT, PT	95 sec	60 sec	140 sec	35 sec
Cartridge size	Single use	75-450 tests	250-750 tests	25-300 tests	Single use
Cartridge life	Two weeks once at room temp	30 days in use	28 days in use	15-30 days in use	
Dimensions/size	3 × 9.2 × 2.8 in 22.9 oz	44 lb	11.5 × 16 × 21.5 inches, 34 lb	9 × 11 × 16 in, 19 lb	8.5 × 3.3 × 2 inches, 1.1 lb
Device memory	5000 patient results, L QC and E QC	80 gigabyte hard drive, 1-yr retention of data	Information unavailable	500 patient test 500 system cycle 500 manual QC unlimited user ID	No memory in meter
Operation temperature	15-40°C	12-32° C	15-32°C	12-28°C	15-30°C
Operation humidity	Up to 90%	5%-85%	5- 85%	Up to 85%	Up to 85%
Operationaltitude	300 – 1000 mmHg	Not applicable	523-800 mm Hg	Up to 7513 ft.	400-835 mm Hg
QC	Automatic QC and Calibration unless glucose test strips use, then liquid QC		Automatic QC and calibration	Automatic QC and calibration	Automatic
Comments	Cartridges must be refrigerated, brought to room temp prior to use May use Abbott Glucose test strips				Data transferred to mobile computer, uses test cards, more analyte cards under development

*Test menu varies depending on cartridge chosen for some devices. For example, iSTAT offers 18 different cartridges with various combinations of parameters.

Glucose itself is very difficult to measure, so it is usually done by indirect methods, whereby glucose is converted enzymatically to a substance that is easily measured. Current blood glucose monitoring systems use one of two methods, reflectance photometry, which measures a colored product or dye, or electrochemistry, which measures electrical current.[6] Hand-held glucose measurement systems consist of a meter and a disposable strip, or in the case of the HemoCue device a cuvette, which is inserted in the meter. A tiny sample of whole blood, between 0.5 and 5 µL, is then applied to the strip, which is impregnated with dry enzymes and coenzymes that allow the analysis to occur. Examples of meters and strips are shown in Figure 20–2.

Glucose meters are approximately 3 × 7 × 2 inches, have a display window, a slot on the top or side for a test strip, a key board for data and selection entry, a battery compartment, a laser window for bar code scanning, and an infrared window for data transfer. They often come with a docking station or base unit for charging, data transfer, or both. Meters have built in memory to store results, quality control, and operator

data. Like other POCT devices, most now have software programs that allow centralized management of competency, operator access, transfer of results to laboratory information systems, and billing programs. Meters allow scanning and in some cases manual entry of patient identification, operator ID, and strip or cuvette bar codes.

Dry reagent glucose strips or cuvettes come in either individual sealed packets or multicontainer jars. The HemoCue cuvettes must be refrigerated until used. Other strips are kept at room temperature. They all have expiration dates, usually contained along with a lot number and calibration information in the bar code information on the package. Quality control levels are run on the meters at an interval that is determined by the testing site, recommended by the manufacturer, using commercially available samples at two to four glucose levels.

Three enzyme systems are currently used in measuring blood glucose: glucose oxidase, glucose dehydrogenase, and hexokinase.[7] Each then uses a coenzyme to create an end product which either generates electrons and a current, or a colored product, either of which is proportional to the amount

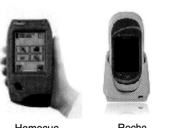
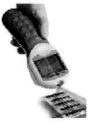
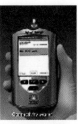
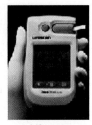

| Hemocue | Roche | Abbott | Nova Biomedical | Lifescan |
| Glucose 201 DM | Accuchek Inform II | Precision PCx | StatStrip | SureStep Flexx |

Figure 20–2   Some of the available glucose meters.

Table 20–2 Factors That Affect Point of Care Blood Glucose Testing

Blood sampling site, arterial/capillary vs. venous
Hematocrit
Peripheral hypoperfusion
Sample processing delay
Substances reported to interfere
  Mannitol
  Maltose
  Xylose
  Galactose
  Acetic Acid
  Acetaminophen
  Severely elevated bilirubin
  Severe lipemia
  Elevated uric acid
  Extremes of Pao_2, particularly glucose oxidase methods

of glucose in the specimen. The HemoCue (HemoCue Diagnostics AB) cuvette adds a step: red blood cells are lysed by saponin so that a true whole blood glucose level is measured. The enzyme system used and the method of measuring the end product are of interest to anesthesiologists because of the potential for interference from other substances in the sample. For example, reactions that use glucose dehydrogenase and pyrroloquinoline quinone (GDH-PQQ) are not glucose specific, and cannot distinguish between glucose, maltose, galactose, or xylose. Maltose is in intravenous immunoglobulin solutions and in peritoneal dialysis solutions, such that blood glucose measurement for those patients with a device that uses the GDH-PQQ method may give falsely high readings. The enzyme system used is described in the package insert that comes with the test strips, and should be a factor considered when choosing a device.

Accuracy Of Point Of Care Blood Glucose Measurements

Accuracy of point of care testing of blood glucose is determined by comparison with samples run in the core laboratory. To obtain approval for a medical device from the Food and Drug Administration), the manufacturer must provide data showing correlation with acceptable standard methods of measurement, but this testing is done under ideal conditions. A number of factors have been shown to affect the accuracy of POCT for glucose, shown in Table 20–2, and many of them can apply to patients undergoing surgery and anesthesia.[8] Importantly, glucose metabolism occurs in red blood cells during transport of a sample from the point of care to the

laboratory, which builds in a variable difference between even very accurate point of care testing, depending on temperature, time of transport, and absolute level of glucose. Manufacturers specify that blood should be tested as soon as possible after collection, and always within 30 minutes.

POCT devices measure glucose on whole blood, whereas laboratories routinely measure glucose in plasma or serum. Plasma values can be as much as 12% higher than whole blood values because of lower water content of red blood cells. Thus most meters mathematically correct the result to simulate plasma, generally calibrated using normal hematocrits. Many meters have been shown to exhibit positive bias (read too high) at lower hematocrits, and negative bias at higher hematocrits.[9] To address this issue, the Multi-Well StatStrip (Nova Biomedical) measures both hematocrit and glucose and corrects for hematocrit interference, though the device only reports glucose.

Though arterial and venous blood can be used with glucose strips, often capillary or fingerstick testing is done because it is convenient and uses less blood. However, hypoperfusion states, such as hypotension, use of vasopressors, and vasoconstriction because of cold have all been shown to introduce error.[10] Because venous blood glucose in the nonfasting state is approximately 8% lower than arterial or capillary blood glucose, meters compensate mathematically for this and require the user to select the type of sample being used. Running a venous sample in the capillary/arterial mode can thus result in falsely high results.

Anesthesiologists should keep in mind that with the exception of the HemoCue device, POCT glucose meters are approved by the FDA as screening devices; they are not approved for the diagnosis of diabetes or determination of treatment. Despite this fact, in most hospitals (and certainly in the hands of diabetic patients at home) POCT glucose meters are used as part of sliding scale insulin administration.

Manufacturers of glucose testing systems continue to work on improvements, particularly in areas of increased accuracy, and most recently, continuous glucose monitoring. Devices which continually measure blood glucose via subcutaneous and intravascular catheters are under development. Table 20–3 shows the specifications for five currently available hand-held glucose monitoring devices.

Hematologic Parameters
Hemoglobin and Hematocrit

Probably the most widely tested parameters at the point of care are the hemoglobin (Hgb) concentration and hematocrit (Hct). They can be measured with hand-held, desk top, and

Table 20–3 Specifications of Five Glucose Monitoring Systems Available in the U.S. for Hospital Point of Care Testing

Device	Abbott Precision Xceed Pro/Precision Pcx Plus Test Strips	Nova Biomedical StatStrip	Lifescan SureStep-Flexx/Sure Step Test Strips	Roche Accu-chek Inform/Comfort Curve Test Strip	HemoCue Glucose 201/ Microcuvettes
Chemistry	GDH-NAD, amperometric	4 well modified glucose oxidase, amperometric	Glucose oxidase amperometric	Glucose dehydrogenase with potassium ferricyanide/PQQ	Saponin hemolysis, GDH/NAD photometric
Reportable range	20-500mg/dL	10-600 mg/dL	0-500 mg/dL	10-600 mg/dL	0-444 mg/dL
HCT range	20%-70%		25%-60%	20-65% for results <200, 20-55% for >200	"Care should be taken when... hematocrit may be extreme"
Sample size	1.2 μL	1.2 μL	10 μL	1.2 μL	5 μL
Operation Temperature	15-40° C	15-40° C	15-40° C	14-40° C	18-30° C
Operation altitude	Up to 7200 ft	Up to 15,000 ft	Up to 10,000 ft	Up to 10,000 ft	Not applicable
Operation humidity	10%-90%	10%-90%	30%-70%	<85%	<90%
Meter memory	2500 results 1000 control test results 6000 user ID	1000 tests 500 QC 4000 user ID	1500 tests 4000 user ID	4000 tests	4000 tests 500 analyzer logs
Report time	20 sec	6 sec	30 sec	26 sec	40-240 sec
Comments		Two well system corrects for HCT		Interference by maltose, galactose	Approved for diagnosis, screening, monitoring, cuvettes must be refrigerated

GDH, Glucose dehydrogenase; NAD, nicotinamide adenine dinucleotide; PQQ, pyrroloquinoline quinone.
Information obtained from meter manuals and strip package inserts.

portable devices using a variety of technologies. Hematocrit is measured using centrifugation and conductometry, and hemoglobin is measured with co-oximetry and other optical methods. Most devices measure one parameter and calculate the other using an algorithm. Table 20–4 shows the specifications for four commonly used devices.

Centrifugation is often considered the gold standard for testing hematocrit. Whole blood is spun at high speed for several minutes to separate red cells from plasma and the buffy coat layer, which contains white blood cells and platelets. The QBC Star (QBC Diagnostics) is a centrifugal hematology analyzer, which contains a single tube centrifuge for mixing and separating blood into various cell populations. The Star glass tube contains dried coatings of acridine orange, heparin, K2EDTA, potassium oxalate, monoclonal antibody, and reagents and when capped contains a float that expands the buffy coat layer and penetrates the red blood cell (RBC) layer. Hematocrit is measured by the width of the RBC band, platelets, and white blood cells (WBCs) by the width of their respective bands using an optical method. Hemoglobin is measured by the depth of penetration of the float into the red blood cell layer, as a measure of density.

Many POCT devices use conductivity of blood to measure Hct, based on the fact that electrical conduction in blood is reduced in plasma as the concentration of red blood cells

increases. Though this methodology is considered accurate in most clinical situations and for physiologically normal patients, accuracy is affected by changes in electrolytes, very high white blood cell counts, use of volume expanders, and most importantly by plasma protein concentration.[11] This effect is of concern in critically ill patients, and especially during and after cardiopulmonary bypass, when some of these conditions routinely occur. Using the conductivity method, low serum protein will falsely lower the reported hematocrit, which may lead to unnecessary transfusion. Some devices give the option of using a "cardiopulmonary bypass mode," which adjusts results based on a constant positive adjustment of hematocrit. Thus it is incapable of adjusting to a variety of protein concentrations. The conductivity method is used by a number of the multianalyte POCT devices, including the i-STAT, the Gem Premier 3000, and the RAPIDpoint 350 (Siemens).

Optical methods, photometry, and spectrophotometry are used to measure Hgb in POCT devices. The HemoCue Hemoglobin Analyzer (HemoCue Diagnostics AB), a widely used POCT device, uses dry reagents in a cuvette. Blood is drawn into the cuvette by capillary action, red cells are disintegrated by sodium deoxycholate, releasing hemoglobin. Sodium nitrite converts Hgb iron from ferrous to ferric to form methemoglobin, which combines with azide to form azidemethoglobin. This photometric chromogen is quantitated

Table 20–4 Specifications of Some Devices Available for Testing Hemoglobin and/or Hematocrit

Device	HemoCue HemoCue 201 DM	QBC Diagnostics QBC Star	Siemens RAPIDpoint 350	IL Gem 4000
Type/size	Hand-held, 0.77 lb	Desk top, 16 × 16 in	Portable, Multianalyte 17 lb	Desk top, Multianalyte 44 lb
Methodology	Modified azidemethe-moglobin/ photometry	Centrifugation/ optical	Conductivity	Co-oximetry
Reportable range	0-25.6 g/dL	5-20 g/dL	10%-70%	5-23 g/dL
Sample size	10 µL	65-75 µL	95-120 µL	150 µL
Operation temperature	18-30° C	16-32° C	15-30° C	12-32° C
Operation altitude	Not applicable	Up to 2000 meters	500-800 mm Hg	Not applicable
Operation humidity	Up to 90%	10%-95%	5%-85%	15%-85%
Meter memory	4000 test results 500 QC results 500 log entries	No memory	64 results	80 gigabyte hard drive storage, 1-yr limit
Report time	15-60 sec	7 minutes	120 sec	95 sec
Comments	Single use cuvette	Measures Hct, Hgb, CBC Single use capillary tube No data management No operator lockout	Rapidpoint 450 Has co-oximetry	Cartridges test 75, 150, 300, or 450 samples, expire 30 days

by absorbance of light at 570 nm and at 880 nm to compensate for turbidity. This method is unaffected by changes in proteins or lipid levels, but air bubbles in the cuvette must be avoided.

Another optical method, used in some multianalyte POCT devices as an integral or optional module and in many laboratory blood gas analyzers, is co-oximetry. Co-oximetry is a spectrophotometric methodology, which measures total hemoglobin, oxyhemoglobin, deoxyhemoglobin, carboxyhemoglobin, and methemoglobin. Co-oximeters hemolyze blood with high frequency vibrations; light passes through the resultant solution. Hemoglobin specific wavelengths are directed onto photodiodes to produce electrical current, which is proportional to the intensity, and therefore to the concentration of various types of hemoglobin. Though high lipids and cell fragments can scatter light and create errors, co-oximetry has been shown to be significantly more accurate than conductivity methods, especially during cardiopulmonary bypass.[12-14]

Coagulation Tests
Prothrombin Time (PT)

The PT is a measure of the extrinsic and common coagulation pathways. Thromboplastin (tissue factor and phospholipids) is added to blood, and the clotting time is measured in seconds. Because of the variability of thromboplastins and monitoring devices, the International Normalized Ratio (INR) was developed. Each reagent is assigned an International Sensitivity Index (ISI), determined by the manufacturer, which is used to calculate the INR.[15] It has been recommended that core laboratory and POCT instruments use reagents with similar ISIs, and correlations with existing lab systems is critical.

Activated Partial Thromboplastin Time (APTT)

The APTT is a measure of the integrity of the intrinsic and common coagulation pathways. It measures the clotting time in seconds when an activator initiates clotting in the presence of a "partial thromboplastin" (phospholipids without tissue factor) and calcium. Different laboratory and POC tests have different normal ranges, and in the case of APTT, there is no INR equivalent. However, because heparin prolongs the APTT, correlations can be done with heparin levels, usually antifactor Xa assays, with normal ranges set to reflect a given heparin level.

A number of POCT devices can be used to measure the PT/INR and the APTT. Most use a single drop of fresh whole venous, arterial, or capillary blood, using a single use cartridge or strip. Methods for clot detection include cessation of capillary or pump-induced movement, alteration in fluorescence, or change in oscillation of magnetic particles.

Activated Clotting Time

Activated clotting time (ACT) is a whole blood coagulation test initiated by contact activation with celite or kaolin. Blood is mixed with the activator, and a timer is started and stopped when a clot forms. Methods of clot detection include pump driven movement of blood through a capillary tube, resistance to movement of a plunger in the sample, displacement of a magnet, or change in oscillation of iron particles. For example, the ACTPlus (Medtronic) instrument detects a clot by moving a plunger through the blood; as a clot forms, it resists the plunger. The Gem PCL (Instrumentation Laboratories) device draws blood back and forth across a light detection window; when a clot forms, blood no longer flows. The i-STAT device measures a thrombin substrate; as blood clots,

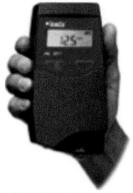 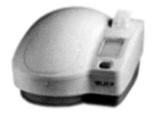

HemoCue Hemoglobin   QBC Diagnostics' STAR
                            hematology analyzer

Figure 20–3   Two devices available for testing hemoglobin.

thrombin cleaves the substrate, releasing a compound that is detected amperometrically.

ACT methods use different activators to detect effects of low dose versus high dose heparin, such that there are both low and high dose cartridges in cartridge based systems. Not all ACTs are equivalent because there is significant interpatient variability in heparin response[16]; in fact this is the reason that ACTs are used during therapy. Celite based results tend to be significantly longer than kaolin based results, even in the same patient, especially when aprotinin is used.[17]

Method validation for ACT testing is challenging because there is no gold standard for comparison. Varying doses of heparin may be added to whole blood to perform linearity tests, and any new technology can be run in parallel with existing technology. For low dose heparin, comparison with APTT may be adequate.[18]

Table 20–5 shows specifications for a number of devices that can be used to measure PT, APTT, and ACT and other coagulation parameters at the point of care.

Platelet Tests

There are several POCT devices that can be used to measure platelet count. One is the QBC Star, which has already been discussed. Another POC hemacytometer is the ICHOR (Helena Laboratories) device, which is an impedance counter. A blood sample passes through an aperture, interrupting a constant electrical current, resulting in an electrical impulse that is amplified and sorted to provide a platelet count.

For a number of reasons there has been intense research on development of platelet function assays for the point of care. In the operating room, platelet dysfunction due to cardiopulmonary bypass, a variety of pathological conditions, and the therapeutic use of glycoprotein IIb/IIIa inhibitors has generated interest in such devices to help guide transfusion therapy. Core laboratory testing of platelet aggregometry is a labor intensive, slow process, that is not useful for many surgical situations.

A number of devices have been developed to measure platelet function. The ICHOR device is usually marketed with the Plateletworks assay system designed to determine the percent of platelet aggregation in fresh whole blood samples. Plateletworks consists of tubes containing aggregation activators, ADP, collagen, or arachidonic acid. A platelet count is determined as described above on native blood, and at the same time on a sample containing an activator. Once platelets

aggregate, they exceed the threshold for size and are no longer counted. The difference between the control and activated tubes represents platelet aggregation.

Another device, the Platelet Function Analyzer, PFA-100 (Siemens), is designed to simulate hemostasis after injury to a vessel. The test cartridge consists of a blood reservoir, a capillary tube, and a collagen coated membrane with an aperture, also coated with ADP or epinephrine. Blood moves through the membrane under a vacuum, and the time to closure of the aperture is measured.

Tests Of Viscoelastic Clot Formation

Several POCT devices are now available to assess multiple aspects of hemostasis. The thromboelastograph, or TEG (Haemoscope) is the best known and most widely used device, particularly for assessing clotting abnormalities during cardiac surgery and liver transplantation. FDA approval is currently pending for the ROTEM (Pentapharm) thromboelastometer, which operates on similar principles.

Both devices produce a graphic representation of clot formation and subsequent lysis. Blood is pipetted into a heated cup, with a pin suspended in the cup. With TEG, the pin is attached to a torsion wire. The cup oscillates back and forth through an arc. As the blood coagulates, fibrin strands form between the walls of the cup and the piston, causing the piston to oscillate in phase with the clot. The motion of the pin is converted by a mechanical-electrical transducer to an electrical signal, which can be monitored by a computer. The resulting hemostasis profile measures the time it takes for the first fibrin strand to form, the kinetics of clot formation, the strength of the clot, and the dissolution of the clot.

The TEG analyzer is a bench top device that must be placed on a level, stable surface. Its dimensions are $25 \times 26 \times 29$ cm, and it weighs 6 kg. QC with lyophilized bovine plasma is performed every 24 hours. The device allows operator lockout, and manual or barcode scanned patient ID. Information from the TEG analyzer is transmitted to a computer via a TEG enabled central computer or remotely. The measured parameters, but not the tracings, can be transmitted to hospital laboratory information systems. Figure 20–4 shows a normal TEG tracing with measurements.

Four parameters are typically measured from a TEG tracing and reported along with the tracing by the TEG software. The R, or reaction time, is the time from placement of blood in the cup until the onset of clot formation, defined as a 1 mm deflection of the trace. It seems to correlate with the APTT, and appears to reflect the intrinsic clotting cascade.[19] The K, or clot formation time, is the time from the initial clot formation to a 20 mm deflection of the tracing, a fixed level of clot firmness. The angle is the maximum slope from initial clot formation to the shoulder of the tracing, a measure of clot strengthening. The MA, or maximal amplitude, is the width of the tracing at the maximal strength of the clot, and is probably the most widely used TEG parameter. The MA correlates with platelet count and function and fibrinogen concentration.[20] The shape of the trace after achievement of the MA represents fibrinolysis.

When using native whole blood, it often takes 30 minutes to reach the maximal amplitude, and if waiting to assess hemolysis, can take 60 minutes to complete. There are modifications of the standard TEG procedure, including the addition

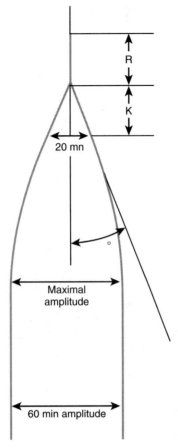

Figure 20–4   TEG trace.

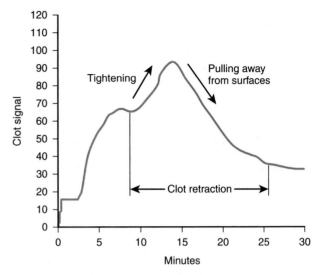

Figure 20–5   Sonoclot Signature.

of kaolin activator to accelerate the test, use of heparinase coated cups and pistons to evaluate for residual heparin after protamine reversal, and use of the Rapid TEG, with the addition of tissue factor to markedly accelerate the test and obtain results in 60 seconds, useful in cases of massive blood loss from trauma. A modification of TEG called platelet mapping is used to monitor aspirin and Plavix effect, but is used only in core laboratories because of the complex sequence of pipetting required.

Perhaps more so than with some other POC tests, training in interpretation of TEG tracings and results is extremely important. Clinical decisions are often made on the pattern of the tracing as it develops. In some centers, the analyzer is placed in or near the OR suite; in others, the analyzer is in the core laboratory. Because of the complexity of analysis of the tracing, some centers transmit the tracing to a central site for interpretation. If fresh whole blood is tested at the bedside, it must be placed in the cup within 3 minutes after blood draw. Citrated blood for transport to a core lab should be placed in the cup after 30 minutes. Some differences in tracings have been reported when citrated blood is used.[21]

The ROTEM device also tests clot formation and stability, again using a cup and pin, but the pin rotates rather than the cup. As the clot forms, the pin's oscillation is reduced, and is measured by a change in the angle of deflection of a beam of light directed at the pin. Citrated blood is always used in the ROTEM, and it can be used immediately. The nomenclature for various measurements of the tracing is different from TEG, though the tracing is very similar. Again,

ROTEM is currently available only for research purposes in the United States.

The Sonoclot Analyzer also measures multiple aspects of the hemostatic system with changes in the viscoelastic properties of blood clots. A plastic probe is suspended and oscillates in whole blood in a heated plastic cuvette containing celite. The probe is attached to a transducer; as a clot forms the impedance to oscillation changes and is translated into a tracing, called the Sonoclot Signature. Figure 20–5 shows an example of a normal Sonoclot Signature.

Parameters derived from the tracing include the lag period before a clot forms, which corresponds to the ACT, the slope of the first wave, which reflects fibrin formation, a plateau which represents platelet incorporation, another upslope, representing completion of fibrin formation, and subsequent downslope, which represents clot retraction. The time to the peak of the tracing is an indicator of platelet count and function. The full Sonoclot® tracing takes approximately 30 minutes to develop, unless hyperfibrinolysis or coagulopathy is present.

Heparin Assays

For many years, the ACT has been used to determine heparin dosing and protamine reversal for cardiopulmonary bypass. However, patients' dose response and clearance of heparin are variable, and ACT does not correlate well with heparin concentrations during bypass.[22] As a result, heparin management devices have been developed that determine a heparin dose response for the individual patient, monitor heparin concentration, and determine a protamine reversal dose.

The HMS Plus (Medtronic) performs a number of tests, including whole blood heparin concentration using an automated protamine titration method, which allows calculation of a patient specific heparin dose response curve, and calculation of a protamine reversal dose. It also measures high range kaolin ACT. The heparin dose response cartridge contains six channels, each with kaolin and various concentrations of heparin. A fresh whole blood sample, before heparinization, is added; clotting times are measured; and a dose response slope is calculated. The heparin assay cartridge has channels

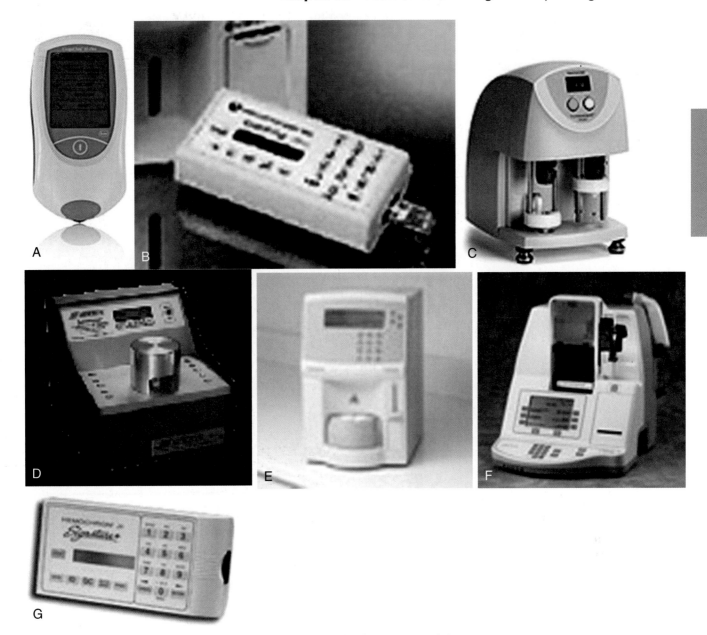

Figure 20–6   Some devices available for testing coagulation parameters.

containing identical amounts of dilute thromboplastin and varying amounts of protamine. Blood is added to the cartridge and clotting times are measured. Using the fact that 1.3 mg of protamine neutralizes 100 units of heparin, the amount of protamine in the sample that clots first is used to calculate the heparin level in the sample. If patient characteristics are entered into the device, heparin bolus dose and protamine reversal dose are derived.

The Hemochron RxDx is a drug and monitoring system that can be used with the Hemochron Response (International Technidyne Corp.) coagulation monitoring device. The Response offers a menu of tests, including celite or kaolin ACT, APTT, PT/INR, and protamine dose assay. The RxDx uses the ACT and protamine dose assay to calculate heparin dose response curves and protamine reversal doses. Heparin neutralization after reversal can also be assessed with the protamine dose assay.

Numerous studies have looked at the effect of the use of various tests of hemostasis and protocols on reduction of transfusion of blood products during and after cardiac surgery.[3,23,24] Studies show that hemostasis testing, whether at the point of care or using the core laboratory, does not reduce blood loss during cardiac surgery, but does tend to reduce transfusion of blood products, if testing is used with a transfusion algorithm.

Figure 20–6 shows some of the instruments available for testing various coagulation parameters, and Table 20–5 shows specification for a number of devices.

Pregnancy Testing

Preoperative screening for pregnancy is a controversial topic. This discussion is included because some anesthesia departments now routinely test female patients before administration of anesthesia.

Table 20–5 Specifications of Some of the Devices Available for Testing Coagulation Parameters

Device	Tests	Sample	Method
QBC STAR	Hgb, Hct, CBC	Whole Blood	Centrifugation, optical
Helena ICHOR/Plateletworks	Platelet count, aggregation, inhibition	Whole blood	Impedence counter Platelet activator
Roche Diagnostics CoaguChek XS Plus	PT/INR	Capillary or fresh venous	Capillary blood movement, optical
Medtronic ACT Plus	High range ACT Low range ACT Heparinase ACT Recalcified ACT	Native or citrated blood	Optical detection of change in plunger motion
Instrumentation Laboratories Gem PCL Plus	PT, PTT, ACT	Fresh whole blood, citrated option for PT PTT	Optical detection, blood drawn across window
Abbott i-STAT	ACT	Whole blood	Amperometric detection of product of thrombin substrate
Hemoscope TEG	Thromboelastogram	Whole blood	Mechanical detection of change in cup oscillation
Sienco Sonoclot	Sonoclot Signature trace	Whole blood	Impedence detection of probe oscillation after celite activation
Siemens PFA-100	ADP clot time, Epinephrine clot time	Whole blood	Detection of pressure across aperture with clot
Medtronic HMS Plus	High range ACT Low range ACT Heparin response Heparin assay Protamine reversal	Whole blood	Optical detection of plunger motion
ITC Hemochron Response/RxDx	Kaolin ACT, APTT, PT/INR, protamine dose assay	Whole blood	Optical detection of change in rotating magnet position

Pregnancy tests measure either serum or urine levels of human chorionic gonadotropin (hCG), a glycoprotein hormone produced by the placenta shortly after fertilization. In normal pregnancy, hCG can be detected as early as 7 to 10 days after conception at levels of 5 to 50 mIU/mL.[25]

A number of POCT devices are marketed for use in hospitals and physician offices. Most companies offer a version that is used for testing urine, and an alternative that can be used to test either urine or serum. Because urine concentration is so variable, urine testing should be done on first morning or concentrated urine samples to maximize concentration of the hormone in the sample.

One popular device is the Icon 20 (Beckman Coulter), a small plastic single use disposable device, which may be used to test urine or serum at a level of 20 mIU/mL. It performs a chromatographic immunoassay using mouse anti-CG antibody. A fixed volume sample, approximately 110 µL, is added to the sample well, and migrates by capillary action along a membrane to react with colored conjugate at a test line. A control line shows that the test was performed correctly, and the test line changes color in the presence of hCG. The urine test is read at 3 minutes, the serum at 5 minutes.

Other devices that use a similar method are the Clearview hCG Combo (Inverness Medical Innovations), which allows both urine and serum testing, and the RediScreen Cassette, both of which test hCG at 25 mIU/mL. Permaxim makes the RediScreen Strip as well, which is dipped into urine to a specified depth, and is read the same way as the cassette device.

None of the POC pregnancy tests allow operator lockout or data transfer to information systems. Urine tests are typically CLIA waived (see Regulatory Issues section), while serum tests are not. There are no POC pregnancy tests for whole blood, so use of a blood test would require serum sample preparation with centrifugation.

Regulatory Issues

Laboratory testing, including POCT, is subject to federal, state, and local regulations. It is important for anesthesiologists who perform POC tests to have a basic knowledge of these requirements, so they understand why they are asked to comply with procedures for training, maintenance of competency, performance of QC, and documentation. In addition, anesthesia providers who consider new POCT programs must create an infrastructure to support compliance with regulations. Compliance with regulations is complex enough that many hospitals have a laboratory division devoted to POCT oversight and compliance.

All laboratory testing in the United States is regulated by the Clinical Laboratory Improvements Act of 1988 (CLIA), which was implemented in 1992 and is overseen by the Centers for Medicare and Medicaid Services (CMS).[26] The basic philosophy defined by CLIA is that all laboratory tests must meet a minimum standard of quality, and are subject to the same regulations, no matter where they are performed. Point of care tests and sites are subject to these regulations.

While CLIA sets minimum requirements and CMS inspects sites, POCT sites may, and many do, choose voluntary accreditation through professional organizations deemed to have equivalent requirements. Such organizations include the Joint Commission, the Laboratory Accreditation Program of the college of American Pathologists (LAP-CAP), or the Commission on Office Laboratory Accreditation (COLA).[27-29]

POC testing must be performed under the appropriate CLIA certificate, granted by CMS through an application process biannually. The holder of the certificate for a POCT site may be the central laboratory, covering all institutional testing, or the individual POCT site. CLIA certificates are based on the complexity of testing, and the associated fee is determined by the test volume, specialty of testing, and complexity.

FDA classifies test methods into waived, moderate, and high complexity tests. CMS has combined the latter two into the nonwaived category. POCT sites may obtain a CLIA Certificate of Waiver if only waived tests are performed. If any nonwaived tests are performed, a CLIA Certificate must be obtained and pertinent regulations followed.

Waived test methods are those which are simple, with low probability of error, and include many POC tests, such as glucose testing, urine pregnancy testing, and some hemoglobin and hematocrit tests. Waived tests must be performed on native samples without the requirement for modification or preparation; thus urine pregnancy tests are waived, while blood pregnancy tests, which must be performed on serum, are not. Some of the individual tests performed by multianalyte devices are waived, while others are nonwaived. Since CLIA was implemented in 1992, the number of waived tests has increased dramatically, as manufacturers have simplified and improved technology. A CLIA waiver is considered a selling point for POCT methodology because of less stringent regulatory oversight conferred by waived status.

POCT sites that perform only waived tests are free from federal oversight, except that they are required to obtain a CLIA Certificate of Waiver, and they must follow manufacturers' directions for use of an instrument. There are no requirements for personnel qualifications and training, QC (unless specified as required in the test system instructions), proficiency testing (PT), or routine quality assessment. CMS will not routinely inspect sites performing only waived tests, although it conducts educational, scheduled review visits of 2% of waived testing sites annually. If a hospital is accredited by the Joint Commission, it will inspect even waived testing sites every 2 years. The Joint Commission requirements for waived testing sites include having policy and procedures available, identification of staff responsible for performing and supervising testing, demonstration and documentation of competency, performance of QC, and documentation of results in the patient's clinical record along with reference ranges as appropriate.

POCT sites holding their own CLIA certificates for nonwaived testing must identify individuals with proper qualifications as director, technical consultant, clinical consultant, and testing personnel. Requirements for these positions appear in the CLIA regulations. In some situations in the operating room, an anesthesia clinician may fill several of these roles.

Sites holding CLIA certificates must also develop "standard operating procedures" (SOP), and make them available to all testing personnel for each test performed. The basis for the SOP may be the device manufacturer's product insert or operator's manual, but it must include site specific information.

The site holding a CLIA certificate must implement control procedures to detect errors, and monitor accuracy and precision. For most nonwaived tests, the minimum requirement is two levels of liquid QC per 24 hours unless the manufacturer requires more. This requirement may be met in some cases by internal or process controls of the device, now called equivalent quality control, or EQC, once the site completes its own evaluation of such controls.

Sites must verify performance specifications of each testing method implemented, including accuracy, precision, the reportable range, and reference range, in their own facility and for their patient population. There is also a requirement for participation in a CMS-approved proficiency testing (PT) program for selected analytes. Anesthesiologists who use POCT devices may be asked to participate in PT. Typically, unknown samples are provided by the PT agency, to be tested as if they were patient samples, by operators of the device or test method. Failure of two of three consecutive PT events for a given analyte can result in sanctions or suspension of testing for that analyte.

When more than one method of testing is used for a given analyte under the same CLIA certificate, CLIA requires that method correlations be done at least every 6 months. For example, if PT/INR is performed by a POCT device, and also in the core laboratory, the site must run correlations between the two methods every 6 months. The Joint Commission goes further, requiring correlations across all test sites and CLIA certificates in the entire organization.

Conclusions

Point of care testing is a rapidly growing field. As such, manufacturers continually modify, improve, and upgrade their products, and companies buy, sell, and rename product lines. There are many more devices available on the market than those that have been discussed in this chapter. The hope is that the principles discussed here will allow anesthesiologists to evaluate and compare the various products to best meet their clinical needs.

References

1. Scott, M.G., Heusel, J.W., LeGrys, V.A., et al., 1999. Electrolytes and blood gases. In: Burtis, C.A., Ashwood, E.R. (Eds.), Tietz textbook of clinical chemistry, ed 3. WB Saunders, Philadelphia.
2. Astles, J.R., Lubrsky, D., Loun, B., et al., 1996. Pneumatic transport exacerbates interference of room air contamination in blood gas samples. Arch Pathol Lab Med 120, 642–647.
3. Despotis, G.J., Joist, H., et al., 1997. Monitoring of hemostasis in cardiac surgical patients: impact of point-of-care testing on blood loss and transfusion outcomes. Clin Chem 43, 1684–1696.
4. Udelsman, R., Donovan, P.I., Sokoll, L.J., 2000. One hundred consecutive minimally invasive parathyroid explorations. Ann Surg 232, 331–339.
5. Tang, Z., Louie, R., Kost, G.J., 2002. Principles and performance of point-of-care testing instruments. In: Kost, G.J. (Ed.), Principles and practice of point-of-care testing, Lippincott, Williams & Wilkins, Philadelphia.
6. Clarke, W., Nichols, J., 2001. Bedside glucose testing. Clin Lab Med 21 (2), 308–310.

7. Nichols, J., 2002. Bedside testing, glucose monitoring, and diabetes management. In: Kost, G.J. (Ed.), Principles and practice of point-of-care testing, Lippincott, Williams & Wilkins, Philadelphia.

8. Fahy, B.G., Coursin, D.B., 2008. Critical glucose control: the devil is in the details. Mayo Clin Proc 83, 394–397.

9. Tang Z, Lee JH, et al. Effects of different hematocrit levels on glucose measurements with handheld meters for point-of-care testing. Arch Pathol Lab Med 200;124:1135-1140

10. Desachy, A., Vuagnat, A.C., et al., 2008. Accuracy of bedside glucometry in critically ill patients: influence of clinical characteristics and perfusion index. Mayo Clin Proc 83, 400–405.

11. Myers, G.J., Browne, J., 2007. Point of care hematocrit and hemoglobin in cardiac surgery: a review. Perfusion 22, 179–183.

12. McNulty, S.E., Torjman, M., Wlodzimierz, G., et al., 1995. A comparison of four bedside methods of hemoglobin assessment during cardiac surgery. Anesth Analg 81, 1197–1202.

13. Hopfer, S.M., Nadeau, F.L., Sundra, M., et al., 2004. Effect of protein on hemoglobin and hematocrit assays with a conductivity based point of care testing device: comparison with optical methods. Ann Clin Lab Sci 34 (1), 75–82.

14. Steinfelder-Visscher, J., Weerwind, P.W., Teerenstra, S., et al., 2006. Reliability of point of care hematocrit, blood gas, electrolyte, lactate and glucose measurement during cardiopulmonary bypass. Perfusion 21, 33–37.

15. World Health Organization, 1983. Standardization. W.E.Co.B., 33rd report. WHO technical report series. World Health Organization, Geneva.

16. Mulry, C.C., Le Veen, R.F., Sobel, M., et al., 1991. Assessment of heparin anticoagulation during peripheral angioplasty. J Vasc Interv Radiol 2, 133–139.

17. Despotis, G.J., et al., 1996. Aprotinin prolongs activated and nonactivated whole blood clotting time and potentiates the effect of heparin in vitro. Anesth Analg 82, 1126–1131.

18. Dougherty, K.G., Gaos, C.M., et al., 1992. Activated clotting times and activated partial thromboplastin times in patents undergoing coronary angioplasty who receive bolus doses of heparin. Cathet Cardiovasc Diagn 26, 260–263.

19. Kang, Y.G., Martin, D.J., Marquez, J., et al., 1985. Intraoperative changes in blood coagulation and thromboelastic monitoring in liver transplantation. Anesth Analg 64, 888–896.

20. Tuman, K.J., et al., 1991. Comparison of thromboelastography and platelet aggregometry. Anesthesiology 75, A433.

21. Zambruni, A., Thalheimer, U., et al., 2004. Thromboelastography with citrated blood: comparability with native whole blood, stability of citrate storage and effect of repeat sampling. Blood Coagul Fibrinolysis 15:103-107.

22 Santrach, P., Point of care hematology, hemostasis, and thrombolysis testing. In Kost, G.J. (Ed.), Principles and practice of point of care testing, Lippincott, Williams and Wilkins, Philadelphia.

23. Nuttall, G.A., Oliver, W.C., et al., 2001. Efficacy of a simple intraoperative transfusion algorithm for nonerythrocyte component utilization after cardiopulmonary bypass. Anesthesiology 94, 773–781.

24. Avidan, M.S., Alcock, E.L., et al., 2004. Comparison of structured use of routine laboratory tests or near-patient assessment with clinical judgment in the management of bleeding after cardiac surgery. Br J Anaesth 92, 178–186.

25. Braunstein, G.D., Rasor, J., Adler, D., et al., 1976. serum human chorionic gonadotropin levels throughout normal pregnancy. Am J Obstet Gynecol 126, 678.

26. Public Law 100-578, Section 353 Public Health Service Act (42 U.S.C. 263a) October 31, 1988.

27. Joint Commission. Laboratory accreditation standards, (website): http://www.jointcommission.org. Accessed July 2009.

28. College of American Pathologists (CAP). Laboratory accreditation program, (website): http://www.cap.org/apps/cap.portal?_nfpb=true&_pageLabel=accr editation. Accessed July 2009.

29. COLA. Accreditation manual, (website): http://cola.org/. Accessed July 2009.

Suggestions for Further Reading

1. Kost, G.J. (Ed.), 2002. Principles and practice of point-of-care testing, Williams & Wilkins, Philadelphia, Lippincott.

2. Price, C.P., St John, A., Hicks, J.M., (Eds.), 2004. Point-of-Care testing, ed 2. AACC Press, Washington, DC.

3. Point of care: the journal of near-patient testing & technology, (serial online): www.poctjournal.com.

www.roche.com
www.instrumentationlaboratory.com
www.haemoscope.com
www.sienco.com
http://diagnostics.siemens.com/webapp/wcs/stores/servlet/StoreCatalogDisplay~q_catalogId~e_-101~a_langId~e_-101~a_storeId~e_10001.htm
www.medtronic.com
www.itcmed.com
www.hemocue.com
www.qbcdiagnostics.com
www.abbott.com
www.novabiomedical.com
www.lifescan.com
www.radiometeramerica.com
www.epocal.com
www.helena.com
www.beckman.com
www.permaxim.com
www.clearview.com

Chapter 21

Anesthesia Information Management Systems

Sachin Kheterpal

Technological advancements have revolutionized not only patient monitoring and therapeutic equipment, but also something as fundamental as the anesthesia record itself. The paper anesthesia record, still in use at more than 95% of U.S. hospitals, has been replaced at some institutions by an anesthesia information management system (AIMS). An AIMS is a comprehensive software application that fulfills the clinical, communication, medicolegal, regulatory, and charge capture roles of the paper record. Given their evolving role, AIMS are increasingly being recognized as valuable anesthesia "devices" that may improve patient safety and process efficiency—going far beyond the role of a paper record replacement.

History of Anesthesia Information Management Systems

The first paper anesthesia records were developed and described by the pioneering surgeons Codman and Cushing in 1894. As surgical medical students assigned the task of anesthetizing surgical patients, they established a wager regarding who could minimize the overall complications experienced by their patients. To that end, each began graphically recording patient vital signs during the operation: heart rate, respiratory rate, and temperature (Figure 21–1). Although it is unclear who won the wager,

this seminal effort in anesthesia patient safety reveals a fundamental concept: the anesthesia record's primary role is to improve *patient safety*. Initially, this was perceived to be accomplished purely by recording and evaluating the patient's physiological trend. As a result, some of the earliest efforts were focused purely upon automation of physiological parameter recordings, including a crude yet innovative vital sign recorder that looked similar to a polygraph machine (Figure 21–2). The advent of personal computers in the 1980s was an important turning point in the development of modern day AIMS. Technologically savvy anesthesiologists began to extract real-time digital data elements from the anesthesia machine and physiological monitor and store them on local personal computer storage media. These vital signs were printed out and represented the physiological recording element of a paper anesthesia record.

Next, user data entry devices such as keyboards and proprietary keypads were integrated into the workstation and allowed the anesthesiologist to document elements that could not be automatically recorded using device interfaces: clinical interventions, procedures, observations, and medications. This virtual document combining physiological and device information with user entered elements could then be printed out and replace the paper anesthesia record. This paper record replacement gave rise to the term *anesthesia record keeper* (ARK) and reflected the state of AIMS until the mid to late 1990s. Beginning

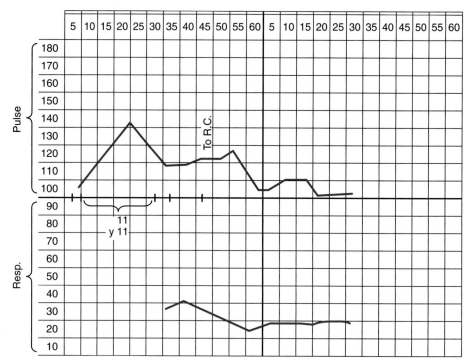

Figure 21–1 A schematic of the early anesthesia records maintained by famed neurosurgeons Codman and Cushing.

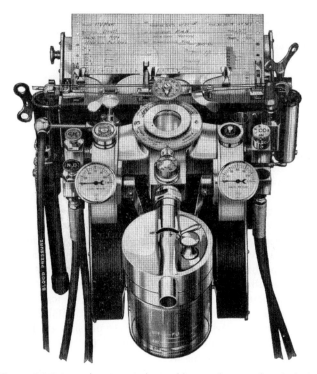

Figure 21–2 An early automated record keeper that transferred physiological information from patient monitoring device to a piece of paper.

in the late 1990s and year 2000, AIMS evolved from paper anesthesia record replacements to true information systems. Leveraging the explosion of healthcare information technology, AIMS began to integrate with other clinical information systems and incorporate more perioperative documents. Most recently, AIMS have developed into workflow management solutions, the source of critical reporting data, and alerts and reminders regarding clinical or administrative elements.

Point-of-Care Software

In general, modern AIMS software can be grouped into three broad categories: traditional client-server, web-based, and handheld. Each type of software implementation leverages a unique information technology infrastructure. The decision to implement a given type of point-of-care software must incorporate cost and functionality criteria.

The first group of point-of-care AIMS software is the ubiquitous client-server architecture. Before the advent of web browsers, most modern software required a variety of files to be installed on each local workstation. These files provided the instructions for how the software should behave, display information, and interact with the user. The primary interaction between the workstation (known as the client) and the location of the patient data (known as the server) was the exchange of data. A balance of duties exists between the client and server computers; hence, the term *client-server application*. Unfortunately, this type of software provides distribution and maintenance challenges for an institution's information technology staff. Because most of the instructions for the application's behavior are stored locally in files on the workstation, the files must be updated on all workstations by the information technology staff. As clinical information technology offerings expand, client-server applications may become victim to unintentional interactions between two applications that share a common file. Updates to the file by one vendor could have an impact on another vendor's application. However, new management and automation tools allow upgrades to be sent to the client workstations through the network and enable careful version checking for the files shared across vendors. Most importantly, the development tools for client-server software are extremely mature and allow advanced user interface development. They have progressed through multiple generations of improvement and offer a very robust development environment with very detailed control over the workstation itself. Historically, client-server applications have been more capable of leveraging unique point-of-care hardware, such as barcode readers and radiofrequency tags.

Web-based software uses web browsers to perform the display function and stores the application instructions in a more centralized location, known as a web or application server. Rather than distributing instruction files to every point-of-care workstation, most of the application logic is stored on the centralized web server. Ubiquitous web browsers that are already installed on the point-of-care workstation then interpret these instructions from a specific web server. The workstation interacts with the web server not only for data, but also for display instructions, validation rules, and business logic. When a vendor offers software upgrades, files can be updated on only a limited number of centralized web servers. Web software is especially advantageous when the workstations that access the system are extremely large in number or in unpredictable locations. For example, access to an operating room schedule from hundreds of surgeons' offices may be best enabled by web software. Because the development tools available for web-based software are not as mature as those for client-server development, user interfaces and robustness are less advanced. This drawback is rapidly being mitigated through extensive efforts by the software industry. A more challenging drawback can be inconsistency between the web-browser software and the instructions on the web server. Some advanced capabilities and instructions might require a specific browser version or vendor. In addition, easier access to the application is associated with increased security risk; therefore, security concerns may be heightened.

The latest software tools blur the dichotomy between client-server and web-based applications. Using technologies that maintain a centralized store for the instructions, they also copy software that interprets the instructions to individual workstations. This decreases dependency on the browser vendor and version. Decreased dependency on the browser also enables more advanced user interfaces and complex business logic to be run efficiently.

Finally, some software is designed specifically to run on mobile, hand held devices that have unique requirements for ergonomics, speed, and screen size. The widely variant user interfaces of a desktop computer and hand held PocketPC or iPhone demand that software be designed specifically for the mobile device, even though it might be similar to that run on a desktop. A combination of all three types of software is possible and may actually optimize the speed, usability, and cost of the system.

Point-of-Care Hardware

Most potential customers recognize the importance of choosing the right software model and vendor, and they recognize the difficulty of this task. However, choosing the correct *point-of-care hardware* remains a very challenging decision that is often overlooked by customers. The workstation bears a number of point-of-care demands. Given the increasing healthcare industry focus on nosocomial infections, the institution's infection control leadership must review the potential point-of-care hardware. Stationary, mounted hardware must be capable of being cleaned as part of the routine housekeeping process during patient turnover. Typical cleaning agents could harm hardware not designed for the point-of-care environment. Hence, water-resistant keyboards that lack crevices capable of housing infectious materials are often chosen. One should also confirm that the hardware is reliable in difficult environments. Certain clinical situations (burn surgery or pediatric operating rooms) warrant a room temperature outside the typical operating range of a standard workstation.

Although they are mounted, stationary workstations are routinely moved by maintenance and housekeeping staff. Exposure of the equipment to this level of maneuvering should be considered when evaluating the necessary durability. In addition, a small footprint is helpful to minimize the space consumed by the information system in already cramped patient care areas. Finally, regardless of which hardware is chosen, it must be mounted or secured in an economical and effective manner. Although the price of workstations continues to plummet due to the commoditization of computer hardware, simple mounting arms and carts remain relatively expensive items that often surpass the cost of the workstation itself. In addition, the AIMS workstation display can be mounted on either side of the anesthesia machine, each with its own advantages and disadvantages. Mounting on the left side (near the head of the operating table) allows the user to interact with the AIMS display while looking at the patient and surgical field. Theoretically, this enables vigilance and may enable real-time documentation. Alternatively, the AIMS display can be mounted on the right side of the anesthesia machine. Proponents of this ergonomic choice note that the head of the bed is an already-overcrowded area with multiple IV poles, infusion pumps, ancillary monitors, and additional devices. The addition of another piece of hardware near this sterile area exacerbates an existing ergonomic challenge, possibly reducing patient safety. Displays mounted on the right side of the anesthesia machine can be articulated toward the head of the bed during anesthesia induction to enable real-time documentation and then articulated back to a natural position during maintenance of anesthesia. Figures 21–3 and 21–4 demonstrate these two alternative approaches.

Despite these healthcare-specific point-of-care hardware demands, most current AIMS can be deployed on any standard, modern personal computer. However, this flexibility brings with it an overabundance of options. In addition, each point-of-care—advanced testing clinic, preoperative holding room, operating room, offsite procedure site, imaging suite, PACU, ICU, or general care floor—presents its own challenges and opportunities for the information technology department. Potential customers may wish to work with the healthcare-specific division of a general computer hardware manufacturer. Furthermore, vendors' user groups are invaluable sources of advice and experience that can substantially reduce frustration, cost, and project delay. Unfortunately, access to this resource typically occurs only after installation. Though the highly competitive computer hardware industry offers many pricing options, the initial capital costs must be balanced with the long-term operating maintenance expenses associated with each hardware option.

Many AIMS implementations depend upon the familiar touch-screen user interface of modern physiological monitors. This application paradigm is familiar to many anesthesiologists and may reduce the initial training effort required. In addition,

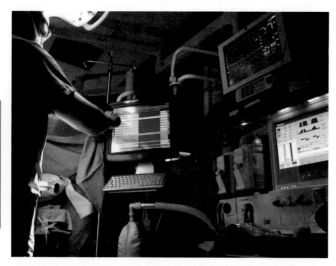

Figure 21–3 The anesthesia cockpit with an anesthesia information management system mounted on the left side of the anesthesia machine.

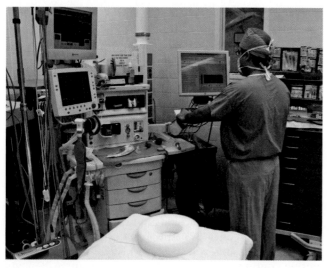

Figure 21–4 The anesthesia cockpit with an anesthesia information management system mounted on the right side of the anesthesia machine.

touchscreen-focused interfaces that decrease the need for a keyboard or mouse may be more sustainable in the tight confines of the operating room. The additional space consumed by a keyboard and mouse is valuable real estate competing with other anesthesia devices. However, elimination of the keyboard and mouse often proves difficult because of the stringent user interface demands placed upon software dependent upon a touch-screen user interface. All buttons, scroll bars, and action areas must be "touchable" with a finger rather than stylus or pointing device. Furthermore, since most AIMS implementations also install other applications upon the point of care workstation (enterprise electronic mail, web browser, medical reference), a keyboard and mouse is necessary for these cross-industry applications that do not assume a touchscreen.

Some vendors offer unique functionality that requires vendor-specific hardware. Proprietary hardware such as special keyboards, entry keypads, or syringe pumps can be specialized for the AIMS feature set. Even if proprietary hardware is not required, some advanced functionality could require

hardware such as barcode readers or radio-frequency sensors, and a typical information technology department is not familiar with this equipment or comfortable supporting it. The value of the advanced functionality must be assessed in terms of the potentially high initial cost, ongoing maintenance effort, and information technology training requirements. Optimistically, these issues will wane as AIMS and other point-of-care information systems increase their market penetration.

Functional Components of an Anesthesia Information Management System

Much like an anesthesia machine has discrete functional components that work together to create a complete medical device, an AIMS is also a complex system of functional modules and systems working together to create a complete patient care "device." Consideration of the individual components comprising a complete AIMS allows one to consider the variant levels of functionality available. More importantly, absence of one of these components at a given implementation allows us to consider the impact and capabilities of a given AIMS implementation.

Figure 21–5 is a hierarchical rendering of a comprehensive AIMS. At its core, a modern AIMS is based upon a functioning physiological device interface, intraoperative record keeper functionality for user-entered documentation, basic operating room schedule integration, and some type of outbound rendering of the final anesthesia record itself. The next level of application maturity and functionality is shown in the next concentric circle. This incremental maturity may reflect incorporation of clinical areas upstream or downstream of the operating room itself—the required preoperative anesthesia history and physical (H&P) or compulsory postoperative inpatient visit or outpatient phone call. Alternatively, this advanced functionality may include more comprehensive uses of the intraoperative data such as a quality improvement reporting module or richer user interface such as minor procedure documentation templates.

The most advanced AIMS implementations extend beyond the intraoperative anesthesia period and could be considered perioperative clinical information systems. Postanesthesia care unit nursing documentation, preoperative clinics, preoperative nursing assessments, and comprehensive acute pain service documentation by physicians and nurses are incorporated into some comprehensive AIMS implementations. Alternatively, an advanced AIMS may contain functionality that goes beyond the typical medical purpose of the anesthesia record: automated research infrastructure, preoperative and postoperative patient trackers and workflow managers, and alerts and reminder systems.

Automated Physiological Device Interfaces

Integrating the physiological monitor and device data from point-of-care devices is a critical element of a perioperative clinical information system. The frequent vital signs and

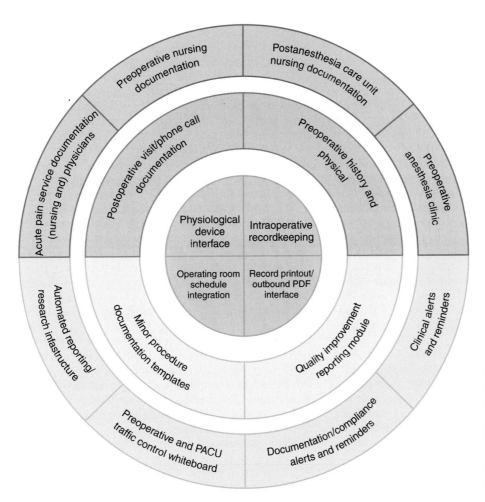

Figure 21–5 A schematic demonstrating the variety of functional components of an anesthesia information management system. The features common to most modern anesthesia information management systems are shown at the core of this figure. More comprehensive components are demonstrated as concentric circles of advancing functionality.

device settings collected in the operating room and postanesthesia care unit warrant an efficient means of transferring digital data from these devices to the computerized clinical record. Commonly interfaced devices include physiological monitors, anesthesia machines, gas analysis monitors, and ancillary monitors such as level of consciousness and continuous cardiac output. Less commonly interfaced devices include heart-lung bypass machines, infusion pumps, and digital urimeters.

A fundamental question raised by AIMS implementations is the desired sampling rate of the *automated device interfaces.* Although the standard of care in paper anesthesia records is the recording of heart rate and blood pressure every 5 minutes (via graphing) and other elements every 15 minutes, an AIMS allows extremely granular data recording. Most commercially available AIMS support recording of continuous values every 15 seconds—far more granular than in the paper record. The vast majority of current AIMS implementations chooses to only store values every 60 seconds for medical record purposes. An important issue raised by this sampling rate is which mathematical function should be used to "filter" continuous data to the desired interval—median, most recent value, or mean. In a paper anesthesia record, this "filtering" is performed by anesthesiologists as they choose to record certain values while excluding others, a process known to be less accurate than an AIMS automated interface.

A second important issue is the management of monitoring artifacts in an automated device interface environment. Artifacts due to clinical issues (i.e., electrocautery interface, noninvasive cuff occluding flow to an invasive arterial catheter) or intervention (arterial blood gas sampling occluding flow to an invasive arterial catheter) are typically ignored by the anesthesiologist when recording values in a paper record. However, AIMS generally do not perform any automatic artifactual filtering due to medicolegal and technical issues. As a result, spurious blood pressures or heart rates may be present throughout the record. Although many anesthesiologists fear a litigious practice environment and the potential liability associated with these values, these concerns are contradicted by actual experience. The illegible, error prone, and interpretation-based paper record may represent a higher risk than automatic recording of completely defensible clinical artifacts. The veracity of the AIMS device data may be its greatest asset and offer legal protection in establishing the true observed physiological parameters during an adverse clinical event. The acuity of perioperative clinical events demands that the anesthesiologist focus on therapy and diagnosis over documentation; as a result, paper anesthesia records suffer from a retrospective documentation limitation that becomes painfully apparent during legal proceedings.

Technical Infrastructure for Automated Physiological Device Interfaces

To enable the remote viewing of waveforms, many physiological monitoring implementations from the leading vendors have included a "monitoring network," which carries vital-sign information to central viewing stations. These networks can be leveraged to interface device data into the AIMS. Using a centralized interface server, information is copied from the monitoring network to the AIMS database server—the source of the anesthesia intraoperative record data. Because each vendor's monitoring network uses a slightly different language to transmit the device data, it is critical to ensure that the interface server is capable of interpreting a given monitoring vendor's protocol. If the physiological monitors already display data from other devices, such as the anesthesia machine, ventilator, gas analyzer, or ancillary monitors, the monitoring network will probably also contain information from these additional devices. Connecting these ancillary devices generally requires some type of integration device in each operating room. In this situation, the interface server may fulfill all of the device integration requirements (Figure 21–6, *A*).

If ancillary devices such as an anesthesia machine or alternative monitors cannot be integrated into the monitoring network, a distributed strategy may be necessary. Most devices offer an outbound data port. Specifically, an RS-232 port can be used to connect the medical device to another processing device. This processing device can be a local workstation that is running device integration software or dedicated device integration equipment. In either case, the device's information is temporarily stored locally and then forwarded to the centralized database storage server. If the local PC is used to perform the device integration work, it can also serve as the AIMS workstation used by the anesthesia provider. The device integration software can run silently in the background (Figure 21–6, *B*). This local mechanism of device integration can be used for nearly any device that is not capable of connecting directly to a network: heart-lung bypass machines, infusion pumps, and even bench lab testing equipment.

Finally, if a monitoring network cannot be implemented for either cost or technical reasons, the primary physiological monitor and all ancillary devices can be integrated locally using device integration software (Figure 21–6, *C*).

The AIMS vendor is responsible for developing device integration software that can translate between the device's unique communication protocol and the vendor's data storage mechanism. Maintaining an expansive and up-to-date library of supported devices can prove challenging. In fact, many vendors have chosen to outsource the development of these specialized software libraries to companies that exclusively focus on device interfaces.

User-Entered Documentation

Although automated device interfaces relieve much of the monotonous documentation burden, many elements of the intraoperative anesthesia record require user-entered documentation in the paper or AIMS environments. Fundamental documentation such as provider "signatures," medication administration, fluid documentation, intubation details, surgical events, and time events all require manual entry.

Although every patient and anesthetic record is unique, there are a variety of similarities among anesthesia records for a given anesthetic technique and surgical procedure. For example, all general anesthesia cases involving endotracheal intubation demand the documentation of an induction agent (intravenous or inhalational), use or omission of neuromuscular blockade, intubation aid (direct laryngoscopy, video laryngoscopy, etc.), laryngeal view and intubation difficulty, and endotracheal tube type and size. These induction elements can be organized into documentation templates within an AIMS user interface for general anesthesia cases. Much like the traditional paper record allowed anesthesiologists to "fill in the blanks" in specific sections (Figure 21–7), AIMS can offer documentation templates (Figure 21–8). This ability to template AIMS documentation applies to various anesthesia techniques (endotracheal intubation, neuraxial blockade, emergence, and extubation) and surgical procedures (cardiopulmonary bypass, liver transplantation). These templating efforts result in a more efficient documentation, standardized documentation for reporting and billing purposes, and the substrate for clinical alerts and reminders.

Given the limited number of medications typically administered in the operating room, AIMS typically include a selection list of medications for documentation. These medications can be part of a template or can be searched within a list of medications. The medication information is typically stored with a structured medication code that may enable advanced functionality such as allergy checking.

Many user-entered documentation elements are not easily templated. Given the wide variety of comments seen in hand-written paper anesthesia records, some mechanism to allow users to enter comments in an AIMS is also necessary. Typically, a free-text "comment" option allows the user to simply type in any phrase or clinical documentation they desire. Although this flexibility is important to user acceptance, excessive usage of the free-text option results in a less standardized, searchable, or consistent anesthesia record. As a result, most AIMS implementations attempt to decrease the need for prose free-text documentation by creating structured selection lists for common miscellaneous comments.

For example, although a user may be able to type in a comment of "tourniquet up," it may be preferable to create a structured, searchable selection for this comment. The structured element may include pick-lists regarding the extremity involved and the pressure setting. For example, an AIMS may offer the option of "Tourniquet placed on _____ and set to _____ mm Hg" where the "____" sections represent selectable options. By transforming this free-text opportunity to a structured element, several important clinical and documentation goals are achieved. First, a standard of documentation is established: the site and pressure of the tourniquet should be documented, not just the presence of a tourniquet. Secondly, because each structured element in an AIMS has a codified identifier associated with it, future quality assurance and research efforts are facilitated because the identifier can be the target of a query rather than a free-text entry. Finally, if the AIMS offers clinical alerts and reminders, a structured tourniquet element could be associated with a timer event that reminds the user to inform the surgeons of 60 minutes of tourniquet time.

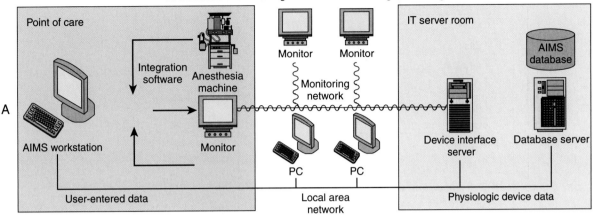

Architecture 1: Monitoring network + device integration using monitor

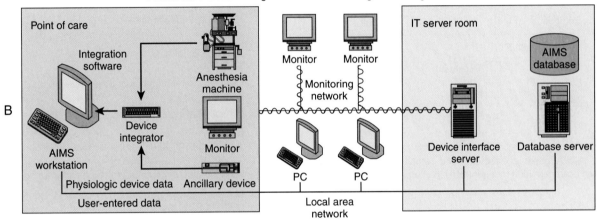

Architecture 2: Monitoring network + device integration using AIMS workstation

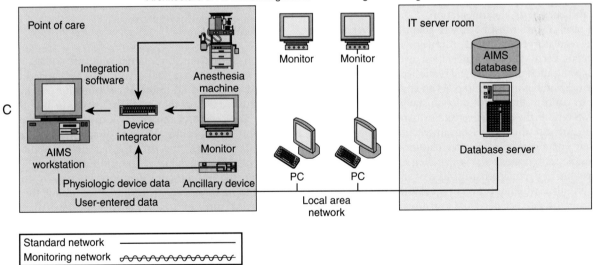

Architecture 3: No monitoring network – All integration using AIMS workstation

| Standard network | —————————— |
| Monitoring network | ~~~~~~~~~~~~~~~~ |

Figure 21–6 Three variant technical and networking architectures for physiological device integration with an anesthesia information management system.

Staff and Billing Documentation

Although the anesthesia record was originally designed as a patient safety "device," it has evolved into a document with many more pragmatic purposes. One of the most important roles it serves is the legal evidence of staff presence for regulatory and professional billing purposes. Just as in a paper record, an AIMS must incorporate the ability for anesthesia providers to attest to their role in the perioperative period—be it as the attending physician that started the case, relieved another attending, or as the anesthesia resident or nurse

Induction

- ☐ Mask # _____
- ☐ Easy   ☐ Difficult
- ☐ Airway # _____
- ☐ Oral   ☐ Nasal
- ☐ ETT # _____
- ☐ Oral   ☐ Nasal
- ☐ DL view _____
- ☐ LMA
- Blade # _____
- Length @ teeth _____
- Cuff (ml) _____ ☐ BIL BS
- ☐ Difficult (note on chart)

Intubation	☐ Easy	☐ Difficult

- ☐ Existing trach/ETT
- ☐ Topical   ☐ Transtrach
- ☐ Awake   ☐ DL   ☐ F. optic
- ☐ RSI   ☐ DLT   ☐ L wand
- ☐ Blind   ☐ Jet   ☐ Stylette

Figure 21–7 A paper anesthesia record sample demonstrating the structured documentation for endotracheal tube placement.

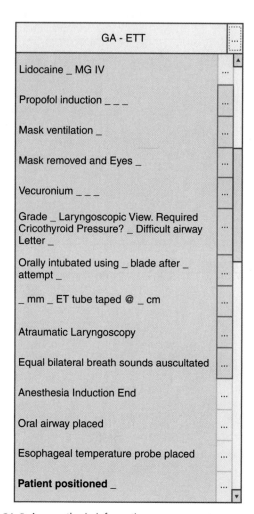

Figure 21–8 An anesthesia information management system template for induction of general anesthesia. Each step of a typical anesthetic induction, and the expected documentation, is available for facile, structured documentation.

anesthetist for a portion of the case. Although the federal government is a major payer at most hospitals, each state and institution has specific requirements for attestation statements and anesthetist documentation.

As a result, AIMS must be able to adapt to the varying and evolving regulatory requirements placed upon the anesthesiology department. Each AIMS implementation involves configuration of the specific attestation statement requested by an institution's compliance and billing leadership. As an end user, one must be careful to confirm that the attestation statement generated by the AIMS reflects the care delivered. Furthermore, each institution may increase the level of documentation required by the end user. For example, some sites require that the attending anesthesiologist repeatedly document their episodes of physical presence during the maintenance phase of anesthesia.

The anesthesia billing process requires the documentation of not only the care provided and individuals providing it, but also key times when the services were initiated and completed. Anesthesia start and anesthesia end must be documented clearly and consistently, a major challenge in the paper medical record environment. Automated reminders in an AIMS can greatly facilitate record completeness and accuracy. However, each AIMS implementation must ensure that no systematic "upcoding" or increased billing is implemented. Regulatory oversight agencies may consider automated measures that systematically increase charges to be fraudulent. The focus must be on systems and processes that increase the accuracy of documentation, whether this results in a decrease or increase in charges.

The increasing adoption of electronic medical records has brought the term "*electronic signature*," or "e-sig," into the medical vernacular. Fundamentally, an "e-sig" within an AIMS consists of two major concepts: first, a successful user ID and password combination submission, and, second, a user-entered action that states he or she is now the attending or anesthetist of record for a case. In the case of minor procedures (i.e., epidural blood patch or invasive monitoring access), the "e-sig" attests to the fact that they supervised or performed the procedure in question.

Given the unique considerations created by concurrency checking in anesthesia professional fee billing, the transition to an AIMS may be a major change for departmental billing staff. Because AIMS may contain point-of-care alerts that warn the clinician if they attempt to supervise an excessive number of cases concurrently, the number of final concurrent errors detected and managed by billing staff may be decreased. This can significantly decrease the work effort to correct concurrency errors. In addition, if the final medical record output of the AIMS is electronic (as opposed to a printout placed in the paper medical chart), corrections needed to the record can be communicated and performed electronically. This eliminates the need to transport a paper anesthesia record from the point of care to the billing staff and then to clinician's office. The increased efficiency in the charge capture and submission has real financial benefits. However, if the AIMS does not contain basic point-of-care concurrency checks and alerts, the transition from a paper process to an electronic process may result in documentation errors that increase the billing staff work burden.

Alerts and Reminders

Although the initial transition from paper anesthesia records to an AIMS may be a lateral shift rather than leap forward, the financial and human resource cost of an AIMS demands that progress justify the initial investment. A major functional component of AIMS that can be used to create a return on investment is *alerting and reminder infrastructure.*

Clinical alerts can be used to improve the process of care or the safety of care itself. The high acuity of the operating room environment combined with the efficiency demands placed upon providers creates a high-risk clinical situation. For example, medications are administered without the typical checks and balances created by an order entry, pharmacy verification, and order fulfillment process. The anesthesiologist must integrate multiple sources of information—patient, family, surgeon, laboratory system, dictations, radiology, and the physiological monitors—to make effective and safe decisions. The most basic of clinical alerts is the documentation template itself, as discussed earlier. By listing out the recommended documentation and clinical steps for a procedure, the AIMS reminds the anesthesiologists of the standardized clinical protocol. Much like nursing pathways in the intensive care unit or general floor, these guidelines do not mandate a specific care pattern, but simply remind the clinician of the standardized process. For example, an anesthesia induction template may contain an element for the administration of cefazolin as surgical site infection prophylaxis before incision.

Next, if an element is not documented within a certain time frame, a more intrusive alert can be delivered to the user via an on-screen prompt, sound alert, or alphanumeric page. Different vendors and institutions have implemented a variety of alerts using their AIMS or the data created by AIMS. In many instances, the alerting systems are not commercialized products, but innovative custom applications written by the customer itself. Some vendors offer configurable alert writing and triggering modules that enable institutions to customize the criteria and impact of alerts.

Independent of the architecture used to create the triggers, each institution may identify a clinical or administrative problem that warrants the use of an alerting system. Many of the clinical alerts used in current AIMS are based upon national perioperative pay-for-performance measures. For example, because the timely administration of preoperative antibiotics for surgical site infection prophylaxis is a national standard, many AIMS implementations have incorporated real-time alerts to increase compliance. At the same time, a variety of institution-specific clinical experiences can result in clinical reminders implemented as a patient safety net. For example, some institutions have incorporated automated alphanumeric preoperative paging for abnormal laboratory values to ensure that abnormal preoperative laboratory tests are noted and managed by the perioperative team. The AIMS can integrate across the scheduled anesthesia and surgical providers, patient laboratory values, and paging system to send prospective alerts the day before surgery to the surgical and anesthesia team. This may reduce the likelihood that critical coagulation studies, blood type antibodies, or electrolyte abnormalities are resulted but not managed.

Many AIMS implementations use automated alerts and reminders to improve compliance with documentation and administrative standards. The anesthesia literature has many examples of on-screen alerts, alphanumeric paging, and electronic mail alerts that are sent to providers to ensure appropriate documentation of key billing elements such as provider sign-in, anesthesia start or end, or minor procedure notes. The literature has demonstrated significant and sustained improvements in days from clinical activity to billing and actual reimbursement. In many cases, these financial benefits are used to justify the capital and operating expenses associated with a comprehensive information technology implementation. However, each prospective customer must ensure that a robust return on investment analysis establishes an accurate current state and confirms that the proposed AIMS implementation has the technical capabilities necessary to deliver on the promise of alert-based process improvement.

Anesthesia History and Physical

Medicolegal, clinical, regulatory, and reimbursement guidelines demand that every procedure involving anesthesia personnel be accompanied by a preoperative *anesthesia H&P* distinct from the surgical H&P. The anesthesia H&P is a comorbidity and airway examination focused evaluation that does not delve into the minute details of the primary disease process, unless there are systemic effects. As a result, although the typical internal medicine or surgical H&P is focused on the history of present illness, the anesthesia H&P is focused on the past medical history and its potential impact on the patient's ability to tolerate the planned surgery and anesthetic.

As a result of this unique clinical approach, the anesthesia H&P presents an automation challenge to many AIMS implementations. In fact, many of the longest tenured AIMS implementations do not include an electronic anesthesia H&P. Instead, this document is completed on paper and a few essential elements are reentered in the AIMS by the anesthesiologist: ASA physical status, allergies, and medications. The absence of an electronic, integrated anesthesia H&P in an AIMS limits the ability of clinical alerts and reminders to offer patient context sensitive feedback and recommendations. In addition, some of the process and efficiency gains of an electronic record are degraded by the need to locate and collate a paper anesthesia H&P for billing and reporting purposes.

However, just as the intraoperative anesthesia record in most AIMS has evolved, so too has the ability to document an H&P. As a result, many recent implementations have incorporated an electronic anesthesia H&P in the initial AIMS go-live. The usability, efficiency, and configurability of this component are essential to its success. For example, an excessively detailed and time-consuming H&P will be much more laborious than a paper record when delivering care to a healthy ASA 2 patient undergoing an elective knee arthroscopy. However, an excessively simplistic and text-driven component requires lengthy and difficult free-text entry when anesthetizing an elderly ASA 4 patient with multiple medical problems. Striking a balance between these documentation extremes—some pick-list and some free-text entry—is the challenge faced by all H&P implementations. Unlike the intraoperative anesthesia record, the usability, user interface, and configurability of the H&P component varies widely among vendors and implementations. This functional component should be reviewed and assessed in great detail before vendor selection or implementation.

In some cases, an institutional electronic medical record may be used to complete the anesthesia H&P—replacing the AIMS H&P functionality and components. Typically, enterprise information technology or medicolegal leadership exerts influence upon the anesthesiologists and demands the use of an integrated institutional H&P rather than an AIMS H&P. Although this does result in an H&P more effectively integrated into the patient's longitudinal electronic medical record, it typically eliminates the integration of comorbidity information into the intraoperative record keeper's alerts and reminders. Furthermore, users must interact with multiple application user interfaces and still need to double document certain elements such as ASA physical status and allergies. To decrease these disadvantages, some interfaces or integration may be developed.

Reporting for Quality Improvement, Compliance, or Research Purposes

Robust reporting is also an important element of most AIMS implementations. Many justifications for the return on investment are based on the clinical, operational, and financial improvements offered by analysis across patients. The ability to quickly and easily retrieve key metrics about a perioperative process allows for evidence-based change initiatives. However, the technical complexity of reporting requires foresight and planning. In addition, the paucity of standardized anesthesia efficiency metrics within the industry itself challenges vendors attempting to create reusable standardized reports for multiple institutions.

Reports can be categorized into standardized and ad hoc. Standardized reports are usually built into the AIMS and are based on industrywide indicators: case volume, cases by anesthesia type, cases per provider, billable units. These reports are easily created on a regular basis without substantial effort. Perioperative process reports and indicators are more prevalent than clinical indicators because surgery scheduling and management systems are much more widespread than AIMS. To prevent wasted effort, project planning must ensure that the reports sought from the AIMS are not already offered by another existing information system. Ad hoc reports are unique reports that answer specific clinical, operational, or *quality improvement* questions at a given institution. They may require considerable technical expertise and an understanding of the clinical data and its accuracy.

During the vendor and application selection process, the customer must clearly understand the limitations of the ad hoc reporting tools available. In many situations, the flexibility and ease of ad hoc reporting is improved by the implementation of a separate reporting database. Although the transactional database may be optimized for application functionality, reliability, and performance, it may not be the optimal data structure for reporting. A separate reporting database, housed on a distinct physical server may be a necessary luxury for certain customers. Off-the-shelf reporting tools can be directed against denormalized reporting databases. These robust tools increase an institution's flexibility by creating independence from the AIMS vendor's offerings.

It is important that customers not assume that all collected data can be the source of easy cross-patient reports. For example, although the system may document the type of endotracheal tube type and size, it might be difficult to create a report on the type of endotracheal tube only. It may be necessary to decompose a comprehensive clinical element into more discrete reportable elements. Trade-offs are necessary between reporting flexibility and ease of use by the end user. Discrete content often requires more selections by the end users. During the planning and implementation of the clinical content, the vendor and institution must discuss the type of reports envisioned. However, many institutions cannot predict their future reporting needs because of the dynamic research and clinical environment. As a result, a content-development philosophy that balances reporting and ease of use should be assumed.

Finally, the configurability of the system can impact the ease of reporting. To make content customizable and configurable while maintaining fast response times, one might need to abstract the clinical concepts and data so that certain data describe what data are stored in other tables. This content-describing data are known as metadata. Conversely, systems with very robust reporting may limit the configurability because the reporting tools assume specific content and concepts. The configurability reporting trade-off must be considered carefully and should factor in the decision of which AIMS to purchase.

Configurability

Ever-changing clinical standards, medical technology, and regulatory requirements demand that an AIMS be easily configured after the system is implemented. Changing pressure from groups such as The Joint Commission and Center for Medicare and Medicaid Services requires that the information system be able to adapt its screens, questions, and process flow. Some aspects integral to the information system might require specific application logic updates from the vendor. In this case, the vendor must provide an upgrade to the institution to implement the change. These upgrades must be carefully coordinated with the institution's information technology department. Other changes may simply be content or configuration settings that are stored in the database or other content-defining files. These settings can be changed more easily. In either case, it is important to understand how content and basic configuration changes are managed.

Some vendors require that only vendor-supplied staff are able to make the changes. Although this policy may improve the robustness of the changes and free the department from such worries, it also makes the department dependent on the vendor's time lines and cost demands. If the vendor offers configuration tools that can be used by the institution's staff, it is essential that the tools be easy to use and that the staff be adequately trained. Such internal training allows the institution to make changes without waiting for the vendor but does consume some internal staff resources. During the vendor selection process, it may be prudent to specifically identify which aspects of application behavior and content the vendor must change and which are configurable by the institution, as these issues will have a significant impact on the system's use and user satisfaction soon after go-live.

Integration with Institutional Medical Record Systems

Although AIMS had historically resided as stand-alone departmental systems within the institutional information technology environment, the increasing use of enterprise *electronic medical records* has brought the days of parochial departmental solutions to an end. Integration with the enterprise medical record can be both inbound and outbound.

Some AIMS attempt to integrate institutional electronic sources of data into the AIMS user experience. Data essential to the usability of the AIMS are seamlessly integrated into the AIMS database. For example, most modern AIMS implementations have a patient demographics and scheduling interface operational as part of the initial go-live. Other sources of data—such as laboratory results, medical record dictations, radiology images, and exam results—may be helpful to the anesthesiologist as they deliver care. As a result, comprehensive AIMS implementations attempt to integrate these sources of clinical information into the user experience. There are two methods for this "integration:" (1) data interfaces that colocate AIMS data with these ancillary sources in the AIMS database and (2) application context integration that allows the user to switch between the AIMS application and institutional electronic medical record applications that contain the information. Data integration results in a superior and more seamless user experience, but demands significant information technology investments to develop and maintain data interfaces that send data to the AIMS. Application context-sharing integration results in a less seamless experience. However, it may achieve the end user functional requirement of facilitating access to the institution's clinical information from within the AIMS application. The application context-sharing integration decreases or eliminates the need to have the user authenticate to multiple applications and select the patient multiple times. Although many institutional information technology departments appear to prefer application context-sharing because it eliminates data redundancy, it is unclear whether the information technology effort or cost is actually decreased compared with data integration.

Given that the output of an AIMS—the anesthesia record—is an important medicolegal document and integral part of the medical record, outbound "integration" into the medical record is also essential. A crucial decision made in each AIMS implementation defines what is the final medical record copy of the anesthesia record: a paper printout or the virtual electronic rendering of the final anesthesia record. If the institutional definition of the medical record is still limited to a paper-only definition, the AIMS implementation must result in a paper record printout. This is due to not only medicolegal concerns, but also the clinical need for access to the anesthesia record by downstream clinicians. However, if the institutional medical record policy incorporates electronic medical records, a virtual anesthesia record that is accessible from the enterprise electronic medical record satisfies both medicolegal and clinical needs. In many cases, a virtual anesthesia record is easier to develop, produce, and maintain than a paper printout. Although a given operation's anesthesia record should theoretically be "complete" at the end of the operation, practical experience demonstrates that missing or inconsistent billing and clinical information is still corrected in a notable proportion of records. Provider electronic signatures, clinical documentation essential to billing (ASA status, etc.), and inconsistent documentation (arterial line tracing without a note indicating invasive catheter placement) may require clarification or correction after the day of surgery. If a paper printout is the final medical record definition, placement of an updated paper record into the patient chart requires significant resources, similar to the current paper process. However, a virtual anesthesia record that is updated eliminates the need to find and update specific physical versions of the patient's medical record. This virtual anesthesia record can be a rich text document or a PDF file viewable from the institutional electronic medical record.

In some settings, the institutional medical record may incorporate discrete data elements from the anesthesia record. For example, rather than just integrating a virtual view of the AIMS output, the general floor or intensive care unit electronic record may wish to receive a discrete, granular record of the fluid input and output during the operation. Essential elements of the anesthesia H&P, if completed within the AIMS, could be integrated into an enterprise electronic medical record. Items such as allergies, home medications, height, and weight may be recorded by the anesthesia provider first and sent to the enterprise electronic medical record for downstream use.

AIMS Redundancy Infrastructure and Failover

As electronic medical records evolve from helpful software applications to mission-critical "medical devices," providers and processes become increasingly dependent upon them. Outside the perioperative environment, the "point of care" is a flexible concept that is capable of moving from patient bedside to nursing station to hallway to conference room. However, the anesthesiologist's clinical role demands continuous physical presence at a very specific place—the anesthesia cockpit. As a result, workstation failure at this point of care is a challenging IT event. If a specific workstation is disabled due to device or software issues, it must be evaluated and repaired immediately. Momentary failures lasting less than 10 or 15 minutes can be handled via patience and temporary paper charting that is then transcribed into the AIMS. Longer workstation failures may require the transition to a paper record for the remainder of the case, a challenging medical record result.

Beyond the individual workstation, networking or database server failure results in a systemwide failure that can have significant impact. Generalized cross-industry IT redundancy improvements have resulted in significant gains for AIMS vendors: hot-swap clustered database servers, storage area networks, redundant power supplies, and dual network interface cards virtually eliminate susceptibility to single-point failure at the database server level. Network uptime is maximized using advanced diagnostic tools detecting packet loss before failure, redundant routers and bridges, and prophylactic hardware upgrades. As a result, network outages are typically rare and ephemeral at most modern hospitals sophisticated enough to implement an AIMS. However, network and database failures are still possible. Various vendors have implemented variant strategies to deal with these system or workstation level failures. They range from focusing on preventing failure to creating complete local and remote redundancy (Figure 21–9). Clearly, an optimal solution leverages the network when it is available, yet allows the user to continue documenting and accessing information when the network or database server

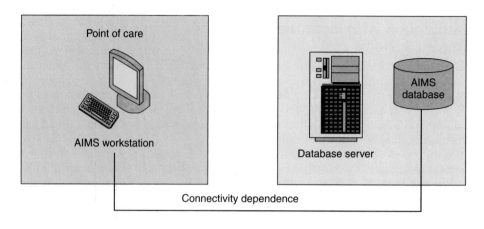

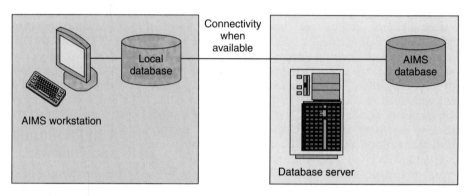

*Record locked to workstation

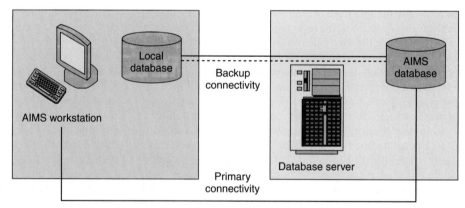

*Record locked to workstation

Figure 21–9 Variant technical options for redundancy and failover of point of care hardware and network connectivity.

fails. However, the infrequency of this scenario combined with the software development costs for vendors allow other less redundant options to be feasible or even desirable.

The Future of Anesthesia Information Management Systems

Vendor Environment

Although best-of-breed vendors that focus on departmental systems still represent the majority of current AIMS implementations, enterprise electronic medical record vendors are engaged in aggressive product development efforts in the AIMS space as well. Although these vendors historically partnered with best-of-breed vendors or simply did not offer perioperative solutions, they are now attempting to implement first generation applications at development partner sites. The hyperacute operating room environment, unique ergonomic challenges, automated physiological device interfaces, and distinct perioperative workflow offer significant challenges to enterprise vendors. However, their experience managing the variant roles of the electronic medical record and relationships with information technology leadership will be used to make inroads into the AIMS market space. More importantly, the specialty of anesthesiology is evolving from an operating room practitioner to a perioperative, critical care, and pain management physician and administrator. Unless AIMS keep pace with this evolution, the clinical and documentation needs of anesthesiologists will outstrip the rich intraoperative record keeper history of AIMS.

Decision Support and Integration with Physiological Monitors

The entire field of *decision support* in clinical informatics is undergoing a major evolution. Enterprise provider order entry systems that have attempted to incorporate decision support functionality have failed to deliver on the promise of fundamental shifts in patient safety or resource use. Although some AIMS have rudimentary decision support capabilities, they may be considered little more than alerts and reminders (discussed earlier). Advanced decision support that incorporates evolving evidence based medicine and patient comorbidities into real-time clinical recommendations is absent from currently commercially available AIMS. As the field of decision support matures and perioperative evidence-based medicine gains a stronger foothold in routine clinical practice, AIMS may be able to infuse evidence-based medicine into the AIMS user experience. Commonly encountered clinical situations, such as postoperative nausea and vomiting, optimization of perioperative myocardial ischemia risk, uncontrolled postoperative pain, and postoperative respiratory insufficiency, may be areas ripe for AIMS-driven decision support.

As decision support matures, the current clear divide between a physiological monitor (with real-time waveforms for ECG, Spo_2, etc.) and AIMS console may blur. The next generation of physiological devices will struggle to differentiate themselves based upon increasingly commoditized parameters, alarm algorithms, information technology specification, and cost. Integration of baseline patient information into the physiological monitors may be the next "game-changer," creating a unique opportunity and role for the AIMS.

Standardization of Anesthesia Information System Content and Data Extracts

One of the greatest challenges facing each AIMS implementation is the configuration and customization required at each site. Although a given vendor's system may already be implemented at several sites, the clinical content (medication lists, H&P elements, physiological parameter definitions, postoperative outcomes) is often reconfigured at each site. The absence of a national standard "anesthesia record" in the paper or electronic realm is a major limitation to the adoption and functional advancement of AIMS. National quality effort such as the American Society of Anesthesiologists' Anesthesia Quality Institute and Committee on Performance and Outcome Measures may spur the standardization necessary. In addition, the culture of anesthesiologists adopting AIMS must change as well. Variation from national standards should be driven by clinical or operational needs rather than personal or institutional idiosyncrasies. In addition, any necessary customization must be used as feedback to national standards so that they can be informed of evolving clinical needs.

Until such standardization occurs, it will be difficult to use AIMS data to compare quality across institutions or to study infrequent events. Aggregation of AIMS data across facilities has been a hope since the first implementations, but there has been very limited success thus far. Compounding the variable clinical content across AIMS implementations is the lack of a standardized data extraction structure. Some progress has been made to incorporate anesthesiology concepts into international medical lexicons such as the Systematized Nomenclature of Medicine - Clinical Terms (SNOMED-CT). However, this very detailed work has not created the higher level metadata structures necessary to leverage the anesthesiology terms.

Summary

An AIMS can be a crucial component of the anesthesiologist's cockpit. The technical underpinnings of AIMS continue to mature as software and hardware capabilities evolve. Its ability to integrate information from and to institutional sources of patient data is consistent with the anesthesiologists evolving patient care and process role. A well-functioning AIMS is an integrated set of functional software components suited to the process needs of a given anesthesiology department and institutional information technology department. The decision to implement specific components significantly affects the ability of an AIMS to serve as a workflow tool with smart alerts and reminders. The future of AIMS will be influenced by the maturation of the clinical information industry and vendor and the development of national anesthesia documentation standards.

References

1. Beecher, H.K., 1940. The first anesthesia records (Codman and Cushing). Surg Gynecol Obstet 71, 689–693.
2. Blum, J.M., Kheterpal, S., Tremper, K.K., 2006. A comparison of anesthesiology resident and faculty electronic evaluations before and after implementation of automated electronic reminders. J Clin Anesth 18, 264–267.
3. Edsall, D.W., Deshane, P., Giles, C., et al., 1993. Computerized patient anesthesia records: less time and better quality than manually produced anesthesia records. J Clin Anesth 5, 275–283.
4. Elmasri, R., Navathe, S., 2004. Fundamentals of database systems, ed 4. Pearson/Addison Wesley, Boston.
5. Gibby, G.L., Paulus, D.A., Sirota, D.J., et al., 1997. Computerized pre-anesthetic evaluation results in additional abstracted comorbidity diagnoses. J Clin Monit 13, 35–41.
6. Kheterpal, S., Gupta, R., Blum, J.M., et al., 2007. Electronic reminders improve procedure documentation compliance and professional fee reimbursement. Anesth Analg 104, 592–597.
7. Kheterpal, S., Tremper, K.K., O'Reilly, M., et al., 2004. A perioperative information system: technical considerations and tradeoffs. Semin Anesth Perioper Med Pain 23, 125–132.
8. McKesson, E.I., 1934. The technique of recording the effects of gas-oxygen mixtures, pressures, rebreathing and carbon-dioxide, with a summary of the effects. Anesth Analg 13, 1–7.
9. Muravchick, S., Caldwell, J.E., Epstein, R.H., et al., 2008. Anesthesia information management system implementation: a practical guide. Anesth Analg 107, 1598–1608.
10. Lubarsky, D.A., Sanderson, I.C., Gilbert, W.C., et al., 1997. Using an anesthesia information management system as a cost containment tool. Description and validation. Anesthesiology 86, 1161–1169.
11. Monk, T.G., Sanderson, I., 2004. The development of an anesthesia lexicon. Semin Anesth Perioper Med Pain 23, 93–98.
12. O'Reilly, M., Talsma, A., VanRiper, S., et al., 2006. An anesthesia information system designed to provide physician-specific feedback improves timely administration of prophylactic antibiotics. Anesth Analg 103, 908–912.

13. Reich, D.L., Wood R.K., Jr., Mattar, R., et al., 2000. Arterial blood pressure and heart rate discrepancies between handwritten and computerized anesthesia records. Anesth Analg 91, 612–616.

14. Reich, D.L., Krol, M., 2004. Using AIMS data for quality improvement and research. Semin Anesth Perioper Med Pain 23, 99–103.

15. Spring, S.F., Sandberg, W.S., Anupama, S., et al., 2007. Automated documentation error detection and notification improves anesthesia billing performance. Anesthesiology 106, 157–163.

16. Stonemetz, J., Ball, M.J., Hannah, K.J., et al., 2009. Anesthesia informatics. Springer, New York.

17. Vigoda, M.M., Lubarsky, D.A., 2006. The medicolegal importance of enhancing timeliness of documentation when using an anesthesia information system and the response to automated feedback in an academic practice. Anesth Analg 103, 131–136.

18. Weinger, M.B., Herndon, O.W., Gaba, D.M., 1997. The effect of electronic record keeping and transesophageal echocardiography on task distribution, workload, and vigilance during cardiac anesthesia. Anesthesiology 87, 144–155, discussion 29A–30A.

19. Sandberg, W.S., Sandberg, E.H., Seim, A.R., Anupama, S., Ehrenfeld, J.M., Spring, S.F., Walsh, J.L., 2007. Real-time checking of electronic anesthesia records for documentation errors and automatically text messaging clinicians improves quality of documentation. Anesth Analgesia 106(1), 192–201.

20. Epstein, R.H., Dexter, F., Ehrenfeld, J.M., Sandberg, W.S., 2009. Implications of event latency on anesthesia information management decision support systems. Anesth Analgesia 108(3), 941–947.

21. Ehrenfeld, J.M., Sandberg, W.S., 2010. Managerial and clinical decision support in the digital operating room. Int. J. Comp. Assisted Radiol. Surgery 5(1), S194–S195.

Further Reading

Muravchick, S., Caldwell, J.E., Epstein, R.H., et al., 2008. Anesthesia information management system implementation: a practical guide. Anesth Analg 107, 1598–1608. *This is a readable peer-reviewed manuscript regarding the opportunities and challenges of AIMS implementation, written from a variety of viewpoints. By aggregating the implementation experiences of users of several different AIMS systems, this reading offers a more balanced and usable primer on implementation.*

Stonemetz, J., Ball, M.J., Hannah, K.J., et al., 2009. Anesthesia informatics. Springer, New York. *An authoritative and detailed book regarding business, technical, implementation, and clinical issues surrounding AIMS. Although sections are clearly geared toward a technical reader, most chapters are usable by anyone with a role in the AIMS purchase, decision making, implementation, research, or maintenance. The chapters are authored by experts in the field, and it offers a fresh, updated view of the state of the industry.*

Ehrenfeld, J.M. 2009. A guide to anesthesia information management systems. Anesthesiology news, Sept 35, 9.

Ehrenfeld, J.M., 2010. The impact of information management systems on anesthesia practice. Anesthesiol News 36 (Aug), 8.

Chapter 22

Pediatric Considerations

Rebecca N. Lintner and Robert S. Holzman

Specialized pediatric equipment is a recent phenomenon during the relatively short history of modern anesthesia. Parity of standards for pediatric and adult breathing systems was not established until 1963 by the American Society of Anesthesiologists and 1967 by the International Anesthesia Standards Committee.[1]

Intravenous Infusion Equipment

Intravenous (IV) infusions are started for almost all anesthetized children, with the occasional exception of very short procedures such as myringotomy and tube placement or selected examinations under anesthesia. Intravenous administration sets most useful for pediatric patients usually have a method of quantifying and limiting the amount of fluid delivered; graduated drip chamber IV sets ("Buritrol") are most commonly used. Pumps designed to deliver precise quantities of intravenous medications and provide continuous infusion for regional anesthesia are common in the pediatric operating room and are useful for total intravenous anesthesia techniques. Programmability of the pump for calculations in micrograms per kilograms per minute or conveniently available conversion tables are urged for practical daily use.

Intravenous filtering systems, whether for blood or air, should be readily available as the incidence of small ventricular septal defects or patency of the foramen ovale is not rare in the first year of life. Moreover, survivors of early cardiac surgery or children with palliated or unrepaired congenital heart disease with residual intracardiac communications may present for "routine" surgery. Small volume microaggregate filters have been developed but may lead to significant red cell destruction.[2,3]

Anesthetic Gas Delivery Systems

Breathing Circuits

The circle anesthesia system or variations of Ayre's T-piece[4] (Table 22–1) are the most common breathing circuits for pediatric patients (Figure 22–1). For years, variations of the T-piece were recommended for children weighing less than 10 kg because of the decreased resistance to spontaneous breathing, the better "feel" of the rebreathing bag in the hand of the anesthetist, and the faster anesthesia induction and emergence times at higher fresh gas flows. Improvements in machine components such as lower resistance valves, reduced dead space at connections, improved CO_2 absorbent canister design, and the availability of capnography and changes in philosophy favoring controlled pulmonary ventilation in small children have rendered these arguments less durable.[5,6] Likewise, less soluble inhalation agents such as sevoflurane make the influence of the breathing circuit less of an issue.

Normocarbia with a Mapleson breathing system is the result of a dynamic relationship between the fresh gas flow and the minute ventilation. When the fresh gas flow is high enough that rebreathing does not occur, the $Paco_2$ is determined by the minute ventilation. When the minute ventilation is significantly greater than the fresh gas flow, it is the fresh gas flow that becomes the principal determinant of the $Paco_2$.

Table 22-1 Comparison of Breathing Systems Useful in Pediatric Anesthesia

	Advantages	Disadvantages
Valveless, Variable F_ICO_2 Systems (Rebreathing and Non-Rebreathing)	1. Simplicity 2. Lightweight and non-bulky (minimizes drag on mask or endotracheal tube, and risk of extubation 3. Durable (no moving parts) 4. Rebreathing results in retention of heat and moisture; in co-axial systems, inspired gas is heated and humidified by warm expired gases.	1. Use of high fresh gas flows is wasteful, results in heat and humidity loss, increased pollution. 2. Optimum fresh gas flow may be difficult to confirm empirically; settings are best adjusted with end-tidal CO_2 or blood gas analysis. 3. Lowering of fresh gas flow is hazardous, as normocarbia is dependent on the relationship between fresh gas flow and minute ventilation. 4. Scavenging can be difficult with Mapleson systems with APL valve located near the patient. 5. Air dilution can occur with the Mapleson E (T-piece). 6. May not be suitable for patients with a dramatically increased minute CO_2 production, such as MH, or altered respiratory quotient.
Circle Systems (0 F_ICO_2 Systems with valves)	1. Low fresh gas flows (low flow anesthesia, closed circuit) can be used. 2. Normocarbia is a function of minute ventilation only, not fresh gas flow. 3. Is suitable for patients with a dramatically increased minute CO_2 production, such as MH, or altered hyperalimentation, or altered respiratory quotient	1. Complex construction composed of many parts that may (potentially) fail. 2. More difficult to clean. 3. Bulky, heavy system which may affect drag on mask and endotracheal tube, and may result in kinking or extubation if unsupported. 4. Minute volume must be carefully controlled to prevent hyperventilation.

Rapid respiratory rates may result in a higher F_IO_2 because of the decreased time available for fresh gas inflow to wash out alveolar gas from the expiratory limb of the breathing system. Fresh gas flow rates for controlled and spontaneous ventilation with or without rebreathing have been validated with this system.[7-11]

Bain and Spoerel's modification of the Mapleson D circuit[12] resulted in a coaxial breathing system with the fresh gas inflow hose within the exhalation limb. Verification of the integrity of the fresh gas inflow hose relies on the Pethick test,[13] when a distended rebreathing bag collapses because fresh gas flow in the inner tube creates a Venturi effect in the outer tube. The Pethick test is not foolproof because the turbulence created by the rapid flow from the oxygen flush valve may not result in an adequate Venturi effect, and the bag may not collapse.

Cold, anhydrous anesthetic gases delivered to a breathing circuit adversely affect mucociliary transport and contribute to a higher incidence of tracheal tube obstruction because of accumulated dried or thickened secretions. Controlled partial rebreathing in Mapleson D or Bain systems can achieve an airway humidity of 24 to 26 mg H_2O/L within 30 minutes[14] without the use of external humidifiers or heat and moisture exchangers. Another alternative is low flow or closed circuit anesthesia using the circle absorption system (see Chapter 4).

Alveolar ventilation is influenced by the compression volume of the breathing circuit in relation to the tidal volume of the patient. Breathing circuits with large compression volumes will be "ventilated" far in excess of the volume delivered to the patient, which can become a significant consideration for small infants. Many pediatric circle systems are not only shorter, but also have a smaller radius of curvature of the tubing, which, according to LaPlace's Law, renders them less distensible and thus further decreases compression volume.

Another important consideration for small children is the dead space of the breathing system. Dead space only exists when fresh and exhaled gases are mixed (i.e., at the Y-piece). Dead space no longer exists when fresh and exhaled gases are completely separated. The dead space of the Y-piece in a circle system can be decreased by the addition of a median septum (Figure 22–2). The dead space of an elbow in a Mapleson D system can be decreased by the addition of a fresh gas delivery port within the elbow, such as the Norman elbow (Figure 22–3).

Anesthesia Machines

There is no specific "pediatric" anesthesia machine; its design and checkout are identical whether used to anesthetize children or adults.[15] Many anesthesia machines are equipped to provide air or nitrogen through the addition of a compressed air flowmeter and cylinder yolk for those circumstances when nitrous oxide-oxygen mixtures or 100% oxygen are to be avoided, for example, when anesthetizing premature or expremature infants, for prolonged abdominal surgery or procedures with a higher risk of accidental air embolism such as craniofacial reconstruction.

The proper size rebreathing bag for children may be calculated as a volume approximately equal to the patient's vital capacity, or three times the tidal volume. The same calculation is applicable for the doubly open (Boothby-Lovelace-Bourbillion) rebreathing bags used on the Jackson-Rees modification of the Ayre's T-piece.

Anesthesia Ventilators

Current anesthesia machine ventilators are typically pneumatically and electronically powered, ascending bellows, time-cycled, constant flow, and electronically controlled. The lungs

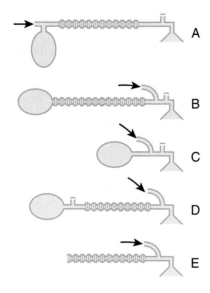

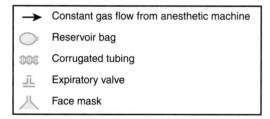

Figure 22–1 Mapleson's classification of the T-piece system.

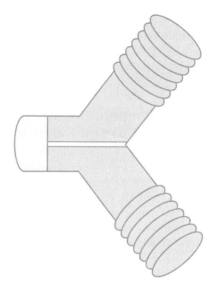

Figure 22–2 Median septum to functionally decrease the dead space in the Y-piece of a circle system.

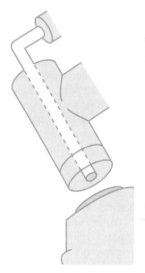

Figure 22–3 Norman elbow.

of most children can be ventilated very well with such ventilators, notwithstanding differences in compressible volume of the ventilator bellows and breathing circuit. The availability and skilled application of appropriate clinical and instrument monitoring are crucial. The use of a pediatric bellows (300 mL maximum tidal volume) will lessen the compression volume of the bellows itself (4.5 mL/cm H_2O compared with 1 to 2.5 mL/cm H_2O).[16]

Controlled ventilation is now much more precise for small patients. Machines now adjust for fresh gas flow and circuit compliance; recent models also allow sampling of the tidal volume measurement at the airway rather than at the expiratory valve, allowing for a better estimate of true tidal volume. Previously, tidal volume was usually measured at the expiratory valve. Thus the measured volume was not only the exhaled gas but also the gas compressed in the circuit during the previous inspiration.

Pediatric anesthesiologists have traditionally preferred pressure-controlled ventilation. Using a preset pressure and assessments such as $ETco_2$ and chest wall excursion, the anesthesiologist was assured of adequate ventilation with a reduced risk of barotrauma. Stayer et al found that flow generated on inspiration did not reach the set peak pressure when using short inspiratory times in a ventilator without constant pressure or piston-driven bellows.[17] In addition, changes in chest wall compliance can greatly influence delivered tidal volume during pressure controlled ventilation, therefore, close attention must be paid to changes in $ETco_2$ and chest wall excursion.

Newer ventilators adjust for fresh gas flow and circuit compliance. In Drager machines the fresh gas is not

continuously supplied during the expiration phase and is decoupled from the patient by a valve. Therefore, fresh gas flow does not influence the tidal volume during the inspiratory phase.[18] Additionally the Drager Apollo ventilator measures the compliance of the breathing circuit during the initial check and compensates for it so as to deliver accurate tidal volumes. The Aisys by General Electric also measures circuit compliance and allows for compensation during the initial check. Some older ventilator models such as the Datex-Ohmeda Smartvent and the GE Avance do not have circuit compliance compensation but allow for flow sensors at the inspiratory valve, thus offering better volume control and measurement. If the ventilator has a decoupling mechanism and circuit compliance compensation, the anesthesiologist should feel comfortable using volume-controlled ventilation since this newer generation of ventilators is less influenced by fresh gas flow and circuit compliance. For the compliance compensation to be accurate, however, machine checkout must occur with each new circuit placed on the machine. Even with the new advances, examination of chest wall excursion, $ETco_2$ and blood gas analysis remain the gold-standard tools for assessing the adequacy of pulmonary ventilation.

Temperature Control

Equipment for Temperature Monitoring
(also see chapter 19, patient warming devices)

Body temperature may be measured at a variety of sites. The skin temperature reflects the extent of peripheral perfusion rather than the core temperature. The temperature of the pulmonary artery's blood can generally be regarded as the core temperature, although even the pulmonary artery may not provide "accurate" core temperature measurements during a thoracotomy or a sternotomy, especially when cold cardioplegia solutions are administered. Also, during a rapid blood transfusion, the pulmonary artery's temperature may not reflect the core temperature of vital organs. Temperature measured at the distal third of the esophagus, the nasopharynx, and the tympanic membrane correlates well with pulmonary artery blood temperature. The temperature measured at the nasopharynx and tympanic membrane correlates well with temperature at the hypothalamus, and these measurements have special applicability during periods of decreased perfusion when induced hypothermia may be used protectively such as low-flow cardiopulmonary bypass and deep hypothermic circulatory arrest. The nasopharyngeal temperature is less accurate as a measure of brain temperature. The axilla may be a particularly important monitoring site for patients with suspected malignant hyperthermia because it drains blood from several large muscle masses. The rectal temperature is not as accurate a measure of a patient's core temperature as was once thought since the probe may be insulated by feces. Also, cooler blood returning from the patient's lower extremities may alter the measured rectal temperature. Conversely, heat-producing organisms in the gut may artifactually increase the rectal temperature. Sublingual sites are subject to the temperature-altering effects of the patient's respiratory gas flow and any liquids that have been consumed. Urinary temperature correlates well with the core temperature when the flow of urine is high, but when the flow of urine is low, the cool blood returning from the lower extremities may lower the temperature.

Maintenance of the Normothermic State
Thermostat Control of the Ambient Operating Room Temperature

A neutral thermal environment is that temperature range at which a patient's oxygen consumption and heat production at rest is minimal, yet the core temperature remains normal. As the environmental temperature decreases below this range, the body's homeothermic strategy is to increase oxygen consumption and produce heat. If the operating room can be warmed while anesthesia is being induced, it will limit redistribution hypothermia. The operating room may then be cooled once the patient is adequately covered with drapes and blankets and rewarmed at the procedure's end. When the operating room's temperature is greater than 21° C, most adult patients will not become hypothermic. Infants and neonates, however, may require ambient room temperatures that are higher, approximately 26° C, to remain normothermic.[19]

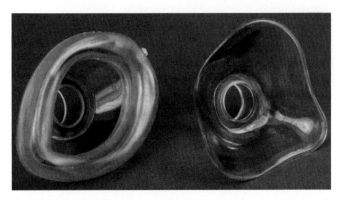

Figure 22–4 A cushioned face mask *(left)* and a Rendell-Baker-Soucek mask *(right)*. The decreased dead space of the Rendell-Baker-Soucek mask provides an advantage for infants and children who are breathing spontaneously, whereas a tight mask seal is more easily obtained with the cushioned mask.

Intravenous Fluid Warming

The infusion of cold intravenous fluids, blood, or blood components may contribute substantially to the development of hypothermia. The temperature drop attributable to such infusions depends upon the volume of the infusate, the size of the patient, the initial temperature of the patient and the infusate, and the time over which the infusion is administered.

In an effort to prevent hypothermia, blood may be warmed before rather than during a transfusion. This is referred to as *pretransfusion warming*. This may be accomplished by placing the blood in a temperature-regulated warm water bath, by mixing the blood with saline that has been brought to normal body temperature, by wrapping the blood in a temperature-controlled warm water mattress or warm air blanket, or by placing prefilled syringes in an infant incubator. These methods must be used with great caution since blood may be contaminated by pathogens or damaged by overheating. *In-line warming devices* heat the fluids by passing them through modified intravenous tubing placed in either a water bath or between two electrically heated metal plates. The degree of heat transfer to the fluid is dependent upon the fluid's flow rate, the initial fluid temperature, the warmer's temperature, and the heat transfer capabilities of the plastic bags and tubing. Some in-line warming devices improve the heat transfer by using a countercurrent mechanism. There is a risk of conducting an electrical current through the warming fluid's path when using water bath fluid warmers and so these devices should be properly isolated electrically. Dry-heat fluid warming devices consist of two heated plates through which a plastic bag of varying design is placed. The blood or other fluid to be infused runs through channels in the plastic bag, and heat is transferred to it from the metal plates.

The Prevention of Patient Heat Losses Via The Respiratory System: The Effect of the Breathing System

As water evaporates, cooling occurs. Such evaporative cooling of an anesthetized patient's airways may be prevented by the humidification of the inspired gases; however, this will have a minimal effect on the body temperature of an anesthetized adult or a large child. The major reason for warming and humidifying the inspired gases delivered to anesthetized patients is to prevent the desiccation of the airway's epithelium and the inspissation of secretions and to preserve normal mucociliary function. Since lower fresh gas flows may be used with a semiclosed circle anesthesia system rather than with the Mapleson system, heat and moisture may be better preserved in the former[20,21] (see Chapter 4).

Devices for Airway Heating and Humidification

Active Airway Warming Systems

The active heating and humidification of respiratory gases may not prevent cooling of an adult patient's body, but there may be an advantage to such heating for preserving normothermia in small infants and neonates.[22] However, anesthesia circuit leaks, inadvertent hyperthermia, and bacterial contamination concerns have made kettle type of heating systems largely obsolete.

Passive Airway Warming and Humidification Systems

Passive airway warming and humidification systems are variously referred to generically as "heat and moisture exchangers" (HMEs) or "artificial noses" and are constructed of materials such as wool, foam, or methylcellulose, which are usually contained within a clear plastic cylinder. Condensation of expired water vapor occurs as the exhaled, humidified gases contact the cooler membrane's surface. As the water vapor changes its phase from a gas to a liquid, heat is transferred to the membrane's surface. During the subsequent respiratory cycle, the heat is transferred from the membrane to the inspiratory gas, vaporizing the water. The result is the partial conservation of the heat and moisture of the patient's respiratory gases. For maximum efficiency, passive airway heating and humidification devices should be inserted while the patient is still relatively warm.

The Use of Blankets for Passive Patient Warming

Ordinary cloth blankets provide a means of passive thermal protection for patients by decreasing radiative and convective heat losses. Furthermore, they may reduce conductive heat losses if placed between the patient and a colder surface such as the operating room table. The effectiveness of a blanket in the prevention of a patient's heat loss is directly proportional to the amount of the body's surface area that is covered. An important strategy in conserving a child's body heat is to cover the head with a blanket or a hat since the head may account for as much as 50% of the body's total heat loss.[23,24] If a hat is placed on a patient's head, however, care must be taken to assure that the nares and mouth are not covered since exhaled gases may accumulate under the hat if a cuffless endotracheal tube is used. The accumulation of gases, such as oxygen and nitrous oxide that support combustion, under plastic or paper drapes, may increase the risk of a catastrophic fire, especially if lasers are used.

Blankets for Active Patient Warming

Thermal water mattresses may be used to either warm or cool a patient. They may be helpful in cooling a patient who has been inadvertently overheated, is febrile, or has developed malignant hyperthermia. For the maintenance of a patient's body temperature, heated water mattresses are usually set to a temperature of 38° to 40° C. Heating blankets are most effective when they are placed on *top* of the patient where they can decrease convective heat losses. Burns may occur if a heating blanket is left in contact with the patient's skin for a prolonged period of time, especially if there is poor blood flow to that area of skin. A layer of protective cloth, such as a cloth blanket or a sheet, should be used to diffuse the heat and to insulate the patient from direct contact with the warming element.

Forced-Air Convective Patient Heating Systems

Forced-hot-air convection is the most effective way of preventing the heat losses of an anesthetized patient. These devices can also effectively transfer heat and warm a hypothermic patient. The heat is initially transferred convectively from the air to the surface of the body, and then to the core by the patient's own blood flow. The blanket is composed of polyethylene bonded to a tissue paper laminate. The warm air circulates in tubes formed by the interface of the plastic and paper. The tissue paper laminate contains slits through which the heated air may escape. A thermostat controls the temperature of the heated air circulating in a forced air patient heater. A forced air patient warming device can also be used to cool a patient by directing ambient operating room air over the patient at a high flow rate. Burns are rare with these devices, nevertheless, care should be taken to prevent the wrong side of the heating blanket from contacting the patient. Also, if the perfusion of the skin is limited (such as in a hypovolemic patient or a patient with minimal subcutaneous tissue), the heat may not be adequately dissipated. Heavy blankets should not be placed on top of a forced-air heating device's covers since they may direct a jet of warmed air into direct contact with the patient's skin.

Radiative Patient-Warming Devices

Infrared radiation is helpful when the patient is undraped, during the surgical preparation and the emergence from anesthesia. In the postanesthesia care unit, radiative heaters may also reduce shivering. Care must be taken to prevent burns by keeping the heating element at least three feet from the patient. Radiative heating lamps should be kept clear of plastic intravenous fluid bags and other combustible materials.

Noninvasive Monitoring

Precordial and Esophageal Stethoscopes

Stethoscopy remains the simplest, least expensive, and most risk-free monitoring method for the cardiorespiratory system. Proper placement of the chest stethoscope over the precordium reveals the regularity of the heart rate, presence and intensity of heart tones and murmurs, and confirms the presence and quality of breath sounds. An irregular heart rate, air embolism, right mainstem intubation, or abnormal breath sounds may also be appreciated. As a monitoring device during induction, much has been made of heart tone assessment through progressive levels of anesthetic depth. Experienced pediatric anesthetists tend to favor this qualitative method, although quantitatively, changes in heart tones may not be appreciable until over a 50% reduction in cardiac output has occurred.[25,26] Similarly, the presence of breath sounds does not quantitate the adequacy of gas exchange like a pulse oximeter or a capnograph. Furthermore, "ventilation" via the esophagus in children may very well sound like breath sounds when chest auscultation is performed.[27-29]

Electrocardiography

Infants, especially neonates, tolerate bradycardia poorly because of the limited stroke volume response to changes in heart rate. Although tachycardia is generally tolerated much better, it may also be a significant indicator of hypovolemia. The diagnostic evaluation of rapid or slow heart rates must also include variable degrees of heart block, supraventricular or ventricular tachycardias, and pre-excitation syndromes such as the Wolff-Parkinson-White syndrome or the persistence of fetal and neonatal accessory conduction pathways. Rarely, electrolyte disturbances such as potassium and calcium abnormalities may also be detected by ECG analysis. Patients with congenital heart disease may show ischemia.[30] For these reasons, the ECG must always be displayed during pediatric anesthesia.

Noninvasive Blood Pressure

An automatic blood pressure apparatus compares two sequential cardiac cycles, with the averaged pairs of oscillations analyzed to produce the displayed systolic, diastolic, and mean arterial pressure. Errors can arise due to patient movement, irregularities of heart rhythm, or external influences such as extrinsic compression of the cuff by operating room personnel. If these events occur, then cardiac cycles continue to repeat, prolonging the determination until two comparable cycles are recorded at a given inflation pressure. This may result in discomfort in awake children or microvascular injury in anesthetized children. In general, the width of the cuff bladder should be 0.4 to 0.5 times the circumference or 120% of the diameter of the extremity. The length of the bladder should be at least twice the width of the extremity.[31-33] As a practical solution, we apply the largest cuff that will fit the blood pressure measuring site, typically the upper arm.

Pulse Oximetry

Pulse oximetry has become a standard of practice and is arguably the most important safety monitor currently. Pulse oximeters rarely function well in the active, nonanesthetized small child because motion artifacts prevent the accurate determination of pulsatile blood flow. Undue delay of an anesthetic induction while waiting for a "baseline" may, however, make the child more anxious. Therefore, these monitors should be placed during or following anesthetic induction in extremely anxious and upset preschool children.

The pulse oximeters in clinical use in the operating room measure functional saturation (the percentage of oxyhemoglobin in relation to the sum of oxyhemoglobin and deoxyhemoglobin), but they do not measure abnormal hemoglobins such as carboxyhemoglobin or methemoglobin. Fetal hemoglobin,

skin color, and bilirubin or tissue thickness do not usually affect pulse oximeters. Because of their absorbance properties, intravenously administered dyes such as methylene blue and indocyanine green can cause errors in pulse oximeter readings. Care should be exercised in pulse oximeter probe placement when the ductus arteriosus is still patent. If the measured oxyhemoglobin saturation is intended to approximate cerebral oxygenation, then *preductal* placement (i.e., right hand or ears) is desirable. *Postductal* placement of the oximeter probe in a neonate will reflect oxygen saturation delivered to tissues distal to the ductus arteriosus and may be extremely helpful as a guide to persistent pulmonary hypertension of the newborn.

Many clinicians choose to reuse the disposable probes, but caution applies as such reuse may result in fatigue of the thin light-emitting diode wires, which may in turn cause an electrical shock or burn to the patient. The mismatching of a probe and an oximeter unit from different manufacturers may also result in a burn.[34]

Ultrasound Technology (also see Chapter 15, Ultrasound and Fluroscopy for Regional and Vascular Access)

Ultrasound technology is emerging as an important technique for pediatric line placement and regional block. The ability to visualize the internal jugular or subclavian vein for central line placement decreases the number of attempts and the risk of arterial puncture. When used for regional blocks, ultrasound allows visualization of the nerve sheath, showing the spread of local anesthetic and safe injection. Previous block techniques using a nerve stimulator did not allow for such accuracy and comprehensiveness.

Transcranial Doppler cerebral blood flow measurement is an evolving technology, which has been used to examine the relationship of cerebral perfusion to cardiopulmonary bypass, particularly for circulatory arrest techniques in small infants and the putative effect of various anesthetics on the cerebral circulation in children. Venous air embolism has been detected with regularity during craniectomies in infants undergoing craniosynostosis surgery and liver transplantation, and a posterior chest wall Doppler probe can be effective for venous air embolism monitoring in infants.[35] Moreover, transthoracic, transesophageal, and intraoperative epicardial echocardiography have made important contributions to the evaluation of the adequacy of surgical repair and the detection of occult cardiac anomalies before definitive repair.

Invasive Monitoring

More frequent use of invasive cardiovascular monitoring has been a major trend in the care of high-risk children over the last 20 years. The response time is particularly important for producing pressure wave fidelity in patients with rapid heart rates, like children. Low dead space noncompliant tubing is best for measuring physiological pressure signals.

Intraarterial Monitoring

Twenty-four gauge catheters are available for cannulating the peripheral arteries of small infants or children, otherwise, 22-gauge or 20-gauge catheters are used. Technical concerns important in pediatrics include familiarity with the normal range of blood pressures and an understanding of alternative insertion sites in addition to the radial artery. These sites include the dorsalis pedis or posterior tibial arteries, the femoral or axillary arteries, and the umbilical artery. In this case, the location of the catheter tip should either be high (above the diaphragm) or low (level of L3 or below) to avoid flushing into the renal circulation, with the catheter location confirmed before the anesthetic. Nevertheless, complications are rarely associated with umbilical arterial catheters. Special considerations that may influence the site of the arterial catheter's placement include children who have a patent ductus arteriosus or coarctation of the aorta, or those who have undergone a Blalock-Taussig shunt with compromise of the ipsilateral subclavian artery.

Central Venous Pressure

The technique used for central access in children does not vary much from that used for an adult; "high" and "low" approaches in the neck have both been advocated. The internal jugular vein is generally encountered in a more cephalad position in infants. Rao suggested a "low" approach (supraclavicular at the level of the sternoclavicular joint) based on the more predictable central venous anatomy that occurs the closer one gets to the central circulation.[36] J-wire techniques, similar to those used for adults, can also be used, although the internal jugular vein is often more predictably cannulated than the external jugular vein. In general, the internal jugular vein is preferred for short term monitoring and for cardiac surgery whereas for prolonged use (chemotherapy, parenteral alimentation), the subclavian approach with tunneling is preferred because of increased security, patient comfort, and a lower infection rate.

Femoral vein cannulation is another route frequently chosen for central or emergency access in children because of the predictable bony anatomic landmarks of the pubic tubercle and the anterior superior iliac spine and its location medial to the femoral artery. In the operating room the main concern about femoral lines is their lack of intraoperative visibility.

Umbilical central venous cannulation is usually accomplished by the neonatologist, in which case preoperative confirmation of the catheter's location is important. Catheter tip location within the liver may be associated with portal vein thrombosis or hepatic necrosis. The umbilical catheter is only for short-term use or as a temporary measure until adequate peripheral or central access is established.

Pulmonary Artery Pressure

Pulmonary artery catheters are infrequently placed in children due to the relative health of their coronary circulation. Exceptions include children with known coronary insufficiency or anomalous coronary arteries, cardiomyopathy, or storage diseases due to inborn errors of metabolism. Other candidates for pulmonary artery catheters include children who have pulmonary hypertension as a primary problem or secondary to severe cardiac or respiratory dysfunction with cor pulmonale and/or right heart failure. Balloon flotation pulmonary artery catheters may not "float" with the same efficiency in children with lower cardiac outputs, and fluoroscopic guidance may be needed. Patients with repaired or unrepaired congenital heart disease should be approached with caution; an aberrant pulmonary artery catheter course or incorrect interpretation of data may result. Such children should have pulmonary artery catheters inserted only under fluoroscopic guidance, preferably in conjunction with a pediatric cardiologist.

Transesophageal Echocardiography

Although used mainly during cardiac surgery to evaluate abnormal anatomy or the adequacy of the surgical reconstruction, there is little doubt that the use of transesophageal echocardiography (TEE) will increase inside and outside the cardiac operating rooms in a fashion analogous to adult anesthetic practice. The biplane TEE is now available with an infant probe; the adult probe can be used in children greater than 10 to 12 kg. Intracardiac air can be recognized easily by TEE. A prior history of esophageal atresia with tracheoesophageal fistula or a reconstructed esophagus may contraindicate the use of a transesophageal probe.

Routine and Special Airway Equipment

Mask

As a rough guide, the tidal volume of infants and children is approximately 6 mL/kg or three times the dead space, a ratio similar to that of adults. The tidal volume of a spontaneously breathing 6-month-old is therefore approximately 45 mL. Because available cushion-seal masks have dead spaces from 50 to 80 mL, physiological dead space may increase dramatically. The anesthetist's fingers must not depress the submental tissue in small children as the tongue will be forced against the hard and soft palate and may produce upper airway obstruction. Although the faces of most infants are similar with regard to mask fit, children with craniofacial anomalies such as Apert and Crouzon syndromes, choanal atresia, or more severe forms of frontonasal dysplasia may present special challenges for obtaining a good mask seal. The mask fit in these patients may be considerably more difficult than the laryngoscopy or tracheal intubation, as their branchial arches tend to develop normally. Occasionally, children with midface hypoplasia should have their cheeks supported by dental rolls placed between the gingiva and buccal mucosa.

Oral Airway

Oropharyngeal airways should be available in the full range of sizes. An oral airway that is too small will displace the base of the tongue inferiorly toward the pharynx whereas an airway that is too large may reach to the laryngeal inlet and cause trauma and/or laryngeal hyperactivity and laryngospasm. Correct airway size can be assessed by a careful external examination of the child and estimation of the distance from the teeth to the base of the tongue. Although it is now common practice to insert an oral airway convex to the tongue surface ("upside down") and then rotate it, one should recognize that this maneuver may scrape the hard palate, traumatize the tonsils and/or adenoids, and push the tongue caudally. A less traumatic alternative is to use a tongue depressor to displace the tongue to the floor of the mouth, and then insert the oral airway with its concave side to the tongue surface. Oral airways are often used as "bite blocks" to prevent the clenching of teeth on the endotracheal tube. Such a practice is a particular hazard in children between 5 and 10 years of age who may have loose deciduous teeth. Oral airways are responsible for up to 55% of dental complications.[37] Furthermore, an oral airway used as a bite block in long cases may cause tongue necrosis or edema, uvular edema, or lip damage. A dental roll placed between the upper and lower molars will also prevent clenching while minimizing dental trauma.

Nasal Airway

Nasopharyngeal airways are generally constructed from red rubber or polyvinyl chloride and are available in various sizes. They may be softened in warm water, lubricated with water-soluble or lidocaine jelly, and gently inserted transnasally. However, nasal airways may traumatize the turbinates or adenoids of young children. Also, care must be exercised when using nasopharyngeal airways in children with a bleeding diathesis or congenital abnormalities of the midface such as choanal atresia or frontonasal dysplasia. The appropriate length for the nasopharyngeal airway may be estimated from the distance between the auditory meatus to the tip of the nose and the size of the airway may be estimated from the calculated endotracheal tube size converted to French size (approximately the internal diameter in millimeters multiplied by four, or the external diameter in millimeters multiplied by three).

Laryngeal Mask Airway (LMA)

Although originally thought that pediatric-sized laryngeal mask airways (LMA) might not function adequately due to differences in airway anatomy, this fear proved to be unfounded (see Table 22–2). The No. 1 LMA, which is a miniaturized version of the adult LMA, was designed to fit small infants until they reached a weight of 6.5 kg. It has worked satisfactorily even in premature infants of 1 kg, in newborn resuscitation, and in airway maintenance for infants with upper airway congenital anomalies (e.g., Pierre-Robin, Goldenhar, Treacher Collins, and Schwartz-Jampel syndromes). In these difficult intubating conditions, it has been used throughout the whole procedure or as a conduit for endotracheal intubation. Frequently, the endotracheal tube can be easily directed through an LMA without fiberoptic laryngoscopy.

Flexible LMAs in sizes 2, 2.5, and 3 are also available for pediatric use. The cuff is similar to a standard LMA but the airway tube is wire-reinforced, longer, and more flexible—allowing it to be positioned away from the surgical field. Although the flexibility of the tube is advantageous for positioning, it is more difficult to insert, may dislodge more easily, and biting can occlude it. Moreover, the flexibility of this LMA does not allow the rotation technique for insertion. Adenoidectomy or even tonsillectomy can be performed with the flexible LMA as the cuff prevents soiling of the glottis and the trachea by blood and secretions from above. If tracheal intubation is planned via a LMA, a standard LMA is a more logical choice in children because it is shorter and has a larger diameter, whereas in adolescents or adults, the intubating LMA (Fastrach) can be used.

Table 22–2 **Recommended LMA Size**	
Size 1	Neonates and infants up to 5 kg
Size 1.5	Infants 5-10 kg
Size 2	Children 20-30 kg
Size 2.5	Children 20-30 kg
Size 3	Adolescents more than 30 kg and young adults

Endotracheal Tube

The majority of pediatric airway management involves endotracheal intubation. Polyvinylchloride remains the most popular material for endotracheal tubes, although other materials continue to be used and newer technologies are evolving. For example, Weiss et al have reexamined design requirements of pediatric endotracheal tubes, including cuff placement below the cricoid cartilage, thus requiring a smaller, more distally placed cuff. Among other features, with polyurethane replacing the polyvinylchloride cuff, the sealing pressures for children are in the range of 6 to 14 cm H_2O.

Estimates of the appropriate endotracheal tube size and length for pediatric patients are given in Table 22–3. The formulas are based either on age or direct examination of the patient. When selecting endotracheal tubes for children, one should keep in mind that the presence of a deflated cuff adds about 0.5 mm to the tube's external diameter. In addition, since nitrous oxide enters the closed air space of a cuff when the valve on the pilot tube is competent, the intracuff pressure should be monitored and maintained at less than 25 mm Hg, or the valve should be rendered incompetent during long cases. A variety of endotracheal tubes are available for special needs, including preformed nasal (for oral surgery and dental restorations) and angled oral (Ring-Adair-Elwyn or RAE) endotracheal tubes. Wire-reinforced or anode tubes may be particularly useful for head and neck surgery cases.

Since Koka's seminal report, an air leak around an endotracheal tube has been strongly advocated for the prevention of postintubation croup in infants and children less than 10 years of age.[39] Clinicians' abilities to recognize an air leak are variable, but if a cuffless tube is chosen, a reasonable leak (between 20 and 30 cm H_2O) should be maintained following endotracheal intubation to minimize the risk of postintubation croup, atmospheric pollution, or failure of the ventilated volume to return through the exhalation limb of the breathing circuit. Cuffed endotracheal tubes are advantageous for certain abdominal or thoracic procedures, and patients with pulmonary pathology who have poor lung compliance. Accordingly, the use of a cuffed endotracheal tube should be individualized. Children easily susceptible to croup during viral illnesses of the respiratory tract may benefit from tracheal intubation with a smaller tube, as long as the lungs can be ventilated adequately.

Endotracheal tubes are available with and without a hole in the wall opposite the bevel. Those without the hole are known as Magill tubes whereas those with the hole (the Murphy eye) are called Murphy tubes. The Murphy eye was originally designed to provide an alternate pathway for gas flow if the end-hole of the endotracheal tube was occluded. There are potential disadvantages of the Murphy eye, however, including a tendency for the accumulation of secretions and impaired passage of stylets, catheters, and bronchoscopes. If such an

Table 22–3 Calculations for Endotracheal Tube Size and Length for Pediatric Patients

Age	Weight (kg)	ID (mm)	Length (OT) (cm)	Length (NT) (cm)
Premature	<1	2.5	7-8	9
Premature	1-2.5	3	8-9	9-10
Newborn	2.5-3.5	3	9-10	11-12
3 m	3.5-5	3.5	10-11	12
3-9 m	5-8	3.5-4	11-12	13-14
9-18 m	8-11	4-4.5	12-13	14-15
1.5-3 yr	11-15	4.5-5	12-14	16-17
4-5 yr	15-18	5-5.5	14-16	18-19
6-7 yr	19-23	5.5-6	16-18	19-20
8-10 yr	24-30	6-6.5	17-19	21-23
10-11 yr	30-35	6-6.5	18-20	22-24
12-13 yr	35-40	6.5-7	19-21	23-25
14-16 yr	45-55	7-7.5	20-22	24-25

ID, Internal diameter; OT, orotracheal tube; NT, nasotracheal tube.
Table adapted from Motoyama EK. *Smith's anesthesia for infants and children,* St Louis, Mosby, 1990.
Calculations for estimating the ID of an endotracheal tube:
$\frac{16 + age\ (yr)}{4}$ (from reference (44))
(Patient age (yr)/4) + 4 (from reference (45))
The diameter of the fifth finger
Calculations for estimating the length required for an orotracheal tube:
Height (cm)/10 + 5 (from reference (46))
Weight (kg)/5 + 12
Advance the endotracheal tube 30 times the internal diameter from the alveolar ridge (228)
(Patient age (yr)/2) + 12 (from reference (44))
Insert the endotracheal tube to the first or second black line marked on tube
Advance the endotracheal tube into a bronchus, then withdraw it, 2 cm (not recommended for routine cases)

object becomes stuck in the Murphy eye, the entire assembly may have to be removed, resulting in unnecessary extubation. Nevertheless, we tend to use endotracheal tubes equipped with a Murphy eye in our patients, favoring the notion (particularly in small tube sizes) that blood and secretions potentially obstructing the end-hole of the tube pose a greater risk.

Stylets are frequently used to provide rigidity and malleability for endotracheal tubes, particularly in infant sizes when the walls of the tube are thinner than in adult sizes. However, the increased rigidity provided by a stylet can result in greater tissue trauma. Stylets should be properly sized for each endotracheal tube, and well lubricated so that they slide easily no matter how the endotracheal tube is bent.

Laryngoscopes

Most standard laryngoscope blades are available in sizes for premature infants (00), neonates (0), infants (1), children (2), and small (3) and large (4) adults. However, many of the specialty blades are not. Due to the anatomic characteristics of the pediatric airway, straight blades (with tip deflection) of a C/D-shaped cross-sectional design are traditionally preferred over curved blades in neonates, infants, and preschool-age children.

Rigid Fiberoptic Laryngoscope—The Bullard Laryngoscope

The Bullard laryngoscope (Figure 22–5) is a rigid curved blade available in neonatal, pediatric, and adult sizes. A working channel and two fiberoptic bundles for lighting and

viewing are integrated into the blade. A stylet is mounted on the laryngoscope, parallel to the blade. The working channel is useful for oxygen insufflation during intubation of the trachea in a spontaneously breathing patient. To insert the laryngoscope, it is held parallel to the body axis and the tip of the blade is guided into the mouth. The curve of the blade is rolled around the tongue along the palate and pharynx through an angle of approximately 90 degrees until the handle is perpendicular to the body axis. At that time, the tip of the blade lies posterior to the tongue and along the laryngeal side of the epiglottis. Mild vertical pull is exerted on the laryngoscope, at which time the glottis can usually be seen through the fiberoptic bundle.

Anterior Commissure Laryngoscope

Anterior commissure laryngoscopes require a fiberoptic external light source. In addition, thin, long (e.g., bronchoscopy) forceps need to be available. The 15-mm connector is removed from the endotracheal tube, and the laryngoscope is inserted. With the epiglottis lifted directly from the laryngeal surface, the tip of the laryngoscope should be placed at the glottic opening. The endotracheal tube is inserted through the tubular laryngoscope blade. Although direct visualization of the glottis is usually lost at this point, correct positioning and the tubular structure of the blade safely guide the tube into the trachea. Using the forceps, the tube is held in place while the laryngoscope is removed over the tube and forceps (Figure 22–6). The endotracheal tube connector is then replaced and the tube position verified.

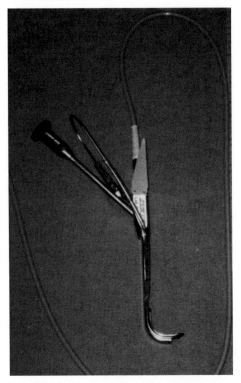

Figure 22–5   Pediatric Bullard laryngoscope.

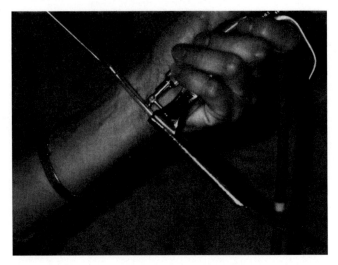

Figure 22–6   Infant anterior commissure laryngoscope. After inserting the endotracheal tube through the anterior commissure laryngoscope into the trachea, the laryngoscope is removed over the tube while holding the tube with a long pair of forceps.

Fiberoptic Laryngoscopy and Bronchoscopy

The flexible fiberoptic laryngoscope or bronchoscope may be used to evaluate the upper or lower airway, verify or guide endobronchial tube placement, aspirate secretions, or facilitate intubation of the trachea for those patients who cannot be intubated with conventional laryngoscopy. Pediatric fiberscopes are generally smaller than adult fiberscopes and not all fiberscopes in small sizes are designed for biopsies, suctioning, or insufflation. They may also be limited in tip excursion in comparison to larger scopes. Many pediatric fiberoptic tracheal intubations are done with volatile anesthetics, allowing the patient to breathe spontaneously. In such cases, a Patil-Syracuse or a similarly designed mask with a grommet through which a fiberoptic laryngoscope may be passed is very useful. Ultrathin fiberscopes can accommodate an endotracheal tube to 2.5-mm inner diameter, and their use compares favorably with standard laryngoscopy.

The Lighted Stylet and Other Techniques

The lightwand, or lighted stylet, now manufactured in smaller sizes, is a useful device for the difficult pediatric airway. It is best used in the spontaneously breathing patient, either sedated with topical anesthetic or anesthetized but breathing spontaneously with deep inhalation anesthetic. Patients whose tracheas were found extremely difficult to intubate by conventional means were intubated without difficulty using the lighted stylet.[40] The pediatric optical telescope, typically inserted through a rigid bronchoscope for examination of the airway, may also be used for difficult intubations. An endotracheal tube is threaded over the telescope, and with the aid of a laryngoscope to visualize the base of the tongue and as much of the larynx as possible, the optical telescope may be used (through either direct vision or by connection to a video

monitor) to visualize the larynx. The endotracheal tube is then advanced into the trachea. Further advances in optical stylets include the Bonfils Retromolar Intubation Fiberscope (Karl Storz Endoscopy, Culver City, Calif.), the Shikani Optic Stylet (Clarus Medical LLC, Minneapolis), the StyletScope (Nihon Kohden Corp., Tokyo) the Video Optical Intubation Stylet (VOIS, Acutronic Medical Systems AG, Baar, Switzerland), and the Levitan FPS Scope (Clarus Medical LLC, Minneapolis). The Bonfils is a nonmalleable scope while the Shikani has a distally malleable stylet. It can accommodate a size 2.5 endotracheal tube in its pediatric version.

Rigid video laryngoscopes display an image of the larynx in the eyepiece or on a video screen mounted on the handle or displayed remotely. Rigid laryngoscopes without an endotracheal tube guide have the advantage that the endoscopist does not have to align the axes of the scope and the trachea to advance the endotracheal tube. Those laryngoscopes now being introduced into pediatric practice include the Glidescope (Verathon, Inc., Bothell, Wash.). Because the larynx is not in the line-of-sight, the Glidescope should be used with a stylet. In addition, the technique is different than that used for conventional laryngoscopy, in that the approach is in the midline and the larynx is not viewed directly transorally but rather on the video screen display. Antifogging solutions are not required because a charge-coupled video chip covered by a heated glass window is incorporated into the blade, making it fog resistant.

Respiratory Gas Monitoring

The ASA's Standard for Basic Anesthetic Monitoring mandates the use of continual monitoring of expired carbon dioxide. Artifactual widening of the alveolar-arterial CO_2 (A-aCO_2) gradient is a particular problem with children because of the use of uncuffed endotracheal tubes and aspiration flow rates that may exceed the maximum expiratory flow rate of the patient. The accuracy of ETCO_2 measurements depends on the respiratory frequency (f), variations in the aspiration flow rate, the sampling site (whether distal or proximal airway), and the type of capnometer. As f increases in both aspiration and flow-through systems, measured values of inspired CO_2 increase in the Bain and circle breathing systems. The $ETCO_2$ decreases as f increases in circle anesthesia systems, but it remains constant in Bain systems. Parabolic distortion of CO_2 "plugs" traversing long-sampling catheters probably makes up a significant percentage (8% to 36%) of the elevated baseline in aspiration capnography, depending on f and breathing circuit type.[41] In patients less than 6 kg, differences have been found in the accuracy of $ETCO_2$ measurement at the distal end of the endotracheal tube compared with the proximal end, the proximal sidestream connector, and the Y-piece of the ventilator. Alterations in tidal volume made less of a difference than alterations in respiratory rate in comparing $ETCO_2$ to capillary CO_2.

The flow rate for gas sampling in children should not be reduced out of concern for the volume aspirated. A faster sampling rate *enhances* the accuracy of measurement because the response time is decreased, and at higher respiratory rates, an artifactually lower $ETCO_2$ and higher inspired CO_2 is avoided. Strategies that enhance the accuracy of capnography in children include a fast sampling rate and distal airway sampling.

The dilution of exhaled gases with fresh gas devoid of CO_2 may occur while using high flows in nonrebreathing systems such as the Mapleson D, Jackson-Rees modification of Ayre's T and the Bain circuit. The degree of dilution depends on the relationship between the fresh gas flow rate, the aspiration sampling rate, and the expiratory flow rate of the patient. Sample dilution may also be seen when endotracheal tubes in small children have a very low leak (i.e., <10 cm H_2O) because exhaled gas is preferentially vented around the endotracheal tube rather than through its lumen. Sampling within the endotracheal tube or at the endotracheal tube connector generally helps with this problem. Although sampling within the tracheal tube has the advantage of better accuracy, the sampling port can easily become obstructed by secretions or humidity.

$ETCO_2$ measurements for children with cyanotic congenital heart disease tend to be lower in the presence of reduced pulmonary blood flow or right-to-left shunts. The $A-aCO_2$ gradient will be wider in these cases. The $ETCO_2$-$PaCO_2$ differences measured in children with acyanotic-shunting and mixing congenital heart lesions are stable intraoperatively, although patients with mixing lesions may demonstrate large individual variations. In children with cyanotic-shunting congenital heart lesions, the $ETCO_2$-$PaCO_2$ gradient is not stable, and $ETCO_2$ cannot be used to reliably estimate the $PaCO_2$.[42] This may also be true for children with pulmonary disease, in whom the large differences between $PaCO_2$ and $ETCO_2$ are comparable to those observed in children with cyanotic congenital heart disease.[43]

The interpretation of the capnograph waveform is generally reliable although there are several specific situations worth special mention. First of all, when using a cuffless endotracheal tube with a leak, an incomplete, nonsquare wave capnograph trace may be produced. In addition, pediatric patients, when ventilated with nonrebreathing systems at partial rebreathing flows will demonstrate a double hump (rebreathing CO_2 and $ETCO_2$) on the capnograph trace, with an elevated baseline. Thirdly, respiratory rate, frequently higher in pediatric patients, may result in baseline elevation of the $FICO_2$. Finally, the maximum expiratory flow rate of the patient may be far less than the sampling flow rate of the capnography system; therefore the patient's $ETCO_2$ will have a tendency to be washed out and artifactually lowered. This can be compensated for by

large, tidal breaths, a throat pack to seal the escaping patient gases around the endotracheal tube, intratracheal sampling with a thin catheter, proximal airway sampling at the 15-mm connector, or a decrease in respiratory rate.

This chapter has considered routinely used equipment from the "pediatric" point of view and some specific equipment modifications uniquely suited to infants and children. For the occasional practitioner of pediatric anesthesia, consistency, familiarity with the equipment used daily, and constant vigilance are probably the key features for safety.

References

1. Rendell-Baker, L., 1992. History and evolution of pediatric anesthesia equipment. In: Pullerits, J., Holzman, R. (Eds.), Anesthesia equipment for infants and children, Little, Brown, Boston.
2. Longhurst, D.M., Gooch, W.M., Castillo, R.A., 1983. In vitro evaluation of a pediatric microaggregate blood filter. Transfusion 23, 170–172.
3. Schmidt, W.F., Kim, H.C., Tomassini, N., et al., 1982. RBC destruction caused by a micropore blood filter. JAMA 248, 1629–1632.
4. Mapleson, W.W., 1954. The elimination of rebreathing in various semiclosed anesthetic systems. Br J Anaesth 26, 323–332.
5. Ledbetter, J.L., Rasch, D.K., Pollard, T.G., et al., 1988. Reducing the risks of laryngoscopy in anaesthetised infant. Anaesthesia 43, 151–153.
6. Spears, R.S., Yeh, A., Fisher, D.M., et al., 1991. The "educated hand": Can anesthesiologists assess changes in neonatal pulmonary compliance manually? Anesthesiology 75, 693–696.
7. Bain, J.A., Spoerel, W.E., 1973. Flow requirements for a modified Mapleson D system during controlled ventilation. Can Anaesth Soc J 20, 629–636.
8. Bain, J.A., Spoerel, W.E., 1975. Prediction of arterial carbon dioxide tension during controlled ventilation with a modified Mapleson D system. Can Anaesth Soc J 22, 34–38.
9. Bain, J.A., Spoerel, W.E., 1977. Carbon dioxide output and elimination in children under anaesthesia. Can Anaesth Soc J 24, 533–539.
10. Jonsson, L.O., Bain, J.A., Lese, R., 1990. Predicted normocapnia in infants and children using the Bain circuit with controlled ventilation. Acta Anaesthesiol Scand 34, 257–262.
11. Spoerel, W.E., Aitken, R.R., Bain, J.A., 1978. Spontaneous respiration with the Bain breathing circuit. Can Anaesth Soc J 25, 30–35.
12. Bain, J.A., Spoerel, W.E., 1972. A streamlined anaesthetic system. Can Anaesth Soc J 19, 426–435.
13. Pethick, S., 1975. Letters to the Editors. Can Anaesth Soc J 22, 115.
14. Rayburn, R.L., Watson, R.L., 1980. Humidity in children and adults using the controlled partial rebreathing anesthesia method. Anesthesiology 52, 291–295.
15. Morrison, J.L., 1993. FDA anesthesia apparatus checkout recommendations. Newsl Am Soc Anesthesiol 1994, 25–26.
16. Binda, R.E.J., Cook, D.R., Fischer, C.G., 1976. Advantages of infant ventilators over adapted adult ventilators in pediatrics. Anesth Analg 55, 769–772.
17. Stayer, S., Bent, S., Skjonsby, B., et al., 2000. Pressure control ventilation: three anesthesia ventilators compared using an infant lung model. Anesth Analg 91, 1145–1150.
18. Rupp, K., Holzki, J., Fischer, T., et al., 1999. Pediatric anesthesia. Lubeck, Germany, Dräger Medical.
19. Bennett, E.J., Patel, K.P., Grundy, E.M., 1977. Neonatal temperature and surgery. Anesthesiology 46, 303–304.
20. Chalon, J., 1980. Low humidity and damage to tracheal mucosa. Bull N Y Acad Med 56, 314–322.
21. Sessler, D., 1994. Temperature monitoring. In: Miller, R. (Ed.), Anesthesia, ed 4. Churchill Livingstone, New York.
22. Bloch, E., Ginsberg, B., Binner, R.J., et al., 1992. Limb tourniquets and central temperature in anesthetized children. Anesth Analg 74, 486–489.
23. Hess, D., Kacmarek, R., 1994. Technical aspects of the patient-ventilator interface. In: Tobin, M. (Ed.), Principles and practice of mechanical ventilation, McGraw-Hill, New York.
24. Sessler, D.S.M., 1993. Heat loss in humans covered with cotton hospital blankets. Anesth Analg 77, 73–77.
25. Petty, C., 1987. We do need precordial and esophageal stethoscopes. J Clin Monit 3, 192–193.
26. Webster, T., 1987. Now that we have pulse oximeters and capnographs, we don't need precordial and esophageal stethoscopes. J Clin Monit 3, 191–192.

27. Birmingham, P.K., Cheney, F.W., Ward, R.J., 1986. Esophageal intubation: a review of detection techniques. Anesth Analg 65, 886–891.

28. Caplan, R.A., Posner, K.L., Ward, R.J., et al., 1990. Adverse respiratory events in anesthesia: a closed claims analysis. Anesthesiology 72, 828–833.

29. Sum-Ping, S.T., Mehta, M.P., Anderton, J.M., 1989. A comparative study of methods of detection of esophageal intubation. Anesth Analg 69, 627–632.

30. Bell, C., Rimar, S., Barash, P., 1989. Intraoperative ST segment changes with myocardial ischemia in the neonate: a report of three cases. Anesthesiology 71, 601–604.

31. Kimble, K.J., Darnall, R.A.J., Yelderman, M., et al., 1981. An automated oscillometric technique for estimating mean arterial pressure in critically ill newborns. Anesthesiology 54, 423–425.

32. Park, M.K., Menard, S.M., 1987. Accuracy of blood pressure measurement by the Dinamap monitor in infants and children. Pediatrics 79, 907–914.

33. Perloff, D., Grim, C., Flack, J., et al., 1993. Human blood pressure determination by sphygmomanometry. Circulation 88, 2460–2470.

34. Murphy, K.G., Secunda, J.A., Rockoff, M.A., 1990. Severe burns from a pulse oximeter. Anesthesiology 73, 350–352.

35. Soriano, S.G., McManus, M.L., Sullivan, L.J., et al., 1994. Doppler sensor placement during neurosurgical procedures for children in the prone position. J Neurosurg Anesthesiol 6, 153–155.

36. Rao, T.L.K., Wong, A.Y., Salem, M.R., 1977. A new approach to percutaneous catheterization of the internal jugular vein. Anesthesiology 46, 362–364.

37. Clokie, C., Metcalf, I., Holland, A., 1989. Dental trauma in anaesthesia. Can J Anaesth 36, 675–680.

38. Weiss, M., Hartmann, K., Fischer, J., et al., 2001. Use of angulated video-intubation laryngoscope in children undergoing manual in-line neck stabilization. Br J Anaesth 87, 453–458.

39. Koka, B.V., Jeon, I.S., Andre, J.M., et al., 1977. Postintubation croup in children. Anesth Analg 56, 501–505.

40. Holzman, R.S., Nargozian, C.D., Florence, F.B., 1988. Lightwand intubation in children with abnormal upper airways. Anesthesiology 69, 784–787.

41. Badgwell, J.M., Kleinman, S.E., Heavner, J.E., 1993. Respiratory frequency and artifact affect the capnographic baseline in infants. Anesth Analg 77, 708–712.

42. Lazzell, V.A., Burrows, F.A., 1991. Stability of the intraoperative arterial to end-tidal carbon dioxide partial pressure difference in children with congenital heart disease. Can J Anaesth 38, 859–865.

43. Lindahl, S.G., Yates, A.P., Hatch, D.J., 1987. Relationship between invasive and noninvasive measurements of gas exchange in anesthetized infants and children. Anesthesiology 66, 168–175.

44. Cole, F., 1957. Pediatric formulas for the anesthesiologist. Am J Dis Child 94, 472.

45. Penlington, G.N., 1974. Endotracheal tube sizes for children. Br J Anaesth 29, 494–495.

46. Morgan, G.A., Steward, D.J., 1982. Linear airway dimensions in children: including those from cleft palate. Can Anaesth Soc J 29, 1–8.

Chapter 23

Anesthesia Equipment Outside of the Operating Room

Sergio D. Bergese, Erika G. Puente, and Gilat Zisman

General Considerations

Anesthesiologists routinely provide care to patients in locations remote from the operating room (OR) or alternate sites. In some academic practices, the proportion of "out-of-OR" (OOOR) anesthetics approaches 40%. The remote site should be interpreted as a place that is located distant from where the main operating room headquarters is located, now considered routine sites of care. Nevertheless, these remote locations present additional challenges for the anesthesia provider, since it is not uncommon that detailed protocols for provision of anesthesia care are not in place and specialized equipment is not readily available.

Intuitively, patient safety while delivering anesthesia is enhanced by the standardization and reliability built into the environment where the delivery of anesthesia is taking place. Such is true in the operating room suite, but is less so in OOOR locations. The circumstances, including unusual physical layout, energy sources, and working conditions encountered in remote sites may challenge the safety of the environment, and it potentially increases anesthetic risk to patients and to some degree, to personnel. It is the responsibility of the anesthesiologist to optimize conditions for patient safety by emphasizing teamwork and following established guidelines, when available, to minimize adverse events.[1-4] Moreover, the anesthesiologist must understand the unique features of each type of remote location and how these impact the function of anesthesia equipment to effectively and safely provide anesthesia wherever it is needed. This latter concept forms the topic of this chapter.

Remote locations can be classified into four main categories, which are outlined in Table 23-1.[1,4]

The American Society of Anesthesiologists (ASA) has published anesthesia care standards and patient monitoring requirements that must be met and uniformly maintained independent of the location where anesthesia care is provided.[4,5]

To provide proper anesthetic care in remote locations, there are three major aspects that need to be taken into consideration by the anesthesiologist before administering anesthesia. This three-step approach involves evaluating the OOOR location, the procedure, and the patient.[6]

The OOOR Location

When considering the OOOR environment, anesthesiologists must take into consideration the need for any special anesthetic and monitoring equipment, room set-up, personnel, and temperature control. They must also be aware of potential radiation hazards and dangers associated with strong magnetic fields, and they must confirm the proper functioning and location of all resuscitation equipment, including a defibrillator, a physiological monitor, suction devices, oxygen source, Ambu bag, and resuscitation drugs.[4,7]

Additionally, it is important that the anesthesiologist becomes familiar with any anesthesia machines that are available in these remote locations, and make sure that the machine is working properly before initiating patient care. Sometimes the machines are older, not used often, or are serviced infrequently. However, these factors must not be allowed to affect their usability. In other words, the anesthesia machines must be maintained and serviced before being used, have standard safety features such as oxygen failure alarms and a minimum gas ratio device, and may have specific electrical requirements

Table 23–1 Classification of Remote Anesthesia Locations

1. Locations not designed specially for providing anesthesia
   - Emergency room
   - Psychiatric wards: electroconvulsive therapy
   - Hospitalization wards: dressing changes, cardioversion

2. Locations with fixed procedural equipment installed
   - CT
   - MRI
   - Interventional radiology
   - Interventional neuroradiology
   - Radiation therapy

3. Specially designed ORs outside of the main operating room headquarters
   - Dental surgery
   - Outpatient surgery
   - Obstetric unit
   - Burn unit

4. Specialized diagnostic/interventional suites
   - Gastrointestinal endoscopy
   - Cardiovascular (EP, catheterization laboratory)

CT, Computed tomography; *MRI*, magnetic resonance imaging.

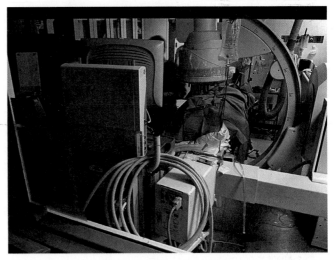

Figure 23–1 Anesthesia provided in an invasive radiology procedure room, as viewed from the control room.

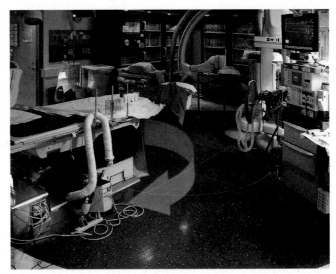

Figure 23–2 Neurointerventional radiology suite with anesthesia care capabilities.

such as grounded power outlets. More fundamentally, the anesthesia machine, if one is provided, must meet minimum standards for usability under the rules applicable in the country where the care occurs.

The various OOOR anesthetizing locations are primarily designed with the needs of the proceduralist in mind rather then the anesthesiologist. Often there are large pieces of equipment that can be in the way of the anesthesiologist, obstructing access to the patient. Also, equipment such as piped-in gases, suction, overhead lighting, and isolated power, which are considered standard in the operating rooms, may not be available in most nonoperating anesthetizing locations. For example, as seen in Figure 23-1, the anesthesia machine is wedged between the procedure table support and the control room window, leaving no space for the anesthesiologist. The anesthesia machine blocks visual communication between the proceduralist and the technologist in the control room. Also of note is that the piped gases are at the opposite end of the room, and that there is an unconnected air line on the anesthesia machine.

These less than ideal situations, as depicted in Figure 23-1, are becoming increasingly unacceptable as OOOR anesthesia matures. Early involvement of anesthesiologists in the design of these facilities to account for safe and effective anesthesia care is essential, but anesthesiologists share the responsibility to assert the perogative to participate in facility design, and equipment specifications and purchasing.

When anesthesiologists contribute to the design of OOOR locations safety issues can be improved. As seen in Figure 23-2, the design of this neurointerventional radiology suite has been improved, but a safety issue remaining is that medical equipment is plugged into a consumer grade "power strip." Some of the positive attributes of the design of this procedure room include:

- The anesthesia machine is positioned away from the head of the bed, which eliminates competition for space around the patient's head during the procedure.

- The procedure table rotates on its pedestal (yellow arrow), bringing the head and airway into easy reach, with the anesthesia machine in its customary location, for induction and emergence.

- The monitor data acquisition unit (lower left) is mounted on the procedure table pedestal rather than the anesthesia machine, so that the patient connection cables do not drape across a gap between the highly mobile table and a fixed anesthesia machine (the data are carried from the acquisition unit and anesthesia machine by a dedicated, fixed cable).

Anesthesia machines, monitors, and anesthesia carts for OOOR procedures are generally housed at or near the actual anesthetizing site. However, in some cases it may be necessary to use portable machines and transport them to the desired location. Not all OOOR anesthetics require an anesthesia machine, as long as the ASA standards for monitoring under anesthesia can be met. For example, infusion pumps, a physiological monitor and a transport ventilator can provide a very credible anesthetic. In either case, transporting equipment increases the possibility of malfunctions due to damage or improper setup upon arrival, increasing the need to assure that all equipment is functional before initiation of the anesthetic care.

Another concern for the anesthesiologist to keep in mind is that OOOR locations are generally less secure than the operating room. Thus, anesthesia carts must easily lock and, ideally, lock automatically when the anesthesiologist is absent. One compromise solution is to use a lock that can be opened by the same proximity card technology commonly used as part of the ID badge that also opens doors. In addition to enhanced security, the OOOR anesthesia cart tends to require a wider variety of supplies than are typically stocked in the main OR carts to account for (sometimes tremendous) distance to the nearest anesthesia supply room. All these supplies must also be accounted for before initiating anesthetic care.

Procedures

Since anesthesiologists are no longer providing anesthetic care only in the operating room, the number of procedures that are carried out in alternate sites that require anesthesia or sedation are increasing exponentially. Examples of procedures most commonly performed outside of the OR include computed tomography (CT), magnetic resonance imaging (MRI), and many interventional radiology procedures, including gastrostomy tubes, nephrostomies, liver biopsies, and transjugular intrahepatic portosystemic shunts (TIPS) procedures. Other examples include interventional neuroradiology procedures, functional brain imaging radiotherapy procedures such as radiation therapy, intraoperative radiotherapy, and radiosurgery. Gastroenterology procedures that may require anesthetic care include upper gastroenterology endoscopy, endoscopic retrograde cholangiopancreatography (ERCP), colonoscopy, and percutaneous endoscopic gastrostomy placement. In the future, weight reduction procedures involving reduction of gastric volume will be performed in the gastroenterology procedure suit. Cardiology procedures that often require anesthesia include cardiac catheterization, radiofrequency ablation of arrhythmogenic foci, cardioversion, and transesophageal echocardiography (TEE). The electroconvulsive therapy conducted in the psychiatry unit also requires anesthetic care.[1]

The key concept, regardless of the location, is that anesthesia care and monitoring must meet the same standards as those applied in the OR. To facilitate and promote quality patient care, the American Society of Anesthesiologists publishes specific guidelines for providing anesthetic care outside of the operating room that apply to all anesthesia care and anesthesiology personnel at any location outside of the OR. These procedures are to be followed in all nonoperating room settings as long as they are applicable to the individual patient or healthcare setting.[5]

The anesthesiologist must adapt to the challenges presented by different room settings, locations, procedures, and specialized equipment used to perform OOOR procedures. The following are but a few examples:

- When working in the **MRI suite,** the anesthesia staff must have specialized training to maintain proper patient safety while surrounded by a strong magnetic field.
- When **iodinated contrast dye** is administered to the patient, close monitoring must be maintained for any adverse reactions.

Table 23–2 Problems That Can Be Encountered at Remote Locations During Anesthesia
Lack of continuous electrical supply
Lack of continuous supply of oxygen and nitrous oxide
Difficulty with storage of drugs and equipment
Difficulty in transport and supply of drugs and equipment
Lack of maintenance of equipment
Lack of skilled assistance

- When anesthesia is given during **cardiac catheterization,** special attention must be paid to the patient's underlying cardiac morbidity.
- When patients receiving **radiation therapy** require general anesthetic, remote monitoring devices must be used during the procedure to protect the anesthesiologist from strong radiation.
- In the **psychiatric unit,** profound physiological changes may occur in patients during electroconvulsive therapy. The heart rate, respiration, blood pressure, and oxygen saturation of these patients must be carefully monitored and controlled by the anesthesiologist.[8]
- While conducting anesthesia in the **radiology suite,** the anesthesiologist must have a good understanding of radiology equipment, radiation safety, and proper safety precautions.

A list of problems that can be encountered at any remote location during anesthesia, including the radiology suite, is summarized in Table 23-2.[6]

To prevent injury to patients during anesthesia, The American Society of Anesthesiologists (ASA) 1994 Guidelines for Non-Operating Room Anesthetizing Locations recommends the following[1,5,9]:

1. Always have a reliable source of oxygen with a full backup E cylinder
2. An adequate and reliable suction source
3. A scavenging system for waste gas
4. Adequate monitoring and anesthetic equipment, including a self-inflating hand resuscitator bag
5. Multiple and safe electrical outlets
6. Appropriate illumination with battery-powered backup (i.e., flashlight)
7. Adequate space for the anesthesia personnel and equipment
8. A resuscitation cart with a defibrillator and emergency drugs and equipment
9. Effective telecommunication
10. Compliance with safety codes of the facility
11. Appropriate postanesthesia management

The Patient

There are several indications for anesthetic care at alternate sites. Patients may be too hemodynamically unstable to tolerate the procedure without homeostatic intervention from an anesthesiologist. They may have a difficult airway, unacceptably raising the risks from accidental oversedation. The

Table 23–3 Contributing Factors Requiring Anesthesia Outside of the OR
Pain management
Children, elderly, or disabled patients that will not follow instructions
Psychiatric disorders: anxiety and panic disorders, claustrophobia
Neurological disorders: movement and seizure disorders, cerebral palsy
Trauma: unstable cardiovascular, respiratory, or neurological status
Patients with significant comorbidities that require monitoring
Difficult airway

Table 23–4 MRI Suite Levels	
Level I	Medical support or physiological monitoring is not required.
Level II	Any level of anesthesia or critical care and monitoring is required.
Level III	Intraoperative setting (iMRI) where anesthesia and patient monitoring are required and are performed in a specially designed operating room (see Chapter 30, Equipment for Neuromonitoring)

patient may be unable to tolerate mild or moderate sedation, or such sedation may be inadequate for a given patient. Finally, the procedure may require prolonged, complete immobility, which can only be achieved under general anesthesia. Some of the most common patient factors for requiring deep sedation, monitored anesthesia care (MAC), or general anesthesia outside of the OR are listed in Table 23-3.[1,4,9,10] Depending on a specific situation, additional equipment such as the airway cart, defibrillating device, or a code cart may be needed.

Locations

Magnetic Resonance Imaging

Magnetic resonance imaging (MRI) technology functions as a diagnostic tool and is increasingly being used on a wider array of patients. This technology provides anatomic, physiological, and metabolic imaging.[3,4]

To codify safe practice for MRI suites, the ASA created a practice advisory for anesthesia care in the MRI environment. The practice advisory categorizes MRI suites into three general levels, according to the level of patient care anticipated (Table 23-4).[11]

The indications for anesthesia in the MRI suite are similar to those listed in Table 23-3. The most common reason for requiring anesthesia in this setting is the patient's inability to follow instructions or stay still for an extended period of time. For this reason these patients (who usually include children, claustrophobic patients, patients with movement disorders, and the mentally challenged) require sedation or general anesthesia under the supervision of an anesthesiologist.[1,3,4,6]

The main concern with the MRI scanner is the strong magnetic field that is always present around the scanner, regardless of whether it is actively scanning. Any ferrous metal-containing object, either equipment or implant will be attracted to the magnetic field of the MRI scanner. The anesthesiologist must take special precautions to ensure that the patient is properly screened for any implanted devices, such as pacemakers, implanted pumps, deep brain stimulators, aneurysm coils, etc. While the scanner is on, additional radiofrequency pulses are emitted that may interfere with the anesthesia monitors and equipment. Wire coils and sheets of metal can absorb the radiofrequency pulses and become very hot, risking patient burns. In turn, the interference between the scanner and the anesthesia equipment and monitors can distort or interrupt the technique or quality of the images.[12] In response to this risk, MRI equipment manufacturers and government regulators recognize the **5-gauss exclusion zone**. This zone is demarked with a piece of red tape on the floor of the MRI suite. Inside this line (i.e., closer to the magnet), attraction of ferromagnetic components within medical devices such as pumps, vaporizers, batteries, and instruments such as clamps and scissors become a very significant risk—both because of aberrant operation and because they become deadly missiles. Thus no ferromagnetic equipment or device should be brought beyond this 5-gauss line.

Figure 23-3 illustrates the 5-gauss exclusion zone and several other gauss lines drawn around a theoretical but typical modern, high-field MRI scanner. The technological drive is to higher and higher magnetic field strength, as this produces faster scans and better detail. However, it means that the fringe fields around the magnets are also increasingly strong.

Equipment can be modified so that it can be used within a range from the MRI scanner and has been designated as "MR-safe." Equipment is categorized as safe, unsafe, or conditional for use in the MRI environment. MRI-*safe* equipment is identified by the American Society for Testing and Materials (ASTM) as having no ferromagnetic parts or radiofrequency interference. MRI-*unsafe* equipment is identified as having ferromagnetic parts or being affected by radiofrequency interference. MRI-*conditional* equipment may be safe in certain locations of the suite depending on gauss line locations, but cannot be identified as having no ferromagnetic parts.[11]

Equipment that is MR-safe has met specific guidelines that indicate that it can be used in the MRI suite without causing any additional risk to the patient. MR-compatible equipment is not only MR-safe but also doesn't interfere with the operation of the scanner or the images produced, or is interrupted by the scanner. The anesthesia machines specially designed as MR-safe or MR-compatible have had their ferromagnetic components replaced to account for less than 2% of their total weight. Modern anesthesia machines that are available are usually made from stainless steel, brass, aluminum, and plastic.[13] Nevertheless, there is still often a prohibition against bringing these machines inside the 400-gauss line. This is much closer to the magnet than the 5-gauss exclusion zone, but reference to Figure 23-3 indicates that it is still likely that an anesthesiologist would want to position the machine inside this line. If brought within the 400-gauss line, some MRI-compatible anesthesia machines will be pulled forcefully against the magnet, risking patient injury. Reportedly, several people are required to remove the machine from the magnet once this attraction has occurred.

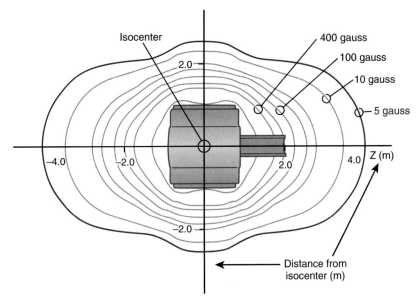

Figure 23–3　The 5-gauss exclusion zone and several other gauss lines drawn around a theoretical but typical modern, high-field MRI scanner.

Not all facilities that perform MRI scanning have MR-safe equipment available, relying instead on clinicians keeping conventional equipment far from the bore. In such settings, it becomes doubly important to maintain an adequate distance between certain equipment and the location where the magnetic field is the strongest.

In addition to protecting patient safety, it is also imperative to ensure the safety of the hospital personnel when interacting with the MR magnet. To guarantee safety and limit MRI-related hazards, the area where the magnet is located can be classified into four different zones, indicating increased hazard areas (Table 23-5).[11]

Once the environment and the patient have been screened and determined to be safe, the anesthesiologist must prepare a plan for providing optimal anesthetic care within this special setting. The anesthesia provider should take into consideration the requirements of the scan and needs of the personnel, the positioning of the equipment within the hazard zones according to whether they are MRI safe and/or MRI compatible, special requirements of the patient or the procedure that is being performed, and location of the anesthesiologist in regard to the scanner. Finally, the anesthesia provider must have an action plan for emergencies.[13]

There is an insignificant amount of ferromagnetic materials found in vaporizers and mechanical ventilators. The nonmagnetic MRI anesthesia machine is compatible with most inhaled anesthetic vaporizers, such as the Tec 5 and Tec 7. *Tec 6 vaporizers designed for desflurane administration are not MRI safe and have not been cleared for the use in MRI environments* (Tables 23-6 and 23-7 and Figure 23-4).

It is recommended that the anesthesia machine be located distally to and on the lateral sides of the magnet. The field strength generated tends to dissipate rapidly to the sides compared with the front of the magnet.[14-16]

One of the most vulnerable signals affected by the high-energy RF pulses generated by the MRI technology is the electrocardiographic (ECG) signaling. This can be decreased, though, by the use of safeguarded cables, telemetry, or fiber-optic machinery.[17] The use of telemetry for ECG eliminates

Table 23-5 MRI Suite Hazard Zones	
Zone I	Free transit area, outside of the MR suite. Common area freely accessible to the general public.
Zone II	Interface between zone I and zone III (restricted). Area where patients are greeted and must always be under the supervision of designated personnel.
Zone III	Restricted area. Access permitted only under supervision and after screening for ferromagnetic objects. Permanently under the influence of the magnetic field.
Zone IV	Magnet room. Within zone III, generates the surrounding magnetic field.

the use of wires (Figure 23-5). The ECG electrodes must be nonmagnetic or "MRI-safe" to protect the patient from potential injuries and should be placed carefully to minimize MRI-related artifacts.[14] Special shielded nonmagnetic MRI pulse oximeters are also available (Figure 23-6).

The FDA reported in a recent public health advisory the risk of burns from transdermal drug patches with metallic backings during MRI scans. It has also been described that neurosurgical patients have an increased risk for postoperative nausea and vomiting (PONV), and the use of some antiemetics that are available in transdermal patches (e.g., scopolamine) is increasingly popular for these patients. These patches can contain metal components, may overheat during the scan, and cause skin burns in the immediate area under the patch. It is important to identify patients who may be wearing a patch before introduction into the OR, or have the anesthesiologist choose an alternative medication with a different mode of delivery.[18]

Another consideration for high-field MRI environments is the acoustic noise that can be generated from the magnet during a scan. The noise increases proportionally to the field of magnet. Simple measures ensure hearing safety and provide comfort to the patient. The placement of foam earplugs

Table 23–6 Compatibility of Anesthesia Vaporizers With Their Use in the MRI Setting

Anesthesia Vaporizers	Manufacturer	MRI Compatible
Vapor 19 (Dräger)	Drägerwerk AG & Co.	✓
Vapor 2000 (Dräger)	Drägerwerk AG & Co.	✓
Dräger D-Vapor**	Drägerwerk AG & Co.	X
Tec 4*	GE Healthcare	✓
Tec 5*	GE Healthcare	✓
Tec 7***	GE Healthcare	✓
Tec 6**	GE Healthcare	X
Tec 6 Plus**	GE Healthcare	X
Aladin Cassette	GE Healthcare	✓ Except for desflurane
Penlon PPV*	Penlon, Inc.	X
MAQUET 950	Maquet, Inc.	✓ Except for desflurane

*Isoflurane
**Desflurane
***Sevoflurane

Table 23–7 Compatibility of Anesthesia Workstations With Their Use in the MRI Setting

Anesthesia Workstations	Manufacturer	MRI Compatible
Fabius GS (Dräger Medical AG)	Drägerwerk AG & Co.	X
Fabius MRI	Drägerwerk AG & Co.	✓
Apollo (Dräger Medical AG)	Drägerwerk AG & Co.	X
Aisys (GE)	GE Healthcare	X
Aestiva/5 with 7900 ventilator (GE)	GE Healthcare	✓
Datex-Ohmeda ADU	GE Healthcare	✓
Avance (GE)	GE Healthcare	X
Julian	Drägerwerk AG & Co.	X
Narkomed 6400	DRE, Inc.	X
DRE Integra SP II	DRE, Inc.	✓

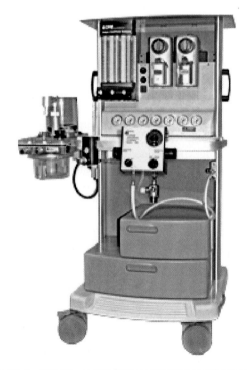

Figure 23–4 DRE Integra SP II (MRI-compatible) anesthesia machine.

is sufficient. Both the patient and staff may benefit from the use of earplugs, as long as this does not interfere with the ability of the staff to hear and communicate with the physician or respond to emergency situations.

Finally, in addition to the patient, all hospital staff should complete a detailed MRI compatibility examination and also be adequately trained when required to work within an MRI setting.[11,19]

Projectile Risk

The projectile risk of ferrous metal in the strong magnetic field deserves special attention. Any ferrous object becomes a missile in the strong magnetic field always present in the MRI scanner. Common objects such as anesthesia carts, IV poles, hospital beds and stretchers, and compressed gas tanks become deadly if accidentally brought into the MRI scanner room. MRI-compatible anesthesia machines have oxygen, air, and nitrous oxide tanks made of aluminum; this is in contrast to standard E cylinders that are highly ferromagnetic. Thus standard E cylinders should never be brought into the MRI suite. Figures 23-7 and 23-8 show the "projectile effect" of MRI magnets on items containing ferromagnetic materials. In Figure 23-7, a standard ferromagnetic E cylinder is inside the MRI scanner. Patients have been killed by projectile gas cylinders in the MRI scanner. In Figure 23-8, a (heavy) hospital bed has been pulled into the MRI

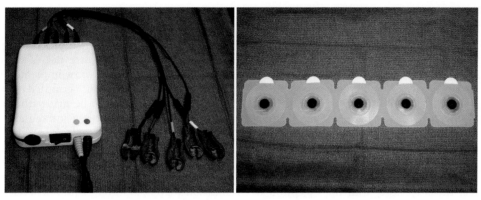

Figure 23–5   Telemetric ECG and MRI nonmagnetic ECG electrodes.

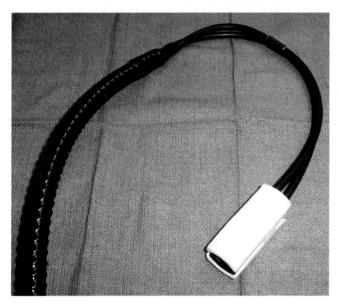

Figure 23–6   Pulse oximeter with shielded cables.

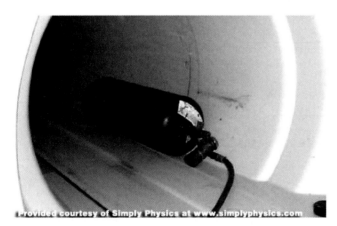

Figure 23–7   An example of the missile or projectile effect of MRI magnets on items containing ferromagnetic materials.

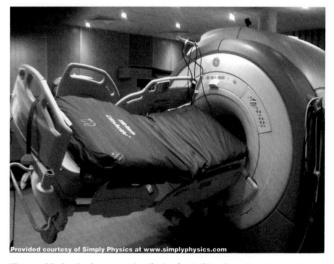

Figure 23–8   Bed as a projectile in the MRI suite. *(From Simply Physics. (website): www.simplyphysics.com.) Accessed* 31 March 2010.

scanner. Note that no part of this multihundred pound bed remains in contact with the floor.

Additional issues that may be confronted during MRI scanning under anesthesia include the lack of accessibility to the patient, lower room temperature of the MRI suite (to prevent excessive heating of the MRI equipment and due to the fact that the magnet is made superconducting by cooling with liquid helium), increased level of noise from the scanner, and fewer staff who are prepared or trained to provide anesthesia assistance or emergency care.

Monitoring

Patients undergoing an MRI scan under anesthesia must be monitored according to the ASA standards for basic anesthetic monitoring, and if used within zone IV, all monitors should be MRI-safe. Distance monitoring should also be available in zone III during the times when the anesthesia provider is not within zone IV (Figure 23-9). Some special considerations when monitoring the patient are listed in Table 23-8.[3,10,11] MRI-safe patient monitoring equipment is commercially widely available. One of many examples is the MRI Non-Magnetic Tesla Guard Vital Signs Monitor that is approved for 3T magnets (Figure 23-9). Basic configurations include monitoring of an electrocardiogram (ECG), pulse oximetry, and blood pressure (invasive and noninvasive). Other options include measuring anesthetic agent concentrations and end-tidal CO_2. The monitor offers wireless data transfer and has an integrated safety sensor that measures the magnetizing force. It can operate on a battery up to 180 minutes.

Airway Management Equipment in the MRI

Standard anesthesia equipment carts used in the operating rooms are not safe and should never be used inside the MRI; instead, plastic MRI-compatible anesthesia carts should be used. Conventional laryngoscopes and laryngoscope blades are not ferromagnetic, but they must contain lithium batteries made from low magnetic materials. Conventional batteries are not safe. Blades and handles made entirely of plastic materials are also available. Equipment containing lithium batteries can be safely used outside of the 5-gauss line, but the risk is increased beyond this line. Standard plastic endotracheal tubes are safe, with the exception of metal reinforced tubes, which should not be used. Endotracheal tube stylets must be nonferromagnetic, usually made of aluminum.

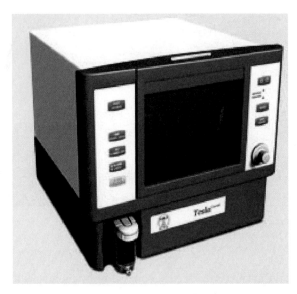

Figure 23–9 MRI Nonmagnetic Tesla Guard vital signs monitor. *(From MRIequip. MRI Nonmagnetic Tesla Guard vital signs monitor (website):* http://www.mriequip.com/store/pc/viewPrd.asp?idproduct=940&idcategory=98.) *Accessed* 31 March 2010.

Other Equipment in the MRI

Other monitoring equipment such as esophageal stethoscopes and Swan Ganz catheters are not MRI-safe. Patients with AICDs, pacemakers, and most implanted biological pumps and devices are generally not permitted to undergo MRI scanning. Stethoscopes should be made from nonferromagnetic materials, and both single-use and reusable MRI-safe stethoscopes are commercially available. Defibrillating devices are not considered MRI-safe, and the patient must be removed from the MRI suite before such devices are used.

Additional equipment considerations include safe use of infusion pumps, warming equipment such as blood warmers and forced-air patient warming devices, ear protection devices, and nerve stimulators. There are currently no warming devices or nerve stimulators specifically designed for use in the MRI suite. An example of an MRI compatible syringe pump is the MRI syringe pump from Harvard Apparatus (Figure 23-10). It can be used for drug delivery and tracer studies, and it combines a two syringe pump mechanism, constructed of nonferromagnetic metal, with an up to 60-foot cable connection to the pump electronics control box.

Alternatively, standard infusion pumps can be used with long infusion tubing routed through a waveguide (Figure 23-11). This has the advantage of using what is presumably the hospital standard pump—familiar to the anesthesiologist—and, in modern practice, likely to include the safety features of a "smart" pump (see Chapter 17). The pump is situated at the anesthesiologist's station in the control room, and the tubing routed through the wave guide (lower left of the photograph) connects to the IV infusion near the patient.

Several other features of a well-designed MRI anesthesia workstation are evident in Figure 23-11. An MRI-compatible anesthesia machine is positioned outside the 400-gauss line, visible through the window. The flow tubes are visible from the MRI control room, as are the ventilator bellows. An anesthesiologist is at the patient's head in this image. In the control room, a slave display of the anesthesia monitor is near the infusion pump. Importantly, the emergency quench control is easily within reach (*top left*). This allows the magnet to be quenched by instantaneously dumping the liquid helium coolant up a stack. This immediately removes the magnetic field, but destroys the MRI scanner.

Table 23–8 Special Considerations When Monitoring a Patient During MRI

Blood Pressure	MRI-compatible or MRI-safe monitors. Automated oscillometric blood pressure monitoring avoids electromagnetic interference. Conventional disposable transducers may function adequately outside the 5-gauss line for invasive blood pressure monitoring.
ECG	ECG morphology may be altered by small induced voltages from blood flowing perpendicular to the magnetic field and may be distorted by RF artifact during scanning. Only MRI-compatible ECG pads should be used. Spike artifacts ≅ R waves create difficulty in identifying ischemic changes or interpreting arrhythmias. Special MRI-compatible electrocardiographic leads minimize induced RF currents.
Ventilation	Positioning of the patient within the magnet renders impossible to visualize the patient's face and chest directly during scanning. Respiratory capnography is available in MR-compatible systems.
Oxygenation	Severe burns may be caused by the induction of current within a loop of wire. MR-specific pulse oximeters use fiberoptic cables that do not overheat and cannot be looped.
Temperature	Body temperature may fluctuate. It may increase as a result of heating caused by the magnet field or decrease from the cool environment in the MRI suite to protect the superconductors

Computed Tomography

Computed tomography (CT) scanning is a noninvasive and painless diagnostic test that is used in a wide variety of patients, and it has become an indispensable tool for the diagnosis of certain pathologies. This technology is commonly used for diagnostic and/or treatment purposes mostly when dealing with intracranial, thoracic, or abdominal pathologies.[1,3,4,6] Computed tomography also provides guidance to allow a new category of procedures used for the treatment of disease. Interventional CT procedures, known as stereotactic-guided procedures, are techniques that allow for the sampling of tissue with needle biopsy or the drainage of fluid collections with needle aspiration.[4,20]

Most of the time, CT scans can be performed without the assistance of an anesthesiologist. There are, however, two broad categories of patients that require anesthetic care during their scan: those that need to be sedated or those that are critically ill with physiological instability. The types of patients that need to be deeply sedated or anesthetized to tolerate a CT scan have essentially the same characteristics as patients requiring an anesthetized MRI scan (Table 23-3). The urgent or emergent patients that are to be scanned may arrive to the radiology suite already intubated and accompanied by an anesthesiologist or anesthesia care provider. These patients usually need to be scanned immediately due to a complication that arose during or after an interventional procedure or surgery, or as a consequence of trauma. Due to the emergent nature of the environment surrounding these patients, organization and communication are paramount and essential in delivering proper anesthetic care to the patient during the scanning.[20,21]

There are several issues that may arise while providing anesthesia care in the CT suite. The anesthetic machine, if available, may be older and used infrequently. Also, the anesthetic medications, equipment, gases, and anesthesia assistance may be very minimal in these remote locations. During the scan, the anesthesiologist will usually not have direct access to the patient and must stay outside of the scanning area, or he or she must wear protective lead shielding to be in more direct contact with the patient. The scanning table upon which the patient lies moves quickly and forcefully through the scanning gantry during the scan. Extra vigilance must be maintained to ensure that breathing circuit apparatus, monitoring cables, or infusion lines have not been interrupted or disconnected during the movement during the scan. Visual alarms should be used when available since audible alarms might not be heard. Finally, the temperature of the CT scan room is usually kept below 20° C and care must be taken so that the patient is sufficiently warm.[1,6,20]

Interventional Neuroradiology

Interventional neuroradiology (INR) is a rapidly expanding area of radiology, with the procedures used to treat patients with neurovascular diseases (Table 23-9) and to deliver therapeutic drugs and/or devices via endovascular access.[4] The most common INR procedures performed include treatment for brain aneurysms and arteriovenous malformations, and embolizations of neoplasms.[22] Stenting of carotid and other arterial lesions is increasing in importance.

Anesthesiologists need to be able to provide care to the patient in a field where radiological imaging such as high-resolution fluoroscopy and high-speed digital subtraction angiography are used while maintaining radiation safety for both the patient and the anesthesia staff. To maintain a safe environment, extension tubing for monitor and infusion lines, protective lead garments, clear lead screens, and console areas for monitoring patients from a distance should be implemented.[22,23]

Also, it is important to properly position the anesthesia equipment closer to the patients' feet or off to the side to allow more mobility for the neuroradiologist and the imaging equipment around the patient's head. See Figure 23-12 for an example.

Here, near optimal access for imaging devices to the patient's head is achieved, albeit by placing the anesthesiologist behind the proceduralist's monitors.

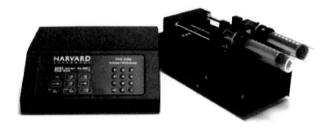

Figure 23–10   MRI-compatible syringe pump, Harvard apparatus. *(From Harvard Apparatus. (website): www.harvardapparatus.com.) Accessed 31 March 2010.*

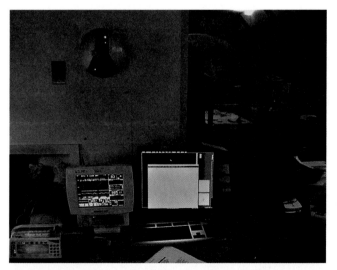

Figure 23–11 An MRI-compatible anesthesia machine is positioned outside the 400-gauss line, visible through the window. The flow tubes are visible from the MRI control room, as are the ventilator bellows.

Table 23–9 Classification of Diseases Amenable to Endovascular Treatment
Emergent or elective
Hemorrhagic or occlusive
Definitive, adjunctive, or palliative

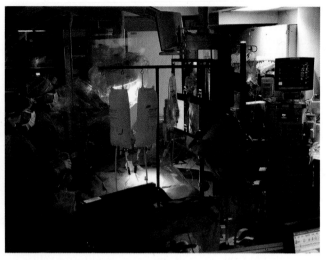

Figure 23–12 Anesthesia equipment arranged for mobility for patient and operating staff.

All of the anesthesia IV lines, monitoring lines, and airway connections should be long and loose enough so that they are not accidentally disconnected during imaging. Since a large amount of radiographic contrast and heparinized flush is used during the procedure, a large volume of fluids is also administered to the patient. To increase patient comfort and maintain fluid dynamics, a bladder catheter is required for most procedures.[4,6,22]

Cardiovascular Suite

Anesthesia in the cardiac catheterization suite can be extremely difficult at times due to the patients' unstable condition and their concurrent myocardial disease. To avoid excessive intravenous fluid administration, it is helpful to use a minidrip. Also, ECG monitors need to be adjusted to be able to detect pacemaker spikes in patients that have one. Many of these patients have a low ejection fraction and may need invasive arterial blood pressure monitoring.[4,6,7] Additionally, all other general considerations for OOOR anesthesia care apply, particularly with respect to protecting personnel from radiation exposure.

Radiation Therapy

To precisely deliver radiation therapy to a specific target, the primary goal of anesthesia is to keep the patient immobile. During gamma knife procedures, anesthesia is provided by either sedation or general anesthesia to place a head frame, followed by an MRI and/or CT scan procedure. After the scan, maintenance of anesthesia is provided while awaiting the data collection/interpretation, and transportation to the gamma knife suite. During cyber knife procedures, radio-opaque markers need to be surgically implanted under either sedation or general anesthesia. During the marker implantation, the anesthesia equipment, tubing, and wires must be kept away from the robot arm, while the anesthesia providers must monitor the patient from outside of the room through video monitoring. Due to the high amount of radiation that is emitted during these procedures, the suite

is heavily shielded and has a lead or iron door that can take up to 60 seconds to open. The patient must be closely monitored by video monitors because of the decreased access to the patient.[3,6,7]

The Psychiatric Unit

In the psychiatric unit, an anesthesiologist is usually only needed to assist during the conduction of electroconvulsive therapy (ECT). ECT is used for the treatment of severe depression and other affective disorders, bipolar depression, and schizophrenia after pharmacotherapy therapy has failed. The goals of the anesthesiologist are twofold. First, anesthesia must provide neuromuscular blockade to prevent body injury from the seizure activity. Also, anesthesia must make the patient briefly unconscious for the application of the electrical stimulus for the induction of the seizure.

There are several additions to the standard anesthesia practice in ECT procedures. To monitor motor activity during the seizure, a second blood pressure cuff is used on the lower part of the leg or arm and is inflated before the administration of the neuromuscular blocking agent. After induction, anesthesia is administered and the patient is rendered unconscious, and the cuff is inflated above the arterial pressure to prevent distal perfusion, essentially acting as a tourniquet. The ECT electrodes and a bite block are also placed on the patient at this time. Some anesthesiologists tend to hyperventilate the patient with the Ambu bag to create a state of hypocapnia, which lowers the seizure threshold. It is usually not necessary to intubate most patients during ECT procedures.

Further Reading

Landrum, A.L., 2006. Anesthesia for sites outside the operating room. Adv Anesth 24, 163–175.

Gross, W.L., Gold, B. (Eds.), 2009. Anesthesia outside the operating room. Anesthesiol Clin 27(1), 1–184. *Comprehensive text.*

ASA. Practice advisory on anesthetic care for magnetic resonance imaging. A report by the American Society of Anesthesiologists task force on anesthetic care for magnetic resonance imaging. Anesthesiology 110, 459–479. *Recent compendium of expert opinion and recommendations to guide virtually all aspects of anesthesia care in the MRI suite; arguably the most hazardous of all OOOR locations.*

References

1. Tan, T.K., Manninen, P.H., 2000. Anesthesia for remote sites: general considerations. Semin Anesth 19, 241–247.
2. Frankel, A., 2009. Patient safety: anesthesia in remote locations. Anesthesiol Clin 21 (1), 127–139.
3. Stoelting, R.K., Miller, R.D. (Eds.), 2007. Basics of anesthesia, ed 5. Churchill Livingstone, Philadelphia.
4. Souter, K.J., et al., 2006. Anesthesia provided at alternate sites. In: Barash, P.G., et al., (Eds.), Clinical anesthesia, ed 5. Lippincott-Raven, Philadelphia.
5. ASA. ASA guidelines statement on nonoperating room anesthetizing locations. standards and practice parameters (website): http://www.asahq.org/publicationsAndServices/sgstoc.htm. Accessed 12 September 2009.
6. Stensrud, P.E., 2009. Anesthesia at remote locations. In: Miller, R.D. (Ed.), Miller's anesthesia, ed 7. Churchill Livingstone.
7. Landrum, A.L., 2006. Anesthesia for sites outside the operating room. Adv Anesth 24, 163–175.
8. Van De Velde, M., Kuypers, M., Teunkens, A., et al., 2009. Risk and safety of anesthesia outside the operating room. Minerva Anestesiol 75, 345–348.
9. Hausman, L., Russo, M., 2009. Anesthesia in distant locations: equipment, staffing, and state requirements. Int Anesthesiol Clin 47, 1–9.

10. Dorsch, J.A., Dorsch, S.E., 2008. Equipment for the magnetic resonance imaging environment. In Understanding anesthesia equipment, ed 5. Lippincott Williams & Wilkins, Philadelphia.

11. ASA, 2009. Practice advisory on anesthetic care for magnetic resonance imaging. A report by the American Society of Anesthesiologists task force on anesthetic care for magnetic resonance imaging. Anesthesiology 110, 459–479.

12. Bergese, S.D., Puente, E.G., 2009. Anesthesia in the intraoperative MRI environment. Neurosurg Clin N Am 20, 155–162.

13. Gillies, B.S., Lecky, J.H., 1997. Anesthesia for nonoperative locations. In: Barash, et al., (Eds.), Clinical anesthesia, ed 3. Lippincott-Raven, Philadelphia.

14. Trankina, M.F., 1998. Neurodiagnostic procedures. In: Cucchiara, R.F., et al., (Eds.), Clinical neuroanesthesia, ed 2. Churchill Livingstone, New York.

15. Tan, T.K., Goh, J., 2009. The anaesthetist's role in the setting up of an intraoperative MR imaging facility. Singapore Med J 50 (1), 4–10.

16. Lipson, A.C., Gargollo, P.C., Black, P.M., 2001. Intraoperative magnetic resonance imaging: considerations for the operating room of the future. J Clin Neurosci 8 (4), 305–310.

17. Kraayenbrink, M., McAnulty, G., 2005. Neuroanesthesia. In: Moore, J.A., Newell, D.W. (Eds.), Neurosurgery: principles and practice, Springer-Verlag, London.

18. US Food and Drug Administration. Public health advisory: risk of burns during MRI scans from transdermal drug patches with metallic backings (website): http://www.fda.gov/Drugs/DrugSafety/PostmarketDrugSafety InformationforPatientsandProviders/DrugSafetyInformationforHeathcare-Professionals/PublicHealthAdvisories/ucm111313.htm Accessed 12 September 2009.

19. Kanal, E., Barkovich, A.J., Bell, C., et al., 2007. ACR guidance document for safe MR practices. AJR Am J Roentgenol 2007 188, 1–27.

20. Bryson, E.O., Frost, E.A., 2009. Anesthesia in remote locations: radiology and beyond. Int Anesthesiol Clin 47 (2), 11–19.

21. Bell C. Anesthesia in the MRI suite, Clin Window (serial online): http://www.clinicalwindow.net/cw_issue_10_article1.htm#. Accessed 27 August 2009.

22. Varma, M.K., Price, K., Jayakrishnan, V., et al., 2007. Anaesthetic considerations for interventional neuroradiology. Br J Anaesth 99 (1), 75–85.

23. Taylor, W., Rodesch, G., 1995. Recent advances: interventional neuroradiology. BJM 311, 789–792.

Chapter 24

Provision of Anesthesia in Difficult Situations and the Developing World

Deborah J. Harris, John A. Carter, John Hodgson, and Necia Williams

The provision of anesthesia in modern, well-equipped operating rooms is dependent on sophisticated electronic equipment that requires an uninterrupted supply of both electricity and compressed gases. Such equipment is not readily transportable, although it may be moved within a hospital facility. There are many locations throughout the world where anesthesia is administered to facilitate surgery, examinations, or other forms of treatment outside this generally accepted "safe" environment.

The following are examples of locations and situations away from hospital operating rooms where anesthesia may be required, and where simpler or alternative means of providing anesthesia may need to be employed:

- Within hospitals away from operating rooms:
  - Emergency department
  - Radiology department (MRI, CT, interventional radiology) (See Chapter 23);
  - Radiotherapy department
  - Cardiac catheterization and electrophysiology laboratories
  - Endoscopy suite
  - Intensive care unit
  - Coronary care unit (e.g., for cardioversion)
  - Psychiatric unit (e.g., for electroconvulsive therapy)
- Site of an accident or major disaster
- The battlefield
- Developing countries:
  - Hospitals, medical centers
  - Self-contained visiting surgical teams

All of these situations are remote from the relatively safe, comfortable, and familiar operating room anesthetic environment, and the following problems may be encountered to a greater or lesser degree:

- Lack of continuous electricity supply
- Lack of continuous supply of oxygen and nitrous oxide
- Difficulty with storage of drugs and equipment
- Difficulty in transport and supply of drugs and equipment
- Lack of maintenance of equipment
- Lack of skilled assistance
- Lack of control of environment
- Financial restrictions

Where possible, on grounds of safety, patients should be transferred to medical facilities capable of providing the appropriate level of care. For example, electroconvulsive therapy for psychiatric patients with severe aortic stenosis and depression would be better managed (from their cardiac status) in the operating suite of the main hospital rather than in a room off the psychiatric ward. Nonessential surgery should not be undertaken at the site of a major disaster or on the battlefield, and the use of local, regional, or sedative techniques should be considered where appropriate.

The overriding principle in providing anesthesia under any of these conditions should be to use a simple, safe technique, familiar to the practitioner. To reduce complexity and prevent the potential administration of a hypoxic gas mixture and reducing the need for scavenging (and for many other well-rehearsed reasons), there is a case for avoiding the use of nitrous oxide entirely. Training and practice in such techniques are invaluable for the time when they may be required. Even within a modern operating room environment, a "difficult situation" may arise due to failure of a sophisticated electronic anesthetic workstation, a major power cut with failure of back-up generators or a disruption to piped gas supply. The use of total intravenous anesthesia (TIVA) and a self-inflating bag with a separate oxygen cylinder, combined with practical clinical monitoring, will allow adequate and safe anesthesia in such a situation, and a flashlight may be the most essential item of additional equipment.

Difficult Situations Within Hospitals

Sites away from the operating rooms often have anesthetic equipment that is used only occasionally. Piped oxygen and suction facilities may be absent. The equipment in such areas must be maintained and checked adequately, with basic monitoring meeting the standard recommended by the American Society of Anesthesiologists.[1] All modern anesthetic machines in use in the United States should be incapable of delivering a hypoxic mixture. There must be immediate access to resuscitation equipment and drugs, and a means of summoning additional assistance (i.e., telephone or intercom). The anesthesiologist and his or her assistant should have sufficient experience and be familiar with both the environment and the equipment.

Some specific problems posed to patients, medical attendants, and equipment within particular areas are listed below. More detailed discussion of equipment considerations for MRI, CT, and radiotherapy suites can be found in Chapter 23.

Radiology Departments

- Ionizing radiation risk
- Long procedures (e.g., coiling of intracerebral aneurysms)
- Low levels of lighting
- Restricted access to patient or patient's head
- There may be a requirement to stop ventilation briefly to prevent image blurring.

Radiotherapy Suites

- Intense ionizing radiation requiring patient isolation from the medical attendants
- Closed-circuit television or glass-liquid-glass window to view patient causing color and image distortion
- Multiple frequent treatments over a few weeks
- Radiotherapy applicators may obstruct access to the patient's head

Magnetic Resonance Imaging (MRI)

- Intense magnetic field with the ability to cause equipment made of ferromagnetic material to be attracted at projectile velocity into the scanner. There is, however, a rapid decrease in field strength with distance.
- Electrical inductance—potential thermal injury from electrical conducting leads

- Electromagnetic interference leading to equipment malfunction (e.g., syringe drivers)
- Noise from vibration of switched gradient coils—ear protection for patients
- Theoretical risk of hypoxia if quenching of the superconducting magnets with cryogenic gases (usually helium) occurs. Quenching may occur as a fault condition or be initiated for emergency shutdown of the magnet.

These factors pose risks to patients and potential occupational hazards to staff. Patients and staff must be screened before access is granted to an MRI scanner to exclude ferromagnetic implants such as aneurysm clips or pacemakers. Anesthetic equipment taken into the vicinity of the MRI scanner must be MR-compatible.[2]

Remote Anesthesia

Anesthesia for MRI, radiotherapy, and some radiological procedures may necessitate the anesthesiologist and the bulk of the anesthetic equipment being remote from the patient. This may be either to ensure all ferromagnetic equipment is outside the magnetic field or to remove anesthetic personnel from ionizing radiation.

- TIVA may be employed using long infusion lines on pumps, which must be able to cope with the increased resistance to flow caused by the increased length. This usually means setting to maximum the pressure limit for sensing an occlusion.
- Although sedation may be sufficient for some patients, the airway may need to be secured with a laryngeal mask airway (LMA) or tracheal tube.
- Intermittent positive pressure ventilation through a long co-axial breathing system, such as a 9.6 to 10 m Bain circuit and Nuffield Penlon series 200 ventilator, has been shown to provide safe anesthesia.[3] With this system, there is an increase in the static compliance in proportion to the length of the tubing. This is caused by expansion of the breathing hose and compression of the volume of gas during positive pressure ventilation and will result in a lower tidal volume being delivered than is set on the ventilator. This is insignificant in adults. In children, if a Newton valve is used, the ventilator becomes a pressure generator, and the increased resistance and compliance of the long system results in the pressure delivered being significantly less than that selected (23% less with a 10 kg child). This compares with a 6% to 11% reduction when using a long rubber Ayre's T-piece.[4]
- The capnography signal is delayed due to the length of the sampling line but provides a guide for adjustment of the tidal volume.

Major Accidents and Disasters

These may occur in any part of the world at any time and are by definition unexpected. All medical services should have a plan to deal with major disasters. A typical approach is to have a mobile medical team that can be rapidly deployed to the disaster site and a receiving hospital capable of dealing with the retrieved casualties. In the event of the number of casualties overwhelming the initial response, there should be a means of either escalating the number of teams or hospitals deployed. In developing countries, there may be a need to seek international assistance. Many countries have teams available for worldwide deployment at short notice. Particular problems encountered include:

- Unfamiliar territory
- Unfriendly environment
  - Extremes of hot and cold and altitude, even in normally temperate climates
  - Dark, wet, cramped conditions
- Unfamiliar injuries
  - Blast and crush injuries
  - Delayed extrication
- Risk to rescuers:
  - Nuclear, biological, or chemical incidents
  - Terrorism
  - Fire, explosion risk
  - Continuing disaster (e.g., earthquake)
  - Unstable buildings

The predominant anesthetic contribution to a major disaster is resuscitation and stabilization before transfer to the receiving medical facility. Exceptionally, to aid extrication of casualties, amputation of trapped limbs may be required. This is best achieved using ketamine, either intravenously or intramuscularly. Equipment for intubation, self-inflating bag, fluid, and cannulas for intravenous fluid resuscitation should be available. Oxygen and Entonox (mixture of nitrous oxide 50% and oxygen 50%) should be used cautiously in such conditions because they support and accelerate combustion of flammable materials, and although the latter has excellent analgesic properties, it may not be suitable in very cold conditions or in the presence of a head injury or pneumothorax.

The Battlefield

Mobile field hospitals are deployed as close to the battlefront as safety will allow and receive casualties who may have had pressure dressings applied and airways secured in the field, or possibly have had first-aid treatment at a battalion aid station or equivalent. In addition to military casualties from both sides of the conflict, there are frequently civilian casualties, which may include children. This poses a problem if pediatric equipment is not available. Large numbers of casualties may arrive simultaneously and require triage on arrival. In some, immediate surgery is required as part of the resuscitation process. Some of the features of military anesthesia are as follows:

- Equipment must be portable and durable
- Oxygen cylinders or concentrators are usually readily available
- Cost constraints for drugs and equipment are minimal
- Resupply can often be difficult, especially if supply lines are cut or the area of operation is a truly austere and hostile environment with little existing infrastructure

Electricity is required for lighting, monitoring, suction, heating, and refrigeration (for blood storage and some drugs) and usually will be supplied from generators that must be of sufficient power to cope with maximum demand. Vital equipment should have an independent battery back-up to allow for continued use in the event of power failure. Sensitive equipment should have surge protection to limit voltage spikes from erratic power supplies.

Draw-over anesthesia is the most suitable inhalational technique for use in the field. It can be employed for both spontaneous and controlled ventilation, is not dependent on compressed gases, and requires only light portable equipment. The basic equipment required comprises:

- Nonrebreathing valve
- Self-inflating bag
- Low-resistance vaporizer
- Means of giving supplemental oxygen (T-piece, length of tubing to use as oxygen reservoir and source of oxygen [i.e., cylinder or concentrator]).

The Ohmeda Portable Anesthesia Complete, or PAC (Figure 24–1), is the draw-over vaporizer currently in use by the U.S. military. The PAC is a calibrated, temperature compensated, flow-over, low resistance vaporizer, which is designed for use in austere environments where economy of size and simplicity are essential. It is designed for use with nonrebreathing type of circuits and is classified as "agent nonspecific,"[5] although it is generally used with isoflurane. It is important that when using the PAC the dial setting is not relied upon as an absolute indicator of the true vaporizer output. Gas analyzers can be used to determine actual vaporizer output. The difference between the dial setting and true output varies based on ventilation or ventilator type, and minute ventilation.[6] In the combat environment often simply verifying that anesthetic gas is being delivered by quickly sniffing the end of the circuit is all that is possible. IV adjuncts and monitoring physiological parameters can then help ensure proper depth of anesthesia.

Besides its ease of use and portability, the vaporizer is also extremely durable and requires low maintenance, which is particularly valuable in austere environments that often lack medical equipment maintenance support. The contents will not spill if the vaporizer is accidentally inverted or dropped; however, if the vaporizer is inverted, it must be kept upright for a few minutes before use to allow any agent that has entered the bypass or control mechanism to drain back into the chamber, otherwise very high concentrations of vapor may be initially delivered. It is recommended that the vaporizer should be drained for transport. The PAC, when in use in the austere military setting, is commonly paired with a portable ventilator while maintaining the draw-over configuration. The ventilator currently used by the U.S. military is the Uni-Vent Eagle Model 754 Portable Ventilator, which is commonly used by civilian EMS and critical care transport professionals (Figure 24–2). Capnography, end-expired agent concentration monitoring, and pulse oximetry, if available at the field hospital, will help enable safe anesthesia to be provided with such equipment. In addition to the ventilator, the military also uses the impact 326 Ultra-Lite continuous and programmable intermittent suction system (Figure 24–3). The PAC, due to its size and therefore limited components, is not approved for routine use in the United States. This causes difficulty in attempts to gain experience with the equipment in the modern hospital environment where more advanced equipment is the standard. There are, however, courses available to demonstrate the use of the draw-over apparatus, using highly sophisticated anesthetic simulators. There are also more advanced field-ready anesthesia machines that may be used in some military deployment settings. Currently the Fabius Tiro M by Drager (Figure 24–4) is in use by the U.S. military, although other machines can still be found. The advantage of the Tiro M over the draw-over type of system

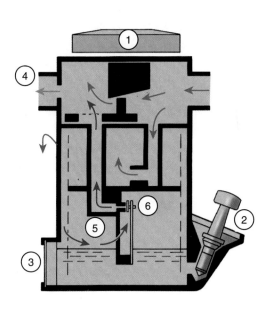
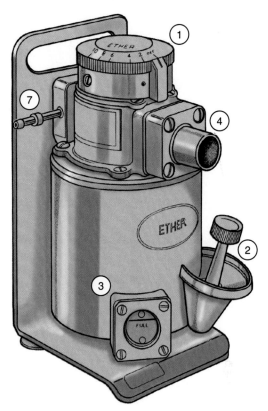

Figure 24–1   PAC (portable anesthesia complete) vaporizer (Ohmeda). *(1)* Concentration control, *(2)* filling port for ether, *(3)* ether-level gauge, *(4)* outlet and one-way valve, *(5)* vaporizing chamber, *(6)* thermocompensator valve, *(7)* port for oxygen enrichment. *(Reproduced with permission of WHO from Dobson MB. Anaesthesia at the District Hospital, Geneva, World Health Organization, 1980.)*

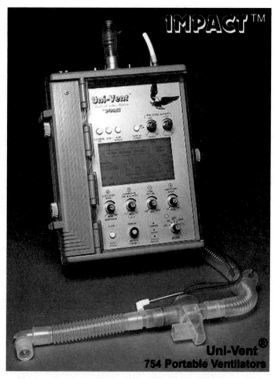

Figure 24–2   Uni-Vent 754 Portable Ventilator. *(From Glacier County EMS. (website): http://www.glacierems.com/impact_uni-vent-754_.jpg.)*

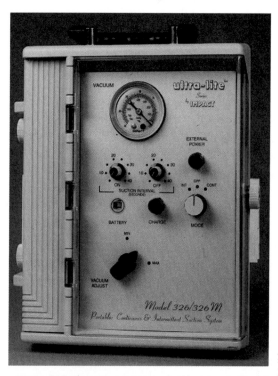

Figure 24–3   326 Ultra-Lite continuous and programmable intermittent suction system. *(From JD Honigberg International. (website): http://www.jdhmedical.com/Impact/326.jpg.)*

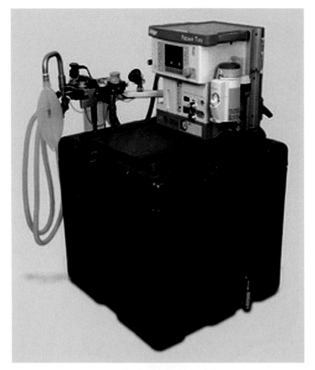

Figure 24–4   Fabius Tiro M by Dräger. *(From Dräger. (website): http://www. draeger.com/media/productSelector/m-resultview1/fabius_tiro_m_MT-0961-2007_us.jpg.)*

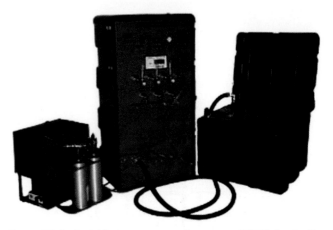

Figure 24–5   Portable oxygen generation system (POGS), by On Site Gas Systems. *(From On Site Gas Systems (website): http://www.onsitegas.com/images/pogscase.jpg.)*

is significant. Although a more complex machine, the Tiro M uses an electronically controlled, piston-driven ventilator, which decreases fresh gas usage and the air entrainment capability allows the ventilator to continue to function in the absence of fresh gas flow.[7] The Tiro M is easily set up and is transported in a military grade shipping container, which doubles as a workstation and machine stand. The Tiro M has a familiar interface from which to supply anesthetic care in a more controlled and elegant manner, taking full advantage of the oxygen sensor, multiple ventilation modes, and clear display of circuit pressure.

One of the most essential pieces of gear to the military field hospital is the oxygen generator. Although some may argue that otherwise healthy individuals can tolerate room air during controlled ventilation, those with the most significant injuries require supplemental oxygen. This requirement is met in field units with the use of the Portable Oxygen Generation System (POGS) by On Site Gas Systems (Figure 24–5). The U.S. military uses two variations of the system, the POGS-10 and the POGS-33, each capable of delivering up to 93% oxygen at 10 L or 33 L/min, respectively. These systems essentially compress room air, filter out nitrogen, and store the remaining oxygen in a reservoir for delivery to the patient. There is also a booster assembly that can be used to fill small oxygen tanks, thus maintaining consistent supply of oxygen for use in patient transport.

Nuclear Biological Chemical (NBC) Capability

Under conditions of NBC warfare, mobile military operating rooms are designed, by the use of air filters, to provide a protected environment. For additional patient protection, an NBC filter may be placed on the end of the inlet tubing of the breathing apparatus, and if an oxygen concentrator is used as the source of supplemental oxygen, this can also be provided with an NBC filter.

Equipment for Other Battlefield Anesthetic Techniques

Total intravenous anesthesia is also advocated for military anesthesia because it can simplify equipment requirements. Ketamine/midazolam and propofol/alfentanil (either combination with vecuronium added for controlled ventilation) have been used very successfully and requires little more than a self-inflating bag and oxygen source, together with an infusion bag (or syringe) with the mixed combination of drugs, and an infusion pump if available.[8]

Abnormal Ambient Pressures

Altitude

It may be necessary to use anesthetic equipment at low ambient pressures, as in the transfer of patients by aircraft and in high-altitude locations. The highest human habitation is at about 5,000 m or 16,000 feet, giving an atmospheric pressure of about 400 mm Hg. Commercial aircraft, however, usually have cabin pressure maintained at 640 mm Hg minimum, which is equivalent to 5,000 feet, despite flying at heights of more than 30,000 feet. To provide safe anesthesia, a knowledge of the altered performance of anesthetic equipment at different ambient pressures is essential.

- *Vaporizers.* Saturated vapor pressure is a function of temperature, not ambient pressure. Hence, the concentration delivered by a vaporizer is inversely proportional to the ambient pressure as the vapor pressure takes up a higher proportion of the ambient pressure at altitude, and a lesser proportion under hyperbaric conditions. However, the partial pressure of the agent, which determines the clinical effect remains constant. Therefore, when vaporizers are used at a given setting, the anesthetic will be delivered at a constant potency or effect, regardless of concentration changes with altitude (or depth). A vaporizer set at 1% at sea level will deliver 1.7% at 15,000 feet, but the clinical effect will be unaltered.

- *Flowmeters.* The reduction in gas density at altitude results in under-reading of variable orifice, constant differential pressure flowmeters. The error is about 20% at 10,000 feet. Under hyperbaric conditions, these flowmeters will overread.[9]
- *Venturi type of oxygen masks.* These will entrain less air at altitude and so deliver higher concentrations of oxygen. A 35% mask will deliver approximately 41% oxygen at 10,000 feet.
- *Ventilators.* Volume- or time-cycled ventilators may be preferable to pressure-cycled ventilators, but capnography and other monitoring will assist in adjusting ventilator settings under these conditions.
- *Pressure gauges.* These are calibrated at sea level and so overread at altitude. The error is negligible because the pressures measured are so much greater.
- *Gas analyzers and capnography.* Gas analyzers measure the partial pressure of the gas under test but are calibrated in percentage at sea level. They will, therefore, underread at high altitude. Reduction of atmospheric pressure may also affect capnography in the following ways:[10]
  - Pumping of gas through sample chamber
  - More powerful pump may be required to maintain flow rates
  - Calibration inaccuracies may occur; this may be corrected by recalibration at altitude
  - Fall in barometric pressure may be electronically sensed as a gas leak within the monitor

Hyperbaric Chamber and Anesthetic Equipment

A brief synopsis of some issues specific to high ambient pressure environment is given below:

- Gas diffusion into gases or liquids causes bubbles on decompression. Rapid decompression with gas expansion may result in breakages of sealed and, particularly, glass containers.
- Oxygen-rich environment under hyperbaric conditions increases the risk of fire; normally nonflammable materials may become flammable.
- During decompression, humidity increases, causing water condensation.
- The combination of increased water vapor and metallic walls and equipment increases the risk of electrocution and short circuits.

Most anesthetic equipment is at best untested under these conditions, and at worst dangerous. The following issues should be considered:

- Batteries—risk of bursting or leaking.
- Endotracheal tube cuffs should be liquid filled.
- Intravenous lines must be primed without air.
- Chest drains must be vented to chamber air through flutter valves (not bottles, as water seals may be problematic, particularly during rapid transition to different pressures).
- LCD monitor screens may crack or break due to gas bubbling out of solution during rapid decompression.
- Pressure transducers may malfunction.

- Simple minute volume divider ventilators may function better than other types of ventilators.
- Defibrillators are extremely hazardous due to the risks of electrocution and fire (see previous discussion). The metal floors and walls of the chamber mean that patient and operator are permanently earthed. Sparking may be disastrous under hyperbaric conditions in an atmosphere that may be contaminated with additional oxygen from the patient.

Developing Countries

There are two extremes of conditions that may be met in providing anesthesia in developing countries. The anesthesiologist may be totally dependent on the equipment, drugs, and personnel provided within the healthcare system of that country, or they may be part of a visiting team that is totally self-contained. Visiting teams may be very operation-specific (e.g., Project Orbis, Operation Smile, and other eye or cleft palate teams), or they may have a much wider remit. These teams usually have rigid preassessment protocols, ensuring that standard operations are carried out on fit patients, enabling the greatest good to be done to the largest number of people.

Some visiting teams may bring everything they need to perform a certain number of standard operations and anesthetics (in which case the equipment may be very similar to that for battlefield anesthesia [i.e., OMV based draw-over or TIVA]), although others opt to mainly use local equipment, adding only their own disposable equipment.

"District Hospital"-Based Anesthesia

Many small hospitals in developing countries rely on non-medically qualified assistants to deliver anesthesia under the supervision of the doctor, who will also be performing the surgery. Under these conditions, anesthetized patients are more likely to be intubated to ensure a secure airway. Most anesthesiologists in developing countries work in larger hospitals, but even here they may be responsible for the training and supervision of medical assistants giving anesthesia. Many such hospitals, large and small, will have storerooms, which have become graveyards of anesthetic machines and other equipment donated by well-meaning organizations or countries, without consideration for spare parts or expertise needed for their maintenance. There will often be continuous flow (Boyle's) machines, discarded as the necessary compressed medical gas supply is absent or erratic. In addition, such machines may not have antihypoxia devices and vaporizers may be outdated, unserviceable, or grossly inaccurate. For all these reasons, local anesthetic techniques (nerve blocks, spinals, and epidurals) should be used where appropriate.

Draw-Over Apparatus

The unreliability of supply of pressurized gases favors the use of air with supplemental oxygen when available and draw-over type vaporizers. A combination of the EMO vaporizer or the OMV (calibrated and used for both halothane and trichloroethylene), together with a means of inflation such as a manual resuscitator or Oxford bellows, a Ruben, Ambu E, or similar nonrebreathing valve, and a facemask or endotracheal connector and tube, may be the most practical equipment for safe anesthesia under these circumstances. The facility for giving supplementary oxygen, using a T-piece and reservoir tubing is desirable.

Various arrangements of draw-over apparatus are shown in Figure 24–6, and the working principles of the commonly available draw-over vaporizers, both in the United States and other countries, are shown in Figures 24–7, 24–8, through 24–9.

Supplemental Oxygen

Medical oxygen may be available in cylinders, but these may not follow international standards of cylinder identification, and apparently full cylinders may be found to be empty. Industrial oxygen may be available, but be aware that there may be an increased level of impurities in such supplies. Up to 95% high-quality oxygen may be obtained from an oxygen concentrator. Oxygen concentrators are relatively maintenance-free but require a source of electrical power to run a compressor and a switching device. A concentrator the size of

a small domestic fridge will produce an inexhaustible supply of oxygen at the rate of about 4 L a minute.

Ventilators Suitable for Developing Countries
Manley Multivent Ventilator

This ventilator was developed by the late Roger Manley, specifically for use in developing countries (Figure 24–10).[11] It differs from most other gas driven ventilators in that the volume of gas required to drive the ventilator is only one tenth of the patient's minute volume. Furthermore, if the driving gas is oxygen it may be automatically collected and used to supplement the inspired oxygen concentration. Used in this way, set at a minute volume of 4 L/min, an E size oxygen cylinder containing 680 L would drive the ventilator and supply 35% oxygen in air for a period of 28 hours. The ventilator consists of a weighted beam, attached at one end to a fulcrum and at the other end to the top of the bellows. The beam is pushed upwards by the driving gas under

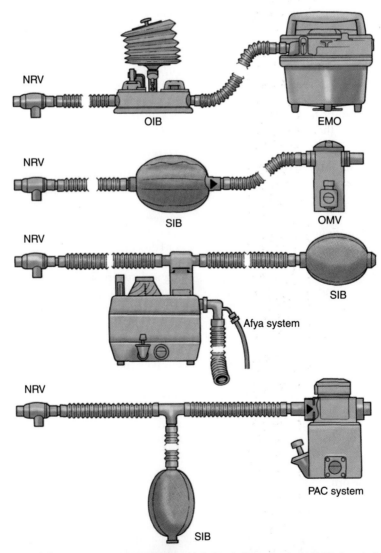

Figure 24–6 Several arrangements of drawover apparatus: OIB, Oxford inflating bellows (Penlon); EMO, Epstein Macintosh Oxford ether vaporizer (Penlon); NRV, nonrebreathing valve (e.g., Ruben); SIB, self-inflating bag (Laerdal, Ambu, etc.); PAC, portable anesthesia complete (Ohmeda). *(Reproduced with permission of WHO from Dobson MB. Anaesthesia at the District Hospital, Geneva, World Health Organization, 1980.)*

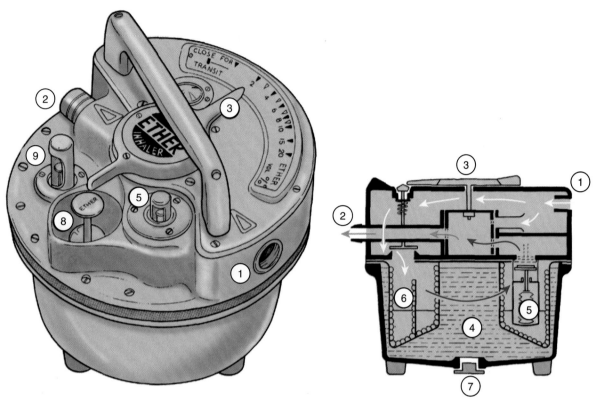

Figure 24–7 EMO vaporizer. *(1)* Inlet port, *(2)* outlet port, *(3)* concentration control, *(4)* water jacket, *(5)* thermocompensator valve, *(6)* vaporizing chamber, *(7)* filling port for water, *(8)* filling port for anesthetic, *(9)* anesthetic-level indicator. *(Reproduced with permission of WHO from Dobson MB. Anaesthesia at the District Hospital, Geneva, World Health Organization, 1980.)*

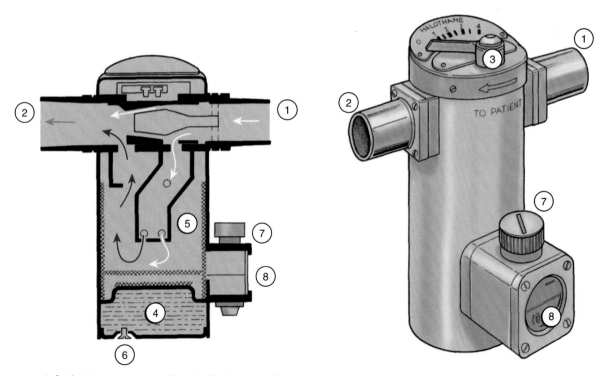

Figure 24–8 Oxford miniature vaporizer (OMV). *(1)* Inlet port, *(2)* outlet port, *(3)* concentration control, *(4)* heat sink, *(5)* vaporizing chamber, *(6)* filling port for water, *(7)* filling port for anesthetic, *(8)* anesthetic-level indicator. *(Reproduced with permission of WHO from Dobson MB. Anaesthesia at the District Hospital, Geneva, World Health Organization, 1980.)*

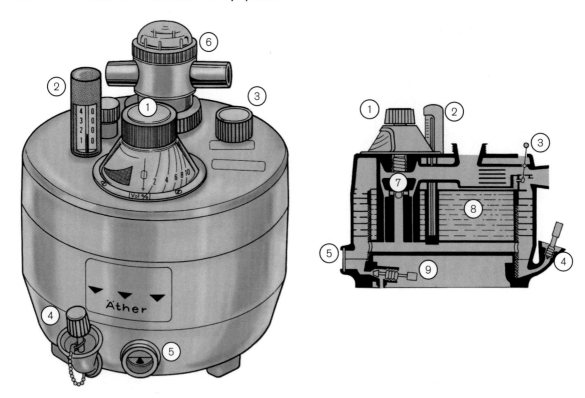

Figure 24–9 Afya vaporizer (Dräger). *(1)* Concentration control, *(2)* thermometer, *(3)* on/off control, *(4)* filling port for ether, *(5)* ether-level gauge, *(6)* outlet and one-way valve, *(7)* vaporizing chamber, *(8)* water-filled heat reservoir, *(9)* drainage port for ether. *(Reproduced with permission of WHO from Dobson MB. Anaesthesia at the District Hospital, Geneva, World Health Organization, 1980.)*

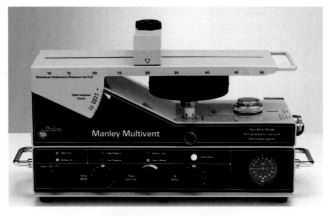

Figure 24–10 Manley Multivent. *(Photo courtesy Penlon Ltd, UK.)*

a pressure of at least 140 Kpa acting on a piston. When the set tidal volume is reached, the flow of driving gas is interrupted and the weight of the beam compresses the bellows, delivering the mixture of anesthetic gases to the patient. The economy of driving gas is achieved by the relative distances of the piston and the bellows to the fulcrum. Should the supply of pressurized gas fail completely, the bellows can be operated manually.

Combination Anesthetic Equipment

A number of ingenious machines incorporating an oxygen concentrator, oxygen cylinders, a ventilator, and vaporizers, which can be used in either draw-over or continuous flow

mode, assembled on a mobile trolley, have been produced. The advantage of such equipment is that it is permanently assembled and available and recognized as the complete versatile anesthetic machine. If monitoring equipment is available, this can be incorporated as well. Two examples of these are the "Glostavent" (Figure 24–11), which was developed by Roger Eltringham in Gloucester, UK,[12] and is based on the Manley Multivent Ventilator, and the "Fentolator" developed by Paul Fenton in Malawi.[13]

Finally, the other essential piece of equipment is suction apparatus. In areas where electricity supply may be unreliable, it is advisable to have manual or foot-operated suction apparatus.

Essential Equipment to Pack

When going to work as an anesthesiologist in a developing country, there is a limit to the amount of equipment that can be taken. Excess baggage is currently charged a significant fee on most airline flights, although many airlines may waive charges if contacted in advance and charitable status is established. Examples of equipment to take include:

- Bodok seals
- Assorted connectors and adaptors
- Basic airway equipment—self-inflating bag, mask, guedel airways, laryngoscope (including spare batteries and bulbs)
- Stethoscope
- Peripheral nerve stimulator needles, nerve stimulator, and batteries

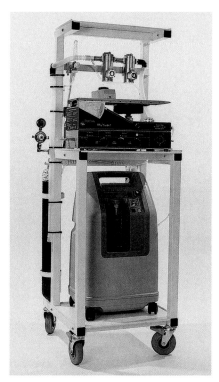

Figure 24–11 Glostavent anaesthetic machine. *(Supplied by Dr. Roger Eltringham.)*

- Selection of emergency drugs, relaxants, and local anesthetics, preferably in plastic ampules (special permission is required to take controlled drugs across international borders)
- Rolls of adhesive tape

Monitoring

The minimum standards of monitoring for safe anesthesia have been recommended by the American Society of Anesthesiologists. These include:

- Pulse oximetry
- Electrocardiogram
- Arterial blood pressure
- Capnography and gas analysis

In developing countries, various local factors may make this ideal difficult to attain, in particular:

- Capital cost of equipment
- Reliable power source
- Availability of disposables—electrodes, transducers, etc.
- Maintenance of equipment
- Transportability of equipment
- User ability to interpret results

In the absence of electronic equipment, relatively safe anesthesia may still be achieved using minimal equipment and observations, for example:

- Precordial stethoscope
- Sphygmomanometer
- Finger on pulse
- Patient's color (mucous membranes)
- Capillary refill time
- Other clinical observations

However, in remote situations, there is no doubt that both the safety and quality of anesthesia depend upon the ability of anesthesiologists to adapt techniques and equipment appropriate to the local resources, and to their skill and attention to respond rapidly to clinical signs where monitoring may be minimal by comparison with standards of practice in the developed world.

Further Reading

Dobson, M.B., 1988. Anesthesia at the District Hospital. World Health Organization, Geneva.

Ezi-Ashi, T.I., Papworth, D.P., Nunn, J.F., 1983. Inhalational anesthesia in developing countries. The problems and a proposed solution. Anesthesia 38, 729–747.

Magee, P.T., Tooley, M., 2004. The physics, clinical measurement and equipment of anesthetic practice. Oxford University Press, Oxford.

References

1. ASA. The American Society of Anesthesiologists standards for basic anesthetic monitoring (website): http://www.asahq.org/publicationsAndServices/standards/02.pdf. Accessed April, 15, 2010.
2. ASA, 2009. Practice advisory on anesthetic care for magnetic resonance imaging: a report by the American Society of Anesthesiologists task force on anesthetic care for magnetic resonance imaging. Anesthesiology 110, 459–479.
3. Sweeting, C.J., Thomas, P.W., Sanders, D.J., 2002. The long Bain breathing system: an investigation into the implications of remote ventilation. Anaesthesia 57, 1183–1186.
4. Jackson, E., Tan, S., Yarwood, G., et al., 1994. Increasing the length of the expiratory limb of the Ayre's T-piece: implications for remote mechanical ventilation in infants and children. Br J Anaesth 73, 154–156.
5. Walter Reed Army Medical Center. (website): www.wramc.army.mil/patients/healthcare/surgery/anesthesiology/pages/trainingguidlines.aspx.
6. Hawkins, J.K., Ciresi, S.A., Phillips, W.J., 1998. Performance of the universal portable anesthesia complete vaporizer with mechanical ventilation in both drawover and pushover configurations. Mil Med 163, 159–163.
7. Dräger, Fabius Tiro M (website): http://www.draeger.com/US/en_US/products/medical_therapy/anesthesia_workstations/ane_Fabius_M.jsp.
8. Restall, J., Tully, A.M., Ward, P.J., et al., 1988. Total intravenous anaesthesia for military surgery. A technique using ketamine, midazolam and vecuronium. Anaesthesia 43, 46–49.
9. McDowall, D.G., 1964. Anaesthesia in a pressure chamber. Anaesthesia 19, 321–336.
10. Pattinson, K., Myers, S., Gardner-Thorpe, C., 2004. Problems with capnography at altitude. Anaesthesia 59, 69–72.
11. Manley, R., 1991. A new ventilator for developing countries and difficult situations. World Anaesth Newsl 5, 10–11.
12. Eltringham, R.J., 2001. Fan Qui Wei. The Glostavent—an anesthetic machine for difficult situations. ITACCS; Spring/Summer 38–40.
13. Fenton, P.M., 2003. Inhalation anesthesia in developing countries: the problems and a proposed solution - 3. Anaesth News 191, 8–9. www.aagbi.org/_news_2003.html .

Chapter 25

Prevention of Infection: Disinfection and Sterilization of Equipment

Arnold J. Berry

Patients and healthcare providers expect that surgical and invasive diagnostic or therapeutic procedures will not lead to infection. In the United States, there are more than 45 million surgical and invasive procedures performed annually, and lapses in infection control procedures may have devastating consequences producing patient morbidity or mortality. Based on estimates made by the Centers for Disease Control and Prevention (CDC), healthcare-associated infections (HAI) are one of the top 10 causes of death in the United States and produce a significant financial impact on the healthcare system.[1,2]

Proper disinfection or sterilization of equipment is critical for preventing healthcare-related infection. The description of a recent outbreak of infection after thoracic surgery clearly illustrates the importance of adherence to accepted protocols.[3] Seven patients having thoracic or cardiac anesthesia developed *Pseudomonas aeruginosa* pneumonia or bronchitis within several days after surgery. Investigation of several possible sources indicated that bronchoscopes used by anesthesiologists for placement of double lumen endotracheal tubes had not been properly disinfected after use. Inadequate cleaning of the used bronchoscopes and a problem with the automated equipment used for disinfection resulted in residual bacterial contamination of the bronchoscopes after processing. The pathogens remaining on the inadequately disinfected scopes were subsequently transmitted to several patients. Identification and correction of the flaws in the cleaning and disinfection processes terminated the outbreak.

The Spaulding Classification of Equipment for Disinfection and Sterilization

Infection control practitioners have used a classification scheme proposed by Earle Spaulding for determining appropriate disinfection and sterilization of patient care equipment. This approach has been generally accepted by the CDC and is contained in their most recent guidelines.[1] Spaulding categorized devices as critical, semicritical, and noncritical corresponding to the risk of infection associated with its use. The greatest risk for infection is associated with contaminated critical items because these are devices that enter the patients' sterile tissue or vascular system. Examples of critical devices include surgical instruments and vascular or urinary catheters. Semicritical items are those that contact mucous membranes or nonintact skin and include the majority of devices used in respiratory therapy and anesthesiology. Examples of semicritical items include the following: laryngoscope blades, esophageal stethoscopes, suction catheters, oral and nasal airways, and laryngeal mask airways. Noncritical items are devices that either do not touch the patient or contact only intact skin, but not mucous membranes and do not enter sterile tissues. Noncritical patient care items include devices such as blood pressure cuffs, pulse oximeter probes, and electrocardiogram (ECG) cables. Environmental surfaces can be considered noncritical items and include hospital beds and stretchers, the surface of the anesthesia machine, and laryngoscope handles. Since intact skin should provide an effective barrier to most pathogens, noncritical items are associated with a lower risk of infection, but they can serve as an environmental reservoir for pathogens. Because noncritical items are frequently touched by healthcare workers, secondary transmission of pathogens can occur to patients via contaminated hands or gloves.

Cleaning

A reduction in the number of microorganisms or their complete elimination from medical devices occurs along a spectrum, from cleaning through disinfection to sterilization. Cleaning is simply the physical removal of organic and inorganic material from devices and the surfaces of equipment. This can be accomplished by using water and detergents or enzymatic products to manually scrub and mechanically loosen the unwanted contaminating material. Cleaning may be used as a lower order process on noncritical items, but it is a mandatory step before disinfection or sterilization since the effectiveness of these higher order processes is compromised when residual inorganic or organic materials limit the active ingredients from contacting the device's surfaces (Figure 25–1). Decontamination is the process of removing pathogenic organisms from items before discarding or to make them safe to handle.

Disinfection

Disinfection can be used to eliminate most or all pathogenic micro-organisms, except bacterial spores or prions, from medical devices. Disinfection occurs across a range, from low level to high (Table 25–1). The level of disinfection is determined by several factors: the type and quantity of microbial contamination; the specific germicide, including its concentration and the exposure time; the physical nature of the object; the presence of a biofilm (a tightly adherent mass of bacteria and accumulated material); and the temperature and pH of the disinfection process[1] (Table 25–2). Low level disinfection processes kill most vegetative bacteria, some fungi, and some viruses. Intermediate level disinfection kills the previously mentioned groups and most viruses and mycobacteria. High level disinfectants will eliminate all micro-organisms, except bacterial spores and prions. It is important to realize that disinfectants are chemicals and processes designed to kill micro-organisms but are intended only for application to inanimate objects. Chemicals used as disinfectants must be evaluated and cleared for medical use by the U.S. Food and Drug Administration (FDA). In contrast, antiseptics are germicides that are intended for use on living tissue, mucous membranes, or skin, and these substances are regulated by the U.S. Environmental Protection Agency (EPA).

Sterilization

Sterilization is the process that eliminates all micro-organisms and can be performed using either physical or chemical methods. Some chemicals commonly used for high-level disinfection can also produce sterilization under specific conditions (Table 25–3).

Disinfection of Healthcare Devices

With an understanding of the terminology of the Spaulding classification system, a matrix for appropriately processing medical equipment can be more easily understood. Critical

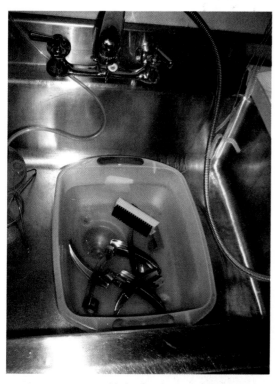

Figure 25–1 Laryngoscope blades for cleaning. Before disinfection or sterilization, equipment must be cleaned to remove blood, secretions, and other organic matter.

Table 25–1	The Order of Resistance of Microorganisms and the Level of Disinfection or Sterilization Required for Inactivation
Most Resistant	**Required Level of Disinfection or Sterilization***
Prions (Creutzfeldt-Jakob disease)	Prion reprocessing
Bacterial spores (*Bacillus atrophaeus*)	Sterilization
Coccidia (*Cryptosporidium*)	
Mycobacteria (*M. tuberculosis*)	High-level disinfection
Nonlipid or small viruses (polio, Coxsackie)	Intermediate-level disinfection
Fungi (*Candida, Aspergillus*)	
Vegetative bacteria (*S. aureus, P. aeruginosa*)	Low-level disinfection
Lipid or medium-sized viruses (HIV, herpes, hepatitis B)	
Most susceptible	

*Level of disinfection or sterilization inactivates all microorganisms in the class and those classes listed below it.

Modified from Figure 1 in Rutala WA, Weber DJ, Healthcare Infection Control Practices Advisory Committee. *CDC guideline for disinfection and sterilization in healthcare facilities, 2008*, CDC (website): http://www.cdc.gov/ncidod/dhqp/pdf/guidelines/Disinfection_Nov_2008.pdf; Accessed February 23, 2009.

items must be sterile and can either be purchased as sterile, single-patient use devices or may be reusable items that must be cleaned and sterilized between uses. Semicritical items must be sterile or require high-level disinfection. Most anesthesia airway equipment is considered semicritical and should undergo either high-level disinfection or sterilization. Because of the materials used and the difficulty sterilizing the long, narrow lumens, most bronchoscopes and endoscopes can only safely undergo high-level disinfection between patient use (see later discussion). Noncritical items should undergo cleaning or low level disinfection between patient use. This can be accomplished with disinfectant wipes to remove

organic material including blood and secretions from external devices such as ECG cables and environmental surfaces (e.g., the work surfaces of anesthesia machines or drug carts) that may become soiled and are touched by healthcare providers.[4]

Cleaning of equipment with detergents or enzymes is a critical part of the preparation process before disinfection or sterilization. Preferably, used items are soaked or rinsed before blood, tissue, or body substances dry on the instrument surface or in its channels (Figure 25–1). Once secretions are dried, they become more difficult to remove. Although cleaning is often done by hand, there are several types of mechanical cleaning machines to automate the process.

Since they are made of materials that are stable during high temperatures, most surgical instruments undergo heat or steam sterilization. An increasing number of medical devices are made of less durable materials such as plastics and require low temperature sterilization. Traditionally, ethylene oxide gas sterilization has been used for heat-sensitive medical equipment, but more recently, many low temperature sterilization systems are available to sterilize devices that would be harmed by high temperatures. These low temperature sterilization techniques include the use of hydrogen peroxide gas plasma, peracetic acid immersion, and ozone.

The most widely used method for sterilization has been saturated steam under pressure in an autoclave (Figure 25–2). Depending on the instrument being sterilized and the specific organisms that are to be eradicated, the autoclave processing cycle can be regulated by several parameters, including the amount of steam, pressure, temperature, and time. To confirm the effectiveness of the sterilization process, indicators are placed with the instruments in the autoclave.

Some materials, delicate electronics, or the optics used in various devices are harmed by the extreme conditions produced during the process of steam sterilization. These items require low temperature sterilization techniques. One of the oldest of these sterilization techniques uses ethylene oxide (ETO), a flammable, explosive gas. There are several limitations associated with the use of ETO sterilization, including a lengthy cycle time and toxicity to patients and personnel. Additionally, after sterilization, the devices must be aerated to remove residual ETO, which may be absorbed into the materials of the device. Acute exposure to ETO can result in skin and mucous membrane irritation while chronic exposure can produce neurological dysfunction, neuropathy, increased

Table 25–2 Factors Affecting the Efficacy of Sterilization

Factors	Effect
Cleaning	Failure to adequately clean an instrument results in higher bioburden, protein load, and salt concentration. These will decrease sterilization efficacy.
Bioburden	A larger number of microbes require a longer exposure to germicide for complete destruction. The natural bioburden of used surgical devices is 10^0 to 10^3 organisms (primarily vegetative bacteria), which is substantially below the 10^5-10^6 spores used with biological indicators.
Pathogen type	Spore-forming organisms are most resistant to sterilization and are the test organisms required for FDA clearance. However, the contaminating microflora on used surgical instruments consists mainly of vegetative bacteria.
Protein	Residual protein decreases efficacy of sterilization. However, cleaning appears to rapidly remove protein load.
Salt	Residual salt decreases efficacy of sterilization more than protein load. However, cleaning appears to rapidly removal salt load.
Biofilm accumulation	Biofilm accumulation reduces efficacy of sterilization by impairing exposure of the sterilant to the microbial cell.
Lumen length	Increasing lumen length impairs sterilant penetration. May require forced flow through lumen to achieve sterilization.
Lumen diameter	Decreasing lumen diameter impairs sterilant penetration. May require forced flow through lumen to achieve sterilization.
Restricted flow	Sterilant must come into contact with microorganisms. Device designs that prevent or inhibit this contact (e.g., sharp bends, blind lumens) will decrease sterilization efficacy.
Device design and construction	Materials used in construction may affect compatibility with different sterilization processes and affect sterilization efficacy. Design issues (e.g., screws, hinges) will also affect sterilization efficacy.

Modified from Table 10 in Rutala WA, Weber DJ, Healthcare Infection Control Practices Advisory Committee. *CDC guideline for disinfection and sterilization in healthcare facilities, 2008*, CDC (website): http://www.cdc.gov/ncidod/dhqp/pdf/guidelines/Disinfection_Nov_2008.pdf. Accessed February 23, 2009.

Table 25–3 Chemical Agents Used as Chemical Sterilants or as High-Level Disinfectants

- Peracetic acid/hydrogen peroxide
- Glutaraldehyde
- Hydrogen peroxide
- Ortho-phthalaldehyde
- Peracetic acid

STERILIZATION TECHNOLOGIES

- Steam
- Hydrogen peroxide gas plasma
- 100% Ethylene oxide or ethylene oxide with hydrochlorofluorocarbon
- Peracetic acid

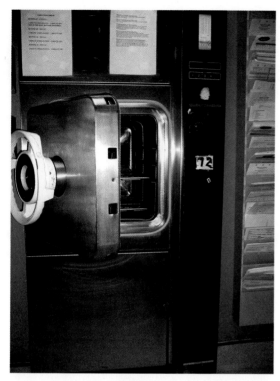

Figure 25–2 Autoclave. Most surgical instruments can withstand the high temperature steam and pressure produced in an autoclave, and therefore this is the most commonly used method of sterilization for these devices.

risk of spontaneous abortion, and cancer. If an ETO-sterilized device is used without adequate aeration, tissue burns may result from contact with patients' skin or mucosa. Because of these disadvantages, newer low temperature sterilization technologies have been developed (Table 25–3).

Either before or after disinfection or sterilization, equipment must be packaged to maintain sterility and prevent contamination. There should also be a clearly identifiable system for designating equipment that has already undergone processing so that it will not be confused with contaminated devices. The sterile or disinfected devices should be stored in an area where they will not become wet or the packaging torn or punctured. The date of processing should be indicated on the packaging and a shelf–life indicated.

Limitations of the Spaulding Classification System

Although the Spaulding classification has been useful, the discovery of new infectious agents such as prions and the introduction of complex, delicate medical equipment has been problematic and has necessitated additional considerations. Prions are the agents producing transmissible spongiform encephalopathies such as Creutzfeldt-Jakob disease (CJD) and are composed of a protein that is extremely resistant to inactivation by standard sterilization processes. Inadvertent human transmission of prion-associated disease has occurred via contaminated neurosurgical instruments used on patients with CJD or the variant forms of the disease. Special sterilization methods are required for instruments that come into

contact with brain, spinal cord, and eyes of patients with or suspected of having prion diseases. Sterilization guidelines for equipment contaminated with prions have been developed by the World Health Organization.[5] Because of the difficulty required to process equipment that has been used on patients suspected of having prion disease, single-use disposable equipment should be used when possible.

Special Considerations for Fiberoptic Endoscopes

Endoscopes with flexible fiberoptic bundles are complex devices that may have one or more small diameter, long working channels and therefore present specific challenges for cleaning and disinfection. Because endoscopes are made of materials that would be damaged by extremes of heat, elimination of pathogens from these devices must be accomplished by processes other than autoclaves that use high temperature and pressure. Fiberoptic laryngoscopes or bronchoscopes, frequently used by anesthesiologists, may become contaminated with blood, respiratory secretions, and respiratory tract pathogens including bacteria, viruses, and mycobacteria. Specific multistep protocols for proper cleaning and high-level disinfection of flexible fiberoptic endoscopes must include leak testing, cleaning, high-level disinfection, drying, and proper storage (Table 25–4). Many healthcare facilities use a combination of manual leak testing and cleaning followed by the use of an automated endoscope reprocessor to ensure that all steps in the disinfection process are followed (Figures 25–3 through 25–7). To facilitate clinical care, the cleaning and disinfection procedures must occur in a timely manner so that the equipment will be readily available.

Considerations for Bloodborne Pathogens and Antibiotic-Resistant Bacteria

Routine high-level disinfection is adequate to eliminate hepatitis B virus, hepatitis C virus, and human immunodeficiency virus (HIV) from medical devices. Some healthcare facilities have heightened concern regarding devices used on patients infected with these pathogens and have modified their disinfection procedures, but this is unwarranted. Additionally, institution of special infection control practices when bloodborne pathogens are suspected is inconsistent with CDC recommended standard precautions. These guidelines are based on the premise that healthcare providers cannot absolutely identify which patients are infected with blood-borne pathogens by history or routine laboratory tests, and therefore, standard precautions should be used with all patients.

Although some bacteria have become resistant to specific antibiotics—for example, methicillin-resistant *Staphylococcus aureus* (MRSA) and vancomycin-resistant *Enterococcus* (VRE)—the antibiotic resistance does not correlate with reduced susceptibility to disinfectants. However, some bacteria do have reduced susceptibility to disinfectants that results from a chromosome mutation or acquisition of new genetic material. Although these organisms have reduced susceptibility to disinfectants, the concentrations of chemicals used in most disinfection procedures greatly exceed the cidal level for these organisms and generally remain effective.

Table 25–4	Steps for Cleaning and High-Level Disinfection of Flexible Endoscopes
Leak testing	Used to detect damaged scopes that have a defect in the external construction that would permit contaminants to enter internal portions of the device.
Clean	Mechanically clean external and internal surfaces with water, detergent, and enzymatic cleaners; channels should also be thoroughly brushed and flushed.
High-level disinfection	Immerse scope in high-level disinfectant and flush channels following the specific requirements for the disinfectant solution; automated endoscope reprocessing devices may be used for this step.
Rinse	Rinse the scope and channels with water (sterile, filtered, or tap depending on the devices used).
Dry	The external surfaces and channels should be rinsed with alcohol and dried with forced air.
Storage	Scopes should be stored by hanging them vertically in a manner that will permit them to remain dry and prevent damage or contamination.

Modified from Rutala WA, Weber DJ, Healthcare Infection Control Practices Advisory Committee. *CDC guideline for disinfection and sterilization in healthcare facilities, 2008,* CDC (website): http://www.cdc.gov/ncidod/dhqp/pdf/guidelines/Disinfection_Nov_2008.pdf. Accessed February 23, 2009.

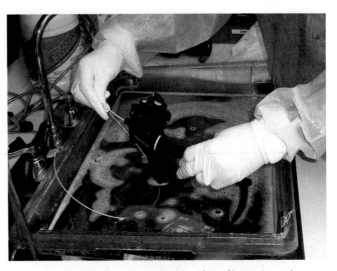

Figure 25–4 Brushing the channels of a fiberoptic endoscope. A flexible cleaning brush with detergent is introduced through the channels of the endoscope to ensure removal of any organic material before the disinfection procedure.

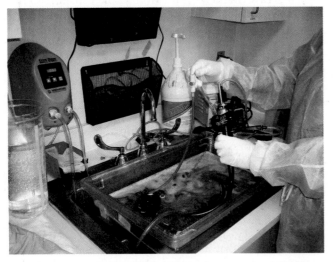

Figure 25–3 Leak testing of fiberoptic endoscope. After initial irrigation of the channels of a fiberoptic endoscope, the device is tested to ensure that there is not a leak in the external casing of the device.

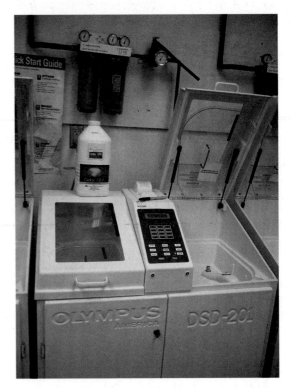

Figure 25–5 An automated endoscope reprocessor. There are several types of automated endoscope reprocessors. The devices are usually specific for the type of scope (bronchoscope, gastroscope) and the disinfecting agent to be used.

Occupational Exposure to Disinfectants

Occupational exposure to some germicide solutions or vapors has been associated with health hazards. Risk of toxicity after exposure depends on the specific chemical, the duration and intensity of exposure, and the route of exposure. Spills of a chemical germicide may result in an emergency situation requiring use of protective clothing and respirators for individuals cleaning the material. Individuals responsible for disinfection of devices may have repeated, chronic exposure to low levels of hazardous substances over a prolonged period. The Occupational Safety and Health Administration (OSHA) has promulgated standards to prevent injury of employees responsible for handling toxic substances. Manufacturers of hazardous chemicals are required to develop data sheets for employees who may be exposed to products via their work.

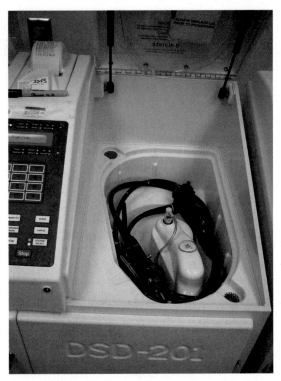

Figure 25–6 Endoscope loaded into the automated reprocessor. After cleaning and leak testing, the endoscope is placed into the automated reprocessor for the disinfection cycle.

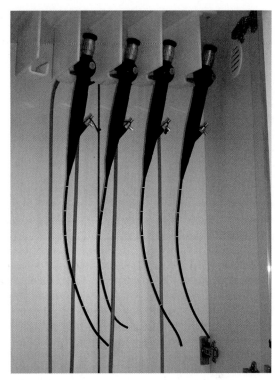

Figure 25–7 Storage of disinfected endoscopes. Disinfected endoscopes must be stored hanging freely in a clean, dry, closed cabinet.

Exposure limits (time-weighted averages) have been set for many substances used for disinfection. Additionally, there are federal limits on disposal of chemical germicides, especially when the substances will reenter the water system. To reduce environmental risks, the microbicidal activity of some chemicals such as glutaraldehyde can be neutralized before disposal.

Federal Regulation of Chemicals Used for Disinfection

In the United States, federal agencies are responsible for regulating chemical germicides. The EPA requires manufacturers to test germicides for microbicidal activity and for toxicity to animals and humans. EPA is responsible for regulation of disinfectants used on environmental surfaces but not for those used to process critical or semicritical medical devices. The FDA regulates chemicals used for high-level disinfection of critical and semicritical devices and antiseptics, the antimicrobials used on living tissue. As part of its duty to prevent infectious diseases, the CDC is responsible for providing scientific evidence and recommendations regarding the safety and efficacy of the chemicals used for inactivating microorganisms in specific clinical situations.

The FDA sets requirements for the antimicrobial activity of sterilants. Tests to demonstrate effectiveness require that low temperature sterilization technologies provide a 6-$\log_{10}$ reduction of microbes on test equipment. It is expected that in most situations, contaminated medical devices have a relatively low number of organisms. After cleaning the bioburden of most devices, it is likely to be less than 10^2 organisms and,

therefore, would be easily inactivated by standard sterilization processes.

Single-Use Devices

Because of the significant cost of equipment, supplies, and personnel required for disinfection or sterilization of medical devices, there may be some instances in which single-use disposable equipment may be preferred. In deciding whether to use single-use equipment or reusable items, it is important to consider costs for procuring, storing, and disposal of single-use equipment. Additionally, the impact of these disposables on the environment (landfills) should be considered.

Some practices have chosen to reuse medical devices intended and labeled as single-use products as a method for reducing costs. The practice of reusing single-use devices creates a series of regulatory and legal issues. The FDA has decided that institutions that reprocess devices labeled as single-use will be considered "manufacturers" and regulated as such.[6] The implication of this is that reused single-use devices must comply with the same requirements as when the equipment was originally manufactured. Since some single-use devices are made of materials that were not intended to be reprocessed, disinfection or sterilization of these items may result in their failure during use. The legal responsibility for sterility and integrity of the reprocessed device falls upon the user rather than the original manufacturer. Because of the complexity of reprocessing equipment intended to be single-use items, some institutions have decided to discontinue the practice. As an alternative, some healthcare facilities have chosen to outsource sterilization of single-use items to third-party reprocessors.

Prevention of Patient Infections Associated with Equipment

Healthcare-associated infections (HAI) remain a significant risk for patients and occur after a break in infection control procedure. Healthcare organizations, the government and regulators, accreditation agencies, medical associations, payers, and consumer advocacy groups are focusing on guidelines to prevent HAI to reduce patient morbidity and mortality and national healthcare costs.[7,8] The most frequent HAI are related to devices and procedures and include central line-associated bloodstream infections (CLABSI), ventilator-associated pneumonia (VAP), catheter-associated urinary tract infections (CAUTI), and surgical site infections (SSI). Increasing incidence of HAI associated with methicillin-resistant *Staphylococcus aureus* (MRSA) and *Clostridium difficile* is resulting in an increased patient morbidity.

Transmission of organisms to produce patient infection requires that the patient be susceptible to the specific pathogen, the viable pathogen be present in the environment, there be a means to transfer the microbe from the environment to the patient, and there be a portal for entry such as a break in the patient's natural barriers such as intact skin. Although pathogens can be found on environmental surfaces throughout the healthcare setting, there must be a mechanism to transmit them to patients. Often this occurs via the hands of personnel or contaminated equipment.[9,10] Intravascular catheters and other invasive devices such as endotracheal tubes provide a portal for entry of pathogens because they transgress natural host barriers.

The CDC and other groups have formulated guidelines to prevent HAI. Since pathogens are commonly found on healthcare workers hands, frequent hand washing is recommended to prevent transmission of disease to susceptible patients.[10] Microbial flora on hands of personnel can be divided into transient and resident. Transient flora colonize the superficial layers of skin, are organisms most likely associated with HAI since they are acquired during contact with patients or contaminated environmental surfaces, but are the most easily removed with hand washing. Resident flora are found in the deeper layers of skin, are harder to remove, but are less likely to be a source for HAI. Indications for hand washing are listed in Table 25–5. Observational studies demonstrate that many healthcare personnel do not wash hands as often as is recommended. Alcohol-based hand rubs should be supplied in patient care locations and operating rooms to encourage frequent hand cleansing, especially when sinks are not available.[11]

Evidence-based guidelines have been promulgated to prevent the most common types of equipment- and surgical-related infections. Recommendations from the CDC and the Healthcare Infection Control Practices Advisory Committee (HICPAC) for preventing CAUTI, CLABSI, and VAP are presented in Tables 25–6, 25–7, and 25–8, respectively.[2,12,13] Additionally, implementation of some recommendations for preventing surgical site infections can best be accomplished with assistance of anesthesia providers.[14] The timely intravenous administration of prophylactic antibiotics will ensure

that serum and tissue levels will be established at incision. Serum glucose levels should be controlled in diabetic patients and perioperative hyperglycemia should be avoided. Operating room doors should be closed during surgery except as needed for movement of equipment or personnel.

Table 25–5 Indications for Hand Washing or Hand Antisepsis

1. When hands are visibly dirty or contaminated with blood or body fluids using either a nonantimicrobial soap and water or an antimicrobial soap and water.
2. An alcohol-based hand rub can be used for routine hand antisepsis in all other clinical situations.
3. Decontaminate hands before having direct patient contact.
4. Decontaminate hands before donning sterile gloves before inserting central venous catheters.
5. Decontaminate hands after contact with a patient's intact skin.
6. Decontaminate hands after contact with body fluids, mucous membranes, nonintact skin, and wound dressings.
7. Decontaminate hands if moving from a contaminated body site to a clean body site during patient care.
8. Decontaminate hands after contact with medical equipment and environmental surfaces in the immediate vicinity of the patient.
9. Decontaminate hands after removing gloves.
10. Wash hands after using the restroom and before eating.

Modified from Boyce JM, Pittet D. Guideline for hand hygiene in health-care settings: recommendations of the healthcare infection control practices advisory Committee and the HIPAC/SHEA/APIC/IDSA hand hygiene task force. Am J Infect Control 2002;30:S1-S46.

Table 25–6 Prevention of Catheter-Associated Urinary Tract Infections

RECOMMENDATIONS FOR APPROPRIATE CATHETER USE

1. Insert catheters only for appropriate indications and leave in place only as long as needed.
2. Do not use urinary catheters for management of incontinence.
3. For operative patients who have an indication for an indwelling catheter, remove the catheter as soon as possible postoperatively, preferably within 24 hours.

RECOMMENDATIONS FOR ASEPTIC INSERTION OF URINARY CATHETERS

1. Ensure that only properly trained persons who know the correct technique of aseptic catheter insertion and maintenance are given this responsibility.
2. Insert catheters using aseptic technique and sterile equipment.

RECOMMENDATIONS FOR PROPER URINARY CATHETER MAINTENANCE

1. Maintain a sterile, continuously closed drainage system.
2. Do not disconnect the catheter and urinary drainage system unless the catheter must be irrigated.

Modified from US Department of Health and Human Services. *HHS action plan to prevent healthcare-associated infections: prevention—prioritized recommendations* (website): http://www.hhs.gov/ophs/initiatives/hai/prevention.html. Accessed April 13, 2009.

Table 25–7 Prevention of Intravascular Catheter-Associated Infections

RECOMMENDATIONS FOR ASEPTIC INSERTION OF VASCULAR CATHETERS

1. Maintain aseptic technique during insertion and care of intravascular catheters.
2. Use aseptic technique including the use of a cap, mask, sterile gown, sterile gloves, and a large sterile drape for the insertion of central venous catheters (CVC) including peripherally inserted central catheters (PICC) and guidewire exchanges.
3. Apply an appropriate antiseptic to the insertion site on the skin before catheter insertion and during dressing changes.
4. Although a 2% chlorhexidine-based preparation is preferred, tincture of iodine, an iodophor, or 70% alcohol can be used.
5. Select the catheter, insertion technique, and insertion site with the lowest risk for complications (infectious and noninfectious [pneumothorax]) for the anticipated type and duration of IV therapy.
6. Use a subclavian site (rather than a jugular or a femoral site) in adult patients to minimize the infection risk.
7. Weigh the risk and benefits of placing a device at a recommended site to reduce infectious complications against the risk for mechanical complications (e.g., pneumothorax, subclavian artery puncture, subclavian vein laceration, subclavian vein stenosis, hemothorax, thrombosis, air embolism, and catheter misplacement).

RECOMMENDATIONS FOR APPROPRIATE MAINTENANCE OF VASCULAR CATHETERS

1. Use either sterile gauze or sterile, transparent, semipermeable dressing to cover the catheter site.
2. Promptly remove any intravascular catheter that is no longer essential.
3. Replace the catheter-site dressing when it becomes damp, loosened, or soiled or when inspection of the site is necessary.

Modified from US Department of Health and Human Services. *HHS action plan to prevent healthcare-associated infections: prevention—prioritized recommendations* (website): http://www.hhs.gov/ophs/initiatives/hai/prevention.html. Accessed April 13, 2009.

Table 25–8 Prevention of Ventilator-Associated Pneumonia

RECOMMENDATIONS FOR ROUTINE CARE OF PATIENTS REQUIRING MECHANICAL VENTILATION

1. Use noninvasive ventilation whenever possible.
2. Use orotracheal rather than nasotracheal intubation when possible.
3. Minimize the duration of ventilation; perform daily assessments of readiness to wean from ventilation.
4. Prevent aspiration by maintaining patients in a semirecumbent position (30-45° elevation of head of bed) unless otherwise contra-indicated.
5. Use a cuffed endotracheal tube with an endotracheal cuff pressure of at least 20 cm H_2O and in-line or subglottic suctioning.
6. Perform regular oral care with an antiseptic solution.

RECOMMENDATIONS FOR APPROPRIATE CLEANING, DISINFECTION, AND STERILIZATION OF VENTILATOR EQUIPMENT

1. Thoroughly clean all equipment and devices to be sterilized or disinfected.
   a. Whenever possible, use steam sterilization or high-level disinfection for reprocessing semicritical equipment or devices that are not sensitive to heat and moisture.
   b. Use low-temperature sterilization methods for equipment or devices that are heat or moisture sensitive.
   c. After disinfection, proceed with appropriate rinsing, drying, and packaging, taking care not to contaminate the disinfected items in the process.
2. Preferentially use sterile water for rinsing reusable semicritical respiratory equipment and devices when rinsing is needed after they have been chemically disinfected; if this is not feasible, rinse the device with filtered water or tap water and then rinse with isopropyl alcohol and dry with forced air or in a drying cabinet.
3. Between uses on different patients, clean reusable components of the breathing system or patient circuit (e.g., tracheal tube or face mask), inspiratory and expiratory breathing tubing, y-piece, reservoir bag, humidifier, and tubing and then sterilize or subject them to high-level liquid chemical disinfection or pasteurization in accordance with the device manufacturers' instructions.

RECOMMENDATIONS FOR APPROPRIATE MAINTENANCE OF VENTILATOR CIRCUIT AND ASSOCIATED DEVICES

1. Drain and discard any condensate that collects in the tubing of a mechanical ventilator, taking precautions not to allow condensate to drain toward the patient.
2. Use only sterile fluid for nebulization and dispense the fluid into the nebulizer aseptically.
3. Use only sterile (not distilled, nonsterile) water to fill reservoirs of devices used for nebulization.

Modified from US Department of Health and Human Services. *HHS action plan to prevent healthcare-associated infections: prevention—prioritized recommendations* (website): http://www.hhs.gov/ophs/initiatives/hai/prevention.html. Accessed April 13, 2009.

Further Reading

Rutala W.A., Weber D.J., Healthcare Infection Control Practices Advisory Committee. CDC guideline for disinfection and sterilization in healthcare facilities, 2008, CDC (website): http://www.cdc.gov/ncidod/dhqp/pdf/guidelines/Disinfection_Nov_2008.pdf. Accessed February 23, 2009. *This CDC document contains detailed recommendations for disinfection and sterilization of medical equipment and is considered the best evidence for infection control practice.*

Boyce, J.M., Pittet, D. 2002. Guideline for hand hygiene in health-care settings: recommendations of the healthcare infection control practices advisory committee and the HIPAC/SHEA/APIC/IDSA hand hygiene task force. Am J Infect Control 30, S1–S46. *These are the most authoritative recommendations on hand washing for healthcare workers. Many observational surveys have demonstrated that healthcare providers do not routinely follow these hand washing recommendations, and this may lead to patient infections.*

References

1. Rutala W.A., Weber D.J., Healthcare Infection Control Practices Advisory Committee. CDC guideline for disinfection and sterilization in healthcare facilities, 2008, CDC (website): http://www.cdc.gov/ncidod/dhqp/pdf/guidelines/Disinfection_Nov_2008.pdf. Accessed February 23, 2009.

2. US Department of Health and Human Services. HHS action plan to prevent healthcare-associated infections: prevention—prioritized recommendations, (website): http://www.hhs.gov/ophs/initiatives/hai/prevention.html. Accessed April 13, 2009.

3. Shimono, N., Takuma, T., Tsuchimochi, N., et al., 2008. An outbreak of *Pseudomonas aeruginosa* infection following thoracic surgeries occurring via the contamination of bronchoscopes in an automatic endoscope reprocessor. J Infect Chemother 14, 418–423.

4. Hall, J.R., 1994. Blood contamination of anesthesia and monitoring equipment. Anesth Analg 78, 1136–1139.

5. WHO 23-26 March 1999. World Health Organization infection control guidelines for transmissible spongiform encephalopathies. Report of a WHO consultation, Geneva, Switzerland (website): http://www.who.int/csr/resources/publications/bse/WHO_CDS_CSR_APH_2000_3/en/. Accessed March 27, 2009.

6. Food and Drug Administration 2000. Enforcement priorities for single-use devices reprocessed by third parties and hospitals. FDA, Rockville, Md.

7. Siegel, J.D., Rhinehart, E., Jackson, M., et al., 2007. Guideline for isolation precautions: preventing transmission of infectious agents in healthcare settings, CDC (website): http://www.cdc.gov/ncidod/dhqp/pdf/isolation2007.pdf. Accessed April 30, 2009.

8. Yokoe, D.S., Mermel, L.A., Anderson, D.J., et al., 2008. A compendium of strategies to prevent healthcare-associated infections in acute care hospitals. Infect Control Hosp Epidemiol 29, S12–S21.

9. Tait, A.R., Tuttle, D.B. 1995. Preventing perioperative transmission of infection: a survey of anesthesiology practice. Anesth Analg 80, 764–769.

10. Boyce, J.M., Pittet, D. 2002. Guideline for hand hygiene in health-care settings: recommendations of the healthcare infection control practices advisory Committee and the HIPAC/SHEA/APIC/IDSA hand hygiene task force. Am J Infect Control 30, S1–S46.

11. Koff, M.D., Loftus, R.W., Burchman, C.C., et al., 2009. Reduction in intraoperative bacterial contamination of peripheral intravenous tubing through the use of a novel device. Anesthesiology 110, 978–985.

12. O'Grady, N.P., Alexander, M., Dellinger, E.P., et al., 2002. Guidelines for the prevention of intravascular catheter-related infections. Centers for Disease Control and Prevention. MMWR 51 (RR-10), 1–29.

13. Tablan, O.C., Anderson, L.J., Besser, R., et al., 2004. Guidelines for preventing health-care-associated pneumonia, 2003: recommendations of CDC and the healthcare infection control practices advisory committee. MMWR 53 (RR-3), 1–36.

14. Mauermann, W.J., Nemergut, E.C., 2006. The anesthesiologist's role in the prevention of surgical site infections. Anesthesiology 105, 413–421.

Legal and Regulatory Issues

Eric T. Pierce

With the increasing complexity of anesthesia equipment, the practitioner is ever more reliant on biomedical engineering, information technology, and regulatory and risk management activities to ensure the safe operation of equipment used in the delivery of anesthesia. Equipment such as anesthesia machines, which were once relatively simple to maintain and troubleshoot, now far exceed most practitioner's technological understanding and require extensive in-servicing to operate and special training to service. This chapter will review some of the legal and regulatory issues relevant to medical device safety.

Product Liability

Equipment failure is the primary cause of the minority of critical events during anesthesia; however, a great deal of attention is paid to this concern. Human error is more frequently the most important causative factor of misadventure, medical or otherwise.[1,2] Focus continues to be placed on equipment malfunction for several reasons. It does appear that it is easier to prevent equipment failure than human error. Practitioners may welcome an opportunity to spread the responsibility for bad outcomes by pointing to the devices on which they depend. Plaintiff's attorneys may also favor including device manufacturers in lawsuits because of their potential "deep pockets." Lastly, there is the view that regulatory guidance encourages device manufacturers and users to maintain a focus on patient safety in a competitive and fast-paced environment. Regardless of the reasons, legal and regulatory constraints will continue to be placed on device manufacturers and the healthcare facilities that use their products, even though equipment is not the primary cause of most anesthesia critical events.

Device manufacturers and users share the responsibility for ensuring the safe operation of medical equipment in the care of patients. The users, including practitioners and healthcare facilities, are responsible for routine maintenance, compliance with manufacturer's product advisories and recalls, and appropriate application of medical equipment as described and defined by the manufacturer. Manufacturers must remain in compliance with FDA requirements, including timely reporting of medical equipment-related patient complications and maintaining manufacturing standards.

Manufacturer's Warranty

Warranties can be classified as either express or implied.[3,4] Express warranties are those with which we are all most familiar and are generally a written promise made by the seller to stand behind the product and correct problems should it fail. Such a warranty creates a strict liability for the seller. The Federal Trade Commission (FTC) requires that written product warranties explicitly contain all the elements listed in Table 26-1.[5] Implied warranties are unstated promises, created by state law, that are based on the common law principle of "fair value for money spent." Almost all states have adopted some form of the Uniform Commercial Code (UCC), which holds that there are implied warranties that are automatically part of every sales transaction.[6] These warranties cover "merchantability" and "fitness for a particular use." A manufacturer may expressly disclaim implied warranties. Such disclaimers must be made conspicuous through means such as bold or large type. Manufacturers are not required to provide express warranties in the United States, but healthcare organizations often require express warranties with a specific duration for products to be considered for purchase.

A product's express warranty, also known as a written warranty, delineates the manufacturer's explicit responsibilities and guarantees that the covered device meets all relevant

Table 26–1   Elements of an Express Warranty
1. Who is covered
2. Length of warranty
3. Description of what is covered and/or excluded
4. Steps for customer to follow in the event of a warranty-related problem
5. Warrantor's response to malfunctions and failures
6. Exclusions and limitations
7. Statement that some states do not allow exclusion and limitations
8. Statement of consumer legal rights
9. Any permitted limitations on length of implied warranties

Table 26–2   Joint Commission's Standards for Hospital Medical Equipment Risk Management
1. Solicit input from those who operate and service equipment in selection and acquisition.
2. Maintain written inventory of all medical equipment or at least selected equipment associated with physical risk (life support). Maintain equipment incident history. Evaluate new equipment before use and determine if it should be on the inventory.
3. Identify and document activities for maintaining, inspecting, and testing for all inventoried medical equipment.
4. Identify and document frequency for inspecting, testing, and maintaining all inventoried medical equipment based on manufacturer's recommendations, risk levels, and recent hospital experience.
5. Monitor and report all incidents in which medical equipment is suspected in or attributed to a death, serious injury, or serious illness as required by the Safe Medical Devices Act of 1990.
6. Document procedures to follow when medical equipment fails, including emergency clinical interventions and backup equipment.

specifications such that it will function properly in the defined environment and fulfills its intended purpose. Warranties also state conditions in which the equipment cannot be expected to function properly and various operating conditions that will invalidate the warranty and thereby reduce the manufacturer's responsibility. Purchasers, users, and patients are all entitled to sue if the terms of the warranty are not met. Manufacturers, distributors, and retailers can all be liable for breach of warranty although the manufacturer is generally most likely to have to pay damages. The other parties become more vulnerable if the manufacturer goes bankrupt.

Express warranties are of two types. Full warranties must meet five criteria specified in FTC regulations, including full money back or replacement, prompt and free repairs, prompt refund if repairs are not fully satisfactory, and customer need only to report the defect and all implied warranties are acknowledged. Limited is the other type of express warranty and must be prominently labeled as such. For example a limited warranty may be good for a limited amount of time or require the customer to ship the product to an approved service center for repair. The distinctions between various forms of warranty vary from state to state and it falls upon the purchaser to read all the products documentation and to understand what is covered (caveat emptor).

Medical Equipment Management

The Joint Commission, formerly known as the Joint Commission on Accreditation of Healthcare Organizations (JCAHO), promulgates standards for the inspection, testing, maintenance, and risk management of medical equipment within the healthcare environment.[7] Each accredited healthcare organization must maintain a program for managing medical equipment to fulfill those standards.

Risk Management and Maintenance

The objective of the Medical Equipment Management Program (MEMP) should be to minimize the risk of using medical equipment in patient care by inspection and routine preventive maintenance. The MEMP should also provide for education and in-service training for those who use and maintain the equipment. The Joint Commission's elements of performance for medical equipment risk management are summarized in Table 26-2 and those for maintaining equipment are summarized in Table 26-3 (see ref. 7, EC.02.04.01

Table 26–3   Joint Commission's Standards for Maintaining Hospital Medical Equipment
1. Perform safety, operational, and function checks before initial use of inventoried medical equipment.
2. Document inspection, testing, and maintenance of all life support equipment.
3. Document inspection, testing, and maintenance of all non-life support equipment on inventory.
4. Conduct and document performance testing of and maintain all sterilizers.
5. Perform and document equipment maintenance and chemical and biologic testing of water used in hemodialysis.

and EC.02.04.03). Note that the Safe Medical Devices Act of 1990 requires healthcare organizations to report all incidents in which medical equipment is thought to be involved in serious injury, illness, or death of a patient (see the Medical Device Reporting section).

Biomedical Engineering Services

Biomedical engineering services can be provided by the manufacturer's service representatives, independent service contractors, and in-house biomedical technicians and/or engineers.

Many manufacturers offer service contracts for purchased equipment often with a choice of levels of service. The level of service will determine the cost, parts, and functions covered and the frequency and timing of visits. Manufacturer's service contracts are particularly useful for highly complex equipment and when a limited number of units are purchased such that the cost of developing and maintaining in-house technical expertise significantly exceeds the cost of service contracts. Independent service contractors can offer contracted services for a broader array of equipment; however, ensuring quality becomes more difficult and they may not be able to obtain manufacturer-approved parts, often a warranty requirement, unless they have been approved and certified by the specific manufacturer. In-house biomedical services offer a number of advantages including rapid response time, ability to observe and troubleshoot problems while the equipment is in use, provide record keeping and timely communication with manufacturers and outside agencies, reduce down-time, and provide staff education and in-service training. In-house biomedical personnel generally attend courses and obtain certification to service equipment in general use. Most healthcare facilities use a combination of service providers, which depends on their size and complexity.

Regulation of Medical Devices

The Center for Device and Radiological Health (CDRH) is the division of the Food and Drug Administration (FDA), which is responsible for development and implementation of national programs to protect the public health in the field of medical devices.[8] The basic framework for these regulatory functions was established in the Medical Device Amendments to the Federal Food, Drug and Cosmetic (FFD&C) Act amended in 1976[9].

The CDRH ensures the safety and effectiveness of thousands of medical devices, from heart pacemakers to contact lenses. Before new devices can be tested in humans or marketed they must be reviewed and approved. The CDRH also collects, analyzes, and acts on postmarketing information about devices in use, sets and enforces good manufacturing practice regulations, monitors compliance and surveillance programs, and provides technical assistance to manufacturers.

Classification of Devices

The FDA has classified about 1700 different types of devices, which are in turn grouped into 16 medical specialty areas referred to as panels. Examples of panel areas include cardiovascular, anesthesiology, and general/plastic surgery. Each device type is assigned to one of three broad regulatory classes (Table 26-4) depending on how much regulatory control is required to ensure its safety and effectiveness.[10]

All three classes are subject to "general controls," which include company registration, medical device listing, manufacturing in compliance with good manufacturing practices (GMP), quality assurance programs, proper packaging and labeling, and submission of a premarket notification [510(k)].[11,12]

For class I devices only general controls apply as they are deemed to have minimal potential for harm. Most class I devices are exempted from 510(k) requirements and some are exempted from most of the GMP requirements. Examples of class I devices include examination gloves and handheld surgical instruments.

Most class II devices have special controls in addition to the general controls, although a few devices in this class are also exempt from the 510(k) requirement. Special controls refer to requirements such as special labeling, guidance

Table 26–4   Medical Device Classes
I. General Controls
With exemptions
Without exemptions
II. Special Controls
With exemptions
Without exemptions
III. Premarket Approval
Preamendments
Postamendments
New transitional

documents and postmarket surveillance. Examples of class II devices include electric wheelchairs and infusion pumps.

Class III devices are the most tightly regulated because they are usually used to sustain human life, prevent serious impairment, or are associated with a serious risk of illness or injury. A scientific review process called premarket approval (PMA) is required for these devices with some exceptions.[13] Examples of class III devices include implantable pacemakers and orthopedic implants.

Transitional class III devices are those that were regulated as new drugs before May 28, 1976, and are now governed by PMA regulations. An example of this category of device is an intraocular lens implant.

Premarket Approval Application

The application process for premarket approval (PMA) by the FDA is designed to ensure safety and efficacy of most class III devices.[13] An approved PMA is analogous to a new drug application (NDA) in that it is essentially a private license to market a particular class III device.

Approval requirements vary depending on whether the device was in commercial distribution before May 28, 1976 (preamendments), or were distributed on or after that date (postamendments). Postamendment devices deemed to be substantially equivalent to preamendment devices are regulated as such. The FDA determines substantial equivalence based on the premarket notification [510(k)]. Devices deemed not to be substantially equivalent to either preamendment or postamendment class I or II devices are considered "new" and are treated as class III. These "new" devices must either obtain PMA or be reclassified into class I or II through an FDA petition process. In some cases, a product development protocol (PDP) can be submitted as an alternative to the PMA process.[14] Clinical studies used to support a PMA, PDP, or a petition to reclassify as a class I or II must comply with the investigational device exemption (IDE) regulations (see discussion below).

Investigational Device Exemption

IDE approved by an institutional review board (IRB) is required to collect clinical safety and effectiveness data on an investigational device.[15] That data can be used in support of a

PMA application or in some cases a 510(k) submission. The IDE must also be approved by the FDA if the device involves significant risk. IDEs can be sponsored by individuals or other entites located within the United States. The sponsor does not actually conduct the research unless an individual serves as a sponsor-investigator and fulfills the obligations of both roles. Sponsors of IDEs are not required to submit a PMA or 510(k), register their establishment, list the device, or use a quality system except for design control requirements while the device is under study.

Good Clinical Practices

Clinical trials conducted on an investigational device with an IDE must follow a body of regulations referred to as good clinical practices (GCP), most of which is included in 21 CFR.[15,16] GCP stipulates the procedures for the conduct of studies including the IDE application, responsibilities of sponsor and investigators, labeling, recordkeeping, and reports. GCP also governs IRBs, informed consent, and investigator financial disclosure and procedures to ensure that the device meets specified design requirements.

Premarket Notification [510(k)]

More than 90% of medical device applications to the FDA are made as premarket notifications, also known as 510(k)s.[12] Most of these are for class I and II devices.

The 510(k) submission notifies the FDA of a manufacturer's intent to market a medical device and must be made at least 90 days in advance. To be granted clearance to market a device, the submitter must demonstrate that the device is at least as safe and effective (substantially equivalent) to one or more legally marketed devices (predicates). If and when the submitter receives an order letter declaring that the device is substantially equivalent, the device can be marketed immediately. Inspection of the manufacturer's facility may occur at any time after 510(k) clearance.

A 510(k) is not required to sell unfinished devices or components to another firm for finished assembly. However, if components are sold to end users as replacement parts, a 510(k) is required. If a device is not being made available commercially, a 510(k) is also not required; but if the device is to be evaluated in clinical trials, an IDE is required. Distributors may market another company's domestically manufactured device without a 510(k) if the device has labeling delineating that relationship. Repackagers, relabelers, and importers are also generally exempted.

Custom devices which are not offered for commercial distribution are exempt from the 510(k). These devices are intended for use by an individual patient or are intended to meet the special needs of a specific physician.

Substantial Equivalence

The 510(k) clearance hinges on demonstration of substantial equivalence (SE) to at least one other legally U.S. marketed device referred to as a predicate.[12,17] To be SE to a predicate it should have the same intended use and technological characteristics. However, if it has different technological characteristics, submitted information cannot raise new questions of safety and effectiveness and must demonstrate that the device is at least as safe and effective as the predicate.

Anesthesia and Respiratory Advisory Committee

There are a number of advisory committees such as the Anesthesia and Respiratory Advisory Committee that provide the FDA with independent advice from outside experts on issues such as drugs, biological products, and medical devices.[18] These committees are composed of a chair, several scientific members, and consumer, industry, and sometimes patient representatives. They provide a valuable resource to the FDA and their nonbinding recommendations are an important component of the agency's decision-making process. Meetings are held one to four times a year.

Medical Device Reporting

Regulation related to medical device reporting is designed to provide the FDA and manufacturers with timely information about significant adverse events involving medical devices.[19] The intention is to quickly identify and correct problems with devices. User facilities must *report within 10 workdays* all device-related deaths to the manufacturer and the FDA. Serious injuries must also be reported within 10 days to the manufacturer or the FDA if the manufacturer is unknown. Facilities must also submit to the FDA a summary of all reports filed within the last year. Manufacturers and distributors also have well-defined reporting requirements.

When an accident occurs, the appropriate safety officer or risk manager should be contacted immediately and all involved equipment should be sequestered as soon as possible. That officer or manager will then follow an established protocol to supervise an investigation. All individuals involved should provide written documentation of their observations of the facts while avoiding judgmental statements and while the events are still fresh in their minds. Sequestered equipment should be evaluated by an independent individual or group taking care to document all dial, button, and alarm settings, photograph the accident setting and involved equipment, and preserve all logged data if applicable.

Medical Device Recall

Medical device recalls are occasionally conducted to remove or correct products that are in violation of laws administered by the FDA or poses a risk to health.[20] Although these recalls are conducted by the manufacturer on a voluntary basis, the FDA can order a mandatory recall under its recall authority. As an alternative, the FDA can also initiate a court action for removal or correction of distributed products that are in violation if a manufacturer is not fulfilling its responsibility to protect the public health and well-being. The FDA conducts a health hazard evaluation and classifies the degree of health hazard (I-III) posed by the device being recalled or considered for recall. For correction or removal of devices in minor violation or not in violation, the manufacturer may conduct a market withdrawal.

Voluntary Standards

The FDA recognizes consensus standards that have been developed by national and international organizations such as the Association for the Advancement of Medical Instrumentation (AAMI), the International Electro-technical Commission (IEC), and the International Organization of Standardization (ISO).[21] The CDRH staff participated in the development of many of these standards, which are used in satisfying portions of premarket reviews and other requirements. A list of currently recognized standards is available on the CDRH website. That site also provides guidance for "Recognition and Use of Consensus Standards."

References

1. Cooper, J.B., Newbower, R.S., Long, C.D., et al., 1978. Preventable anesthesia mishaps: a study of human factors. Anesthesiology 49, 399–406.
2. Cooper, J.B., Newbower, R.S., Kitz, R.J., 1984. An analysis of major errors and equipment failure in anesthesia management: considerations for prevention and detection. Anesthesiology 60, 34–42.
3. Wikipedia. Warranty (website): http://en.wikipedia.org/wiki/Warranty. Accessed November 4, 2009.
4. US Legal. Warranty law and legal definition (website): http://definitions.uslegal.com/w/warranty-law. Accessed June 17, 2009.
5. Federal Trade Commission. Warranties, consumer protection, 2001 (website): http://www.ftc.gov/bcp/edu/pubs/consumer/products/pro17.shtm. Accessed November 13, 2009.
6. Wikipedia. Uniform commercial code (website): http://en.wikipedia.org/wiki/Uniform_Commercial_Code. Accessed on November 14, 2009.
7. The Joint Commission, E-dition. Hospital accreditation requirements (website): http://e-dition.jcrinc.com. Accessed November 9, 2009.
8. US Food and Drug Administration. About the center for devices and radiological devices (website): http://www.fda.gov/AboutFDA/CentersOffices/CDRH/default.htm. Accessed November 13, 2009.
9. US Food and Drug Administration. Medical device amendments, Federal Food, Drug and Cosmetic Act. http://www.fda.gov/RegulatoryInformation/Legislation/default.htm. Accessed November 16, 2009.
10. US Food and Drug Administration. Device classification (website): http://www.fda.gov/MedicalDevices/DeviceRegulationandGuidance/Overview/ClassifyYourDevice/default.htm. Accessed November 11, 2008.
11. US Food and Drug Administration. Good manufacturing practices, 1996 (website): http://www.fda.gov/downloads/MedicalDevices/DeviceRegulationandGuidance/PostmarketRequirements/QualitySystemsRegulations/MedicalDeviceQualitySystemsManual/UCM122806.pdf. Accessed November 16, 2009.
12. US Food and Drug Administration. Premarket notification (510k) (website): http://www.fda.gov/MedicalDevices/DeviceRegulationandGuidance/HowtoMarketYourDevice/PremarketSubmissions/PremarketNotification-510k/default.htm. Accessed May 17, 2009.
13. US Food and Drug Administration. Premarket approval, PMA (website): http://www.fda.gov/MedicalDevices/ProductsandMedicalProcedures/DeviceApprovalsandClearances/PMAApprovals/default.htm. Accessed November 16, 2009.
14. US Food and Drug Administration. PMA application methods, product development, protocol (website): http://www.fda.gov/MedicalDevices/DeviceRegulationandGuidance/HowtoMarketYourDevice/PremarketSubmissions/PremarketApprovalPMA/ucm048168.htm. Accessed November 16, 2009.
15. US Food and Drug Administration. Investigational device exemption (website): http://www.fda.gov/MedicalDevices/DeviceRegulationandGuidance/HowtoMarketYourDevice/InvestigationalDeviceExemptionIDE/default.htm. Accessed November 16, 2009.
16. US Food and Drug Administration. Good clinical practices: 21 CFR (website): http://www.fda.gov/ScienceResearch/SpecialTopics/RunningClinicalTrials/ucm155713.htm. Accessed November 16, 2009.
17. US Food and Drug Administration. Guidance for industry and for FDA staff: use of standards in substantial equivalence determinations, 2000 (website): http://www.fda.gov/MedicalDevices/DeviceRegulationandGuidance/GuidanceDocuments/ucm073752.htm. Accessed November 16, 2009.
18. US Food and Drug Administration. Advisory committees (website): http://www.fda.gov/AdvisoryCommittees/default.htm. Accessed November 13, 2009.
19. US Food and Drug Administration. Medical device reporting for manufacturers (website): http://www.fda.gov/MedicalDevices/DeviceRegulationandGuidance/GuidanceDocuments/ucm094529.htm. Accessed November 16, 2009.
20. US Food and Drug Administration. Medical device recalls (website): http://www.fda.gov/MedicalDevices/Safety/RecallsCorrectionsRemovals/ListofRecalls/default.htm. Accessed November 16, 2009.
21. US Food and Drug Administration. Standards, medical devices, 2009 (website): http://www.fda.gov/cdrh/stdsprog.html. Accessed November 13, 2009.

Further Reading

Pisano, D.J., Mantus, D.S. (Eds.), 2008. A guide for prescription drugs, medical devices, and biologics, ed 2. Informa Healthcare USA, New York.
Medical Devices and Systems 2006. In: Bronzino, J.D. (Ed.), The biomedical engineering handbook, ed 3. CRC Press, Boca Raton, Fla.

Chapter 27

Physical Principles

Paul D. Davis

The art of anesthesiology is essentially practical. For this reason anesthesiologists must have an understanding of the physical aspects of the apparatus they use, not only to use it efficiently but also to understand its limitations and to use it safely. Many avoidable accidents and near misses have occurred as the result of the misuse of equipment or misinterpretation of measurements because the anesthesiologist did not understand the basic principles concerned.

One of the problems facing the medical profession today is the clinician's inability to discuss his or her requirements with the engineer in terms that they both understand. This problem occurs not only with the development of new equipment but also with the discussion of faults and difficulties with existing equipment.

This chapter is therefore devoted to the basic physics of gases, liquids, vapors, and solids and to the principles of modern control systems, which are increasingly a part of the latest anesthetic machines. Where reference is made to units of measurement, the International System of Units, known as the SI System (Système International d'Unités), is generally used (see Appendix).

States of Matter

An understanding of the physical principles applicable to the practice of anesthesiology can begin with a consideration of the differences between three states of matter: solid, liquid,

and gas. The difference between these states is best explained by considering the effects of the interactions between the atoms and molecules of which they are made. Atoms or molecules are subject to forces of attraction known as Van der Waals forces, which act to hold individual atoms or molecules near to each other.

In a solid, these intermolecular forces cause the molecules to maintain a fairly fixed position relative to each other. Although the kinetic energy of the molecules causes them to move about a mean position, these mean positions are fixed and may form a regular geometric structure or lattice. When a solid is heated, the kinetic energy of the molecules increases, so the range of movement about this mean position increases and the volume of the solid increases as expansion occurs.

As more heat is added to the solid, the range of movement of the molecules eventually becomes sufficiently great to disrupt the fixed structure and the molecules are able to move past each other. The solid has changed state to become a liquid. Nevertheless, the kinetic energy is insufficient to overcome the intermolecular forces completely and the molecules remain close to each other. Because the molecules remain near each other in a solid or a liquid, matter in either of these states is not easily compressed.

As more heat is added to the liquid, the kinetic energy of the molecules increases until the intermolecular forces are no longer sufficient to hold the molecules near each other.

The state changes to the gaseous state, in which the molecules move freely throughout the volume in which they are contained. Because of the large distances between molecules in the gaseous state, matter in this state is comparatively easily compressed.

Heat and Temperature

Relationship Between Heat and Temperature

The internal energy of an object is composed of the kinetic and potential energies of the molecules of which it consists. Transfer of heat energy to or from an object alters this internal energy. The temperature of an object determines the direction in which a transfer of heat energy occurs, the energy being transferred from the object with the higher temperature to the object with the lower temperature. Objects at the same temperature are in thermal equilibrium and no transfer of energy occurs.

Temperature Scales

Temperature scales are based on fixed temperatures that can be reproduced by appropriate physical conditions. Two of these fixed temperatures are needed to define a temperature scale.

The SI unit of temperature is the Kelvin (K). The lower fixed point used to define the Kelvin scale is the temperature at which no further heat energy can be extracted from any object. This point is often referred to as the *absolute zero* of temperature and the Kelvin temperature as *absolute temperature*. The upper fixed point is the triple point of water, which is the temperature at which ice, water, and water vapor exist in equilibrium (Figure 27–1). The temperature range between these fixed points is divided into 273.16 equal parts; thus the Kelvin is defined as 1/273.16 of the temperature of the triple point of water.

This rather strange definition of the Kelvin arises from its relationship to another temperature scale, the degree Celsius (°C) scale, the latter based on the freezing and boiling points of water, which are given the values 0° C and 100° C, respectively. The Celsius temperature is now defined by the relationship:

$$\text{temperature (K)} = \text{temperature (° C)} + 273.15$$

Thus the temperature of the triple point of water is 0.01° C and a difference of 1 K is identical to a difference of 1° C.

Heat

The SI unit of energy is the joule (J), although an alternative unit, the calorie (cal) is sometimes used specifically for heat energy. As the calorie is a rather small quantity of heat energy, the energy available from food is often quoted in terms of kilocalories and the symbol Cal is used to represent kilocalories. The relationship between these various units is:

$$1 \text{ calorie (cal)} = 4.187 \text{ joule (J)}$$

$$1 \text{ calorie (Cal)} = 1 \text{ kilocalorie (kcal)} = 1000 \text{ calories}$$

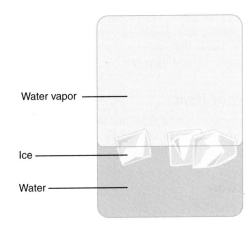

Figure 27–1 A sealed vessel containing water vapor, water, and ice in equilibrium at the triple point of water.

Water vapor

Ice

Water

Heat Capacity and Specific Heat Capacity

Objects differ in the temperature change produced by the gain or loss of a given quantity of heat energy. For example, a large object made of the same material as a small object exhibits a lesser change in temperature than the small object. Objects of the same mass but made of different materials generally also differ in the temperature change produced by the same change in heat energy. The change in heat energy and temperature are related by the *heat capacity* of the object:

$$\text{change in heat energy} = \text{change in temperature} \times \text{heat capacity}$$

To be able to compare different objects and different materials, the term *specific heat capacity* is used. The specific heat capacity, also referred to as the *specific heat*, is the quantity of heat energy required to change the temperature of 1 kg of a substance by 1 K. The units are therefore J kg^{-1} K^{-1}.

For example, it takes 4200 J of energy to raise the temperature of 1 kg of water by 1° C. Therefore the specific heat capacity of water is 4200 J kg^{-1} K^{-1}. In comparison, it takes 910 J to raise the temperature of 1 kg of aluminum by 1° C. Therefore, the specific heat capacity of aluminum is 910 J kg^{-1} K^{-1}.

Latent Heat

A comparatively large alteration in the kinetic energy of molecules occurs when a substance changes state; moreover, this change of state occurs at a fixed temperature that depends on the pressure. In the case of the transition from solid to liquid, this is the *melting point* and in the case of liquid to gas, the *boiling point*. The addition of heat energy is needed for the change of state to occur, even though this change takes place at a fixed temperature. The energy is needed to increase the kinetic energy of the molecules sufficiently to overcome the forces of attraction between them and is known as the *latent heat*. These processes occur in reverse when heat energy is removed from a substance. The transition from gas to liquid is termed the *dew point*, and the transition from liquid to solid, the *freezing point*.

The heat required to melt a solid is known as the *latent heat of fusion*. For ice this is 333 kJ kg^{-1} at 0° C and normal atmospheric pressure. The heat required to vaporize a liquid is called the *latent heat of vaporization*. For water, this is

2257 kJ kg^{-1} at 100° C and normal atmospheric pressure. It is noteworthy that considerably more heat is required to vaporize a liquid than to raise its temperature from room temperature to its boiling point.

Transfer of Heat

Heat may be transferred from one object to another or from one part of an object to another by the processes of *conduction*, *convection*, and *radiation*.

Conduction

In conduction, heat energy diffuses along an object from molecule to molecule. For example, metals such as copper are good conductors of heat, whereas glass and expanded polystyrene are poor conductors. Very poor conductors of heat are termed *thermal insulators*.

Convection

If part of a fluid is heated, it expands and becomes less dense than the fluid surrounding it. Being free to move, it rises, and as it travels upward, its place is taken by the cooler, denser fluid from around it, which in turn is heated and rises. There is, therefore, a constant rising stream of fluid above the source of heat. These currents are known as convection currents (Figure 27–2), and the heat energy is carried by them.

Radiation

The transfer of radiated heat energy does not require the source of heat to be in contact with any other object. The rate at which heat energy is radiated is described by Stefan's law:

$$P = seAT^4$$

where s is Stefan's constant, e is the emissivity, A is the area of the radiating surface, and T is the absolute temperature. The emissivity, which ranges from 0 to 1, quantifies the difference in emission from surfaces at the same temperature. A matte black surface, for example, has a greater emissivity than a reflective white surface, so the rate at which it radiates energy is greater under the same conditions.

Stefan's law shows that the net transfer of heat between two objects at different temperatures is proportional to the difference between the fourth power of their temperatures (i.e., P a $T_1^4 - T_2^4$). Even though the ambient temperature is comparatively high, heat can still be lost to a cooler object through the radiation of heat energy.

Because of its dependence on temperature, radiated heat energy can be used as the basis of temperature measurement techniques.

Properties of Ideal Gases

As is the case with all substances, the smallest particle of a gas that can exist separately is a molecule, or in the case of some gases such as xenon, an atom. Gas molecules are in constant motion, moving in all directions and rebounding from each other and from the walls of the space in which they are confined. It is the change in momentum resulting from the

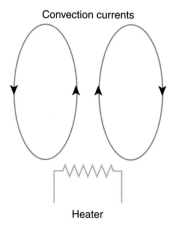

Figure 27–2 Convection currents above a heater; the *arrows* show the movement of fluid.

collisions of gas molecules with the walls that appears as the pressure of the gas.

The physical properties of gases under certain conditions of temperature and pressure approximate those of a collection of noninteracting particles of negligible size that undergo collisions with each other and the walls of the container in which they are situated. These properties are known as the properties of an ideal gas. The state of such a gas in a closed container can be described by four variables: the volume of the container, the number of molecules of gas present, the temperature, and the pressure. These variables are related by several gas laws, which describe the behavior of an ideal gas.

The Gas Laws

Boyle's Law

Boyle's law states that, at constant temperature, the volume of a fixed mass of gas is inversely proportional to its pressure:

$$V \alpha \frac{1}{P} \text{ or } PV = k_B \text{ where } k_B \text{ is a constant}$$

Charles' Law

Charles' law states that, at constant pressure, the volume of a fixed mass of gas is proportional to its absolute temperature:

$$V \alpha T \text{ or } \frac{V}{T} = k_C \text{ where } k_C \text{ is a constant}$$

Gay-Lussac's Law

Gay-Lussac's law states that, at a constant volume, the pressure of a fixed mass of gas is proportional to its absolute temperature:

$$V \alpha T \text{ or } \frac{P}{T} = k_G \text{ where } k_G \text{ is a constant}$$

Combined Gas Law

These three gas laws can be combined to give the following relationship for a fixed mass of gas:

$$\frac{P_1 V_1}{T_1} = \frac{P_2 V_2}{T_2}$$

where P_1, V_1, and T_1 are the pressure, volume, and temperature in one set of conditions and P_2, V_2, and T_2 are the corresponding quantities in a second set of conditions. The temperature, T, must be expressed on the absolute scale as a Kelvin temperature. The above formula may be used to calculate the results of a change of pressure, temperature, or volume of a fixed mass of gas.

Standard Temperature and Pressure

Because the volume of a given mass of gas depends on temperature and pressure, comparison of gas volumes is easier if any given gas volume is converted to the volume it would have at a standard temperature and pressure. The standard temperature and pressure (STP) normally used are 0° C and 760 mm Hg (273.15 K and 101.325 kPa).

Avogadro Hypothesis

The Avogadro hypothesis states that under conditions of constant pressure and temperature, equal volumes of gases contain equal numbers of molecules.

Mole

The SI unit for an amount of any substance is the mole. The mole is the amount of substance that contains as many elementary entities as there are atoms in 0.012 kg of carbon-12. For example, the elementary entities may be atoms, molecules, ions, or electrons. The number of elementary entities in one mole is known as Avogadro's number, the value of which is 6.022×10^{23}.

Avogadro's Law

Avogadro's law states that under conditions of constant pressure and temperature, there is a direct relationship between the volume and number of moles for an ideal gas:

$$V \alpha \, n \text{ or } V = k_A n \text{ where } k_A \text{ is a constant}$$

Molar Volume

The molar volume is the volume occupied by one mole of an ideal gas at STP; its value is 22.414 L.

Ideal Gas Law

The gas laws described above can be combined to produce an equation of state for an ideal gas as follows:

$$PV = nRT$$

where R is the molar gas constant. Its value can be calculated by:

$$R = \frac{PV}{nT} = \frac{\text{standard pressure} \times \text{volume}}{\text{moles} \times \text{standard temperature}} =$$

$$\frac{\text{standard pressure} \times \text{molar volume}}{\text{standard temperature}} =$$

$$\frac{101.325 \text{ Pa} \times 0.022414 \text{ m}^3}{273.15 \text{ K}} = 8.314 \text{ Pa m}^3/\text{mole K}$$

Dalton's Law and Amagat's Law

A vessel may be occupied by more than one gas, in which case the total pressure within it is the sum of the pressures exerted independently by each of the gases. Each gas is said to exert a partial pressure. The pressure exerted by a vapor or a gas in a closed space, at a given temperature, is independent of the pressure of other vapors or gases provided they have undergone no chemical reaction with each other. When several vapors or gases having no chemical reaction with each other are present in the same space, the pressure exerted by the mixture is the sum of the pressures that would be exerted by each of its constituents if it was separately confined in the same space.

Dalton's law states that the pressure of a gas mixture is equal to the sum of the partial pressures of the gases of which it is composed.

Amagat's law states that the volume of a gas mixture is equal to the sum of the volumes of all its constituents which are at the same temperature and pressure as the mixture.

Dry Gas Correction

The addition of water vapor to a mixture of gases reduces the partial pressures of those gases if the total pressure of the mixture remains the same. It may be necessary to correct for this effect when determining partial pressures in humidified mixtures; for example, those present in alveoli. Suppose that end-tidal carbon dioxide concentration is measured in a dry gas mixture; the concentration in the alveoli will be lower because of the presence of water vapor in the mixture. The corrected value can be calculated as follows:

partial pressure of CO_2 in alveoli

= partial pressure of CO_2 in dry gas

$$\times \frac{\text{atmospheric pressure} - \text{partial pressure of water vapor}}{\text{atmospheric pressure}}$$

Graham's Law

The kinetic energy of a gas is dependent on its temperature and the kinetic energy is also proportional to the molecular weight and the velocity of its molecules. So for two different gases at the same temperature, which therefore have the same kinetic energy:

$$\text{kinetic energy} = \tfrac{1}{2} \, m_1 v_1 = \tfrac{1}{2} \, m_2 v_2$$

thus

$$\frac{v_1}{v_2} = \frac{\sqrt{m_2}}{\sqrt{m_1}}$$

This leads to Graham's law, which states that the rate of diffusion of a gas is inversely proportional to the square root of its molecular weight.

Properties of Real Gases

The properties of real gases differ from those of ideal gases because of the finite size of the molecules and the existence of intermolecular forces between them, but divergence from the behavior of ideal gases becomes important only under conditions in which the molecules are close together. These conditions occur chiefly at lower temperatures and higher pressures. The values of temperature and pressure at which divergence from the behavior of ideal gases becomes apparent differ from one gas to another.

Vapor Pressure

A substance in the gaseous state and in contact with the same substance in the liquid or solid state is known as a vapor. The molecules in the solid, liquid, or gaseous state do not all have the same kinetic energy. The more energetic or less energetic of the molecules may move between states until an equilibrium is established, with as many molecules changing state in one direction as those changing in the reverse direction (Figure 27–3).

The pressure at which the gaseous state is in equilibrium with either the liquid or solid state, or with both, is known as the *saturated vapor pressure* (SVP) and is a function of temperature. The boiling point of a liquid is the temperature at which the saturated vapor pressure is equal to the atmospheric pressure, so the boiling point of a liquid depends on the ambient pressure. Since atmospheric pressure depends on altitude, the boiling point is depressed as altitude increases.

Critical Temperature

A substance in the gaseous state at a pressure less than the saturated vapor pressure cannot be in equilibrium with the same substance in the liquid state; the liquid evaporates until the saturated vapor pressure is reached or until no more liquid remains. Conversely, if the pressure of a vapor is increased, liquefaction begins when the saturated vapor pressure is reached. The substance then exists as a vapor, a liquid, or a mixture of both. However, above a certain temperature, known as the *critical temperature*, liquefaction does not occur; thus it is not possible for the liquid state to exist above this critical temperature.

The relationship between pressure, volume, and temperature is usually displayed as a set of isotherms (i.e., a set of curves representing the properties of the gas at constant temperature). Figure 27–4 shows isotherms for nitrous oxide. Each isotherm shows the relationship between pressure and volume at a given temperature. Nitrous oxide may exist as a liquid or a vapor below the critical temperature of 36.6° C; above this critical temperature it may exist only as a gas. It follows that if a gas is stored below its critical temperature as a mixture of liquid and vapor, determination of the contents of its container cannot be made from the pressure within. If a gas is stored above its critical temperature, the quantity of gas will be proportional to the pressure inside its container. An example is oxygen, which has a critical temperature of −118°C, and is therefore in its gaseous state at room temperature. The *critical pressure* is the pressure that is required to liquefy a gas at its critical temperature.

The Poynting Effect

A mixture of 50% nitrous oxide and 50% oxygen is marketed under the name Entonox. A full cylinder of Entonox typically contains these gases at a pressure of 137 bar. According to

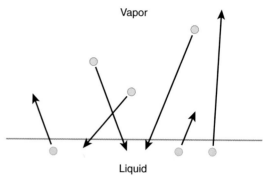

Figure 27–3 Movement of molecules between liquid and vapor states in equilibrium.

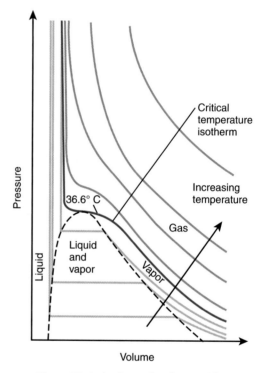

Figure 27–4 Isotherms for nitrous oxide.

Dalton's law, the partial pressure of the nitrous oxide in the cylinder should be 68.5 bar (i.e., ½ of 137 bar). Since the saturated vapor pressure of nitrous oxide at 20° C is less than this, being approximately 52 bar, one might expect liquid nitrous oxide to form when a cylinder is filled to this pressure, and an Entonox cylinder at room temperature to contain liquid nitrous oxide, but this is not the case. An effect known as the Poynting effect, or overpressure effect, alters the pressure at which liquid nitrous oxide forms in the mixture.

If a cylinder is partially filled with liquid nitrous oxide, inverted, and then further filled from a high pressure source of oxygen, an unexpected phenomenon occurs. This may be viewed through the glass observation window of a high pressure rig. The bubbles of oxygen diminish in size as the gas is partially dissolved in the liquid nitrous oxide through which it passes. Simultaneously, the volume of the liquid nitrous oxide diminishes as it evaporates and mixes with the oxygen. Eventually, the cylinder, filled to a pressure of 13.7 MPa (137 bar), contains mixed oxygen and nitrous oxide, both in the gaseous state. Cooling of the cylinder and its contents does eventually result in the condensation of nitrous oxide at a temperature known as the pseudocritical temperature. The value of this temperature depends on the pressure of gas in the cylinder, but can be as high as −5.5° C, so precautions concerning use of cylinders of the mixture in cold conditions are necessary.

Adiabatic Processes

Work has to be done to compress a gas and the energy expended is converted into heat. If the process is adiabatic (i.e., there is no exchange of heat with the surroundings), the temperature of the gas rises. In some circumstances, such as the compression-ignition (diesel) engine, the compression is sufficiently rapid to cause a considerable rise in temperature, resulting in ignition of the fuel vapor. In the same way, if part of an anesthetic apparatus were to contain oil, grease, or some other flammable material and were to be subjected to a sudden rise of pressure in the presence of oxygen, as when a cylinder were turned on suddenly, an explosion could occur. For this reason all apparatus using high pressure oxygen must be free of oil, grease, or other flammable material. Pressure gauges are fitted with a constriction in the inlet to reduce the shock wave that occurs when a cylinder is turned on.

The Joule-Kelvin Principle (Joule-Thompson Effect)

Conversely, when a gas expands, it does work and the temperature drops. Under normal circumstances in anesthetic practice, the expansion of a gas leaving the cylinder is not sufficiently rapid to cause a great fall in temperature. The fall in temperature is, for example, much less than that due to the latent heat of vaporization, which is the main cause of cooling of cylinders of nitrous oxide when in use.

Behavior of Molecules of Solids and Liquids

The molecules of a solid or a liquid attract each other. They may also be attracted by the molecules of another substance. The mutual attraction between molecules of a substance is termed *cohesion*, and their attraction to those of another substance is called *adhesion*.

Surface Tension and Capillary Action

The intermolecular forces that cause liquid molecules to remain near each other (cohesion) result in a measurable tension in the surface of a liquid. The phenomenon is known as *surface tension*.

The intermolecular forces of adhesion acting between molecules of water and the glass wall of a water or saline manometer are greater than the forces of cohesion between water molecules. As a result, the attraction of the water molecules to the molecules in the wall that are above the surface of the liquid has two effects: the surface of the water forms a concave surface at its edge called a *meniscus* and the height of the water in the manometer increases. This is known as *capillary action* (Figure 27–5). The force of adhesion acting at the walls of the

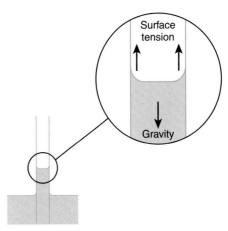

Figure 27–5 Capillary action in a tube of water as a result of surface tension resulting from intermolecular forces.

tube is balanced by the force due to gravity acting on the mass of water contained in the volume that has risen above the level of water outside the manometer; the narrower the tube, the further the water rises up it.

Capillary action is the principle that causes liquid anesthetic agent to rise up the wick in a vaporizer. The wick dips into the liquid agent, the liquid rises up the wick, and a larger surface area is obtained from which vaporization may occur.

The Behavior of Fluids

Fluid Flow

The factors affecting fluid flow through a tube are described by the equation:

$$\text{flow} = \frac{\text{pressure difference}}{\text{resistance}}$$

It is important to distinguish between volume flow and mass flow, since the same volume flow results in a higher mass flow if the pressure of a gas is increased.

The SI unit of pressure is the pascal (Pa) and the units of volume flow are meter^3/second, so in this case, the units of resistance are Pa s m^{-3}. When units other than SI units are used, resistance is typically measured as cm H$_2$O s l^{-1} for values encountered in anesthetic practice. Various physical properties affect the flow of fluid through tubes; some of these are properties of the tube itself, and others are properties of the fluid, such as density and viscosity.

Viscosity

Viscosity arises from friction between layers of fluid, which are moving relative to each other. Although molecules in a particular layer of fluid are moving randomly in different directions, they have an average momentum in the direction of motion of the fluid layer of which they are part, and this momentum is greater for a faster moving layer than for a slower moving one. Random motion causes molecules to transfer from one layer to another, and this results in the transfer of momentum between layers (Figure 27–6). The molecules that move from the faster to the slower moving layer tend to increase the

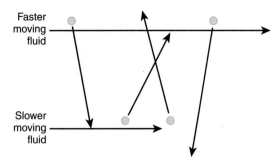

Figure 27–6 Molecules transfer momentum between layers of fluid moving at different rates.

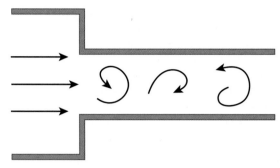

Figure 27–7 Laminar flow becoming turbulent at a sharp change in tube diameter.

speed of the slower layer and vice versa. This results in friction between the layers and the phenomenon of viscosity. The SI units of viscosity are Pa s (pascal seconds).

Types of Flow

The flow of gases or liquids can be one of two types: *laminar* or *turbulent*. In laminar flow, the fluid flows steadily in one direction; in turbulent flow, it swirls in eddies. Turbulent flow occurs at higher fluid velocities than laminar flow. The probability of turbulent rather than laminar flow occurring in a tube can be determined by calculating an index known as the Reynolds number:

$$\text{Reynolds number, } R = \frac{v\rho d}{\eta}$$

where v is the linear velocity of the fluid, ρ is the density, d is the diameter of the tube, and η is the viscosity. Empirical measurements with cylindrical tubes show that transition between laminar and turbulent flow occurs when the Reynolds number is about 2000. If the Reynolds number exceeds 2000, turbulent flow is likely to be present; if the Reynolds number is below 2000, the flow is likely to be laminar. It can be seen from this formula that for a fixed set of conditions there is a critical velocity at which the Reynolds number has the value 2000. When the velocity of the fluid exceeds this critical value, the character of the flow is likely to change from laminar to turbulent (Figure 27–7). This critical velocity applies only for a given fluid in a given tube. Turbulent flow is often present where there is an orifice, a sharp bend, or some other irregularity, which may cause a local increase in velocity and hence an increase in Reynolds number to a value greater than 2000.

Since the volume flow (F) in a cylindrical tube can be represented by the formula:

$$F = \frac{v\pi d^2}{4}$$

which may be arranged as

$$vd = \frac{4F}{\pi d}$$

by substituting vd in Equation 1, the Reynolds number for this type of flow can be represented as

$$R = \frac{4F\rho}{\pi d\eta}$$

This shows that, for the same volume flow (F), the Reynolds number becomes smaller and laminar flow more likely as the diameter of a tube increases.

Laminar Flow

The behavior of laminar flow (Figure 27–8) in a tube is described by the equation due to Poiseuille:

$$\text{flow} = \text{pressure drop} \times \frac{\pi r^4}{8\eta l}$$

where η is the viscosity, l the length of the tube, and r the radius of the tube. From this equation it can be seen that for a given pressure gradient along a tube, flow is dependent on the fourth power of the radius. Similarly, therefore, comparatively small changes in the diameter of a tube will affect the pressure drop noticeably; for example, a reduction of only 16% in the diameter of a tube doubles the pressure drop across it. Figure 27–8 shows the velocity profile of laminar flow in a tube; the velocity is greatest in the center and decreases toward the edges.

Turbulent Flow

Although the resistance can be calculated easily for laminar flow, this is not the case for turbulent flow. The analysis of turbulence is highly complex and the most important point to note is that the resistance is no longer independent of flow, so it is not possible to quote the resistance to flow of a particular item without specifying the flow itself under turbulent conditions.

Flow Through an Orifice

In contrast to a tube, the length of which is by definition much greater than its diameter, an orifice is an aperture, the length of which is less than its diameter.

Flow through an orifice (Figure 27–9) is described by the equation:

$$\text{Flow rate} \propto d^2 \sqrt{\frac{\Delta P}{\rho}}$$

where d is the diameter of the orifice, ΔP is the pressure difference across it, and ρ is the density of the fluid. It is found, however, that if flow through an orifice reaches the speed of sound in the fluid, the rate of mass flow ceases to depend on the downstream pressure (i.e., it depends on the upstream pressure only).

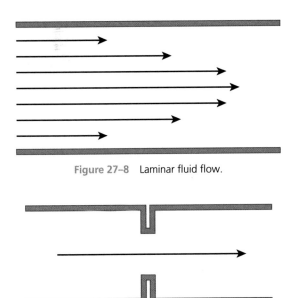

Figure 27–8   Laminar fluid flow.

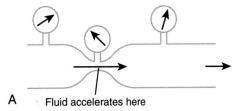

A   Fluid accelerates here

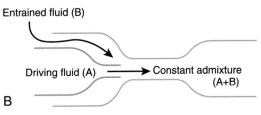

Figure 27–10   **A,** The Bernoulli effect and **(B)** a venturi.

Figure 27–9   Gas flow through an orifice.

Bernoulli's Law, the Bernoulli Effect, and the Venturi

There are three contributions to the energy of a moving fluid: the potential energy due to its pressure, the kinetic energy due to its movement, and the potential energy due to the force of gravity on it. If its total energy does not change, Bernoulli's law applies:

$$P + \tfrac{1}{2}\rho v^2 + \rho gh = constant$$

where P is the pressure, ϱ the density, v the fluid velocity, g the acceleration due to gravity, and h the vertical height of an element of fluid.

If the fluid is not moving, $v = 0$, so the equation becomes

$$P + \rho gh = constant$$

indicating that the pressure at the base of a column of fluid is proportional to its height and its density. This relationship is the basis of fluid manometers.

For the case of fluid moving through a horizontal tube, the equation becomes

$$P + \tfrac{1}{2}\rho v^2 = constant$$

If the fluid flows through a tube which has a constriction within it, the velocity increases as the fluid passes the constriction. Bernoulli's law indicates that the pressure P falls as the velocity increases. A constriction with an entry and exit in which the diameter changes gradually, and which maintains laminar flow, is known as a venturi; the reduction in pressure as the fluid passes through the venturi is known as the Bernoulli effect. When the gas emerges from the constriction into the wider portion of the tube, the linear velocity of flow decreases and the pressure increases again (Figure 27–10, A). The pressure may rise to a level almost as high as that before the constriction, the extent of this rise being dependent on the design of the tube and the constriction.

If a side branch is added to the tube at the venturi, the reduction in pressure causes fluid from the branch to be entrained by the main stream (Figure 27–10, B).

Further Reading

Kuhn, K.F., 1996. Basic physics: a self-teaching guide, ed 2. John Wiley , New york.

Davis, P.D., Kenny, G.N.C., 2003. Basic physics and measurement in anaesthesia, ed 5. Butterworth Heinemann, Edinburgh.

Davey, A.J., Diba, A., 2005. Ward's anaesthetic equipment, ed 5. Elsevier, Philadelphia.

Basic Physics of Electricity

Paul D. Davis

Electric Charge

Electricity arises from the physical properties of the elementary particles that comprise atoms and molecules. Some of these particles possess a property known as *electric charge*, of which there are two forms: a positive form and a negative form. An attractive force occurs between particles of opposite charge and a repulsive force between particles of similar charge.

Atoms comprise a positively charged nucleus surrounded by negatively charged electrons. The aggregate charge on the complete atom is normally zero because the total charge of the electrons is the same magnitude as that of the nucleus, but of opposite sign. Atoms may become charged, however, if electrons are added or removed. Such electrically charged atoms are known as *ions*. Some compounds, such as sodium chloride, dissociate into charged ions when they dissolve in water. The ions may then move through the solution as carriers of charge.

Electrons may also transport charge by moving from one atom to another through a material, but materials differ in the degree to which electrons can readily move through them. In *insulators*, electrons do not move, but remain fixed in position; in *conductors*, they move more readily; in *semiconductors*, their freedom of movement is more dependent on temperature than in conductors.

The SI unit of charge is the *coulomb* (C), which is equal to 6.2×10^{18} times the charge possessed by a single electron.

Static Electricity and Electric Potential

Electrons can be added to an insulator or removed from it, for example, by friction with a different material, and when this takes place, the net charge due to the excess or deficit of electrons tends to remain on the insulator. This accumulation of charge is known as *static electricity* because the position of the charge is normally fixed.

Although the usual SI unit of energy, the joule (J), can be used to quantify the change that takes place when the charge is moved, a different quantity, the electric potential, is normally used. The electric potential, V, is related to the potential energy (E) and the charge (Q), by the relationship: $V = \dfrac{dE}{dQ}$

The SI unit of electric potential is the *volt* (V). An alternative term, voltage, may be used to describe the size of an electric potential.

In some circumstances the electric potential produced by static electricity may amount to thousands of volts. The rate of change of potential with distance is the potential gradient. Although air is normally an insulator, a potential gradient of sufficient magnitude can ionize air molecules, thereby causing the air to conduct, resulting in the occurrence of a spark. The energy contained in the spark may be sufficiently great to ignite a flammable mixture.

Electric Current

Electric current is the flow of electrically charged particles such as electrons or ions. It occurs when an electric potential exists across a conductor or a conducting fluid. The SI unit of electric current is the *ampere* (A), which is equal to a flow of one coulomb of charge per second through any cross-section of the conductor. Current density is current flowing across a unit area; its units are therefore A m^{-2} (Figure 28-1).

Current, which flows in one direction through a conductor at a fixed rate, is known as *direct current* (DC). Current, which changes direction periodically, is known as *alternating*

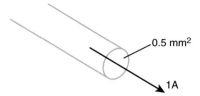

Figure 28–1   Comparison of current and current density; a current of 1 A flows through a conductor with a cross-sectional area of 0.5 mm², so the current density is 2 A mm⁻².

current (AC). An electric current may have both a direct and an alternating component. The waveform of alternating current may be of any shape, but the sine wave is the most fundamental form because all other waveforms can be constructed from a combination of sine waves of appropriate frequencies, amplitudes, and phases. The range of sine wave frequencies of which any waveform consists is known as the frequency range of the waveform.

An electric circuit consists of a source of potential and one or more electrically conducting paths connected to the source that allow current to flow.

Resistance and Ohm's Law

Materials are characterized by their electrical resistance (R), which measures the potential difference (V) required to produce a certain direct current flow (I). The relationship is given by Ohm's law: $I = \dfrac{V}{R}$

The SI unit of resistance is the *ohm* (O).

Heating Effect of Electric Currents

The power converted into heat, or some other form of energy, when electric current flows through a resistance is given by

$$P = V \times I$$

The SI unit of power is the *watt* (W). The heating effect of electric current is the principle used by the fuse, the electric component used to disconnect a supply of electricity if an excessive current flows. Under normal conditions, the current flows through the fuse without producing any noticeable effect, but when the current flow is excessive, the power converted into heat is sufficient to melt the conductor and interrupt the flow of current.

Root Mean Square (RMS) Values

The instantaneous value of an alternating current varies throughout its cycle. It is more convenient to use a single number to specify the value of an alternating current, and it is common to employ the value of direct current that would produce the same heating effect as the alternating current.

Since the heating effect depends on the power, *P*, this is represented by

$$P = VI \text{ (see previous discussion)}$$

and as $V = IR$, (Ohm's law),

$$\text{therefore, } P = I^2R.$$

To obtain the equivalent direct current, the square of the alternating current is averaged over one complete cycle (Figure 28-2), giving the mean square value. The equivalent direct current is then the square root of this and is known as the *root mean square* (RMS) value. A similar procedure is used to derive the RMS voltage of an alternating potential. The RMS voltage of the US main supply, for example, is 220 V, although the peak voltage occurring during the cycle is 170 V.

Capacitance

If an electric charge is added to one of two adjacent conducting surfaces, an equal and opposite charge arises on the other conducting surface. This ability of an object to hold electric charge is the property known as *capacitance* (C). It is measured by the relationship between the charge on the conductors (Q), and the potential between them (V), as follows:

$$\text{capacitance, } C = \frac{Q}{V}$$

The SI unit of capacitance is the *farad* (F). The two conductors form a capacitor (Figure 28-3), and the capacitance between them increases as the distance between them decreases.

An alternating potential applied across a capacitor results in the charges on the two parts of the capacitor alternating. The movement of charges to and from the conductors comprising the capacitor constitutes an alternating current. Although no charge crosses the gap between the two surfaces forming the capacitor, there is an apparent flow of current through the capacitor, which is known as the *displacement current*.

Energy Stored in a Capacitor

The energy stored in a capacitor is a function of the potential and the charge. As the potential across a capacitor rises, it takes more energy to add the same amount of extra charge, so the total energy is not simply the product of the charge and potential. It can be shown that the stored energy, *E*, is represented by the equation:

$$E = QV \text{ (coulombs of charge} \times \text{volts)}$$

and since $Q = CV$ (capacitance × volts)

$$E = \tfrac{1}{2}CV^2$$

A capacitor is used to store the electric energy required to produce the current pulse employed in cardiac defibrillators. Since the electrical resistance of the skin is high, the stored potential must be in the kilovolt range. As the energy required may be hundreds of joules, the capacitor typically has a value in the microfarad range. Because of the high voltage, care is needed during the operation of the equipment.

Variable Electric Current

The flow of a variable current in an electrical circuit produces interesting phenomena (*inductance, reactance,* and *impedance*) not seen when a constant current flows. These are caused by the type of electromagnetic field created adjacent to the electrical circuit by the variable current (see Electric and Magnetic Fields section). Such effects include: the following.

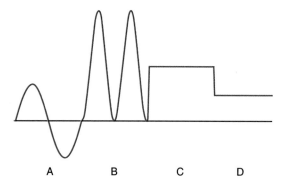

Figure 28–2 Derivation of root mean square values; **(A)** original waveform, **(B)** point-by-point square of amplitude, **(C)** average over one cycle of squared values, **(D)** square root of average (RMS value).

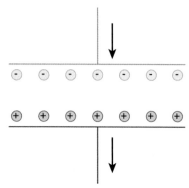

Figure 28–3 Principle of the capacitor; arrows indicate the flow of electrons that produce the change of charge on the capacitor.

Inductance

Conductors in an electric circuit passing a variable current possess a property known as inductance, which controls the rate of change of current when a voltage is applied across the conductor according to the relationship.

Inductance increases if a conductor is wound into a coil, with more turns in the coil, producing greater inductance. A component of this type is known as an inductor. Because an inductor controls the rate of change of current in a circuit, it can be used to regulate the form of the current pulse produced by a defibrillator.

Two adjacent conductors or coils possess *mutual inductance*, a property which results in a changing current in one inducing a current in the other. This property is used in transformers (see later discussion), the components of which cause an alternating voltage at the input to be changed to a different alternating voltage at the output. Note that there is no change in frequency here.

Transformers

A transformer is made by winding two coils of wire around a ferromagnetic material (core). A changing current passing through the primary coil creates a changing magnetic field in the core. This magnetic field induces a current flow in the secondary coil. The voltage output in the secondary coil is determined by both the voltage input to the primary coil and the ratio of the number of windings (*turns*) of the two coils.

If the number of turns of the two coils is identical, then the voltage output will be the same as the input. However, if the secondary coil has more windings, the voltage output will be greater (step up transformer Figure 28-4, *A*) and vice versa (step down transformer Figure 28-4, *B*).

In a well-designed transformer, the power output will be similar to the input. Therefore, if the secondary voltage is greater than the input, then the secondary current flow must be less, according to the formula:

$$\text{Power in Watts (W)} = \text{Volts (V)} \times \text{(I) current flow}$$

Reactance

The opposition to alternating current flow resulting from capacitance and inductance is called reactance. The relationship between the sine wave current flowing to and from a capacitor and the voltage across the capacitor is known as *capacitive reactance* (X_C), and is a measure of the resistance to current flow resulting from capacitance. It is measured in Ohms and is defined as

$$\text{reactance, } X_C = \frac{V}{I} = \frac{1}{2\pi f C}$$

where f is the frequency of the current and voltage, and C is the capacitance. The phase of the current is 90 degrees in advance of the voltage. It can be seen that, for a given voltage, the current increases as the frequency or capacitance increases (Figure 28-5).

For an inductor, *inductive reactance* (X_L), again measured in Ohms, is described by the formula:

$$\text{reactance, } X_L = 2pfL$$

where L is the inductance. An increase in frequency or increased inductance will result in an increase in reactance.

Impedance

Many components of electric circuits possess resistance, capacitance, and inductance, although typically one of these properties will be more apparent than the others. The term impedance is used as a measure of the sum of all of these properties that resist the flow of an alternating current. The unit of impedance is the ohm (Ω):

$$\text{impedance, } Z = \frac{\text{voltage}}{\text{current}}$$

Because impedance includes reactance in addition to resistance, its value is a function of frequency; similarly, the phase difference between voltage and current is also a function of frequency.

Electrodes, Cells, and Batteries

When a metallic conductor is placed in a liquid or solution containing ions, a double layer of charges forms at the interface between the conductor and the electrolyte (Figure 28-6). A negatively charged layer at the surface of the conductor develops adjacent to a positively charged layer in the electrolyte. These charged layers are the origin of an electric potential difference between the conductor and the electrolyte, which

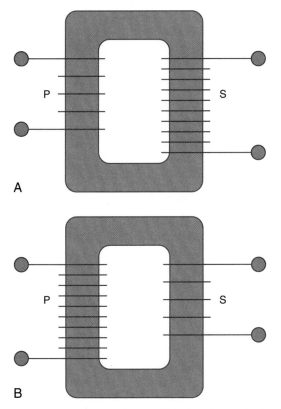

A

B

Figure 28–4 **A,** Step up transformer: (*P*) is the primary winding, and (*S*) is the secondary winding. **B,** A step down transformer.

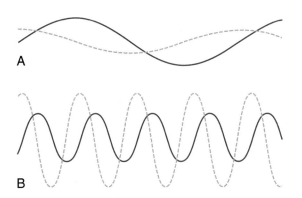

A

B

Figure 28–5 Sine wave current and voltage in a capacitor and their dependence on frequency; the *dashed lines* illustrate current and the *solid lines* voltage. **A,** Low frequency. **B,** High frequency.

is characteristic of the particular conductor and ions present. The interface between the conductor and electrolyte is said to be *polarized*. The combination of a conductor immersed in an electrolyte is known as a *half cell* or *electrode* and the characteristic potential difference between the conductor and solution, when no current is flowing, is known as the half cell or electrode potential. An electrode can be used as a means of making an electrical contact to a solution.

If two half cells with different characteristic potentials are placed in series, the resulting potential difference can be used to drive an electric current through an external circuit, the arrangement being known as a *cell*. Several cells can be placed in series to form a *battery*.

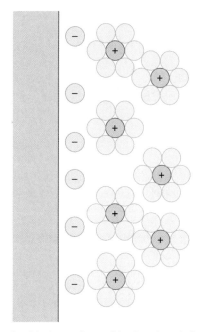

Figure 28–6 Double layer; the positive ions in solution are shown surrounded by water molecules.

Electric currents in the body are generally ionic currents (i.e., they comprise the movement of ions such as Na^+ and Cl^- in solution. Biological potentials measurable on the surface of the body, such as the electrocardiogram (ECG), electro-encephalogram (EEG), electromyogram (EMG), and others, result from the flow of these ionic currents. By contrast, in monitoring equipment, the flow of electric current comprises the movement of electrons through solid materials such as metallic conductors and nonmetallic semiconductors. An electrode is used to convert the ionic currents in the body into electronic currents, which can be amplified, processed, and displayed. The half cell potential of the electrode is usually many times greater than the potential to be measured, which may be a source of artefact in the measurement.

Electrodes possess a property known as *polarization resistance*, which is the change in voltage across the electrode produced by a specific change in current flowing through it. The change in voltage results from a change in thickness of the double layer. If the polarization resistance is high, the change in thickness of the double layer as current flows is greater than if the polarization resistance is low. Electrodes that are particularly suitable for monitoring the small potentials (Figure 28-7), which comprise biopotentials, have a low polarization resistance. This avoids the signal being obscured by changes in the polarization voltage. These changes occur when the thickness of the double layer alters due to current flow or to displacement of charges in the layer when the electrode moves relative to the solution with which it is in contact.

Thermistors

Thermistors are resistors, the resistance of which changes with temperature. Two types are available: those in which the temperature change is positive as temperature increases and

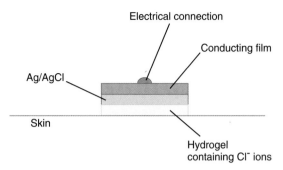

Figure 28–7 Sequence of layers in a typical silver, silver chloride ECG electrode, an example of a system exhibiting low polarization resistance.

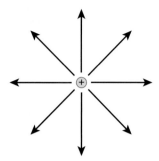

Figure 28–8 Representation of the electric field produced by a positive charge; the arrows show the direction of the force that would be experienced by another positive charge.

those in which it is negative. Thermistors may be used for temperature measurement.

Electric and Magnetic Fields

The term *field* is used to describe how a physical quantity varies with position (i.e., a particular physical quantity has a definite value throughout a region of interest and this value may vary with position). Static electric charges produce an *electric field* (Figure 28-8). Moving electric charges produce an additional field of a different kind, known as the *magnetic field*.

Electric current and magnetism are linked. An electric current results in a magnetic field, and a changing magnetic field induces an electric current in any conductor present in the field. The latter principle, known as electromagnetic induction, is the basis of electricity generators used, for example, to generate the main electricity supply.

Electromagnetic Field and Electromagnetic Radiation

An alternating current produces changing electric and magnetic fields, changes which move outward from the conductor carrying the current with a characteristic speed. The combination of the two fields is known as the *electromagnetic field* and the changing field is known as *electromagnetic radiation*. The speed of propagation of this field is the speed of light, light itself being electromagnetic radiation of a particular range of wavelengths.

Electromagnetic Induction

The phenomena of displacement currents, mutual inductance, and electromagnetic induction can result in a current in one conductor producing a current in another conductor. Although this phenomenon has practical applications, it can also interfere with the monitoring of biological potentials. The magnitude of both electric and magnetic fields decreases as the distance from the current producing them increases, so moving sensitive equipment away from possible sources of interference should reduce the amount of this interference.

The magnitude of the current induced in an electric circuit by a magnetic field is proportional to the area of the circuit perpendicular to the field and to the rate of change of the magnetic field. Thus, high frequency fields, such as those

produced by electrosurgical equipment, are likely to be an important source of interference. The interference can be reduced by decreasing the area of the loop, ensuring that ECG leads are closer together, for example.

Electronics and Control Systems

Electronics in any more than the broadest of terms is outside the scope of this book. However, some basic points will be elucidated so that the terms used in this book and when discussing modern medical equipment may be understood.

Analog and Digital Electronics

Almost every area of medical technology incorporates modern electronic techniques. The reason for this is that logic and computing power of great complexity and reliability is now feasible and economical. Electronic techniques may be subdivided into two broad groupings, namely *analog* and *digital*, both of which are employed in most equipment.

In analog circuits, the values of current and voltage are continuously variable; in digital circuits, these values are limited to discrete steps, the total number of which is usually a power of two. The reason for the use of digital circuits and for their dependence on the power of two arises from the fact that it is comparatively easy to store a value of voltage or current as on or off, but much more difficult to store an exact value for any length of time. It is also easier and more accurate to perform arithmetic and logic functions with discrete values than it is with continuously variable values. The resolution of a voltage that takes only the values zero and one is poor, but by the use of many such circuits, the resolution can be improved. With 10 such circuits, for example, 2^{10} different integers (i.e., any integer between 0 and 1023) can be stored, and the resolution improves to better than 0.1%.

Whereas the numbering system that uses the 10 digits 0 to 9 is known as the decimal system of arithmetic, the numbering system that uses only the digits 0 and 1 is known as the binary system. The conversion of numbers between the decimal and binary systems is illustrated in Table 28-1. The word *bit* is an abbreviation of binary digit.

Almost all modern electronic instrumentation and control systems use a combination of analog and digital circuits. The inputs to electronic processing systems are usually analog voltages. They may be biopotentials such as the ECG or EEG, or a voltage generated by a transducer. An analog signal is converted into digital form using a circuit known as an

Table 28–1 Conversion Between Decimal and Binary Systems								
	BINARY							
	MSB							**LSB**
Decimal	2^7	2^6	2^5	2^4	2^3	2^2	2^1	2^0
0	0	0	0	0	0	0	0	0
1	0	0	0	0	0	0	0	1
2	0	0	0	0	0	0	1	0
3	0	0	0	0	0	0	1	1
4	0	0	0	0	0	1	0	0
5	0	0	0	0	0	1	0	1
6	0	0	0	0	0	1	1	0
7	0	0	0	0	0	1	1	1
8	0	0	0	0	1	0	0	0
9	0	0	0	0	1	0	0	1
10	0	0	0	0	1	0	1	0
200	1	1	0	0	1	0	0	0
255	1	1	1	1		1	1	1

MSB, Most significant bit; *LSB*, least significant bit.

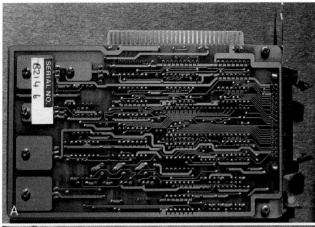
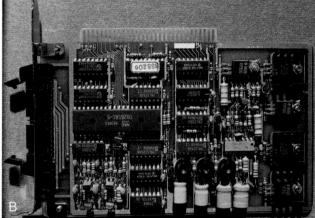

Figure 28–9 Printed circuit board. **A,** The track side. Printed circuit board. **B,** The component side. Note there are conductive tracks on both sides of the board. The components may be conventionally attached to the board by passing their leads through holes in the board and then soldering the connection to make it permanent. Surface mount components are now also used that have shorter connections that are soldered to the same surface of the board as the component is mounted.

analog to digital converter (ADC), which converts an analog input into the nearest discrete value. The performance of an ADC is determined in part by the number of output bits it generates. A 12-bit ADC, for example, produces a number between 0 and $2^{12} - 1$ (i.e., 4095), so its full-scale resolution is approximately 0.025%. A *digital to analog converter* (DAC) has the reverse function of converting a signal in a digital form into an analog form.

Microprocessor Systems

Microprocessors used in electromedical equipment use similar technology and techniques to personal computers. Several different integrated circuits are used to perform various functions within the complete microprocessor system. The central processing unit (CPU) carries out mathematical and logic functions but requires other circuits to perform additional functions. Input and output (I/O) circuits provide the interface between the microprocessor and external functions. The CPU cannot carry out any functions without a program or software, which may be held in *read only memory* (ROM). The contents of ROM cannot be altered by the microprocessor and are retained when power is removed from the system. In much electromedical equipment, software upgrades are normally performed by changing the module that contains the software.

Microprocessors also use memory that can be altered by the CPU. It is said to be volatile because this form of memory, *random access memory* (RAM), is cleared by the disconnection of the power supply. It is used by the CPU for temporarily storing data and for making calculations.

As microprocessor systems use the binary numbering system, it is necessary to use multiple connections between each of the integrated circuits (ICs), and these connections are usually referred to as *buses*. There are three buses in a microprocessor system: a *data bus*, which carries the actual data being manipulated; an *address bus*, which carries the addresses of the data stored in the memories; and a *control bus*, which, as the name implies, carries the control and timing signals. Synchronism is maintained by a crystal-controlled clock or oscillator.

Because of the complexity of the interconnections involved in modern electronics, extensive use is made of printed circuits (Figure 28-9). Once the printed circuit has been designed it has the advantage of ease of economic manufacture without wiring errors and also with high reliability.

Control Systems

The term *control system* may be used when the control of anything is more complicated than, for example, the direct manual manipulation of a valve to control gas flow. A simple example of a control system would comprise a control loop consisting of an actuator, which operates on a valve, a transducer, which senses the flow, and an electronic module, which generates a feedback signal from the transducer to the actuator (Figure 28-10). Such systems are found in ventilators, for example. This seemingly complex system is arranged so that any change in pressure that would cause an alteration in flow may be rapidly and automatically corrected. A separate

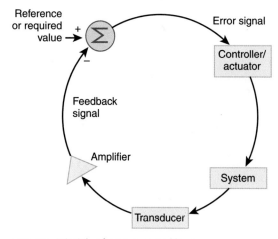

Figure 28–10 Principle of a servo control loop.

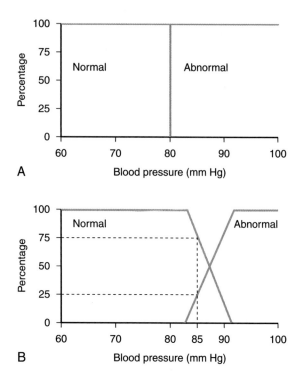

Figure 28–11 Examples of logic sets. **A,** Subdivision of blood pressure into two groups using classical logic. **B,** Subdivision of blood pressures into two groups using fuzzy logic.

input, which may be either manual or from some other part of a larger system, may be arranged to alter the value of the required flow.

Transducers

A transducer is a device that converts one form of energy into another. Most transducers convert an input to an electrical signal, which then undergoes further processing for use to display or record some measurement or to form part of a control system. Many different physical, and in some cases chemical, properties are used in transducers; individual transducers will be discussed in the relevant chapters.

Displays

It is now common practice to use various forms of electronic display in anesthetic delivery machines to indicate gas flow, gas and vapor concentrations, ventilator parameters, and the safety status of the machine. These displays use various forms of *optoelectronic* technology. Optoelectronic displays of simple alphanumerical data may use light-emitting diode (LED) displays or liquid crystal displays (LCD). More complex displays including graphical representations of dynamic pressure and flow require some form of picture display, which may be provided by a cathode ray tube (CRT) or thin film transistor (TFT) display, the latter being a type of LCD display engineered to produce better performance than the simple LCD display.

Fuzzy Logic

In many logical situations, there are just two conditions: on/off, go/no-go, one/zero, yes/no. There are, however, several situations where things are not so clear-cut: for example, at what point is an arterial blood pressure considered as being hypertensive?

Consider a collection of diastolic arterial blood pressure measurements. These can be assigned to two groups (called sets) such as normal (up to 80 mm Hg) or abnormal (above 80 mm Hg). Using classical logic (Figure 28-11, *A*), each value belongs in one group only. This logic becomes unreasonable when 80 mm Hg is interpreted as normal but 81 mm Hg is

abnormal (a difference of only 1 mm Hg). If the data are is now divided into two "fuzzy sets" (Figure 28-11, *B*) where the ordinate (vertical axis on the graph) indicates the relative membership of the group as a percentage, then there is an area of overlap. A given diastolic reading (e.g., 85 mm Hg) will belong in two groups, 75% in the normotensive group and 25% in the hypertensive group. This information can be incorporated into computer programming where an automated response is required. For example, consider an inotrope used to control blood pressure in an automated system. With separation into classical sets, if the pressure were either 1 or 50 mm Hg above a preset limit, the system would switch off. When the pressure dropped below that limit the system would switch back on at the same delivery rate. The pressures would fluctuate greatly. With "fuzzy logic sets" the system would adjust according to the degree (%) of change outside a given value. This has been shown to provide much closer control.

Neural Computing

The origins of neural computing date back to the 1940s but have been overshadowed by advances in conventional computing, especially with the advent of extremely large scale integrated circuits. Neural computing is now rapidly expanding but must not be considered as competitive but rather as complementary to conventional digital computing. The main difference between conventional and neural computing is that conventional computers have to be explicitly programmed, whereas neural computers adapt themselves during a period of training based upon examples with solutions presented to them. Neural computing is so called because the basic unit of the system is similar in function to a neurone (Figure 28–12, *A*). During the training period, the weight applied to any input is

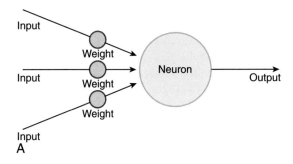

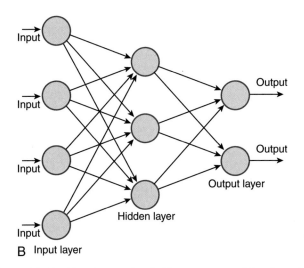

Figure 28–12   Neural networks. **A,** The structure and function of a single neurone. **B,** A typical three-layer neural network.

adjusted to vary the strength of any particular input to the neurone where the decision is made. Neural networks (Figure 28-12) are set up to form a neural computer.

Neural computing has a special role to play in areas of signal processing and data handling involving pattern recognition, for example, in the automatic analysis of the electrocardiogram and electroencephalogram.

Electromagnetic Compatibility

Electrical interference that may affect electromedical equipment is generally of two types: *conducted emissions* that reach the equipment through conductors such as those providing power, and *radiated emissions* that reach the equipment through propagated electromagnetic fields. Conducted interference can be reduced by improving the local quality of the mains electricity supply or by removing interference by electronic means. Radiated interference is more difficult to eliminate in the usual hospital environment.

Electronic equipment may, intentionally or otherwise, emit electromagnetic radiation. When this radiation interferes with the correct operation of other equipment, it is known as *electromagnetic interference* (EMI). Such interference is capable of causing malfunction of electromedical equipment, which may be life threatening in such cases as infusion pumps or ventilators. The effect of EMI on a patient monitor might be to produce artifacts in the display, but its effect on an infusion pump might be to alter the contents of the electronic memory holding the infusion rate.

The likelihood of EMI is a function of the strength of the electromagnetic field generated. Communication equipment

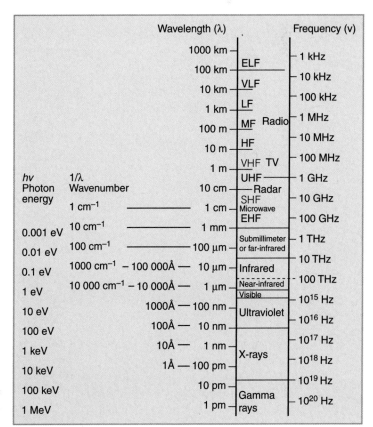

Figure 28–13   The electromagnetic spectrum. *eV,* electron volt, a unit of energy equal to the work done by an electron accelerated through a potential difference of one volt. *Å,* angstrom, a unit of length equal to 10^{-8} cm or 10^{-10} m or 0.1 nm. The ground state diameter of a hydrogen atom is about 1 Å.

devices used in hospitals thus have the potential to interfere with the operation of electromedical equipment. These devices, in decreasing order of field strength (and decreasing likelihood of causing EMI), include emergency services (e.g., police and ambulance) radio handsets, security radio handsets, cell phones, and cordless phones.

Although there are standards that specify the intensity of the electromagnetic field, that should have no effect on various types of electromedical equipment. Communication equipment of all types should not be allowed to come within several meters of medical devices, particularly life support equipment. Users may not realize that cell phones, when turned on, emit pulses intermittently, even when they are not being used. It is also helpful to remember that the electromagnetic field generated (e.g., by a cell phone) decreases by an inverse square law as the distance between the phone and the equipment increases, although reflection within closed spaces such as rooms may diminish the effect of this law.

The Electromagnetic Spectrum

Radio waves, heat, light, and x-rays are all types of electromagnetic radiation and all travel with the same velocity of 3×10^8 m s^{-1} in a vacuum. The various subdivisions of the spectrum have different properties and different methods of generation, absorption, and detection, but may be described by wavelength (λ), wavenumber ($1/\lambda$), frequency (v), or photon energy (hv) (Figure 28-13). A basic grasp of the electromagnetic spectrum helps the anesthesiologist to understand the principles behind the various forms of gas analysis, pulse oximetry, and other monitoring techniques and those of surgical diathermy, radiology, and nuclear medicine with which he or she is likely to come in contact during the course of the working day.

Further Reading

Asbury, A.J., Tzabar, Y., 1995. Fuzzy logic: new ways of thinking in anaesthesia. Br J. Anaesth. 75 (1), 1–2 (editorial).

Gookin, D., Rathbone, A., 1997. PCs for dummies, ed 5. Hungry Minds, New York.

Horowitz, P., Hill, W., 1989. The art of electronics, ed 2. Cambridge University Press, Cambridge, UK.

Medical Devices Agency, 1997. Safety notice MDA SN 9706 mobile communications: interference with medical devices. Medical Devices Agency, London.

Medical Devices Agency. Safety notice SN 2001. 2001(06) update on electromagnetic compatibility of medical devices with mobile communications: TETRA (terrestrial trunked radio system) and outside media broadcasts from hospital premises. Medical Devices Agency, London.

Nickalls, R.W.D., Ramasubramanian, R., 1995. Interfacing the IBM PC to medical equipment. Cambridge University Press, Cambridge, UK.

Sinclair, I., 2002. Electronics made simple, ed 2. Oxford, Newnes, Oxford, UK.

Walters, G., 2000. The essential guide to computing. Prentice Hall, Upper Saddle River, NJ.

Chapter 29

Operating Room Electrical, Fire, Laser, and Radiation Safety

Anuja K. Antony, Chunbai Zhang, and William G. Austen

Electricity and Electrical Safety

Electric current in contact with the human body has direct pathophysiological effects. When electrical current "escapes" from its protective insulation and its intended work pathway, it has potential to cause shock, interference with equipment, or even exploed when combined with flammable/combustible materials present on the body. The most feared of these is electric shock because the ensuing energy delivery to tissues can result in burns, cellular damage, cardiac arrhythmias, and death by electrocution.[1]

In addition to resistant heating of tissues and burning, electrical stimuli can conduct in excitable tissues and result in electrochemical effects. Electrical conductivity will depend on the inherent resistance of individual tissues but can be categorized as follows: high (tendon, bone, fat), intermediate (dry skin), and low (nerve, muscle, blood, mucous membranes).[2]

The severity of electrical injury is dependent on tissue resistance (R), current (I), potential difference (V), current density, current frequency, current pathway, and duration. The thermal energy delivered to the tissues depends on the power dissipated (P), derived from the formula: $V \times I = I^2 R$ or $V = I \times R$, more familiarly known as Ohm's law (also see Chapter 28).[3-5] The body may be considered electrically to be a good conductor (electrolytes) ensconced in insulation (skin, fat). According to Ohm's law, current flow is inversely proportional to impedance. The main impedance is the resistance of the skin, which is variable depending on the skin type (mucous membranes, sole of foot, etc.) and moisture level (dry skin, sweaty skin, wet skin). In addition, the larger the current or the smaller the area over which it is applied, the higher the current density. However, the applied voltage is related to the whole body electrical impedance because higher voltages (>250 volts) result in a drop in the total body impedance irrespective of contact area and pathway of the current.[6]

The electrical current exerts effects on excitable tissues. These effects are dependent on current, time, and current frequency. The commonly used frequencies (line frequency) in the operating room are 50 Hz (UK, Europe) and 60 Hz (United States) and, ironically, are capable of the greatest risk of excitation and damage to human tissues.[1,2] Not surprisingly, given its inherent electrical conduction pathways, the excitable tissue of the heart carries the greatest susceptibility to electrical injury. Cardiac arrhythmias and permanent damage may result. Energy conducted through the heart may result in muscle damage to the heart (vertical pathway) or disturbances in the heart's electrical pathways causing ventricular fibrillation/sudden death (horizontal pathway).[7] Animal studies suggest that a minimum of 100 milliamperes of current applied at 60 Hz may cause ventricular fibrillation.[8] Given this, a very small potential from a stray voltage in the mains can transmit current to the heart causing ventricular fibrillation and electrocution, also known as microshock.

The type of current, alternating (AC) or direct (DC), produces varying effects. Most electromedical devices are powered by AC current for efficiency of power transmission. Alternating current (e.g., power line) consists of current (electron flow) that reverses direction at regular intervals. Direct current (e.g., battery) flows in a single direction. Alternating current carries greater inherent risk of harm than direct current at lower levels of current, and is most dangerous in the 10 to 200 Hz frequency. U.S. current (line frequency) is 60 Hz despite this danger because of its better ability to carry power over long distances than higher frequency current.[1] The current travels from the power station to the substation where it is transformed to line voltage. Current is measured in amperes (A) and represents a flow of 6.24×10^{18} electrons past a specific point in 1 second. Line electric current, typically via a medical equipment source, has the potential to injure the patient and cause electrocution, burns, electrochemical disturbances, and explosion.

The general effects of line supply electrocution (60 Hz) follows:

1 mA—tingling/pain

5 mA—pain

15 mA—tonic muscle contraction/pain

50 mA—respiratory tonic muscle contraction/respiratory arrest

70 to 100 mA—ventricular fibrillation/cardiac arrhythmias/local burns

1000 mA—extensive burning/charring

Direct current tends to produce single muscle spasm, throwing of the victim from the source, blunt mechanical trauma, and heart disturbances. Alternating current induces tetany (continuous muscle contraction), extensive gripping of the power source/conductor by inducing flexion muscle contraction (flexor muscles being stronger than extensor muscles), and local sweating, resulting in lower skin impedance (lowered resistance).

Classes of Electromedical Equipment for Electrical Safety[9,10]

Class I: This type of equipment affords basic protection and includes household equipment. The electrical device has live and neutral leads, which do not come into contact with one another. Additionally, further protection is offered by insulating the metal casing via an earth wire in the plug to the line supply, thereby allowing the casing to be touched by the user. In the event of a fault in the apparatus where current leaks to the casing, the earth connection grounds the leaking current. Fuses are positioned in the live and neutral supply, and in the UK, a fuse positioned in the live lead of the mains plug also melts, disconnecting the circuit in the event of a fault. However, the user loses protection and becomes susceptible to electric shock if the earth lead is faulty.

Class II: This equipment, termed *double-insulated equipment*, has "double insulation" because both the apparatus and casing are insulated. There is no need to earth this type of equipment, and the power cable only has live and neutral conductors with a single fuse.

Class III: This type of equipment operates with a power source that does not exceed 24 volts AC or 50 volts DC. The voltage is called safety extra low voltage or SELV. There is still a risk for microshock. Thus this equipment may contain its own internal power source or connect to the mains supply via SELV transformer or an adaptor.

The following equipment categorization is based on the degree of protection conferred according to the maximum permissible leakage current.

Type B: This categorization defines devices in which the earth leakage current is limited to 0.05 mA in class I equipment and 0.1 mA in class II equipment. Type B classification can be applied to classes I, II, and III equipment or one with an internal power source. These devices may be connected to the patient internally or externally, but are not intended for connection to the heart. They may contain defibrillator protection.

Type BF: These devices are similar to Type B equipment, except that the part applied to the patient is isolated from the other parts of the equipment using a floating (isolated) circuit. The allowed current leakage under single fault conditions must not exceed 1.1 times the rated line voltage applied between the earth and the patient. The maximum AC leakage current under normal conditions is 0.1 mA and 0.5 under a single fault. While Type BF is safer than Type B, direct connection to the heart is still not permitted. These devices may have defibrillator protection.

Type CF: This type of equipment may be class I or II and confers the greatest level of protection against electric shock. Type CF equipment is considered safe for direct connection to the heart as is used for ECG leads and pressure transducers. Allowed current leakage is 0.05 mA per electrode for class I and 0.01 mA for class II equipment. Leakage current resulting from these devices will not cause electrocution. Such equipment may have defibrillator protection.

Isolated or floating circuit—A small isolating transformer is contained within the individual item of medical equipment's internal circuitry. The line circuit is thus earthed, whereas the patient circuit is isolated from the earth and is thus thought of as floating. This safety measure prevents current from flowing between the electrical source and earth.

COELCB (current-operated earth leakage circuit breakers)—These methods of improving patient safety can be connected to an individual item of medical equipment or to the whole operating room. COELCB are also referred to as an "earth trip" or RCCB (residual current circuit breaker). These consist of a transformer with a core that has equivalent numbers of windings of live and neutral wire. A third winding to the coil relays the circuit breaker. The magnetic fields from the two coils cancel one another under normal conditions. However, in the case of a fault, the current generated from the two coils will result in a magnetic field and will cause a current in the third winding "tripping" the circuit breaker. The COELCB are designed to be very sensitive and as little as 30 mA can trip the circuit. These devices are generally less expensive than isolating transformers and similarly decrease the potential for serious shock to the patient.

Methods to Reduce the Risk of Electrocution

- Electrical equipment maintenance and periodic testing
- Avoiding patient contact with grounded objects
- Ensuring equipment compliant with safety standards

Electrosurgery Units[11,12]

Electrosurgery units (ESU), or surgical diathermy, are frequently used in surgery for cutting and coagulation to assist with dissection and to halt bleeding. Surgical diathermy uses current passing through a small amount of tissue to generate the heat needed to carry out these functions. The active electrode consists of high current density with a current passing through a very small area of tissue at the point of contact, as compared with the patient plate, which has low current density with a large conductive area to rapidly conduct away heat to prevent burning. This current density gradient allows for the desired surgical effect. Tissue sensitivity to main frequency electric current decreases at higher frequencies (500,000 to 1,000,000 Hz), allowing the necessary current to pass through the human body and generate the appropriate heat for surgical diathermy without excitation of contractile cells (lowered tissue penetration).

Surgical diathermy frequency (0.4 to 1.5 MHz) is regulated by international standards to certain narrow frequency bands to prevent interference with monitoring devices. A sine waveform for cutting and a modulated waveform for coagulation are used, though a combined waveform (blended mode) is also common. While the risk of electrocution is lowered by the differential impedance provided relative to the current frequency (low impedance to high frequency current of diathermy; high impedance to low frequency current to prevent electrocution), potential burn risk is still a concern and correct lead orientation is critically important to prevent accidental connection of the patient plate to the active terminal.

Two principal types of ESU systems exist: the ground-referenced type and the isolated-generator type. For ground-referenced systems, the electrical current passes through the patient and returns to ground. The grounding is intended to occur through the dispersive plate (pad) placed onto the patient; however, any grounding object can serve as the method of ground return. Given the potential for burns to occur at alternative grounding pathways/sites, many manufacturers no longer rely on ground-referenced ESUs. A safer system incorporates the isolated-generator system where the current return through the dispersive pad to the negative side of an isolation transformer located within the generator. Since the return electrode is not connected or referenced to ground, the current does not return to ground nor does it seek an alternative pathway through other grounded objects (e.g., such as when a conductive material such as metal is in contact with the patient's skin).[12]

In bipolar diathermy, the current flows between the two forceps tips and a patient plate is not needed. The heat generated at both electrodes is equivalent as is the current density and a good coagulation effect is noted. However, the cutting ability of the bipolar diathermy is less effective.

Use of radio frequency diathermy should be avoided in patients with pacemakers. Potential sequelae include cardiac burns and pacemaker malfunction. In these patients, a bipolar cautery, used in locations remote from the heart, provides a safer alternative.

Operating Room Fire and Fire Safety

Obtaining an accurate estimate of the total number of surgical fires in the United States can be trying due to the lack of central reporting mandates and redundancy in reporting agency systems. Fortunately, operating room fires are a relatively infrequent occurrence despite the nearly 50 to 60 million operations that are carried out in the United States each year. In 2007, the ECRI (Emergency Care Research Institute) estimated 550 to 650 incidents of surgical fire in the United States. Of these, the vast majority was due to electrosurgical equipment usage and lasers. The remainder involves other heat-producing sources such as defibrillators, sparking high-speed equipment, and fiber-optic light sources, among others. An oxygen-rich environment and alcohol-based preps contribute to the instigation of a surgical fire. While the majority of fires do not result in injury, nearly 10 to 15 cases are devastating, resulting in serious burn injury to the patient and resultant disfigurement.[13,14]

The traditional model for fire initiation involves three components, termed the "fire triangle," and includes a heat source, a combustible material, and an oxidizer. When a fourth component of the chemical chain is added to create the "fire tetrahedron," an exothermic reaction develops whereby a burning metal reacts with water.

In the operating theater, surgeons, nurses, and anesthesiologists synchronize their efforts to facilitate the successful execution of a safe operation. To accomplish this goal, an intricate interplay of machinery, surgical devices, and chemical components may be involved. In general, surgeons will control potential heat sources, surgical nurses police combustible materials, and anesthesiologists will regulate the oxidizer(s). Therefore a team-based approach with patient safety in mind is critical to prevent fire ignition in the operating room.[15]

Instigation of Surgical Fire

Heat Source

There are numerous sources of heat in the operating room. Surgeons serve as the main source of heat in the fire triangle, usually due to the incorporation of surgical devices or specialized equipment needed for the execution of the particular surgery.

ESU (Electrosurgery Units)

Electrosurgery units, or diathermy, can serve as a source of ignition and fires, and explosion may result; particular attention should be paid in the setting of bowel gas or cleansing solutions. ESUs beget potential hazards in the operating room including fire, burn, shock, and smoke plume. (Burn and shock are discussed earlier in the "Electricity" section.)

Laparoscopic Surgery

In a similar manner to ESU, laparoscopic surgery is associated with several special electrical hazards. The primary ones are insulation failure, direct coupling, and capacitive coupling.[12] Current leakage to the patient may occur from the laparoscopic instrument, resulting in either laparoscopic diathermy malfunction or unintended tissue damage. Stray current may result from insulation break in the diathermy applicator, direct coupling between the active electrode and other organs or metal instruments out of the field of view, or capacitative coupling through intact insulation. Capacitative coupling between a laparoscopic cannula and electrically isolated adjacent tissues can occur, which may be aggravated by smaller cannulas that yield greater capacitance and larger stray current. Insulated instruments and bipolar coagulation help guard against these hazards.

Surgical Plume

Each year, an estimated 500,000 operating room personnel, including surgeons, nurses, anesthesiologists, and surgical technologists, are exposed to laser/electrosurgical smoke. Surgical plumes have contents similar to other smoke plumes, including carbon monoxide, polyaromatic hydrocarbons, and a variety of trace toxic gases. These gases can produce upper respiratory irritation and have in - vitro mutagenic potential. Although no documented transmission of infectious disease through surgical smoke has been reported, the potential for generating infectious viral fragments, particularly following treatment of venereal warts, may exist. The Occupational Safety and Health Administration (OSHA) recommends local smoke evacuation systems, which may improve the quality of the operating field.[16]

Defibrillators

Operating room fires have been reported in defibrillator usage. The source of heat during a defibrillation attempt is typically a spark or electric arc. When there is a poor electrode-chest wall interface, an electric arc may occur during the countershock. A poor interface can also result from paddles that are too large for the chest wall or paddles that extend beyond the conducting electrode cream or conducting gel pads. Electric arcing can also occur when paddles are placed too close to an electrocardiographic electrode. Excessive electrode cream bridges from one paddle to another can also increase the risk for fire, as does a saline-soaked pad placed between the paddle and the patient.[17,18]

Pressure Regulator

When gas is released from a high pressure system to a low pressure system, recompression of the gas can cause an increase of local temperature. When oxygen is in the vicinity, fire or explosion can occur. Aluminum regulators used with high pressure oxygen systems can rarely cause catastrophic combustion in normal usage.[19] Therefore, routine checks of the regulator and updates on product safety from the manufacturers are recommended.

Electrical Faults

In the 1990s, several fires were reported when power plugs were being pushed in or pulled out of the outlet.[20] These were likely due to a "single fault condition"—where a single means for protection against hazard is defective (e.g., a short circuit

between live and applied parts). Today, anesthesia machines and electric surgical equipment can still short circuit and cause operating room fires.

Light Sources

Argon beam coagulators, intense surgical light sources, and endoscopic light systems from a fiber optic system can all serve as sources for heat. Light systems used in the surgical field often need to provide high intensity light through a small diameter device. As the required power densities for the light source are high, they are at risk for overheating. In an environment with a high concentration of oxygen (i.e., during anesthesia induction and emergence), the high power light can serve as a heat source for operating room fires and explosions. To prevent fire, surgical staffs should try to inactivate the power supply whenever possible.

Static Electricity and Sparks

Although operating room static electricity is relatively low in quantity, enough sparking energy can be created to ignite flammable vapors. To prevent unexpected sparks, the floors of operating rooms should be covered with an approved conductive (antistatic) material. Floor conductivity should be tested regularly and records of testing should be maintained by the hospital engineering department. In addition, electrical equipment should be approved by the hospital engineering department before use in the operating room. All mobile electrical equipment should make electrical contact with the operating room floor. Regular checks are needed to ensure proper operation. Likewise, conductive clothing should be worn, and conductive footwear should be required.[21]

Combustible Materials

Combustible material serves as the "fuel" in the fire triangle model. These are any materials that can be burned; they can be in gas, liquid, or solid state.

Endotracheal (ET) Tube

The specific material composition of an ET tube (PVC, red rubber, metallic) determines the risk and characteristics of a tracheal fire. ET tubes are usually penetrated by laser or surgical equipment before ignition. A characteristic of ET tube fire is that the fire usually starts in the inner rim of the penetrated area then spreads along the direction of oxidizing gas.

Polyvinylchloride Tube (PVC Tube)

PVC tubes are products of petroleum-based extractions. They are combustible in an oxidizer-rich environment, usually with an ignition by a laser. Once ignited, PVC tubes can produce a torchlike fire. Increasing positive end-expiratory pressure (PEEP) is thought to decrease the risk of PVC tube fire during laser surgery.[22] Blood, saliva, and mucus covered PVC tubes have a higher risk for fire. Furthermore, rubber-based ET tube may have an advantage over PVC tubes during extubation. Other components of the fire triangle should be avoided when possible (i.e., nitrous oxide or high concentration of oxygen gas). Saline-filled cuff ET tubes may further reduce the risk for fire in the airways.[23-27] Metallic tapes such as aluminum-foil tape and copper-foil tape have been developed to protect combustible endotracheal tubes from the CO_2 laser. Comparatively, the Laser-Guard-wrapped PVC tracheal tube and the Tyco Healthcare/Nellcor Laser-Flex tracheal tube are less reflective of incident CO_2 or KTP laser surgery laser radiation than the copper- or aluminum foil-wrapped red rubber tracheal tubes.[25,28] Laser-Guard helps protect the shafts of combustible PVC endotracheal tubes from direct, high power, continuous CO_2 laser radiation.[25,29]

Red Rubber (RR) Endotracheal Tubes

Sterile disposable PVC ET tubes are now routinely used in surgery. Previously, red rubber (Rusch-Germany) tracheal tubes were used. These tubes were sterilized for reuse, which carried a small a risk of infection. Similar to PVC tubing, RR tubes also pose a risk for operating room fires if penetrated by laser energy in an oxidizer-rich environment. Use of a rubber ET tube may have an advantage over plastic PVC ET tube, with a potentially more rapid extubation in the case of an ET tube fire.[24]

Laser-Resistant Tubes[30]

An appropriate laser-resistant tracheal tube should be used for the procedure (e.g., carbon dioxide [CO_2], neodymium-doped yttrium aluminium garnet [Nd:YAG], Ar, erbium-doped yttrium aluminium garnet [Er:YAG], potassium titanyl phosphate [KTP]). Laser-resistant tubes provide improved safety; PVC and RR tubes can readily ignite in an oxygen-rich environment with continuous laser energy supported by nitrous oxide combustion.[31,32]

The tracheal cuff of the laser tube should be filled with saline and colored with an indicator dye such as methylene blue. Before laser activation, the surgeon should indicate to the anesthesiologist that laser activation is about to occur so that delivered oxygen content can be reduced to the minimum acceptable, nitrous oxide use can be terminated, and ample time can transpire (a few minutes) for reduction of the oxidizer-rich atmosphere. Adding PEEP during CO_2 laser operations on the airway in which laser-resistant tracheal tubes with PVC components are used may decrease the incidence of fire.[33]

Prep Agents[34]

Many prepping agents and certain ointments are flammable. In particular, alcohol-based prepping agents are extremely flammable and vapors from these agents can ignite from a laser or ESU. One should avoid dripping or pooling of residual alcohol-based preps, especially at the umbilicus and suprasternal notch of the patient because vapors trapped under drapes or residual wet draping may ignite with heat or sparks. When prepping with alcohol-based prep, proper technique should be employed to ensure proper drying time and limited exposure of any volatile solution in the operating room. Also, surgical petroleum-based ointment, especially if applied in thin layers, can absorb considerable heat and vaporize. These vapors, after mixing with oxygen, serve as a potential ignitable source. To the contrary, water-based lubricants (K-Y jelly) do not burn and can be used to coat hair as a fire retardant. Similarly, water-based prepping agents (Betadine, Pharmaseal) should be used when possible.

Patients

A patient's body hair, eyelashes, mustache, and eyebrows are all combustible. Water-based lubricant can reduce the fire hazards.

Intestinal Gas

Methane, hydrogen sulfide, and sulfur gas in the GI tract have all been reported sources for combustible gas within the patient's body.[34,35] Care should be taken to reduce the intestinal gases as much as possible by proper preoperative bowel preparation. Oxygen may also diffuse into the GI tract and become a combustible firehazard.

Surgical Products

Surgical drapes, gowns, masks, shoe covers, mattresses, pillows, and blankets can serve as fuels for operating room fires. An oxygen-rich environment may override the fire-resistant properties of surgical products.[36] Sponges, gauze, and ace bandages can also be fuels for operating room fires. However, moistening sponges and gauze with saline reduces the chance for fire. Disposable drapes may be troublesome when caught on fire because they are water repellant. One should consider that fire-resistant drapes are not fireproof.

Gauze, especially with blood, can be very combustible under an oxygen-rich environment.[37,38]

Equipment/Supplies

Other equipment that may become fuel in the operating room include anesthesia components, flexible endoscopes, coverings of fiberoptic cables, gloves, blood pressure and tourniquet cuffs, stethoscope tubing, smoke evacuator hoses, instrument cabinets, disposable packaging material (plastics), and warming blankets (Bair Huggers).

Oxidizing Media
Anesthetic Gases

Older anesthetic gases, such as cyclopropane, ethylene, acetylene, and nonhalogenated ethers (i.e., diethyl ether), are flammable; as are some halogenated volatile agents, such as ethyl chloride and fluoxene.[39] While flammable gases are employed in some cases, most of the halogenated gases currently in use in the United States are not considered flammable.[21] Carbon dioxide, halothane, enflurane, isoflurane, sevoflurane, and desflurane are not flammable, nor is atmospheric pressure nitrous oxide. Mixing these gases with oxygen can alter the mixture's flammability, making fire possible in a clinical setting.[39] Therefore, a routine check of leakage of gas tanks is recommended. Flammable anesthetics should be kept in a National Fire Protection Association-approved central location that is fire-resistant and vented to the outside.[21]

Anesthetic-Proof Equipment

Anesthetic-proof (AP) equipment standards are based on the ignition energy required to ignite the most flammable mixture of air and ether (based on 5 to 25 cm of gas escape from the respiratory system). The temperature should not exceed 200° C.

Anesthetic-Proof Equipment Category G

APG standards are more stringent and based on ignition energy (energy level less than 1 mJ) for 5 cm of gas escape from a respiratory system of the most flammable mixture of air and ether. Temperature should not exceed 90° C.

Oxygen Supply Fire and Nitrous Oxide [40]

Since the introduction of oxygen supplies, the fire incidence in the operating room due to anesthesia gas has increased. Nitrous oxide is a more reactive oxidant and supports combustion more intensely than oxygen.[39] Nitrous oxide should therefore not be used during laser endoscopic surgery.[23]

Faulty assembly of the oxygen regulator can cause serious fire. When oxygen is released from a high pressure to a lower pressure system, the temperature can increase dramatically. With 100% oxygen, this temperature spike can cause fire within the tubing, the regulator seats and seals, or even the metal tank itself. Teflon tape or other hydrocarbon contaminants may potentially cause sparking while under high pressure release from the oxygen tank, inducing a fire. Oxygen-content-lowering devices used in the operating room can reduce the incidence or prevent this type of fire.[41]

Chemical Chain

When a fourth component of the chemical chain is added to create the "fire tetrahedron," an exothermic reaction develops. For example, desiccated Baralyme (CO_2 absorbent) or soda lime can react exothermically with sevoflurane to produce carbon monoxide and flammable organic compounds, such as methanol and formaldehyde. The heat produced accelerates the reaction speed, and at very high temperatures, combustion of the flammable metabolites may occur. Temperatures can reach above 300° C and canister melting and water in the circuit may be observed.[42]

Reported Scenarios

Approximately 21% of the reported fires involve the oropharynx. Forty-four percent of the time, the head, neck, or upper chest were ignited. Other patient surfaces were ignited at a frequency of 26%, while 8% of fires occurred inside of patients.[30,43]

Fire Prevention

Some important safety measures include keeping the Bovie tip in its insulated holster when not in use. Turn down the power of high intensity light sources whenever not in use. Use only protected endotracheal tubes when operating near the trachea.

Use air or air and oxygen mixtures in anesthetic gases. Avoid tenting of surgical drapes to form oxygen-enriched areas (e.g., near a nasal cannula). Decrease oxygen content to lowest acceptable levels.[44,45] Use water-soluble (nonflammable) substances to cover hair and other flammable parts of the body. Use fire-retardant drapes.

Minimizing Combustible Materials

Supraglottic jet ventilation (SJV) is a technique in which adequate oxygenation and ventilation is achieved without using a combustible endotracheal tube during laser surgery. However, there has been a case report of accidental fire caused by other combustible material in the surgical field.[46]

Chemical Chain

As an alternative to Baralyme, Amsorb (carbon dioxide absorbent) can be used. Amsorb remains hydrated and changes color when dehydrated; it does not contain the strong bases necessary to produce carbon monoxide in clinically significant amounts or react exothermically with sevoflurane.[42,47] Routine changing of carbon dioxide absorbent may also reduce the risk of an injurious exothermic reaction.

Fire Safety Plan

A fire safety plan should be adopted and implemented. If a fire is recognized, all unnecessary operating room personnel should leave and notify appropriate authorities, electrocautery should be shut off, and the electrode removed from the area. A fire extinguisher can be used to put out fires in the immediate setting, and, if possible, all oxygen and nitrous oxide should be shut off and the patient extubated as quickly as possible.[12,48] Awareness of surgical suite fire is the key to prevention.[14,49]

A surgical suite primer has been published; appropriate training in fire hazard prevention and proper facility operation and maintenance is critical to ensuring patient and operating room personnel safety.[21,34,50]

- Use separate collection containers for glass, empty ether cans, aerosol cans, disposables, etc., that are not to be incinerated.
- Instruct personnel to report defective equipment.
- Post warning signs where necessary and enforce proper work practices.
- Discuss safe work practices and health hazards with each new worker as part of orientation. This training should be reviewed periodically.

Guidelines for operating room fire safety and hazard prevention are available and should be used accordingly.[51-53]

Lasers and Laser Safety

The increasing popularity of laser use in the operating room demands understanding of its mechanisms, energy delivery, and potential hazards to operating room staff. Laser is an acronym for "Light Amplification by Stimulated Emission of Radiation." Laser energy generates a one wavelength, one color (monochromatic) pure beam of light.

Laser[54]

Laser is a modern technology that converts electric energy into concentrated light energy. Light energy is concentrated by storing it in an enclosed reflective container before release. A laser uses collimated, coherent, monochromatic electromagnetic radiation to achieve the intended surgical goal. Lasers have the inherent ability to cut, coagulate, and/or vaporize tissues, rendering surgery near bloodless.

The power of the energy delivery attributed to a laser is usually described in "watts," or energy (in joules) per unit time of exposure (in seconds). Laser power density is defined as the laser's power per area (in square centimeters). The wavelength of the laser is specified by the medium used for lasing, which may be a solid, liquid, or gas. Stable atoms in the "ground state" of the lasing medium becomes excited to a higher energy state by the photon pumping source and then spontaneously emit a photon of energy as it returns to the ground state, usually in the form of light or radiofrequency energy. Einstein first described the process of adding an additional photon of energy at the correct wavelength to the excited atom to promote "stimulated emission" of two photons of energy, the basis of modern laser technology. As many photons escape back into the lasing medium, a chain reaction of amplification ensues and an intense source of light energy can be generated.

Components of Lasers

Lasers used in clinical settings usually include four components in the apparatus: a delivery system to direct the output of the laser, a power supply with laser control and calibration functions, mechanical housing with interlocks, and associated liquids, solids, or gases as the media for laser operation.[55]

Laser Types

While there are numerous types of lasers, only a dozen or fewer are found in everyday surgical use. The clinical effect of the light energy on human tissues is dependent on the laser's intensity and the frequency of light used. At lower intensities, the laser stimulates cells. However, at higher intensities, cellular activity attenuates, tissue temperature rises, and protein denaturation and photocoagulation occur. To control the thermal energy delivered to tissue, laser pulsing can be carried out to allow for heat dissipation between bursts. "Q switching" refers to the process of storing laser light aliquots for release in bursts of higher energy and shorter duration. With this process, mechanical damage may predominate over thermal damage because of induced vibration. Numerous lasers are available for medical use, the most familiar being CO_2 (carbon dioxide) and Nd-Yag (neodymium: yttrium-aluminum garnet). The carbon dioxide laser (10.6 μm) causes rapid vaporization of intracellular water (absorbs water within 1 mm depth) with energy in the far infrared spectrum; it is mainly used as a vaporizer and bloodless cutter. The Nd-Yag laser uses a solid lasing medium and penetrates at a 3 to 5 mm depth. It produces energy in the near infrared spectrum and maximally penetrates hemoglobin, melanin, and water.

Laser Hazard

Operating room laser usage always carries a risk of accidental injury to OR personnel and patients.[56] Therefore appropriate OR signage (Figure 29–1) should be displayed. A laser source, when not being used, can be accidentally activated (e.g., by stepping on a laser's foot-controlled operating switch). In the setting of potentially flammable surgical drapes and clothing, an accidentally triggered laser can introduce a hazard in the operating room if in the line of clothing, directed toward reflective metal sources, or camouflaged under ignitable surgical drapes. To reduce the prospect of such disastrous occurrences, a surgical laser source should routinely be placed on standby mode when not being actively engaged.

The most common cause of laser-induced tissue damage in humans is thermal. Heat from the laser beam causes biochemical injury by denaturing proteins in the affected body area. The nondivergence of the beam and long range of laser light leaves little protection even when remote from the laser source. A particularly vulnerable portion of the body to the

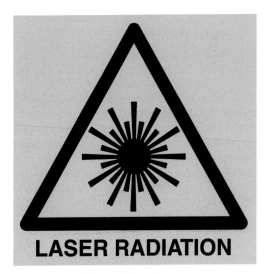

Figure 29–1 Laser radiation warning sign.

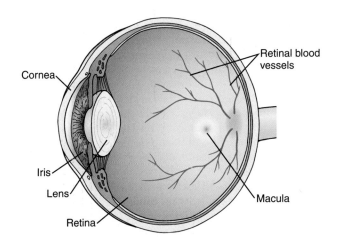

Figure 29–2 Diagram of the human eye. *(From National Eye Institute. Macular hole (website): http://www.nei.nih.gov/health/macularhole/index.asp.) Accessed 20 May 2009.*

laser's thermal damage is the ocular region (Figure 29–2). The specific location of eye injury for a given laser depends upon its output wavelength. Laser light in the visible and near infrared spectrum—400 to 1400 nm—may induce damage to the retina, while wavelengths outside this region (e.g., ultraviolet and far infrared spectrum) are absorbed by the anterior segment of the eye, damaging the cornea and/or the lens. Laser light transmitted to the eye can result in blind spots or even total blindness. The extent of the damage depends on the total energy the body part has suffered under the laser. Therefore protective eyewear in the operating room in the form of goggles, glasses, and shields is crucial to ensure protection against ocular injury, and must be worn at all times during laser surgery. Laser safety eyewear (LSE) is designed to reduce the amount of incident light of specific wavelength(s) to safe levels, while transmitting sufficient light for good vision. Each kind of laser requires a specific type of protective eyewear, and factors that must be considered when selecting LSE include laser wavelength and peak irradiance, optical density, visual transmittance, field of view, effects on color vision, absence of irreversible bleaching of the filter, comfort, and impact resistance.[57]

Laser Classification[55]

Class 1—A class 1 laser system is considered to be incapable of producing damaging radiation levels during normal operation. There are no control measures or other forms of surveillance for class 1 lasers. Some class 1 lasers do emit very weak, nonhazardous beams, but these class 1 laser systems usually have "embedded" higher power lasers, which are only accessible if the interlock safety systems are deliberately opened.

Class 1M—A class 1M laser system is considered to be incapable of producing hazardous exposure conditions during normal operation unless the beam is viewed with an optical instrument, such as an eye loupe or a telescope. Class 1M lasers are also free of any control measures and other forms of surveillance.

Class 2—A class 2 laser system emits in the visible portion of the spectrum (400 to 700 nm) with power up to 1 mW. The means of eye protection is normally done by the aversion responses, which include closure of the eyelid, eye movement, pupillary constriction, or movement of the head to avoid the exposure. The aversion response to a bright visible laser source is assumed to limit the exposure of the retina to 0.25 seconds or less (blink reflex time). Class 2M is potentially hazardous if viewed with certain optical aids.

Class 3R—A class 3R laser system is potentially hazardous under direct or *specular reflection* viewing conditions if the eye is appropriately focused and stable, but the probability of an actual injury is small. This laser is unlikely to pose either a fire hazard or diffuse reflection hazard. Note: an old classification of class 3A should be considered equivalent to class 3R.

Class 3B—A class 3B laser system may be hazardous under direct and specular viewing conditions; class 3B laser is normally not a diffuse reflection or fire hazard thanks to its required laser power limitation: 500 mW for continuous laser sources and 30 mJ for pulse laser sources.

Class 4—A class 4 laser system is a hazard to the eye and skin from the direct beam. It includes any laser systems that emit a higher power than class 3B laser systems. A class 4 laser system poses a diffuse reflection or fire hazard, and may also produce laser-generated airborne contaminants and hazardous plasma radiation.

Nearly all surgical treatment lasers are class 4 because they are designed to deliver laser radiation for the purpose of altering biological tissue. The following section provides information regarding the use of lasers.

Laser Wavelength and the Eye's Response

Different laser wavelengths affect various parts of the human eye and may cause serious injury at high power levels. The following describes these wavelengths and the parts of the eye that are affected.

A. Invisible Ultraviolet
Lasers operating in the ultraviolet spectrum (315 nm to 390 nm) are absorbed by the lens. An *excimer laser* commonly used in eye surgery is a typical ultraviolet medical laser.

B. Visible
Laser radiation in the visible region (between 400 to 700 nm) is absorbed primarily within the retina. An eye can focus a collimated visible beam by as much as 100,000 times. Argon and KTP lasers are typical visible medical lasers.

C. Invisible Near-Infrared
Laser radiation, in the near-infrared region (between 700 to 1400 nm), is also absorbed by the retina. An eye can concentrate a laser beam on the retina as much as 100,000 times. Since the eye does not have an aversion response in the near- or far-infrared portion of the spectrum, the victims usually do not know that they have been overexposed until the injury occurs. This explains why invisible near-infrared lasers are very dangerous.

D. Far-Infrared
Laser radiation in the far-infrared region of 1400 nm to 1 mm and the midultraviolet (180 to 315 nm) primarily affects the cornea. A CO_2 laser is a typical far-infrared medical laser.

Laser-Generated Airborne Contaminants[55]

Lasers used in the OR can vaporize tissue through cellular disruption. Laser-generated airborne contaminants (LGAC) result from laser use and present as an airborne hazard to the surgical personnel. LGAC commonly include: gaseous toxic compounds, bio-aerosols, cellular material, and viruses.

In orthopedics, dentistry, plastic surgery, and other fields, particulates and metal fumes are commonly generated. Some LGAC may cause upper respiratory tract irritation, have unpleasant odors, and incur ocular irritation, particularly when the subject is under a repeated and prolonged exposure. Some LGAC have been shown to have mutagenic and carcinogenic potential. It has also been shown that laser smoke production is a function of increased irradiance levels. Airborne contaminants should be controlled with local exhaust ventilation, personal protective equipment (PPE), or a combination of both.

Training and Credentialing[55]

All surgical and anesthesia personnel working in the presence of class 3B and class 4 health care laser systems should undergo training. All training activities should be documented and retained on file. In all surgical specialties, the laser user should use the laser for its intended purpose within the user's scope of practice, training, and experience.

Radiation and Radiation Safety[58]

Radiation Hazards

Fluoroscopy and mobile radiography account for the vast majority of occupational exposure in the operating room. While many studies have assessed the exposure risk for individual procedures and deemed acceptable safe levels for operating room staff, understanding risks and engaging in safe radiation practices can greatly reduce risk of radiation exposure.[59-62] Implementation of ALARA (as low as reasonably achievable) standards with use of distance, time, and shielding are the standards for operating room radiation safety.[63]

The absorbed dose is defined as the energy per unit mass deposited into tissues and organs of the body. The effective dose concept is employed to account for the different types of radiation and varying biological effects; it is used to estimate risks when different organs receive different amounts of radiation.[64] Because some types of radiation are more injurious than others, rem terminology is used to rectify the differences in biological effect. The NCRP report No. 116 states that annual occupational dose limit for all medical workers should not exceed 50 mSV (5 rem) for the whole body and the lifetime effective dose should not exceed 10 times the medical worker's age in years.[65]

Radiation Prevention

The three main equipment sources of radiation in the operating room are: mobile radiography, dedicated fluoroscopy, and the C-arm or mini-C-arm. Lead aprons, which wraparound and fit properly along with thyroid shields, are required for shielding from radiation in the operating room. Ceiling-mounted lead acrylic face shields, table-side drapes, and mobile "door" type of shields may also add additional protection. Use of protective apparel reduces the effective dose received by the operating room staff. Because of increased risk of radiation scatter to the surgeon and first assistant, particularly to the hands and head and neck region, lead-lined gloves and eye protection should be used when close to the source.[66,67]

Operating room staff may be subjected to radiation exposure by increased scatter. Larger radiation doses and poor beam collimation may result in potentially harmful higher levels of scatter, particularly with prolonged exposure. To assess the different receiver levels of radiation, a pelvic phantom model was used to assess surgeon, first assistant, anesthesiologist, and scrub nurse exposure rates. In this model, the surgeon and first assistant received the highest radiation exposure while the scrub nurse and anesthesiologist positioned farther away received considerably less or no exposure.[68] For procedures requiring two C-arms with long exposure times, shielding is vital for protection as anesthesiologist levels of exposure approach that of the first assistant.[69]

Important ways to reduce radiation exposure include controlling the amount of radiation, increasing the distance from the radiation source, and optimizing the duration and direction of exposure. Use of the lowest effective dose and an experienced fluoroscopic operator facilitate this process. Appropriate training for all operating room personnel should be employed.

In addition to proper shielding, equipment should be checked periodically for radiation leakage. Regular performance of radiation measurements, dosimetric calculations, and performance evaluations of equipment by a qualified radiation safety officer (medical physicist) should be carried out. Radiation measuring devices include dosimeters (photographic emulsion), ionizing chambers (gas-filled radiation detector to measure intensity), and portable survey instruments. Although the surgeon is often the most exposed to radiation, all members of the operating room team should wear a dosimeter on his/her body.[59] Film badges (e.g., thermoluminescent dosimetry, optically stimulated luminescence) are necessary for monitoring of radiation exposure.

Fluoroscopy

Fluoroscopy has become a mainstay for interventional and operating room procedures. In addition to fluoroscopic interventional procedures, pain management procedures and orthopedic procedures requiring fluoroscopy have become increasingly common. While radiation exposure in pain management anesthesia staffs seems to be less than the occupational limit, evidence for long-term effect is still lacking.[70] The use of the C-arm and mini C-arm exposes the operating room staff to higher levels of radiation. When possible, the mini C-arm should be chosen over its larger counterpart to reduce radiation exposure.[71] The major health risks result from long exposure times and high dose rates. Skin injury may result, though it may present in a delayed manner several weeks later.

Radiation-Associated Procedures

Procedures in the operating room where radiation exposure must be considered include:

- Operative cholangiogram
- Endoscopic retrograde cholangiopancreatography (ERCP)
- Bronchoscopy
- Intraoperative angiography
- Vascular surgery/endovascular procedures
- Neurosurgical procedures (cervical laminectomy, fusion, etc.)
- Urological surgical procedures (cytoscopy)
- Orthopedic procedures
- Brachytherapy (sealed-source radiation therapy, "radioactive seeds")
- Intraoperative radiation therapy (IORT)
- Otolaryngology/head and neck surgery

MRI

Advisory guidelines for anesthesiologists with regards to MRI usage are available.[72] All anesthesiologists should have general safety education on the MRI environment and institution-specific features of the MRI facility and equipment. An emphasis on hazards in this environment and monitoring capabilities should be made. Health hazards include noise (high decibel levels) and high-intensity magnetic fields. The necessary precautions required to address the institution's specific field strength and the safety of the MRI scanners should be reviewed. Education should incorporate information regarding ferromagnetic items and implantable devices. A team-based approach with the anesthesia team and radiologists, technologists, and physicists should be used to ensure that safety-training programs are appropriate for the institution.

Further Reading

Buczko, G., McKay, W., 1987. Electrical safety in the operating room. Can J Anaesth 34, 315–322. *We suggest this article because it is a classic summary article of the electrical risks associated with the operating room.*

Lees, D., 2002. Operating room fires: Still a problem? ASA Newsl 66, 33–34. *This article presents the consensus of the anesthesia community regarding the importance of surgical fire safety. A team approach to surgical fire prevention 2006. Understanding the fire triangle. Health Devices 35, 49–53 5-7. This article emphasizes the need for a "team approach" to fire safety in the operating room.*

OSHA. Laser/electrosurgery plume (website): http://www.osha.gov/SLTC/laserelectrosurgeryplume/. Accessed May 20, 2009. *This interactive website demonstrates the laser-generated airborne contaminants as potential hazard.*

Sosis, M., Dillon, F., 1992. Prevention of CO₂ laser-induced endotracheal tube fires with laser-guard protective coating. J Clin Anesth 4, 25–27. *This article demonstrates changing standards for endotracheal tubes to lower the risk for laser-related ETT fire.*

ECRI Institute. The patient is on fire! A surgical fires primer (website): http://www.mdsr.ecri.org/summary/detail.aspx?doc_id=8197. Accessed 20 May 2009. *This website by the ECRI Institute, a leader in operating room safety issues, demonstrates key issues in surgical fire safety.*

Macdonald, A., 1994. A short history of fires and explosion caused by anaesthetic agents. Br J Anaesth 72, 710–722. *This classics article highlights the anesthetic agents used in the 1970s and currently in third world countries. This article may be of benefit to the international audience.*

Castro, B., Freedman, A., Craig, W., et al., 2004. Explosion within an anesthesia machine: baralyme, high fresh gas flows and sevoflurane concentration. Anesthesiology 101, 537–539. *This article highlights potential hazards with anesthetic agents currently in use in the United States.*

Sherer-Statkiewicz, M., Visconti, P., Ritenour, E., (Eds.) 2006. Dose limits for exposure to ionizing radiation. Radiation protection in medical radiography, Mosby, St Louis.

ASA, 2009. Practice advisory on anesthetic care for magnetic resonance imaging: a report by the American Society of Anesthesiologists task force on anesthetic care for magnetic resonance imaging. Anesthesiology 110, 459–479. *This article underscores awareness for MRI-suite personnel because of electromagnetic fields.*

References

1. Buczko, G., McKay, W. 1987. Electrical safety in the operating room. Can J Anaesth 34, 315–322.
2. Magee, P. 2005. Electrical hazards and their prevention, Chapter 25 In Ward's Anaesthetic Equipment, Davey, A., Diba, A. (Eds.).
3. Cromwell, L., Arditti, M., Weibell, F., et al., 1976. Medical instrumentation for health care. Prentice Hall, Englewood Cliffs, NJ.
4. Spooner, R., 1980. Hospital electrical safety simplified. Instrument Society of America, Research Triangle Park, NC.
5. Hoenig, S., Scott, D., 1977. Medical instrumentation and electrical safety: the view from the nursing station. John Wiley and Sons, New York.
6. Beiglemeyer, G., 1987. Effects of current passing through the human body and the electrical impedance of the human body . In A guide to IEC Report 479, Vde Verlag gmbh, Berlin, 1987.
7. Fontanarossa, P., 1993. Electric shock and lightning strike. Ann Emerg Med 22, 378–387.
8. Dalziel, C. F., (Ed.), 1972. Electric shock hazard, IEEE Spectrum 9, 41–50..
9. Al-Shaikh, B., Stacey, S. (Eds.), 2002. Essentials of anesthetic equipment, ed 2. Churchill Livingstone, London.
10. Keynes M. British standard medical electrical equipment part i: general requirements for safety, BS5724: part I (IEC 60101), London, UK, BSI, 1988.
11. Smith, L., Roy, S., 2008. Fire/burn risk with electrosurgical devices and endoscopy fiberoptic cables. Am J Otolaryngol 29, 171–176.
12. Jones, C., et al., 2006. Electrosurgery. Curr Surg 63, 458–463.
13. PA-PSRS., 2007. Patient safety advisory, ECRI Institute & ISMP, Pennsylvania.
14. Lees, D., 2002. Operating room fires: still a problem? ASA Newsl 66, 33–34.
15. A team approach to surgical fire prevention 2006. Understanding the fire triangle. Health Devices 35, 49–53 5-7.
16. OSHA. Laser/electrosurgery plume (website): http://www.osha.gov/SLTC/laserelectrosurgeryplume/. Accessed May 20, 2009
17. Fires from defibrillation during oxygen administration. Health Devices 23, 307–309.
18. Theodorou, A., Gutierrez, J., Berg, R., 2003. Fire attributable to a defibrillation attempt in a neonate. Pediatrics 112, 677–679.
19. Hodous, T., Washenitz, F., Newton, B., 2002. Occupational burns from oxygen resuscitator fires: the hazard of aluminum regulators. Am J Ind Med 42, 63–69.
20. Wald, A., 1994. Short circuit in the operating room. Anesthesiology 81, 260.
21. NIOSH 1998. Recommended guidelines for controlling safety hazards in hospitals. National Institute for Occupational Safety and Health, Cincinnati, OH.
22. Pashayan, A., et al., 1993. Positive end-expiratory pressure lowers the risk of laser-induced polyvinylchloride tracheal-tube fires. Anesthesiology 79, 83–87.
23. Sosis, M., 1987. Nitrous oxide should not be used during laser endoscopic surgery. Anesth Analg 34, 539.
24. Sosis, M., Braverman, B., 1996. Advantage of rubber over plastic endotracheal rapid extubation in a laser fire. J Clin Laser Med Surg 14, 93.
25. Sosis, M., Dillon, F., 1991. Reflection of CO₂ laser radiation from laser-resistant endotracheal tubes. Anesth Analg 73, 338–340.
26. Sosis, M., Dillon, F., 1991. Saline-filled cuffs help prevent laser-induced polyvinylchloride endotracheal tube fires. Anesth Analg 72, 187–189.
27. Wolf, G., Sidebotham, G.W., Lazard, J.L.P., 2004. Laser ignition of surgical drape materials in air, 50% oxygen, and 95% oxygen. Anesthesiology 100, 1167.
28. Walker, P., et al., 2004. Avoidance of laser ignition of endotracheal tubes by wrapping in aluminium foil tape. Anaesth Intensive Care 32, 108–112.
29. Sosis, M., Dillon, F., 1992. Prevention of CO₂ laser-induced endotracheal tube fires with laser-guard protective coating. J Clin Anesth 4, 25–27.
30. E.C.R.I., 2006. Guidance article: surgical fire safety. Health Devices 35, 45–66.
31. Hayes, D., Gaba, D., Goode, R., 1986. Incendiary characteristics of a new laser-resistant endotracheal tube. Otolaryngol Head Neck Surg 95, 37–40.
32. Ossoff, R., 1989. Laser safety in otolaryngology - head and neck surgery: anesthetic and educational considerations for laryngeal surgery. Laryngoscope 99, 1–26.
33. Pashayan, A., San Giovanni, C., Davis, L., 1993. Positive end-expiratory pressure lowers the risk of laser-induced polyvinylchloride tracheal-tube fires. Anesthesiology 79, 83–87.
34. ECRI Institute. The patient is on fire! A surgical fires primer (website): http://www.mdsr.ecri.org/summary/detail.aspx?doc_id=8197. Accessed 20 May 2009.
35. Greilich, P., Greilich, N., Froelich, E., 1995. Intraabdominal fire during laparoscopic cholecystectomy. Anesthesiology 78, 875–879.
36. Goldberg, J., 2006. Brief laboratory report: surgical drape flammability. AANA J 74, 352–354.
37. Ortega, R., 1998. A rare cause of fire in the operating room. Anesthesiology 89, 1608.
38. Wood, D., Hollis, R. 1993. Thermocautery causes a gauze pad fire. JAMA 270, 2299–2300.
39. Macdonald, A., 1994. A short history of fires and explosion caused by anaesthetic agents. Br J Anaesth 72, 710–722.

40. Kalkman, C., Romijn, C., van Rheineck Leyssius, A., 2008. Fire and explosion hazard during oxygen use in operating rooms. Ned Tijdschr Geneeskd 152, 1313–1316.

41. Rinder, C., Dabu-Bondoc, S., Salgar, V., 2005. A device to reduce oxygen accumulation and fire hazard during MAC anesthesia. Anesthesiology 103, A804.

42. Castro, B., Freedman, A., Craig, W., et al., 2004. Explosion within an anesthesia machine: baralyme, high fresh gas flows and sevoflurane concentration. Anesthesiology 101, 537–539.

43. Bruley, M., 2004. Surgical fires: perioperative communication is essential to prevent this rare but devastating complication. Qual Saf Health Care 13, 467–471.

44. Katz, J., Campbell, L., 2005. Fire during thoracotomy: a need to control the inspired oxygen concentration. Anesth Analg 101, 612.

45. Lampotang, S., Gravenstein, N., Paulus, D., 2006. Reducing the incidence of surgical fires: supplying nasal cannulae with sub-100% O_2 gas mixtures from anesthesia machine. Anesth Analg 103 (1048), 51–52.

46. Wegrzynowicz, E., Jensen, N., Pearson, K., 1992. Airway fire during jet ventilation for laser excision of vocal cord papillomata. Anesthesiology 76, 468–469.

47. Laster, M., Roth, P., Eger, E., 2004. Fires from the interaction of anesthetics with desiccated absorbent. Anesth Analg 99, 769–774.

48. Recommended practices for electrosurgery. AORN J 67, 246–250 52-55.

49. Prasad, R., Quezado, Z., St Andre, A., et al., 2006. Fires in the operating room and intensive care unit: awareness is the key to prevention. Anesth Analg 102, 172–174.

50. American Society of Anesthesiologists Task Force on Operating Room Fires, Robert A Caplan, 2008. Practice advisory for the prevention and management of operating room fires. 2008.

51. NFPA, 2003. Fire safety in health care facilities. National Fire Protection Association, Quincy, Mass.

52. NFPA, 2003. Standard for laser fire protection (NFPA 115). National Fire Protection Association, Quincy, Mass.

53. Danne, S., Toth, B., 2005. Fire in the operating room: principles and prevention. Plast Reconstr Surg 115, 73e–75e.

54. Galapo, S., Wolf, G., Sidebotham, G., et al., 1998. Laser ignition of surgical oxygen enriched atmosphere. Anesthesiology 89, A560.

55. OSHA. Use of medical lasers (website): http://www.osha.gov/SLTC/etools/hospital/surgical/lasers.html Accessed May 20, 2009

56. Sliney, D., 1995. Laser safety. Lasers Surg Med 16, 215–225.

57. Bader, O., Lui, H., 1996. Laser safety and the eye—hidden hazards and practical pearls. The American Academy of Dermatology annual meeting, Washington, DC.

58. Chaffins, J., 2008. Radiation protection and procedures in the OR. Radiol Technol 79, 415–428.

59. Otto, L., Davison, S., 1999. Radiation exposure of Certified Registered Nurse Anesthetists during ureteroscopic procedures using fluoroscopy. AANA J 67, 53–58.

60. Lipsitz, E., Veith, F., Ohki, T., 2000. Does the endovascular repair of aortoiliac aneurysms pose a radiation safety hazard to vascular surgeons? J Vasc Surg 32, 704–710.

61. Kumari, G., Kumar, P., Wadhwa, P., 2006. Radiation exposure to the patient and operating room personnel during percutaneous nephrolithotomy. Int Urol Nephrol 38, 207–210.

62. Andersen, P., Chakera, A., Klausen, T., et al., 2008. Radiation exposure to surgical staff during F-18-FDG-guided cancer surgery. Eur J Nucl Med Mol Imaging 35, 624–629.

63. Bushong, S., 2001. Radiation protection procedure, ed 7. Mosby, St Louis.

64. Mahesh, M., 2001. Fluoroscopy: patient radiation exposure issues. The AAPM/RSNA physics tutorial for residents. RadioGraphics, 1033–1044.

65. Harstall, R., Heini, P., Mini, R., 2005. Radiation exposure to the surgeon during fluoroscopically assisted percutaneous vertebroplasty. Spine 16, 1893–1898.

66. Miller, M., Davis, M., MacClean, C., 1983. Radiation exposure and associated risks to operating-room personnel during the use of fluoroscopic guidance for selected orthopedic surgical procedures. J Bone Joint Surg Am 65, 1–4.

67. Singer, G. 2005. Occupational exposure to the surgeon. J Acad Orthop Surg 13, 69–76.

68. Derdeyn, C., Moran, C., Eichling, J., 1999. Radiation dose during intraoperative digital subtraction angiography. Am J Neuroradiol 20, 300–305.

69. Sherer-Statkiewicz, M., Visconti, P., Ritenour, E. (Eds.), 2006. Dose limits for exposure to ionizing radiation. Radiation protection in medical radiography, Mosby, St Louis.

70. Manchikanti, L., Cash, K., Moss, T., et al., 2002. Radiation exposure to the physician in interventional pain management. Pain Physician 5, 141.

71. Giordano, B., Baumhauer, J., Morgan, T., 2009. Patient and surgeon radiation exposure: comparison of standard and mini-C-arm fluoroscopy. J Bone Joint Surg Am 91, 297–304.

72. ASA, 2009. Practice advisory on anesthetic care for magnetic resonance imaging: a report by the American Society of Anesthesiologists task force on anesthetic care for magnetic resonance imaging. Anesthesiology 110, 459–479.

Chapter 30

Neuroanesthesia Equipment in the Intraoperative Setting

Sergio D. Bergese, Gilat Zisman, and Erika G. Puente

Introduction

Recent advances in technology provide monitoring equipment that helps facilitate complex neurosurgical procedures.[1,2] New and innovative methods for assessing neurological function in patients undergoing general anesthesia have been developed. The use of new devices and technologies along with the implementation of the new evaluation methods have allowed clinicians to apply this technology in the operating room for continuous monitoring of neurological function.[3,4]

Neurological Monitoring

Monitoring during neurosurgical procedures requires an advanced understanding of the neuro physiological parameters. Patients with underlying neurological diseases are considered at higher risk for cerebral ischemia when undergoing surgical procedures. Also, patients undergoing neurosurgical procedures tend to have a higher probability of presenting with evidence of past cerebral ischemic events. This risk may be directly associated with the type of neurosurgical procedure performed. It has been established that the use of intraoperative neurophysiological monitoring may improve patient outcome.[2] This also allows physicians to be able to monitor oxygen delivery and to possibly identify intraoperative ischemic events to protect the brain and the spinal cord. Several additional factors increase the likelihood of an undesirable outcome besides the type of surgery, including patient positioning and hemodynamic changes.[3,5]

Monitoring requirements are determined by the type of surgery and the patient's physical status. In most cases, the American Society of Anesthesiologists' (ASA) standard monitors are required. Major intracranial and spinal surgeries may require the application of more invasive monitoring techniques, such as the use of an intraarterial line for invasive blood pressure monitoring when strict hemodynamic control is warranted.[6,7] In less extensive operations, such as ventricular shunt placements, burr-hole biopsies, and minor spinal surgeries, the use of noninvasive blood pressure monitoring techniques may be sufficient. For vascular procedures and in those where major blood loss is possible, added monitoring of central venous pressure (CVP) is recommended. A complete evaluation of each patient and their comorbidities will determine further monitoring requirements. In patients with underlying heart conditions, monitoring of additional cardiovascular parameters, such as pulmonary artery pressures, may be warranted. The selection of placement of a PAC catheter or a central line must be performed to eliminate the possibility of early intervention and treatment in cases of air emboli.[2]

Core temperature monitoring is also recommended during anesthesia. For nonneurosurgical procedures, there are several locations to which the probe may be applied. The most practical site is often the esophagus. An esophageal temperature probe enables the anesthesiologist to monitor not only the core temperature, but also the heart sounds, if the probe happens to include an esophageal stethoscope. In neurosurgical procedures, the esophageal probe may be replaced by a Foley catheter with an incorporated temperature probe. In patients with high urinary output, special attention must be paid to the interference this may cause with the temperature readings.[8]

The effects of neuromuscular blockers should be monitored with a peripheral nerve stimulator to prevent patient movement or coughing. Movement could be catastrophic during neurosurgical procedures.

Patients are often required to be in a head-up or sitting position during neurological procedures, which increases their risk of venous air embolization through open intracranial sinuses. The use of precordial Doppler ultrasonography (PCD) or transesophageal echocardiography (TEE) is advised for the early detection of such complications.[3] It is also possible to use a Bunnegin-Albin catheter to evacuate air from the right heart in these cases.

Monitors Unique to Neurosurgical Anesthesia

The neurophysiologic parameters targeted are usually brain function, blood flow, and metabolism. Monitoring of function is related to the measurement of electrical activity in the brain by means of electroencephalography (EEG), sensory and motor evoked potentials (EPs), and electromyography (EMG). Monitoring of blood flow/pressure is achieved by nitrous oxide wash-in, radioactive xenon clearance, laser Doppler blood flow, and transcranial Doppler sonography. Alternatively, intracranial pressure can be determined by means of intraventricular catheters, fiberoptic intraparenchymal catheters, subarachnoid bolts, and epidural catheters. Lastly, brain metabolism can be measured either through invasive techniques such as placement of intracerebral Po_2 electrodes or noninvasive techniques, such as transcranial cerebral oximetry and jugular venous oximetry. The increased use of these technologies in neuroanesthesia has improved patient care.[1,2]

Requirements for a Nervous System Monitor

For a monitor of the nervous system to have maximum usefulness, it must meet certain requirements. To determine if monitors are useful to be considered as standard of care, sufficient evidence needs to be provided whether these monitors accurately reflect the intraoperative condition of the patient and affect the outcome.

The ideal monitoring device should be one expected to detect alterations in the parameters under observation and reveal any changes in the function, blood supply, or metabolism of the organs involved. Certain requirements should be considered when using a device for neurological monitoring. The monitors should have minimal interference or noise, be able to detect surgical injuries and provide the possibility of repair, and be used in a continuous manner.[1] Some neurophysiologic monitoring is not yet considered standard of care and although it is not routinely performed, many institutions are applying it as a regular practice for numerous surgical procedures.[2]

EEG Monitoring

The cortical electrical activity or electroencephalographic (EEG) activity of the brain consumes nearly 50% of the total brain oxygen and the remainder is consumed by cellular integrity maintenance. When the oxygen supply to the brain is decreased by either hypoxemia or decreased blood flow, the remaining oxygen will be shifted towards cellular maintenance and away from the electrical activity of the brain.[3] Brain monitoring is crucial in the prevention of ischemic or hypoxic damage and can be broadly categorized into monitoring of function, blood flow, or metabolism. An EEG signal reproduces the electrical activity of the brain, which is generated by the pyramidal cells of the cerebral cortex and corresponds to the sum of excitatory and inhibitory postsynaptic potentials that are generated. Therefore the EEG measures the electrical function of the brain indirectly, and it can also indirectly measure the blood flow and anesthetic effects. The EEG is recorded from needles or surface electrodes that are placed on the scalp and forehead.

The waves that are generated in the EEG are classified based on their frequencies as beta, alpha, theta, and delta. Beta waves are high frequency, low amplitude waves between 13 and 30 Hz, which are most active during the awake state. Alpha waves are of medium frequency, high amplitude waves between 9 and 12 Hz, which are seen in the occipital cortex when the eyes are shut, while awake. Theta waves are low frequency waves between 4 and 8 Hz. Delta waves are very low frequency between 0 and 4 Hz and with low to high amplitude. Delta waves are consistent with depressed function consistent with a coma state, which can be caused by anesthesia, metabolic factors, or hypoxia.[2,4]

There are several perioperative applications for the EEG in neuroanesthesia. It can identify if there is adequate blood flow reaching the cerebral cortex during surgical or anesthetic procedures that tend to produce a reduction in flow. The EEG can also perioperatively guide the reduction of cerebral metabolism before the induced reduction of blood flow and it can predict neurological outcomes after brain injury. Other uses for the EEG include identifying consciousness, measuring seizure activity, and identifying stages of sleep or coma state.

Any procedure that increases the risk for ischemia or hypoxia in the brain would potentially benefit from EEG monitoring. Procedures that involve manipulation of the cerebral vasculature, such as carotid endarterectomy or cerebral aneurysm repair, can benefit by the use of EEG in management and risk reduction of intraoperative stroke.[4,9] Deliberate metabolic suppression for cerebral protection during procedures can also be guided by EEG monitoring.[2]

EEG recording is done using an electrode arrangement with bipolar recording due to the fact that there is no electrical neutral area. Both electrodes are active and the recorded signal polarity is dependent on the random designation and not the referential electrode. Common mode rejection, the rejection of the electrical signals that are common to both sites in comparison to the third "ground" electrode, is used to minimize the signal from other electrical activities of the body, such as electromyography and electrocardiography.

The gold standard for EEG recording uses a 16-channel recording with 8 channels for each hemisphere. The electrodes are placed using the International 10-20 system. Due to inaccessibility of the head in general and large parts of the scalp in particular during intracranial surgical procedures, the 16-channel EEG is rarely used during operative procedures. Intraoperative monitoring during craniotomy is usually accomplished with a 2- to 4-channel recording, with computer processing to simplify the recording and interpretation. Most algorithms filter out the high-frequency or 30 Hz activity because it is most likely due to artifact or interference. The raw EEG is then separated using Fourier transformation into component waves, which are then grouped based on their frequency spectrum. This allows the raw EEG recorded in time domain to be displayed in frequency domain. The square of the amplitude of the EEG wave—the power spectrum—can be displayed in several ways. Usually, it is displayed as either compressed spectral array or density spectral array, where either the peaks and valleys or the density of the gray scale represent the power of the spectrum. Another method to process the EEG is the periodic analysis, which tracks and plots each wave as a "telephone pole." The amplitude or power of the wave is represented by the height of the "pole."

To interpret an EEG properly, it is necessary to remember that an EEG is recording the spontaneous activity of the brain and reflects how "awake" or metabolically active the brain is. Electrical activity in the brain is a process that requires energy that is dependent on certain substrates, such as oxygen or glucose. Depression of EEG activity and characteristic changes in the EEG can be seen with reduction in cerebral blood flow, or oxygen or glucose delivery. During an awake-state, the high-frequency and low-amplitude beta waves are most prominent. There is a transient increase in the beta waves with the onset of ischemia or hypoxia, with eventual development of large amplitude theta and delta waves. With the increase in ischemia or hypoxia, the beta waves begin to disappear and there is an appearance of low amplitude delta waves. This progresses to electrical activity suppression with occasional bursts of activity. The onset of irreversible damage can be seen when there is complete electrical silence with a flat EEG.

Monitoring the EEG intraoperatively for the development of delta waves allows the anesthesiologist to be aware of an increased risk of ischemic damage to the brain. EEG has a poor predictive value for brain damage and lacks specificity as a diagnostic test for irreversible damage even though it is sensitive to the ischemic changes. The probability for irreversible damage is increased when there is quicker onset of ischemic EEG changes.

Metabolic depression caused by anesthetic drugs or increasing depth of anesthesia can also cause EEG changes in frequency and amplitude that are similar to those seen with ischemia or hypoxia, though these are reversible.[2,4] Certain inhaled and intravenous anesthetics cause specific EEG changes and are usually dose dependent. Also, hypothermia can cause slowing of the EEG. Due to these influences, the complete clinical picture of the patient should be taken into account with the interpretation of the EEG. Regardless of whether it can be caused by anesthesia or by ischemia, the fast EEG activity is transformed into larger, slower waves, with an eventual decrease in the amplitude of the wave and ultimately the wave becoming flat as metabolic activity decreases.

To simplify EEG interpretation, the anesthetic delivery should ideally be "stable" and not changing during the critical surgical portions of the case. Also, any changes in anesthetic delivery should be communicated to the EEG technician.

The EEG can only provide information of the cerebral cortex function, and not much information on the subcortical brain, spinal cord, or the cranial and peripheral nerves.[4]

Transcranial Doppler

Transcranial Doppler sonography (TCD) noninvasively and continuously measures blood flow velocity in the major vessels in the "Circle of Willis" in the brain, and uses those calculations to make determinations on intracranial hemodynamics. Estimates of cerebral blood flow (CBF) are commonly monitored. Blood flow velocity and actual blood flow are not equivalent, but the two are closely related. By measuring through the thin temporal bone, just over the zygomatic arch with a 2-MHz probe, it is possible to measure the velocity of blood flow in the middle cerebral artery (Vmca). Around 75% to 80% of the ipsilateral carotid blood flows through the MCA.[10] Even though the absolute CBF cannot be measured by the TCD, there is strong correlation between flow velocity

changes and CBF.[11] The TCD can also be used for a qualitative assessment of the intracranial pressure or cerebral perfusion pressure, the detection of air or particulate emboli, and determination of cerebral autoregulation and CO_2 reactivity. An advantage from this is that the basal cerebral arteries do not constrict or dilate as changes occur in the vascular resistance, carbon dioxide tension, or systemic blood pressure. Also, the middle cerebral artery is not considerably constricted or dilated with the administration of intravenous or inhaled anesthetics. The blood flow recorded by the TCD in the MCA represents the velocity in that particular artery. Actual velocity in any other vessel cannot be determined unless the diameter of that artery is established. Therefore, TCD is not used to quantitatively determine CBF, but to evaluate for relative blood flow changes.[12]

TCD can be used to evaluate for cerebral vasospasm, transient ischemic attack, stroke, SAH, syncope, brain death, head injury, and AVM. There are several clinical situations where the use of intraoperative TCD is applicable. During carotid endarterectomies, the TCD can be used for the detection of reduced MCA flow or microemboli caused by particulates or air. TCD also allows monitoring for downstream flow reductions indicating inadequate collateralization during cross-clamping of the carotid artery, the detection of vasospasm, or monitoring for shunt malfunction that can be caused by kinking or thrombosis. There is evidence that the correlation between flow-velocity changes on TCD and EEG changes is strong. When compared with preclamping baseline velocity, a decrease in Vmca of greater than 60% suggests poor CBF and the need to use an intraluminal shunt. TCD technology can also be used for the diagnosis and treatment of postoperative hyperperfusion syndrome, which is seen when patients have constant elevated flow velocities even after the release of carotid occlusion and develop headaches, with eventual development of cerebral hemorrhage. In these cases, by promptly reducing the blood pressure, the ipsilateral flow velocity is normalized and the symptoms are alleviated. Postoperatively, the TCD should be promptly used when clinically significant symptoms develop. It can also be used to evaluate for a postoperative thrombi or an intimal flap to prevent the progression of a stroke, or during cardiac surgical cardiopulmonary bypass procedures to monitor for symptoms of cerebral hypoperfusion or for cerebral emboli. It is important to remember that paradoxically, an increase in blood flow velocities indicates a decrease in cerebral blood flow in patients with vasospasm and subarachnoid hemorrhage.[4,13]

The knowledge of the anatomy and physiology of the cerebral circulation, the skill, and the experience of the technician and interpreter are important for the accuracy of the interpretation of the TCD. Care must also be taken during intraoperative procedures so as not to interfere with the surgical team or the surgical field. The surgical field can limit the probe placement and the maintenance of the proper probe placement. Also, the thickness of the temporal bone is dependent on age, race, and gender, which can influence the results of the TCD.

Intracranial Pressure Monitoring

Intracranial hypertension is described as the elevation of the pressure in the cranium, which can lead to severe sequelae if it rises too high.[14] An increase in pressure—most commonly

Table 30–1

Increased ICP Mechanism	Description
Mass effect	Deformation of adjacent brain tissue due to brain tumor, infarction with edema, contusions, subdural or epidural hematoma or abscess
Brain swelling	Can occur in ischemic-anoxia states, acute liver failure, hypertensive encephalopathy, pseudo tumor cerebri, hypercarbia, and Reye hepatocerebral syndrome
Increase in venous pressure	Can be due to venous sinus thrombosis, heart failure, or obstruction of the superior mediastinal or jugular veins
Obstruction to CSF flow and/or absorption	Can occur in hydrocephalus, extensive meningeal disease, or obstruction in the cerebral convexities or the superior sagittal sinus

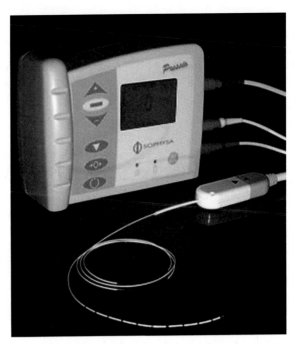

Figure 30–1   Pressio ICP monitor.

due to head injury leading to intracranial hematoma or cerebral edema—can crush brain tissue, shift brain structures, contribute to hydrocephalus, cause brain herniation, or restrict blood supply to the brain.[15] Causes of increased ICP can be classified by type of mechanism, as described in Table 30-1.

According to the American Association of Neurological Surgeons guidelines, intracranial pressure monitoring should be used in the management of patients with a severe traumatic brain injury (TBI), with a Glasgow Coma Scale (GCS) score of 3 to 8 after resuscitation, and an abnormal computed tomography (CT) scan. If an abnormal CT scan of the head shows evidence of a hematoma, contusions, swelling, herniation, or compressed basal cisterns, the risk of increased ICP in this patient population could be around 50% to 60%. In patients with severe TBI, a normal CT scan, and two or more risk factors noted at admission (i.e. over 40 years old, unilateral or bilateral motor posturing, systolic blood pressure (BP) less than 90 mm Hg) the risk of increased ICP could be around 50% to 60%.[16,17]

The treatment for increased ICP depends on the cause. In addition to managing the underlying cause, other factors must be taken into consideration. There is no defined set point at which treatment for increased ICP should be initiated, but levels above 20 mm Hg are usually considered high and are treated.[14] However, it is important to maintain an adequate cerebral perfusion pressure (CPP), which cannot be accurately determined without the use of ICP measurement.

CPP is an indirect measure of cerebral perfusion and is defined as the mean arterial blood pressure (MAP) minus ICP (CPP = MAP − ICP).[18] CPP values below 50 are associated with poor outcomes. The only way to reliably determine CPP, and therefore cerebral hypoperfusion, is to continuously monitor ICP and blood pressure.[18-22] CPP should be maintained within a tight range, typically between 70 to 90 mm Hg. A CPP value that is too high or even too low may lead to secondary brain injury.

Due to the fact that CCP is dependent on the MAP, it is also imperative to maintain blood pressure in a target range that is individualized for each patient, based on their baseline blood pressure, to prevent an increase in CCP during a hypertensive episode. Blood pressure can be lowered using common antihypertensive agents such as calcium channels blockers (CCBs).[23-27]

Monitoring of ICP allows for optimization of CPP and it allows for the prompt treatment of increased ICP to prevent brain herniation. There are several methods for monitoring ICP. The most commonly used is the fiberoptic monitor, which can be inserted at the bedside. The miniature catheter can be inserted in the ventricles, the epidural space, the subdural space, or the brain parenchyma. There are new fiberoptic monitors that can simultaneously measure laser Doppler flow (LDF), Pao_2, $Paco_2$, pH, and temperature. Issues, such as leaking, infection, and drifting that are associated with a fluid-filled system are minimized because the fiberoptic monitor is a self-enclosed electronic system. Another advantage of this system is that the transducer is at the tip of the catheter, so the level of the transducer is no longer a variable (Figure 30–1).

A common alternative technique is to use a ventricular drainage catheter. This technique involves a percutaneous intraventricular catheter that is cannulated into the lateral ventricle through a frontal, occipital, parieto-occipital, or a parasagittal coronal approach. The cannula is attached to a pressure transducer through a fluid column, and the transducer is zeroed at the level of the external auditory meatus. This method is not only reliable for ICP measurements, but it can also be used to measure the intercranial compliance and can be used therapeutically to drain CSF to decrease ICP. On the other hand, this method also presents some risks, including infection and/or injury to the brain parenchyma during cannulation. Patients may also develop cerebral edema that may lead to ventricular collapse, a situation that can pose difficulties in the placement of the catheter or interfere with the catheter's readings.

Another mechanism by which the ICP can be measured uses a subarachnoid screw, similar to a hollow bolt, that when inserted through a twist drill hole in the skull and the dura mater, lies flush against the arachnoid membrane. The increase in pressure against the arachnoid membrane is recorded by the pressure transducer that is also connected to a saline column. This method of ICP measurement is advantageous in that it does not cause direct brain injury with its use, but it cannot be used to drain CSF to alleviate increases in ICP. This method can also present some risks, such as infection, malfunction due to screw dislocation, or brain matter protruding through the hollow bolt.

Other equipment such as transducer tipped catheters, subarachnoid catheters, or epidural sensors can also be used to monitor ICP, but have been shown to be slightly less accurate than the ventricular catheters. Even though these monitors are commonly used in the ICU in the management of patients with head injury, they are used much less often intraoperatively.

Physiological ICP recordings demonstrate a pulsatile wave with a slow respiratory cycle that is superimposed to the biphasic cardiac cycle. Under these conditions, the amplitude of the respiratory cycle is greater than the amplitude of the cardiac cycle. The arterial component, however, has greater amplitude when there is an increase in ICP.[4,6]

There are three pathologic wave forms, "A," "B." and "C," in patients with increased ICP.

The "A" or plateau waves are evident when there are changes that are described in the cerebral blood volume, which leads to a severe pathologic increase in ICP. The "plateau" is caused by a 5-to 20-minute increase of ICP above 40 mm Hg and then a return to baseline. Eventually, the baseline between the plateaus is also progressively increased. In these cases, the patients will exhibit symptoms of headache, loss of consciousness, abnormal motor responses, altered breathing patterns, and papillary signs of clinical deterioration.

"B" waves, which are less clinically important than "A" waves, have a rate of 1 to 2 per minute with amplitude of 20 mm Hg. "B" waves are usually correlated with Cheyne-Stokes type breathing, and may indicate that the patient is at increased risk of intracranial hypertension due to decreased intracranial compliance. Lastly, "C" waves are not clinically significant for any specific pathology.[10]

Intraoperative Magnetic Resonance Imaging (iMRI)

While not an anesthetic monitor per se, intraoperative magnetic resonance imaging (iMRI) deserves mention in a discussion of neuroanesthesia monitoring because of its increasing use and major impact on the conduct of anesthesia. There are significant additional safety implications of iMRI that must be considered. Magnetic resonance imaging (MRI) is a non-invasive technology that has gradually acquired a new role for intraoperative surgical planning and guidance, especially during neurosurgical procedures. Safety and adequate monitoring are the main concerns for the anesthesia provider when introducing the iMRI into the OR setting to accomplish optimal anesthesia management in the iMRI several additional requirements need to be considered.

First, the OR requires special considerations in size and design. The room must be larger than the standard ORs. This will allow enough space to install a MRI machine, a portable shield, if required, and to move the patient in and out of the

MRI core easily. At the same time, a larger room allows the transit of an increased number of hospital personnel, who are required for providing adequate treatment to the patient. The size of the room should allow the incorporation of special "MR-safe" equipment designed to minimize interference from the magnetic field and ensure an adequate distance from the location where this field is the strongest. Since these devices have ferromagnetic properties, maintaining a specific distance from the magnet is required to avoid attraction of these objects.

There are two types of OR designs that could be used. The first, more frequently used with the high-field MRI technology is incorporated into the permanent construction of the OR. This structure is permanent and allocates the OR entirely for iMRI use. The second is a mobile design, which is compatible with most models of low-field MRI scanners. This design requires the use of a portable shield or Faraday cage. This structure renders the OR suitable as two different ORs, with and without the iMRI. The unique design of this portable cage requires a closed shield that collapses into the shape of an accordion when not in use. The bottom of the cage is conformed by a permanent stainless steel floor shield, which is located under the OR table, made out of stainless steel. This particular component of the cage has been discovered to generate artifacts and corrupt MRI images. The shiny finish of the stainless steel plate below the OR table can reflect onto the images, causing artifacts and alterations on image appearance. Therefore, a matte finish is recommended for the floor shield of the Faraday cage to reduce artifact occurrence. Additionally, the bottom of the accordion-shaped shield must have an aluminum type foil wrap that when making contact with the floor will act as an impermeable shield. It is of paramount importance to ensure that the bottom of the Faraday cage surrounding the stainless steel plate is properly positioned to provide adequate sealing of the cage. Devices such as infusion pumps, plasma and LCD displays, physiological monitors, and computers generate a detectable electric noise (EN) trace. This portable Faraday cage has been specially designed to minimize the impact of this low-energy EN on the iMRI.[10]

To achieve high quality readings and decrease the interference with the magnetic field as much as possible, the set-up of the OR in preparation for the scanning is crucial. The set-up usually involves several steps from patient positioning to portable shield preparation to monitoring equipment placement. The anesthesiologist must take into consideration that the use of extension tubing is required. It is also necessary for the patient to have more than one IV access, telemetry ECG monitoring, fiber-optic temperature skin probes, pulse oximeter, blood pressure cuff, and vital sign monitors. All of these must be arranged properly so as to minimize the possibility of moving, interrupting, or disconnecting the breathing circuit, infusion lines, or monitoring cables with the Faraday cage (Figure 30–2).

The extensive preparation requires the involvement of numerous trained hospital staff so that the patient is ready for magnet positioning and scan initiation. Barua et al evaluated the set-up time required for 62 successful iMRI procedures over a 21-month period. It was observed that there was significant decrease of set-up time with increased experience of the staff (Figure 30–3).[11]

Furthermore, there are certain constraints and hazards to consider when incorporating the MRI technology into the OR. These are mainly related to the monitoring equipment,

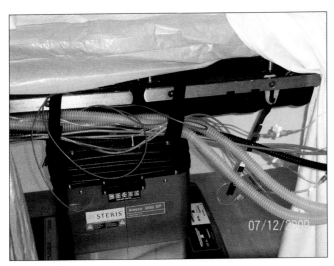

Figure 30–2 Example of arrangement of extended breathing circuit, infusion lines, and monitoring cables arranged so to minimize the possibility of kinking within the Faraday cage.

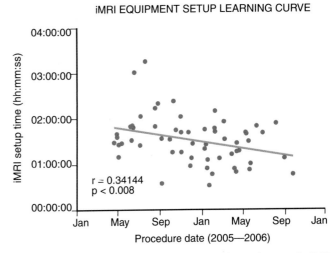

iMRI EQUIPMENT SETUP LEARNING CURVE

r = 0.34144
p < 0.008

Figure 30–3 Learning curve showing a significant decrease in iMRI set-up time with increased training of the staff. *(The Ohio Sate University Medical Center.)*[11]

anesthesia workstation, and infusion devices. According to the monitoring standards of the American Society of Anesthesiologists (ASA), the patient's ventilation, circulation, temperature, and oxygenation should be continuously evaluated throughout the entire procedure. A restriction of the portable iMRI setting is that during the time the patient is inside the Faraday cage, within the bore of the scanner, the patient will not be under the direct visual supervision of the anesthesiologist for the duration of the scan. During this period, it is essential to ensure reliable and accurate monitoring of pulse oximetry (electroencephalographic signaling, if used), blood pressure and temperature control, and continuous ventilatory support in compliance with the ASA standard. Also, IV drug administration, contrast media infusions, inhalation anesthetics, and supplemental oxygen availability and delivery must follow ASA guidelines.[12] The anesthesiologist must also be certain that the appropriate drugs and equipment are readily available in case of encountering unexpected airway or cardiovascular complications.[6]

The crucial role of the anesthesiologist is to promote patient safety by minimizing accidents associated with iMRI technology. To ensure adequate patient safety, the anesthesiologist must perform a detailed MRI compatibility preoperative examination. This examination should include exploring for history of acquired or implanted metallic devices, such as cerebrovascular clips, cardiac pacemakers, stents, bullets, braces, dentures, or even extensive tattoos. These metallic devices may generate image artifacts or move from their place and cause trauma to the patient. They may even heat up and produce severe burns.

The anesthesiologist must ensure that only MR-compatible medical supplies and equipment are present to prevent such complications. This cannot be the sole responsibility of the anesthesia technician. For example, when fastening the endotracheal tube (ET) by inflating the safety balloon, the balloon needs to be drawn away from the patient's face. The safety pilot balloon from the ET has a metallic component (coil spring) that can cause serious burns to the patient's skin. It is also important to reconsider which temperature probes to choose when undergoing iMRI procedures. Frequently used

bladder catheters with incorporated temperature probes or esophageal/rectal temperature probes are metallic and can produce severe local burns. Other temperature probes may produce electrical resistance or electrical potential that may interfere with the MRI imaging. The anesthesiologist must be aware that these catheters must not be used for iMRI and instead be replaced with MRI nonmagnetic thermometers, such as fiberoptic or infrared ones, for core and skin temperature measurement.[8,13-15]

The scanner generates a strong magnetic field that can interfere with monitoring and anesthetic equipment. The MRI technology generates high-energy radio frequency (RF) energy and high-static pulsating magnetic field gradients that are transmitted during the image acquisition. These may affect or cause failure of the electrical, electronic, or mechanical life support and monitoring equipment.[1] At the same time, the monitoring equipment can interfere with the nuclear magnetic signals, leading to poor-quality images.[6]

Special nonferromagnetic equipment has been designed over time to decrease interference as much as possible with the iMRI system and to attempt to obtain the best quality images possible. Unfortunately, this results in considerable cost increments.

Nonmagnetic MRI equipment available includes continuous infusion pumps, which are portable and include rechargeable batteries (Figure 30–4), and vital sign monitors, which usually have an integrated power supply, a safety sensor that measures the magnetic force, and which are compatible with magnets up to 3T. There are also nonmagnetic MRI laryngoscope handles and blades that function with nonmagnetic MRI lithium laryngoscope batteries. It is important to point out that rechargeable batteries should never be recharged in the presence of the electromagnetic field.

Other important aspects to take into consideration when providing anesthesia in the iMRI setting is the length of the different tubing systems required. In order for the IV tubing to reach the patient within the Faraday cage, it is necessary to use extension tubing. Adequately long breathing tubes are also required due to the remote location of the anesthesia machine from the patient (Figure 30–5).

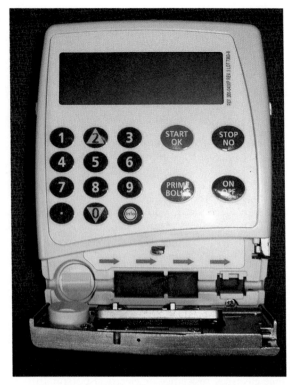

Figure 30–4 Nonmagnetic MRI continuous infusion pump with rechargeable batteries.

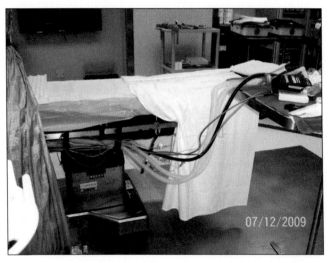

Figure 30–5 Extended anesthesia circuit, including IV tubing with multiple extension, temperature fiberoptic probe, breathing tubes, and pulse oximeter cables.

The IV tubing, temperature fiberoptic probe, the breathing tubes and the pulse oximeter cables and all their extensions should all be introduced into the Faraday cage through a small opening located on the side of the portable shield (Figure 30–6). This extended anesthesia circuit may pose additional challenges for the anesthesia provider to maintain adequate ventilation and administer drugs. The dead space within the extensions creates a time delay upon the administration of volatile anesthetics and drugs before the expected onset of effects can be observed.[10]

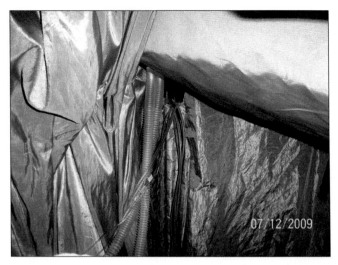

Figure 30–6 Extended anesthesia circuit being introduced into the Faraday cage through a small opening located on one of the sides of the portable shield.

For more on MRI-environment safety considerations and equipment, see Chapter 23, on Anesthesia Equipment Outside of the Operating Room.

References

1. Bendo, A.A., Kass, I.S., Hartung, J., et al., 2006. Anesthesia for neurosurgery. In: Barash, P.G. (Ed.), Clinical anesthesia, ed 5. Lippincott-Raven, Philadelphia.
2. Kinkaid, M.S., Lam, A.M., 2006. Neurophysiologic monitoring. In: Newfield, P., Cottrell, J.E. (Eds.), Handbook of neuroanesthesia, ed 4. Lippincott Williams & Wilkins, Philadelphia.
3. Trankina, M.F., 1998. Neurodiagnostic procedures. In: Cucchiara, R.F. (Ed.), Clinical neuroanesthesia, ed 2. Churchill Livingstone, New York.
4. Fabregas, N., Gomar, C., 2001. Monitoring in neuroanesthesia: update of clinical usefulness. Eur J Anaesthesiol 18, 423–439.
5. Mahla, M.E., 1998. Neurologic monitoring. In: Cucchiara, R.F. (Ed.), Clinical neuroanesthesia, ed 2. Churchill Livingstone, New York.
6. Kraayenbrink, M., McAnulty, G., 2005. Neuroanesthesia. In: Moore, J.A., Newell, D.W. (Eds.), Neurosurgery: principles and practice, Springer-Verlag, London.
7. Drummond, J.C., Patel, P.M., 2009. Neurosurgical anesthesia. In: Miller, R.D. (Ed.), Miller's anesthesia, ed 7. Churchill Livingstone, Pennsylvania.
8. Al-Shaikh, B., Stacey, S. (Eds.), 2007. Essentials of anesthetic equipment, ed 3. Churchill Livingstone, New York.
9. Umamaheswara, G.S., 2002. Neurological monitoring. Indian J Anaesth 46 (4), 304–314.
10. Aaslid, R., Markwalder, T.M., Nornes, H., 1982. Noninvasive transcranial Doppler ultrasound recording of flow velocity in basal cerebral arteries. J Neurosurg 58, 769–774.
11. Alexandrov, A.V., Joseph, M., 2000. Transcranial Doppler: an overview of its clinical applications. Internet J Emerg Intensive Care Med 4 N1.
12. Rommer, B., Bellner, J., Kongstad, P., et al., 1996. Elevated transcranial Doppler flow velocities after severe head injury: cerebral vasospasm or hyperemia?. J Neurosurg 85, 90–97.
13. Dawodu S. Traumatic brain injury: definition, epidemiology and pathophysiology, eMedicine (website): www.emedicine.medscape.com. Accessed October 2009.
14. Graham, D.I., Gennareli, T.A., et al., 2000. Pathology of brain damage after head injury. In: Cooper, P. (Ed.), Head injury, ed 4. Morgan Hill, New York.
15. Bullock, R.M., Chesnut, R.M., Clifton, G.L., 2007. Guidelines for the management of severe traumatic brain injury: indications for intracranial pressure monitoring. J Neurotrauma 24 (1), 37–44.
16. Steiner, L.A., Andrews, P.J., 2006. Monitoring the injured brain: ICP and CBF. Br J Anaesth 97 (1), 23–38.

17. Chambers, I.R., Treadwell, L., Mendelow, A.D., 2000. The cause and incidence of secondary insults in severely head-injured adults and children. Br J Neurosurg 14, 424–431.

18. Rosner, M.J., Daughton, S., 1990. Cerebral perfusion pressure management in head injury. J Trauma 30, 933–940.

19. Chambers, I.R., Treadwell, L., Mendelow, A.D., 2001. Determination of threshold levels of cerebral perfusion pressure and intracranial pressure in severe head injury by using receiver-operating characteristic curves: an observational study in 291 patients. J Neurosurg 94, 412–416.

20. Miller, M.T., Pasquale, M., Kured, S., et al., 2004. Initial head computed tomographic scan characteristics have a linear relationship with initial intracranial pressure after trauma. J Trauma 56, 967–972.

21. Bullock, R.M., Chesnut, R.M., Clifton, G.L., 2007. Guidelines for the management of severe traumatic brain injury: cerebral perfusion thresholds. J Neurotrauma 24 (1), 59–64.

22. Chesnut, R.M., Marshall, L.F., Klauber, M.R., et al., 1993. The role of secondary brain injury in determining outcome from severe head injury. J Trauma 34, 216–222.

23. Marmarou, A., Anderson, R.L., Ward, J.D., 1991. Impact of ICP instability and hypotension on outcome in patients with severe head trauma. J Neurosurg 75, 59–66.

24. Schoon, P., Benito, M.L., Orlandi, G., et al., 2002. Incidence of intracranial hypertension related to jugular bulb oxygen saturation disturbances in severe traumatic brain injury patients. Acta Neurochir (Suppl) 81, 285–287.

25. Tolias C, Sgouros S. Initial evaluation and management of CNS, eMedicine (website): www.emedicine.medscape.com. Accessed December 2009.

26. Czosnyka, M., Pickard, J.D., 2004. Monitoring and interpretation of intracranial pressure. J Neurol Neurosurg Psychiatry 75 (6), 813–821.

Appendix
SI Unit and Conversion Tables
Chetan Patel

SI UNITS

In 1960, the Conférence Générale des Poids et Mesures (11th CGPM), which is the international authority on the metric system, replaced all previous systems with the modern metric system officially named the Système International d'Unités, abbreviated to SI. Over the years, this metric system has been adopted throughout the world and is continually being revised to parallel developments in science and technology.

The SI is founded on seven base units (Table App. 1). Other derived units are defined in terms of the seven base units and, for ease of understanding and convenience, may have special or compound names and their own symbols (Tables App. 2 and App. 3). There are also 20 SI prefixes used to form decimal multiples and submultiples (Table App. 4).

CONVERSION TABLES
French/Gauge

By convention single lumen catheters, like needles, are identified by gauge (G) as a contraction for imperial standard wire gauge (SWG). Multilumen catheters and other larger diameter devices (particularly where there is a noncircular cross section [e.g., double lumen tracheal tubes]) are labeled by French gauge (Fr). French gauge is also referred to as Charriere gauge (CH) after the 19th century Parisian surgical instrument maker and corresponds to the external circumference in millimeters, which approximately equates to three times the maximal external "diameter."

Each lumen of a multilumen catheter is by convention referred to by a nominal gauge (G) derived from the observed flow rate. It should be noted that American wire gauge (AWG) is not the same as SWG.

Table App. 1   The Seven Base Units of the SI

Physical Quantity	Base Unit	Symbol
Amount of substance	mole	mol
Electric current	ampere	A
Length	meter	m
Luminous intensity	candela	cd
Mass	kilogram	kg
Thermodynamic temperature	kelvin	K
Time	second	s

Table App. 2   Examples of SI-Derived Units with Special Names

Physical Quantity	Unit Name	Symbol	Expressed in Base Units
Plane angle	radian	rad	$m\ m^{-1} = 1$
Solid angle	steradian	sr	$m^2\ m^{-2} = 1$
Frequency	hertz	Hz	s^{-1}
Force	Newton	N	$m\ kg\ s^{-2}$
Work/energy	joule	J	$m^2\ kg\ s^{-2}\ (N\ m)$
Pressure/stress	pascal	Pa	$m^{-1}\ kg\ s^{-2}\ (N\ m^{-2})$
Power	watt	W	$m^2\ kg\ s^{-3}\ (J\ s^{-1})$
Electric charge	coulomb	C	$s\ A$
Electric potential difference	volt	V	$m^2\ kg\ s^{-3}\ A^{-1}\ (W\ A^{-1})$
Electric capacitance	farad	F	$m^{-2}\ kg^{-1}\ s^4\ A^2\ (C\ V^{-1})$

Continued

Table App. 2 Examples of SI-Derived Units with Special Names—cont'd

Physical Quantity	Unit Name	Symbol	Expressed in Base Units
Electric resistance	ohm	Ω	m^2 kg s^{-3} A^{-2} [V/A]
Electric conductance	siemens	S	m^{-2} kg^{-1} s^3 A^2 [A/V]
Magnetic flux	weber	Wb	m^2 kg s^{-2} A^{-1}
Magnetic induction	tesla	T	kg s^{-2} A^{-1} (Wb m^{-2})
Inductance	henry	H	m^2 kg s^{-2} A^{-2} (Wb A^{-1})
Luminous flux	lumen	lm	cd sr
Illuminance	lux	lx	cd sr m^{-2}

Table App. 3 SI Units with Compound Names

Physical Quantity	Name of Unit	Symbol
Area	square meter	m^2
Volume	cubic meter	m^3
Speed/velocity	meter per second	m s^{-1}
Acceleration	meter per second squared	m s^{-2}
Density	kilogram per cubic meter	kg m^{-3}
Electric field strength	volt per meter	V m^{-1}
Magnetic field strength	ampere per meter	A m^{-1}
Current density	ampere per meter squared	A m^{-2}
Specific heat capacity	joule per kilogram per kelvin	J kg^{-1} K^{-1}

Table App. 4 The 20 SI Prefixes

Prefix	Symbol	Ordinary Notation	10^x
yotta-	Y	1,000,000,000,000,000,000,000,000	10^{24}
zetta-	Z	1,000,000,000,000,000,000,000	10^{21}
exa-	E	1,000,000,000,000,000,000	10^{18}
peta-	P	1,000,000,000,000,000	10^{15}
tera-	T	1,000,000,000,000	10^{12}
giga-	G	1,000,000,000	10^9
mega-	M	1,000,000	10^6
kilo-	k	1,000	10^3
hecto-	h	100	10^2
deca-	da	10	10^1
		1	10^0
deci-	d	0.1	10^{-1}
centi-	c	0.01	10^{-2}
milli-	m	0.001	10^{-3}
micro-	μ	0.000 001	10^{-6}
nano-	n	0.000 000 001	10^{-9}
pico-	p	0.000 000 000 001	10^{-12}
femto-	f	0.000 000 000 000 001	10^{-15}
atto-	a	0.000 000 000 000 000 001	10^{-18}
zepto-	z	0.000 000 000 000 000 000 001	10^{-21}
yocto-	y	0.000 000 000 000 000 000 000 001	10^{-24}

Table App. 5	French and Gauge Cross Reference (1 inch = 25.4 mm)		
French	**Inches**	**mm**	**Gauge (SWG)**
	0.016	0.406	27
	0.018	0.450	26
	0.020	0.508	25
	0.022	0.559	24
	0.024	0.610	23
	0.028	0.711	22
	0.032	0.813	21
	0.035	0.889	20
3	0.039	0.975	
	0.042	1.067	19
	0.049	1.245	18
4	0.053	1.346	
	0.058	1.473	17
	0.065	1.651	16
5	0.066	1.676	
	0.072	1.829	15
6	0.079	2.001	
	0.083	2.108	14
7	0.092	2.337	
	0.095	2.413	13
8	0.0105	2.667	
	0.109	2.769	12
9	0.118	2.997	
	0.120	3.048	11
10	0.131	3.327	
	0.134	3.404	10
11	0.144	3.658	
12	0.158	4.013	
13	0.170	4.318	
14	0.184	4.674	
15	0.197	5.004	
16	0.210	5.334	

Table App. 6	Useful Conversions
1 meter	= 1.0936 yards = 3.2808 feet = 39.3696 inches
1 kilogram	= 2.2046 pounds = 35.2736 ounces
1 liter	= 0.22 (imperial) gallons = 0.27 (US) gallons = 1.76 pints
1 kilopascal	= 0.146 psi = 7.50 mm Hg = 10.20 cm (100 N m^{-2})* H$_2$O
1 mm Hg**	= 1.36 cm H$_2$O = 133.3 N.m^{-2} ($\equiv$ 0.1333 kPa) = 0.0194 psi
1 psi	= 6.89 kPa = 51.71 mm Hg = 70.33 cm H$_2$O
1 joule	= 107 ergs = 0.239 calories
0 K	= $-$273° C ("absolute zero")
273.15 K	= 0 ° = 32 °F
373.16 K	= 100 °C = 212 °F
K → °C	= $-$273.15
°C → K	= +273.15
°C	= (°F – 32) × 5/9
°F	= (°C × 5/9) + 32

*See Table App. 2: 1 pascal = 1 N m^{-2}
†This unit may also be referred to as torr.

Table App. 7

Symbol	When You Know	Multiply by	To Find	Symbol
LENGTH				
in	inches	*2.5	centimeters	cm
ft	feet	30	centimeters	cm
yd	yards	0.9	meters	m
mi	miles	1.6	kilometers	km
Area				
in^2	square inches	6.5	square centimeters	cm^2
ft^2	square feet	0.09	square centimeters	cm^2
yd^2	square yards	0.8	square meters	m^2
mi^2	square miles	2.6	square kilometers	km^2
	acres	0.4	hectares	ha
MASS (WEIGHT)				
oz	ounces	28	grams	g
lb	pounds	1.45	kilograms	kg
	short tons(2000lb)	0.9	tonnes	t
VOLUME				
tsp	teaspoons	5	milliliters	ml
Tbsp	tablespoons	15	milliliters	ml
fl oz	fluid ounces	30	milliliters	ml
c	cups	0.24	liters	l
pt	pints	0.47	liters	l
qt	quarts	0.95	liters	l
gal	gallons	3.8	liters	l
ft^3	cubic feet	0.03	Cubic meters	m^3
yd^3	cubic yards	0.76	Cubic meters	m^3
TEMPERATURE (EXACT)				
°F	Fahrenheit temperature	5/9 (after subtracting 32)	Celsius temperature	°C

References

1. http://physics.nist.gov/cuu/Units/prefixes.html (07/08/2004)
2. www.arrowintl.com/products/critical_care/faqs2/faq17.asp (02/09/2004)

Index

Page numbers followed by *f* indicate figures; *t*, tables